WOUND CARE PRACTICE

2ND EDITION

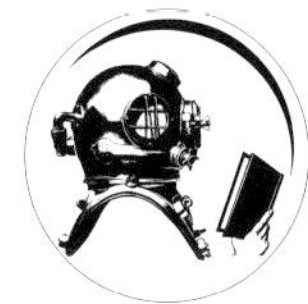

WOUND CARE PRACTICE

2ND EDITION

PAUL J. SHEFFIELD, PhD
Editor

CAROLINE E. FIFE, MD
Co-Editor

BEST PUBLISHING COMPANY

Cover & Layout Design: William Owen
Kelly Phillips

Edited By: James T. Joiner
Kate Lasky

International Standard Book Number-13: 978-1-930536-38-8
International Standard Book Number-10: 1-930536-38-0
Library of Congress Control Number: 2007925867

For more information contact:
Best Publishing Company
2355 North Steves Boulevard
P.O. Box 30100
Flagstaff, AZ 86003-0100 USA

Tele: 928.527.1055
Fax: 928.526.0370
divebooks@bestpub.com
www.bestpub.com

CONTENTS

VOLUME TWO

SECTION 4. PAIN, INFECTION, & ADJUNCTIVE THERAPIES

SECTION 5. COMMUNICATION AND TRUST

SECTION 6. HEALTHCARE DELIVERY

PREFACE

EDITOR

Chronic wounds are a major cause of patient suffering and a profound financial burden to society. The focus of this Second Edition is assessment and management of chronic wounds in a Wound Care Practice. Physicians, podiatrists, nurses, enterostomal therapists, physical therapists, occupational therapists, and other health care professionals will find in this book the principles of modern, moist, interactive wound care, and the application of advanced therapeutic technologies. It represents the combined efforts of 65 authors selected from the basic sciences, clinical sciences, and clinical practice. The reader can examine the principles of managing the wound and treating the underlying cause of pressure sores, vascular insufficiency ulcers, chronic venous insufficiency ulcers, diabetic/ neurotrophic foot ulcers, and other chronic wounds.

Section I defines the Problem Wound. It presents the etiology of a problem wound and thc basic science of wound healing.

Section II describes the Principles of Wound Assessment. It discusses methods used in patient assessment for wound healing and describes specific assessment methods available to the wound care physician. It also addresses the need for evidence-based wound care.

Section III discusses the Principles of Wound Management. It provides general principles of modern wound care and the rationale for medical and surgical management of a wide variety of problem wounds. The authors were asked to write about what works for them in their various wound care practices. Thus, occasionally there are differences in recommended procedures.

Section IV deals with Pain, Infection and Adjunctive Therapies. It addresses nutrition, glycemic control, pain management, wound infection control, wound dressings, and advanced therapeutic methods, including hyperbaric oxygen therapy. It also describes available support services such as physical therapy, occupational therapy, and orthotics. The biochemistry and biophysical basis of the various classes of wound products are presented in depth.

Section V is about Communication and Trust. It addresses the key elements for comforting the patient, as well as the ethical and legal issues that must be dealt with in a wound care practice.

Section VI pertains to Healthcare Delivery. It offers suggestions for creating and managing a modern, comprehensive wound center and how to deal with issues of infection control and latex allergies. There is advice on documentation necessary for facility accreditation and for professional and technical services reimbursement.

The authors were asked to write each chapter as a stand-alone document for clinicians. Thus, there are redundancies pertaining to basic wound physiology, assessment tools, and principles of wound management. Some of the advanced therapeutic options such as negative pressure wound therapy (NPWT) and hyperbaric oxygen (HBO2) therapy are mentioned by several authors as they describe various treatment methods they have found to be useful. The reader will find that the authors have been generous with color photographs, figures, and tables to give a clear image of the wounds and the various assessment and management options. This will be helful to clinicians and medical students alike who read this book to gain a basic understanding of the wound healing process, both at the cellular level and at the bedside.

At the end of each chapter are review questions regarding key points that the reader will find valuable as a self assessment tool while preparing for specialty certification in wound care.

Following the publication of the classic JC Davis & TK Hunt textbook, *Problem Wounds: Role of Oxygen*, in 1988, the first Clinical Management of Problem Wounds Symposium was held in San Antonio, Texas. Subsequently, ten Symposia followed a natural evolution from research-oriented seminars, to clinical management symposia, to case-based workshops, to specific wound care methodologies. In 2002 it became a basic "hands on" course for clinical practice and certification in wound care. It was renamed, *The Wound Care Course*, and become the nucleus of the first edition of *Wound Care Practice* (2004). Most of the contributors to this book have been faculty members of these wound care symposia and courses that were organized by the Senior Editor. Today, because of the wealth of knowledge and growth in wound care technology this second edition of Wound Care Practice has expanded into two volumes.

The editors are grateful to the contributors to this book, who bring their insights and unique experiences to the text and enhance its value both as a readable volume and as an enduring reference.

Paul J. Sheffield, PhD
San Antonio, Texas
Editor

PREFACE

CO-EDITOR

In the 16th century, Ambroise Pare traveled with the French Army as a barber-surgeon. To counteract the purported poisonous effects of gunpowder, the wounds of injured soldiers were scalded with boiling oil. However, at the Battle of Turin, Pare ran out of boiling oil. In hopes of offering some therapeutic intervention for the doomed soldiers, he mixed a potion of egg yolks, turpentine, and oil of roses, thus creating the first controlled clinical trial in wound healing. To his surprise, not only did the soldiers deprived of boiling oil survive, but their wounds healed faster and with less pain. He coined the now famous phrase, "I dressed the wound, and God healed him."

As with all of medicine, the field of wound healing has been a plodding journey, punctuated by periods of enlightment. An understanding of the germ theory led to sterile, dry dressings and frequent antibiotic scrubs. The original work by Dr. George Winter, published in 1962, demonstrated the value of a moist wound environment. Now recombinant DNA technology and genetic engineering hold out the possibility of growing replacement tissues and blood vessels.

As the complexity of the Wound Management field increases, clinicians come to the field from many diverse specialties. The clinical application of wound care crosses most specialty boundaries, as is apparent from a review of the list of contributing authors. Wound healing issues form a continuum. No disease process recognizes specialty "niches" in its clinical manifestations.

This book is an attempt to cross the specialty boundaries and gain insight from all these perspectives. We are deeply indebted to these clinicians, without whom this book, and this specialty would not be possible. Our understanding of the wound healing process continues to evolve. This book is a snapshot of our current level of understanding, thanks to the work and dedication of many. To paraphrase Sir Isaac Newton—If we have seen farther, it is because we have stood on the shoulders of giants.

Caroline E. Fife, MD
Co-Editor

FOREWORD

During my residency, my program director J. Englebert Dunphy, recognized for his interest in wound healing wrote a well-regarded article for the New England Journal of Medicine entitled, "The Fibroblast, an Ally For the Surgeon." By using the word "for," he told me, he meant to carry forward his belief that this valuable ally would be available to us only if we made conditions right. The rest he felt was immutable. Looking back, it was a rebellious streak in me that led me to challenge him. I felt that healing mechanisms, like any other biologic process, can be rationally influenced, rationally slowed, rationally accelerated. (In those days, our sole ambition was to speed it.) I decided to challenge him. If I had fully appreciated the depth of his pessimism, I probably would have left the subject alone in favor of some other project. However, I took the challenge, and sensing my interest, he asked me to take consultations on wound problems. It took only two or three to realize that I had few answers. Protective dressings, casts, debridement, and lots of vitamin C were about all that I had. This state of "cluelessness" led most physicians of that day to avoid wound problems, and hide them behind dry eschars and dressings. One thing, though, warm, wet dressings were in favor. Ironically, they were effective but then fell almost totally out of use for many years. Now warmth is seeing a rebirth. There was cynicism about what warmth does. Does it even get into the tissue? Does it really enhance perfusion? Yes, local heat elevates subcutaneous temperature and with it perfusion and oxygen. Look it up! (Hint: Rabkin).

My first inklings of a real practical progress in wound care came when Hinman and Maibach found that epithelization (note the preferred spelling) could be hastened by keeping wounds moist. Never mind that it was to be another twenty to thirty years before its power was to be fully appreciated. In the 1960's, first Juha Niinikoski, then I, then the two of us together showed the importance of the perfusion and oxygenation of wounds, also a concept that has not yet reached its maximum contribution.

As we all know, antibiotics quickly reached their maximum contribution to wound care. Nevertheless, antibiotics gave great hope at the time. At that time, controversy about prophylactic use polarized the profession. A great deal of print passed through the presses before our current guidelines for prophylactic antibiotics in surgery were finally accepted.

This forward inertia would have run out of steam, I suspect, if the age of rational care, the clinical trial, had not developed on top of the increasing belief that healing could, in fact, be fostered. Trials on pressure garments for "venous wounds," further examination of moisture, protocols on prevention and care of pressure sores, surgical correction of venous and arterial pathologies have led to a discipline that led, in turn, to optimism and development of special expertise. You will find these developments superimposed on advanced understanding of inflammation and vascular pathology in this book.

One great theoretical advance, growth factors, increased industrial participation and funded research like never before. Their discovery multiplied commercial investment in research and centers of excellence, "wound clinics." In a practical sense administration of growth factors has advanced us relatively little, but it did lead to discovery of the value of "radical excision" of chronic wounds—which began as a result of frustration over the failure of growth factors to work and the new belief that "senescent" tissue could not respond to growth factor stimulation.

So, today, we have gathered together a rationale, a fairly tightly knit concept of how healing works, to promise a better day sometime in the not-too-distant future. Although the development of the concept of growth factors, though leading to relatively little in a human clinical level, convinced us ten years ago that if we only knew how to mix and add, suspend and apply, we would find the happier day just around the corner. The joy, though not realistic, has lasted long enough to allow us to reach some real practical advancement. The greatest benefit of the growth factors has been the conviction that their discovery has given us that healing—tissue repair—is, in fact, a malleable process.

This book is different from many others in the sense that it emphasizes assessment or, if you wish, "wound diagnostics." Many wounds fail to heal from inability to cope with natural wear and tear, drying and contamination, local contamination. In these cases, the most important decision is to enhance perfusion or oxygenation. There is often more than one impediment to healing of chronic wounds. There also needs to be an assessment of resources that the victim's body can offer. Perfusion and malnutrition are the major items. An impairment of the normal inflammatory reaction to injury is also one of the most common. Then, of course, there is the need to assess the degree to which antibacterial therapy will advance the course.

Though it has seemed like terribly painful progress, we've gone a long way since vitamin C. The editors of this book have been long interested in the problem of supplying adequate oxygen, and we should compliment them for their pioneering work on being the first, I think, to measure oxygen in chronic human wounds. Paul Sheffield was the first to note that hyper-oxygenation can enhance angiogenesis in human wounds. I predict for this area an interesting near future.

In this book there is a tacit recognition of the history of our recognition of the special properties of oxygen. Forty years ago when Juha Niinikoski started on oxygen, we knew it as an energy substrate and a nutritional substance for collagen production. More recently we began to see it as a source of antibacterial reactive oxygen species, probably the major "internal antibiotic" against organisms that find vulnerability in wounds. There is little or no specific immunity against staphylococcus for instance. Slowly but surely, we have begun to see hypoxia followed by re-oxygenation as a serious problem especially in non-healing wounds due to venous insufficiency and hyperglycemia.*

* High glucose inhibits the enzyme that converts O_2^+ the antibacterial oxidants H_2O_2 and O_2^-.

In the future I think we will find that redox effects that are based on oxygen and lactate constitute a fundamental wound-messaging system. But even at this point, we will have the same problem that has plagued us before. Too little oxygen is obviously bad. Enough oxygen is obviously good, a little more oxygen than normal is almost always helpful, but a lot more is clearly harmful. How do we find the effective range? Can we stay in the effective range? Must we push conditions out of the safe range (hyperbaric) in order to help? We know that inflammation can produce excessive, locally damaging oxidants. Can this flux of oxygen into redox messengers be controlled within the beneficial range? Can we use a combination of antibiotics plus debridement plus moisture retention, plus enhanced perfusion plus supporting oxygen supply to heal wounds that would not otherwise heal? This is the first book that I know to explore the area of oxygen in sufficient detail so that what we know can be exploited in a clinical sense.

Thomas K. Hunt, MD

ACKNOWLEDGEMENTS

Encouragement from Susan and Jim Joiner at Best Publishing Company to produce this book is gratefully acknowledged. In preparing, revising, and editing manuscripts, Suzanne Pack provided excellent technical support.

I am especially thankful for the assistance of Consulting Editor, Caroline E. Fife who is a highly respected wound care specialist at the University of Texas at Houston. She brings a wealth of experience from her wound care practice. As author and consulting editor, she has made major contributions to this book.

Finally, this book is dedicated to Dr. Jefferson C. Davis and—as a surprise—to Dr. Thomas K. Hunt, who introduced the Senior Editor to wound care in the mid 1970s. Dr. Davis was expanding the application of hyperbaric oxygen therapy at the USAF Hyperbaric Center at Brooks Air Force Base, Texas. Dr. T.K. Hunt was the whom of whom when there was no whomer in wound care research. Together, they provided the stimulus for our Center to conduct tissue oxygen studies, which confirmed that respired oxygen was delivered to human wounds and that a course of hyperbaric oxygen therapy elevates basal wound pO_2 as angiogenesis occurs. These pioneers saw the wisdom of adjunctive hyperbaric oxygen therapy to correct severe tissue hypoxia in selected problem wounds, and proposed the creation of wound healing centers. They co-edited Problem Wounds: Role of Oxygen (1988), which was a seminal document, laying the foundation for modern wound care.

DEDICATION

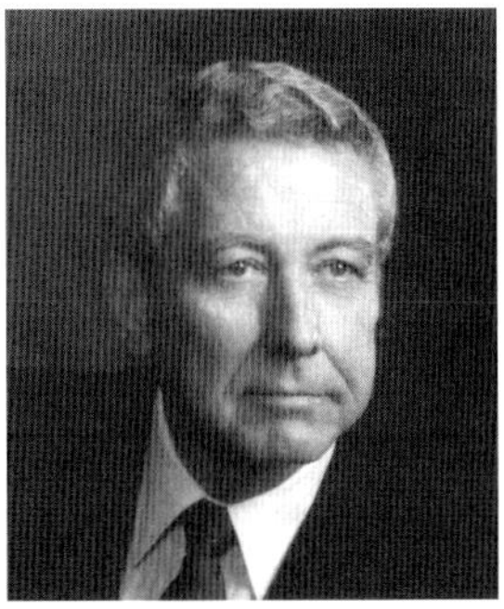

JEFFERSON C. DAVIS, MD

Dr. Jefferson C. Davis was the consummate physician and a pioneer in wound healing and hyperbaric medicine. Through his clinical practice, educational activities, and publications, he inspired several generations of clinicians to provide quality medical service for aviators, divers, and patients with difficult wounds.

Dr. Davis was born December 7, 1932. After receiving his MD at the University of Missouri in 1957, he joined the U.S. Air Force Medical Corps to become a Flight Surgeon. He received his MPH from the University of California and was Board Certified in Aerospace Medicine. In 1974, he founded the USAF Hyperbaric Medicine Center at Brooks Air Force Base in Texas. As the Center's first Director, he created the Davis Hyperbaric Oxygen Protocol for wound healing enhancement. Later, as Medical Director for Medical Seminars' Medicine of Diving Program he taught

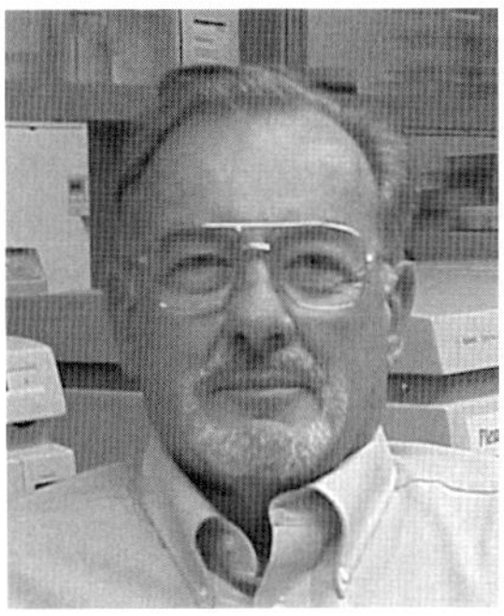

THOMAS K. HUNT, MD

Dr. Hunt is Professor Emeritus and Director of the Wound Healing Laboratory, Department of Surgery, University of California at San Francisco.

Dr. Thomas K. Hunt has devoted over 40 years to serving the wound healing community. He has been an inspiration to researchers and clinicians who advance our understanding of the wound healing process and develop methods to improve healing. Much of what is written in this book is the experience of authors who stand on the academic shoulders of Dr. T.K. Hunt.

Dr. Hunt was born August 6, 1930. After receiving his MD from Harvard Medical School in 1956, he served a brief tour in the U.S. Army Medical Corps. He then completed a Surgical Residency at the University of Oregon Medical School and a Research Fellowship at Western Infirmary, University of Glasgow, Scotland. In 1965, he became Director of the Wound Healing Laboratory at University

DAVIS (continued)

civilian physicians from all medical specialties to treat injured divers.

After retiring from the U.S. Air Force in 1979, Dr. Davis and associates founded International ATMO, Inc, the first known contract provider of wound care and hyperbaric medicine services. He established two successful wound care and hyperbaric medicine services in San Antonio Texas hospitals.

Dr. Davis' collaboration with Dr. T.K. Hunt produced the first hyperbaric medicine textbook, *Hyperbaric Oxygen Therapy* (1977); followed in 1988 with *Problem Wounds: Role of Oxygen*, which is a seminal document in wound healing. He authored over 70 papers and book chapters, and produced 5 books.

Dr. Davis was President of the Aerospace Medical Association, the American College of Preventive Medicine, and the Undersea & Hyperbaric Medical Society. Of all his achievements, he was most proud of being "an old country doctor," and his compassion for every patient's well being was legendary. Dr. Davis lost his battle with cancer in his 57th year on July 30, 1989.

HUNT (continued)

of California at San Francisco where his studies of wound healing mechanisms are legendary. These pioneering studies defined the role of oxygen in healing wounds. Several modern therapeutic modalities for wound healing are based on his scientific findings.

Dr. Hunt was a founding member and first President of the American Wound Healing Society, a founding member of three international professional societies, and President of the American Trauma Society, California Division. He has over 430 publications in the scientific literature and has produced 10 books.

Primary Contributors

RONALD P. BANGASSER, MD, FAAP
Medical Director, Wound Care Department, Redlands Community Hospital, Redlands, California Associate Professor, Loama Linda University, Loma Linda, California

350 Terracina Blvd.
Redlands, California 92373
Direct: (909) 335-4123
Office: (909) 335-5615
Fax: (909) 307-5027
Email: rbangass@epiclp.com

FERNANDO BOCCALANDRO, MD, FACC, FASCAD
Odessa Heart Institute

720 N. Golden
Odessa, Texas 79761
Office: (432) 337-3117
Fax: (432) 337-3448
Email: fernbo@pol.net

GORDON W. BOSKER, MED, CPO, CPED,
University of Texas Health Science Center at San Antonio

7703 Floyd Curl Drive
San Antonio, Texas 78284
Office: (210) 567-5346
Fax: (210) 567-5354
Email: bosker@uthscsa.edu

THOMAS M. BOZZUTO, DO, FACEP, FACHM, ABEM/UHM, FCCWS
Medical Director, Phoebe Wound Care & Hyperbaric Center

Phoebe Wound Care & Hyperbaric Center
803 North Jefferson Street, Suite A
Albany, Georgia 31701
Office: (229) 312-7600
Fax: (229) 312-7605
Email: tbozzuto@ppmh.org

CRAIG L. BROUSSARD, PHD, RN, CNS
Clincial Consultants

4228 Atlantic Road
Port Arthur, Texas 77642
Office: (409) 960-7747
Fax: (490) 962-0949
Email: craigB60@swbell.net

PHILOMENA C. BROUSSARD, PT, MPHA, CERT MDT
Director of Rehabilitation Services and Driector of the Wound Care and Hyperbaric Medicine Center

2809 Denny Avenue
Pasagoula, Minnesota 39581
Email: p_Broussard@srshealth.com

CLIFFORD J. BUCKLEY, MD, FACS
Professor of Surgery, Texas A&M University Health Service Center, College of Medicine Director, Division of Vascular Surgery, Scott & White Memorial Hospital

2401 South 31st Street
Temple, Texas 76508
Office: (254) 724-1647
Fax: (254) 724-3173
Email: cbuckley@swmail.sw.org

GLORIA CHIN, MD, MS
Assistant Professor, Division of Plastic and Reconstructive Surgery, Department of Surgery

University of Florida
Gainesville, Florida 32610-0286
Office: (352) 846-0377
Fax: (352) 846-0387
Email: chinga@mail.surgery.ufl.edu

PEGGY NAKAYAMA COE, BSN, RN, CWOCN, CIC
Wound & Ostomy Nurse—Southwestern Medical Center; Wound Ostomy Nurse Consultant—Quantum, Healthcare Lawton, Oklahoma

Southwestern Medical Center
5602 South West Lee Blvd.
Lawton, Oklahoma 73505
Office: (580) 531-4965
Email: peggy.coe@capellahealth.com

FRANS J. CRONJE, MBCHB (PRET), MSC
President of the South African Wound Healing Association, President of the South African Undersea and Hyperbaric Medical Association, and President-elect of the International Congress of Hyperbaric Medicine. Private practice at the Eugene Marais Hospital Wound Care and Hyperbaric Oxygen Therapy Center. Professor at the University of Pretoria, Faculty of Health Sciences, School of Medicine, Division of Aerospace Medicine, Department of Internal Medicine

AIMEE DENNIS-WAUTERS, MS, RD, CDE
Clinical Dietitian, Diabetes Educator, Diabetes Education Department, Texas Diabetes Institute, San Antonio, Texas

3414 Buckhaven
San Antonio, Texas 78230
Office: (210) 525-1059
Fax: (210) 525-8586
Email: adwauters@hotmail.com

ROBERT F. DIEGELMANN, PHD
Professor of Biochemisty, Anatomy & Emergency Medicine, Virginia Commonwealth University Medical Center

VCU Medical Center—Dept. of Biochemistry; Sanger Hall, Rm 2-007
1101 E. Marshall St.
Richmond, Virginia 23298-0614
Office: (804) 828-9677
Fax: (804) 828-1473
Email: rdieglm@vcu.edu

DUANE A. DIETZ, MD
Wound Treatment Centers of South Texas; Nix Healthcare System; Guadalupe Region Medical Center

414 Navarro, Suite 502
San Antonio, Texas 78205
Office: (210) 223-1145
Fax: (210) 615-7619
Email: hbo2@gvec.net

TIMOTHY A. EMHOFF, MD, FACS
Assistant Professor of Surgery, Tufts University Medical School, Department of Surgery Wound Care and Hyperbaric Medicine Program

WMASS Memorial Medical Center
55 Lake Ave North
Worcester, Massachusetts 01655
Office: (508) 856-1168
Fax: (508) 856-4224
Email: timothy.emhoff@umassmed.edu

JOHN J. FELDMEIER, DO
Toledo Radiation Oncology and The University of Toledo School of Medicine

15044 Kay Circle
Monroe, Michigan 48161
Office: (419) 383-4541
Fax: (419) 383-3040
Email: jfeldmeier@meduohio.edu

HARVEY FERGUSON, JR, RPH, JD, LLM
Gonzales, Hoblit & Ferguson, L.L.P.

One Riverwalk Place
700 N. St Mary's Street, Suite 1800
San Antonio, Texas 78205
Office: (210) 224-9991
Fax: (210) 226-1544
Email: HFerguson@ghf-lawfirm.com

CAROLINE E. FIFE, MD
Associate Professor, Department of Anesthesiology, University of Texas Health Science Center, Houston, Director of Clinical Research, Memorial Hermann Center for Wound Healing & Lymphedema Management

54 N. Brokenfern Drive
The Woodlands, Texas 77380
Direct: (713) 305-2971
Fax: (281) 364-1121
Email: cfife@intellicure.com

DONALD M. GREER, JR., MD
Plastic Surgeon, Private Practice

335 Upper Cibolo Creek Road
Boerne, Texas 78006
Office: (830) 537-3129
Fax: (830) 537-3134
Email: dmgjgmd@earthlink.net

CLYDE O. HAGOOD, JR., MD, FACS (RETIRED)
Emeritus Director of Problem Wound and Hyperbaric Medicine Center—Memorial Hospital, Gulfport, Mississippi

6103 Grande Cove Court
Granbury , Texas 76049-6360
Office: (817) 326-8288
Fax: (817) 326-8288 [Call first]
Email: copdhago1@alltel.net

THOMAS K. HUNT, MD, FACS, FRCS, DMHC
Professor Emeritus, Department of Surgery, School of Medicine, University of California, San Francisco, California

513 Parnassus Ave, HSW 1619, Box 0522
San Francisco, California 94143-0522
Office: (415) 476-1865
Fax: (415) 476-5190
Email: hanlink@surgery.ucsf.edu

CLYDE IKEDA, MD, FACS

1199 Bush Street, Suite 640
San Francisco, California 94109

KHURRAM H. KHAN, DPM
Chief Resident, Department of Orthopedics, Podiatry Division; University of Texas Health Science Center at San Antonio, Texas

7703 Floyd Curl Drive
San Antonio, Texas 78229

PATRICK N. KIMBRELL, MD
Medical Director, Center for Wound Care, Warm Springs Rehabilitation Hospital Clinical Associate Professor, University of Texas Health Science Center of San Antonio

5101 Medical Drive
San Antonio, Texas 78229
Office: (210) 592-5349
Fax: (210) 592-5462
Email: wound_doc@juno.com

DIANE L. KRASNER, PHD, RN, CWCN, CWS, FAAN
Wound & Skin Care Consultant

212 East Market Street
York, Pennsylvania 17403
Office: (717) 812-1734
Fax: (717) 812-0135
Email: dlkrasner@aol.com

VALERIE LARSON-LOHR, MS, APRN, CWCN, CEN, CHRNC
Director, Centers for Wound Care, Warm Springs Hospitals, Diversified Clinical Services

5101 Medical Drive
San Antonio, Texas 78247
Office: (210) 592-5349
Fax: (210) 592-5462
Email: wound_nurse@juno.com

JACK L. LE FROCK, MD, FACP, FIDSA
Medical Director, 3D Dosing Systems Inc.

647 Waterside Way
Sarasota, Florida 34242
Direct: (941) 809-7559
Office: (941) 349-9863
Fax: (941) 309-6304
Email: doclefrock@aol.com

DAVID L. McCORVEY, MD
Guthrie Clinic

130 Centerway
Pine City Corning
New York 14871

CHARLES P. MOUTON, MD, MS
Professor and Chair, Department of Community and Family Medicine, Howard University College of Medicine

520 West Street, NW Room 2400
Washington, DC 20059
Office: (202) 806-6300
Fax: (202) 806-4898
Email: cmouton@howard.edu

HERBERT B. NEWTON, MD, FAAN
Professor of Neurology, Oncology, and Hyperbaric Medicine, Dardinger Neuro-Oncology Center, Ohio State University Medical Center and James Cancer Hospital

465 Means Hole
1654 Uphem Drive
Columbus, Ohio 43260
Office: (614) 293-8930
Fax: (614) 293-6111
Email: newton.12@osu.edu

JEFFREY A. NIEZGODA, MD, FACEP, FACHM
Medical Director, The Center for Comprehensive Wound Care and Hyperbaric Oxygen Therapy, St. Lukes Medical Center, Milwaukee, Wisconsin

5910 Glen Haven Drive
Greendale, Wisconsin 53129
Office: (414) 385-8724
Fax: (414) 525-0490/0491
Email: niezgoda@execpc.com

LIZA G. OVINGTON, PHD, CWS
Associate Medical Director; Johnson & Johnson Wound Management, Somerville, New Jersey

775 South Dogwood Road
Walnutport, Pennsylvania 18088
Office: (610) 760-1304
Fax: (775) 845-9296
Email: lovingt@ethus.jnj.com

RUDY C. PRUNEDA, PHD (ABMM)
Consultant Services, San Antonio, Texas

9114 Serene Creek
San Antonio, Texas 78230
Office: (210) 525-8070
Email: rpruneda@earthlink.net

CHARLES A. REASNER, MD
University of Texas Health Science Center; Texas Diabetes Institute, San Antonio, Texas

University Center for Community Health; Texas Diabetes Institute
701 S. Zarzamora, Mail Stop 12-5
San Antonio, Texas 78207
Office: (210) 358-7402
Fax: (210) 358-7406
Email: Charles.Reasner@UHS-SA.com

JAYESH B. SHAH, MD, CWS
President, South Texas Wound Associates, PA, Medical Director, Southwest Center for Wound Care and Hyperbaric Medicine, Southwest General Hospital, San Antonio, Texas

7500 Bralie Blvd. #104
San Antonio, Texas 78224
Direct: (210) 408-0117
Office: (210) 921-3493
Fax: (210) 921-3533
Email: drshah@wounddoctors.com

KIMBERLY MOREHOUSE SHEFFIELD, MA-LPC
Licensed Professional Counselor (Texas)

Behavioral Health Department
Family Service Associations of San Antonio, Texas
Email: ksheffield@family-service.org

PAUL J. SHEFFIELD, PHD, CASP, CHT
President and CME Program Director, International ATMO, Inc., San Antonio, Texas

Nix Medical Center
414 Navarro, Suit 502
San Antonio, Texas 78205
Office: (210) 614-3688
Fax: (210) 223-4864
Email: psheffield@hyperbaricmedicine.com

J. BENJAMIN SLADE, JR., MD
Northbay Center for Wound Care

131 Blackwood Court
Vacaville, California 95688-1058
Direct: (707) 332-2005
Office: (707) 451-1491
Fax: (707) 455-8353
Email: jslade1515@aol.com

ADRIANNE P. S. SMITH, MD
Medical Director, Kinetic Concepts, Inc., Assistant Professor, University of Texas Health Science Center of San Antonio, Texas

Medical Department
6203 Farinon Drive
San Antonio, Texas 78249
Office: (210) 255-6640
Email: asmith24@satx.rr.com

MELVIN D. SMITH, MD
Associate Director, Methodist Wound Care and Hyperbaric Oxygen Treatment Center, San Antonio, Texas

Methodist Hospital Wound Care and Hyperbaric Oxygen Service
4499 Medical Drive-SL-2
San Antonio, Texas 78229
Office: (210) 575-4497
Fax: (210) 575-4498
Email: msmith11@satx.rr.com

LENA L. SOTO, RN, BSN, MS, CHRN
Operations Branch Chief, Hyperbaric Medicine Division; USAF School of Aerospace Medicine, 2611 Louis Bauer Dr, Brooks City-Base, Texas 78235-5130

25515 Echo Terrace
San Antonio, Texas 78258-6811
Office: (210) 536-3281
Fax: (210) 536-2944
Email: lena.soto@brooks.af.mil

JOHN S. STEINBERG, DPM
Assistant Professor, Department of Plastic Surgery, Georgetown University School of Medicine, Washington DC

3800 Reservoir Rd, Northwest
1-Main-West
Washington, DC 20007-2113
Office: (202) 444-3059
Fax: (202) 444-5391
Email: steinberg@usa.net

MELLICK T. SYKES, MD, MA, FACS
Peripheral Vascular Associates

7950 Floyd Curl Drive, Suite 109
San Antonio, Texas 78229
Office: (210) 692-9700
Fax: (210) 692-9730
Email: mellicksykes@aol.com

MISTY M. VAUGHN, PT, CWS, FCCWS
Comprehensive Therapy Solutions, Owner; American Medical Technologies, Regional Vice President

615 North Main, #102
Euless, Texas 76039
Office: (817) 681-7875
Fax: (817) 685-7243
Email: mistypt@comcast.net

ROBERT A. WARRINER, III, MD, FACA, FCCP, FCCWS, ABPM/UHM,CWS
Executive Vice President of Medical Affairs, Diversified Clinical Services, Jacksonville, Florida; Emeritus Medical Director and Founder, Southeast Texas Center for Wound Care and Hyperbaric Medicine, Conroe Regional Medical Center, Conroe, Texas

1610 Woodstead Court, Suite 460
The Woodlands, Texas 77380
Office: (281) 298-1400
Fax: (281) 298-1570
Email: rwarriner@diversifiedclinicalservices.com

GREGORY R. WEIR, MD
Vascular Surgeon in private practice at the Eugene Maris and Zuid Afrikaans Hospitals in Pretoria; Fellowship in Vascular Surgery, South African College of Medicine; M. Med (Surgery), University of Pretoria

P.O. Box 26091
Gezina, 0031, South Africa
Office: +27123358651
Fax: +27123358651
Email: gweir@vascular.co.2A

LYNDA T. WELLS, MD, DABPM, FRCA
Associate Professor of Anesthesiology & Pediatrics, University of Virginia Health System

Dept. of Anesthesiology
P.O. Box 800710
Charlottesville, Virginia 22908-0710
Office: (434) 924-2283
Fax: (434) 982-0019
Email: ltw6r@virginia.edu

RANDALL D. WOLCOTT, MD
Southwest Regional Wound Care Center, Lubbock, Texas

2002 Oxford Avenue
Lubbock, Texas 79410
Office: (806) 793-8869
Fax: (806) 793-0043
Email: randy@randallwolcott.com

E. GEORGE WOLF, JR., MD
Wound Care and Hyperbaric Medicine, Private Practice

414 Navarro, Suite 502
San Antonio, Texas 78205
Office: (210) 536-3281
Fax: (210) 536-2944
Email: george.wolf@brooks.af.mil

DISCLAIMER

The views expressed by the authors are their own and do not necessarily reflect the opinion of the editors, International ATMO, Inc, or Best Publishing Company.

While the information in this book is consistent with good medical practice, no responsibility can be assumed by the author or the publisher for any injuries or damage of any nature whatsoever, as a result of product failure, negligence, or from the application of any recommendations or ideas contained in this book.

Medicine is an ever-changing field. Standard safety precautions must be followed, but as new research and clinical experience broaden our knowledge, changes in treatment and drug therapy may become necessary or appropriate. Readers are advised to check the most current product information provided by the manufacturer of each drug, device, or equipment to verify the recommended dose, the method and duration of administration, and contraindications.

TRANCUTANEOUS OXIMETRY

To avoid confusion in terminology, in this book TCOM refers to the equipment (transcutaneous oxygen monitoring) or the procedure (transcutaneous oximetry) used for obtaining tissue oxygen values in the skin. PtcO2, aka $TcpO_2$ (transcutaneous oxygen tension) refers to the tissue pO_2 data obtained by TCOM, and is expressed in mm Hg. Although PtcO2 is the technically correct term it is seldom used by government agencies, insurance carriers, or clinicians, who prefer the term TcpO2. Thus, the authors have used PtcO2 and TcpO2 interchangeably in this book.

NOTES

CHAPTER 24

WOUND HEALING IN THE GERIATRIC PATIENT

CHAPTER TWENTY-FOUR OVERVIEW

NOTES

Wound Healing in the Geriatric Patient

Charles P. Mouton, Wayne A. Fredrick, Robert W. Parker

INTRODUCTION

Aging results in changes to overall wound healing in the elderly. It is a major problem for elders with pressure ulcers, venous stasis ulcers and skin tears. These wounds continue to be difficult for patients and clinicians in spite of extensive studies over the last 60 years using various treatment modalities. They cause considerable disability and add millions of dollars to the national health care costs (23). Wound healing has become a fertile ground for plaintiff's attorneys because of the belief that all wounds are preventable and should be healed. Pressure ulcer incidence is now being used as an indicator of quality of care. (Requirements for long term care facilities. Federal Register 1991) Considerable controversy exists concerning our ability to prevent pressure ulcers (5). Most pressure ulcers may be preventable with the most aggressive preventive measures, but there appears to be a limit beyond which prevention is futile (19). Nevertheless, progress is being made in prevention. One study using the Minimum Data Set to study the incidence of new pressure ulcers in over 30,000 nursing home residents, showed a reduction in new stage three and four ulcer from 30% to 22% (5).

Management of chronic wounds in the elderly is still difficult, but there is some consensus on the various treatments. Many roadblocks exist, such as the unfamiliarity of many physicians with the current knowledge of the prevention and management of these wounds, and the competing demands in these frail patients with multiple co-morbidities. The mainstays of therapy are reducing the pressure, friction and shear forces, assessing the wound and choosing a treatment appropriate for the stage of the wound. At the same time the nutrition of the patient is assessed and improved as much as possible while attending to the co-morbid conditions. Nutrition is invariably inadequate in elder patients with chronic wounds. Co-morbid conditions may be the cause of inadequate nutrition. The wound itself may cause cachexia by the production of inflammatory cytokines such as tumor necrosis factor, IL 1 and IL 6. With cachexia, nutritional requirements are increased above basal needs.

With an increasingly expanding elderly population, whose life expectancy is also increasing just as rapidly, we can certainly expect that healthcare for the elderly to come into the spotlight. A major aspect of that care would be the care of wounds. The elderly population over the next decade will prove to be far more active than previous generations. This increase in physical activity will potentially result in more traumatic and orthopedic injuries and increasing needs for wound care. The psychological impact of the decreased mobility associated with the management of chronic wounds is also an area that would need more attention. Chronic venous insufficiency affects ten to thirty five percent of the entire USA population and four percent of people older than sixty five years of age have chronic venous ulcers. Also, among the vulnerable elderly populations, wound care becomes a critical quality care issue.

EPIDEMIOLOGY OF SKIN BREAKDOWN IN OLDER ADULTS

Development of pressure ulcers is a significant problem in the care of frail older adults. An estimated 1.3 to 3 million older adults have a pressure ulcer (8). The overall prevalence of pressure ulcers varies by the setting, a proxy for the degree of frailty. In the outpatient setting, the prevalence of stage II through IV pressure ulcers is 20% (6).

The prevalence of pressure ulcers in homebound elders is 8–29% (20, 21, 27). The annual incidence rate of stage III and stage IV pressure ulcers in home care patients is 0–17% (4). Examining the incidence in the general elderly population, the ten-year incidence of pressure ulcers at stage II or greater for adults age 55–75 years old is 2.2% (18).

Hospitals and long term care settings tend to have higher prevalence and incidence rates. In the hospital inpatient setting, the annual incidence rate for pressure ulcers is 0.4%–38.0% (8). The annual incidence rate in the long term care setting is 2.2–23.9% (8). These higher rates reflect a generally older, more frail population with significant disease co-morbidity and functional impairment. The susceptibility of these older adults to skin breakdown leading to pressure ulcers may be in part due to age related changes in the epidermal and dermal structures.

AGING-RELATED CHANGES IN SKIN

Epidermis

Although controversial, it is generally thought that the epidermis thins with aging. The thickness of the stratum corneum remains unchanged, except for a decrease in water content, and the adhesion between corneocyte decreases (12). The keratinocyte layer tends to display a decreased vertical height (31). The most consistent age-related changes are the flattening of the dermoepidermal interface, effacement of the dermal rete and the decrease in the number of interdigitating papillae; changes which result in decreased nutrient transfer. Melanocytes decrease by 8%–20% each decade after age 30 and the number of Langerhans cells decrease by 58% with aging. The changes in the dermoepidermal intergace predispose older adults to shear injuries and bullae formation, otherwise known as "geri tears." The decrease in Langerhans cells impairs the skin's cell-mediated immunity. Aging also decreases Vitamin D production.

Connective Tissue

Normal human dermis is 70–80% collagen by dry weight with 15 different collagen subtypes (35). Collagen types I, II, and III are the major subtypes that provide tensile properties to the skin (35). Stabilization of this collagen is done by covalent cross-links which are dependent on oxidative deamination of lysine and hydroxylysine.

Elastic fibers make up 2–4 % of the dermis (oxytalan, elaunin, elastin and microfibrillar structures) with elastin predominating at 90% of the elastic fibers. The major source of elastin is from dermal fibroblast and smooth muscle cells. In the extracellular tissue, elastin is stabilized by desmosines. Demosines cross link during the biosynthesis of elastin by the covalent bounding of lysine residues by lsysl oxidase.

Age associated changes in skin are divided into sun-exposed and sun-protected changes. In sun exposed areas (photoaging), aging results in an excessive deposition of elastotic material, basophilic degeneration of collagen and accumulation of glycoaminoglycans. They also undergo fiber disintergration. The elastin content of the dermis increases between 20–80 years of age and the concentration of desmosine is increased fourfold in sun-exposed skin. This material seems to replace collagen in the upper areas of the dermis.

Sun protected areas show a decrease in the number and size of elastin fibers. Results regarding collagen and aging have been conflicting, with some studies showing an increase in collagen concentration and others showing a decrease relative to the total percentage of skin. Also the synthesis of new collagen is decreased with aging as is its solubility. It also becomes more resistant to collagenase and has a lower hexosamine to collagen ratio. Earlier work shows that the total amount of collagen decreases by about 1% per year of adult life (31). The enzyme systems that modify collagen have an age-related decrease in activity thus affecting the cross linking of collagen. In fact, the reduction in propyl hydrolase activity seen in aging is worsened in vitamin C deficiency and hypoxic conditions and is probably the rate-limiting step in collagen production. This age-related reduction in collagen production and the age-related decrease in fibroblast activity could possibly explain the poor wound healing tendency noted in some older adults. As people age, the elastic fibers show increased fragmentation and contain fewer microfilaments. These changes lead to increased laxity and loss of resiliency thus predisposing deeper tissues to injury following trauma.

There are also many age-related changes in the underlying structures. Skin tends to become relatively avascular with a 35% reduction in venule surface area with aging (15). There is also 50% fewer mast cells in older compared to younger adults. Subcutaneous tissue tends to atrophy in the face, hands, feet and shins. However, there is an increased deposition of subcutaneous fat in the waist and thighs.

MUSCULOSKELETAL

Decrease in muscle mass and increase in osteoporosis in the elderly adversely affects the wound healing mechanisms in the overlying connective tissues and epidermis. In elderly patients with chronic ulcers, the incidence of osteomyelitis is increased. Nerve growth factor has been shown to play a role in angiogenesis and the proliferation of keratinocytes. Nerve growth factors also have stimulatory neuro peptides and growth factors which can stimulate the skin healing process of the underlying muscle and bone (10).

PHYSIOLOGY OF WOUND HEALING IN OLDER ADULTS

Wound healing is characterized by four phases: Inflammatory, Migratory, Proliferative, and Remodeling. In the Inflammatory phase, tissue injury results in the release of cellular contents which initiates the clotting cascade. This clotting cascade in turn deposits fibrin at the injured site to form a clot. As this clot is formed, platelet activation causes the activation of the kinin system and release of platelet-derived growth factors. Vasodilatation occurs causing erythema of the wound and causing increased vascular permeability. This increased permeability allows the cellular components of microvascular circulation to enter the wound. Initially, mast cells, polymorphonuclear leukocytes and lymphocytes appear creating an inflammatory infiltrate and releasing a variety of cytokines. In later inflammatory stages, macrophages enter the injured area to clear cellular debris and initiate the healing process. T-lymphocytes stimulate macrophages to produce collagenase, essential to early wound healing. The inflammatory phase typically lasts one week in young adults.

In the Migratory phase, macrophages continue to clear debris and bacteria from the site of injury while fibroblasts migrate to the injured area to initiate wound healing. Various wound growth factors are released that stimulate new in-growth of capillaries. These growth factors include interleukin -1alpha and tumor necrosis factor-alpha. In the proliferative phase, the inflammatory response subsides and the fibroblasts that have migrated into the wound begin to lay down collagen and other matrix proteins and myofibroblasts begin to contract the wound surface area. Fibroblasts reach their peak production after three days. During the first few days large amounts of type III collagen are produced with small amounts of type I collagen. While collagen concentration peaks after nine days, collagen production continues for three weeks and wound contraction continues for several weeks. In the later stages, the resting epithelium is activated at the wound edges and stimulated to migrate over the wound surface.

Re-epithelialization begins with the recruiting resting populations of epidermal cells at the margins of wounds and their migration to the wound center. The extracellular matrix of laminin, fibronectin, and tenascin laid down in the proliferative phase provides the surface from epidermal cells to migrate across. After the surface of the wound is epithelialized (about 3–4 weeks in young adults) with its scar formation, the remodeling phase begins. During the remodeling phase and the late proliferative phase, previously layed down collagen (type III) is broken down and replaced by new collagen, particular over areas on mechanical stress. More collagen cross-linking occurs and the overall wound is strengthened. Vitamin C acts as a proline hydroxylase cofactor and is essential for remodeling and new collagen formation. In about six weeks, overall wound strengths reaches 90% of the original tissue strength.

For in depth discussion of the wound healing process see the chapter by G A Chin et al. entitled, "Biochemitry of Wound Healing in Wound Care Practice."

Wound healing is prolonged in older adults. This prolongation in wound healing has a number of causes that affect each stage of wound healing. In animal experiments, the aging process slows the inflammatory phase. Burn wounds in animal experiments show that peak DNA content in the wound (a measure of inflammatory response) was reached at day 3 for younger animals and at day 7 for older animals (13). Macrophage function, but not the total number of macrophages, seems to be impaired by the aging process. Animal studies by Cohen demonstrate that young mice treated with anti-macrophage serum heal at rates similar to old mice (7). Danon et al. show that even for old mice, wound healing improves significantly when treated with macrophages with the best results seen in those treated with macrophages from young donors (9).

Decreased proliferation of fibroblasts is a well-known feature of aging. In wound healing, the proliferative capacity of fibroblasts was associated with healing rates in young versus old animals (14). Capillary in-growth into wounds is decreased in aging. Yamura and Matsuzawa showed that capillary grew at a rate of 0.189 mm/day in 8–9-week-old rats versus 0.123 mm/day in 59–80 week old rats (36).

The transit time for epithelialization, particularly from the stratum corneum, is increased by 50% to almost 200% in older adults (16, 17). The re-epithelialization of wounds takes nearly twice as long in older adults (28). In experiments using facial dermabrasion, epithelialization occurred in ten days for 25-year-olds versus 21 days for 75-year-olds. Healing time for forearm blisters was 3.6 weeks for young adults versus 5.4 weeks for older adults.

The rate of cellular proliferation, wound metabolism and collagen remodeling are slower in the wounds of older adults. While the amount of collagen synthesis may be unchanged or slightly less in older adults, the quality of the collagen produced and process of collagen degradation and remodeling seems to be impaired (14). With an age-related decrease in tensile strength of healed wounds, the rate of wound dehiscence is increased for older adults, 0.9%, 2.5% and 5.5% for ages 30–39, 50–59, and over 80 respectively (24, 30). This increased dehiscence rate is thought to be due to as decrease in tensile strength in older adults, not a decrease in the amount of collagen produced. The degree of tertiary remodeling through collagen cross-linking seems to be is the most likely cause of the age-related strength differences in wounds.

This is particularly true for elderly patients who have experienced wound dehiscence in abdominal wounds. The decreased skin cell strength and lack of remodeling of the collagen can affect these wounds which rely heavily on skin cell strength to keep them together. In patients undergoing abdominal surgery, there are incidents of wound dehiscence that increased five to ten-fold in elderly patients.

NON-DERMAL AGING RELATED FACTORS

Older adults have a variety of conditions that led to prolonged, poor wound healing. Oxygen is necessary for all stages of wound healing. Ischemia has been shown to decrease mechanical properties of wounds in older animals by 45%–60% (29). In laboratory animals, there is an age-associated decrease in metabolic activity that is associated with a decrease in tissue oxygen consumption (14). Low tissue oxygen tension is probably the single most important factor in slow wound healing. Thus, conditions resulting in poor cardiac output (heart failure, atrial fibrillation, myocardial infarction) or low oxygen carrying capacity (chronic obstructive pulmonary disease, anemia) prolong healing.

Diabetes mellitus affects 11% of older adults over the age of 70 years old. Thus glucose metabolism, which serves as an energy substrate for wound healing, also decreases with age. The effects of impaired glucose metabolism on diabetic older adults are demonstrated by the prolonged healing time in diabetics. Time for complete wound healing is increased 1.5 to three-fold in diabetic elderly compared to elderly without diabetes (34). Diabetes is associated with the premature senescence of cultured dermal fibroblasts and higher level of glucose decreases fibroblast proliferation and inhibits response to platelet–derived growth factor (32). Diabetes also adversely affects microvasculature and osseous structures. Impaired glucose metabolism, impaired insulin utilization, and hyperinsulinemia result in impaired leukocyte function, impaired lipid regulation and its deleterious effects on macrovascular structures, and impaired neurologic function. All of these adverse effects associated with diabetes adversely impact wound healing. Impaired neurological function can also lead to repeated injury of the affected area, hence interrupting the necessary element of wound healing.

Peripheral vascular disease affects 20% of older adults. As a precursor to arterial and/or venous occlusion, peripheral vascular disease diminishes tissue oxygenation thus increasing the risk of ulceration, prolonged healing and tissue necrosis. In addition to its direct effects on tissue oxygenation, peripheral vascular disease is hypothesized as leading to lower capillary pressure thus promoting easier microvascular occlusion (at 12 mm Hg to 32 mm Hg) in the face of sustained surface pressures.

Nutrition intake, particularly fluid and protein balance, is impaired in many frail older adults. About 10% of community-dwelling older adults and one-third or greater of institutionalized older adults have protein-calorie malnutrition. Also, the majority of older adults (67%) report diets that need improvement. Clinically significant malnutrition can be diagnosed by a serum albumin less than 3.5 mg/dl, total lymphocyte count less than 1800/mm^3, and weight loss of greater than 15%. Pre albumin levels are a more sensitive indicator of short term nutritional status, because of its short half-life. Protein-calorie malnutrition leads to decreased visceral protein stores, poor protein balance (indicated by a negative nitrogen balance), altered immune function and further malabsorption leading to poor wound healing (22). Altered immune function decreases the inflammatory response. Decreased protein stores decrease complement and fibronectin, both important in fibroblast proliferation, and decrease clearance of wastes by macrophages. Protein depletion results in decreased fibroblast and collagen production. Trace elements and vitamins are also important for wound healing. Vitamin C is needed for lysine and proline hydroxylation, part of the collagen cross-linking process (3). It is also important for collagen synthesis. Copper, thiamine, riboflavin and pyridoxine are required for collagen cross-linking. Zinc is important for RNA and DNA polymerization, essential for building the wound matrix (3). Zinc is also essential for maintenance of immune function.

MEASURES TO ENHANCE WOUND HEALING IN OLDER ADULTS

Many of the wound care therapies directed at older adults attempt to mitigate the above mention age-related changes in wound healing

Conventional Therapies

A host of conventional therapies are available for wound treatment. Generally there is no evidence that any particular moist dressing is more advantageous than another. Moisture retaining dressings protect the wound surface, reduce bacterial overgrowth and wound infection rates, debride necrotic tissue, and promote granulation tissue.

Electromagnetic Fields

Electromagnetic fields are thought to improve wound healing. These fields have been shown to inhibit bacterial growth in tissue culture and improve the migration and proliferation of fibroblasts. Electrical stimulation has also been shown to increase the expression of transforming growth factor-beta on fibroblasts and collagen synthesis. In small study of venous leg ulcers, Stiller showed that pulsed electromagnetic fields improved healing in 48% of recalcitrant wounds (33). The Agency for Health Care Policy and Research Pressure Ulcer Guideline Committee recommends electrical stimulation for Stage III and IV pressure ulcers that do not respond to conventional therapies (2).

Growth Factors

Several growth factors have been investigated regarding their effect on wound healing. In small trials, human Epidermal Growth Factor (h-EGF) increased healing rates by 15% in partial thickness wounds. Both h-EGF and platelet-derived growth factor (PGDF) increase the tensile strength of wounds in animal studies. In larger clinical trials, the overall success of these factors has been disappointing. One agent, becaplermin gel, a topically applied platelet derived growth factor, showed improved healing rate compared to placebo (48% vs 25%, respectively) and has subsequently received Food and Drug Administration (FDA) approval for use in diabetic ulcers.

Skin Grafts

Meshed autografts accelerate wound healing by reducing the proliferative stress on re-epithelialization. Fatah showed that 100% of meshed areas healed in ten days while 85% of control areas healing in 10–21 days (11). Cultured epidermal allografts from unrelated donors have been used successfully to treat a variety of wounds. In a small study of older adults (63–87 years of age) the healing time for allograft sites was reduced by 7.9 days. Cryopreserved cadaver allografts have been similarly used for burn victims. Composite grafts consisting of a bilayered composite of bovine collagen, allogeneic human fibroblasts, and keratinocytes has improved wound healing rates in diabetic foot ulcers and has been approved by the FDA for treatment of venous stasis ulcers.

Pharmaceuticals

Estrogen may play a role in wound healing. In a small study of elder women, estrogen replacement therapy reversed age-related delays in wound healing.

Pentoxifyline has been shown to improve wound healing in venous ulcers when combined with compression. Gross bacterial infection retards the wound healing process. Although not considered standard conventional treatment, topical antibiotics reduce wound bacterial counts. The AHRQ Pressure Ulcer Guideline (2) committee recommends a two week trial of topical antibiotics in wounds that fail to make adequate progress toward healing in two to four weeks. Systemic antibiotics have improved wound healing in infected wounds. Systemic antibiotics are particularly useful from wound demonstrating signs of cellulites.

Negative Pressure Wound Therapy

Negative Pressure Wound Therapy [e.g., Vacuum Assisted Closure (VAC)] provides a new paradigm that can be used in concert with a wide variety of standard existing plastic surgery techniques. It was originally developed as an alternative treatment for debilitated patients with chronic wounds. It has rapidly evolved into a widely accepted treatment of chronic and acute wounds, contaminated wounds, burns, envenomations, infiltrations and wound complications from failed operations. Two broad mechanisms of action are proposed: removal of fluid and mechanical deformation. Fluid removal both decreases edema–thus decreasing interstitial pressure and shortening distances of diffusion and removes soluble factors that may affect the healing process (both positively and negatively). The relationship of mechanical deformation to increased growth is well known to plastic surgeons, as it is the basis of tissue expansion (25).

Hyperbaric Oxygen Therapy

Hyperbaric oxygen therapy (HBO2) is an important adjunct in the management of problem wounds which exist in chronic oxygen deficiency and in which that local oxygen tension is below optimal for healing. In the treatment of hypoxic and ischemic wounds, the most important effects of hyperbaric oxygenation are the stimulation of fibroblast proliferation and differentiation, increased collagen formation and cross-linking, augmented neovascularization, and the stimulation of leukocyte microbial killing. Ischemic soft tissues also benefit from hyperoxygenation through improved preservation of energy metabolism and reduction of edema (26).

FUTURE DIRECTIONS AND RESEARCH

Most of our understanding of wound healing in older adults arises from surgically created or chemically created wounds. The characteristics of wound healing starting with the inflammatory response to remodeling may be substantially different in wounds created by pressure. Our understanding of the processes of wound healing when tissue damage is initiated through prolonged intracapillary occlusion without an initial disruption of the epithelial surface has been understudied. Until we have a better understanding of these processes at a cellular level, pressure ulcer prevention and treatment will be limited.

REFERENCES

1. Agency for Healthcare Research and Quality (AHRQ) AHCPR Clinical Practice Guideline Number 3: Pressure Ulcers in Adults: Prediction and Prevention. (AHCPR #92-0047: May 1992). Can be ordered at the AHRQ web site (*www.ahrq.gov/news/pubcat/c_clin.htm#clin014*)

2. Agency for Healthcare Research and Quality (AHRQ) AHCPR Clinical Practice Guideline Number 15: Treatment of Pressure Ulcers. (AHCPR #95-0652, Dec 1994). Can be ordered at the AHRQ web site (*www.ahrq.gov/news/pubcat/c_clin.htm#clin014*)

3. Ashcroft ., Horan M, Ferguson M. The effects of ageing on cutaneous wound healing in animals. *Journal of Anatomy* 1995. 187, 1-26.

4. Bergquist S, Frantz R. Pressure ulcers in community-based older adults receiving home health care. *Advances in Wound Care* 1999. 12, 339-351.

5. Brandeis G, Berlowitz D R, Katz P. Are pressure ulcers preventable? A survey of experts. *Advances in Skin & Wound Care* 2001. 14, 244-248.

6. Clark M, Kadhom H M, The nursing prevention of pressure sores in hospital and community patients. *Journal of Advanced Nursing* 1988. 13, 365-373.

7. Cohen B, Danon, D, Roth, G. Wound repair in mice influenced by age and antimacrophage serum. *J Gerontol* 1987. 42, 295-301.

8. Cuddigan J, et al. (eds). National Pressure Ulcer Advisory Panel (NPUAP). Pressure Ulcers in America: Prevalence, Incidence and Implications for the Future. Reston, Va., NPUAP, 2001.

9. Danon D, Kowatch, M, Roth G. Promotion of wound repair in old mice by local injection of macrophages. *Proc Natl Acad Sci USA* 1989. 86, 2018-2020.

10. Demling RH, DeSanti L. Use of extra-cellular wound matrix in treating wounds & burns. *Ann Inter Med* 2003:139:635-641.

11. Fatah MF, Ward CM.The morbidity of split-skin graft donor sites in the elderly: the case for mesh-grafting the donor site. *Br J Plast Surg* 1984 Apr;37(2):184-90.

12. Fenske NA, Lober CW. Structural and functional changes of normal aging skin. *Journal of the American Academy of Dermatology* 1986. 15, 571-585.

13. Forcher B, Cecil H. Some effects of age on the biochemistry of acute inflammation. *Gerontologia* 1958. 2, 174-182.

14. Gerstein AD (1993). Wound healing and aging. *Dermatologic Clinics* 11, 749-757.

15. Gilchrest B A, Stoof J S, Soter N A. Chronologic aging alters response to ultraviolet induce inflammation in human skin. *J Invest Dermatol* 1982. 79, 11-15.

16. Grove GL. Physiologic changes in older skin. *Dermatologic Clinics* 1986. 4, 425-432.

17. Grove GL, Kligman A. Age-associated changes in human epidermal cell renewal. *J Gerontol* 1983. 38, 137-142.

18. Guralnik J M, Harris T B, White L R, et al. Occurrence and predictors of pressure sores in the National Health and Nutrition Examination survey follow-up. *J Am Geriatr Soc* 1988. 6, 7-12.

19. Hagisawa S, Barbenel J. The limits of pressure sore prevention. *Journal of the Royal Society of Medicine* 1998. 92, 576-578.

20. Hanson D S, Langemo D, Olson B, et al. Decreasing the prevalence of pressure ulcers using agency standards. *Home Healthcare Nurse* 1996. 14, 525-531.

21. Langemo D K, Olson B, Hanson D S, et al. Prevalence of pressure ulcers in five patient care settings. *J Enterostomal Therapy* 1990. 17, 187-192.

22. Lipschitz D. Protein caloric malnutrition in hospitalized elderly. *Primary Care* 9[3], 531 543. 1982.

23. Lyder, CH. Pressure ulcer prevention and management. *JAMA* 2003;289: 223-226.

24. Mendoza C, Postlethwait R, Johnson W. Incidence of wound disruption following operation. *Archives of Surgery* 1970. 101, 396-398.

25. Morykwas MJ, Simpson J, Punger K, et al.Vacuum-assisted closure: state of basic research and physiologic foundation. *Plastic Reconstruction Surgery* 2006 Jun;(7 Suppl): 121s-126s.

26. Niinikoski JH. Clinical hyperbaric oxygen therapy, wound perfusion, and transcutaneous oximetry. *World J Surg* 2004 Mar;28(3):307-11. Epub 2004 Feb 17.

27. Oot-Gironomi B. A. Pressure ulcer prevalence, incidence and associated risk factors in the community. *Decubitus* 1993. 6, 24-32.

28. Orentreich N, Selmanowitz V. Levels of biological functions with aging. *Trans NY Acad Sci* 1969. 231, 992-1012.

29. Quirinia A, Viidik A. The influence of age on the healing of normal and ischaemic incisional wounds. *Mechanisms of Ageing and Development* 1991. 58, 221-232.
Ref Type: Journal (Full)

30. Sandblom P, Petersen P, Muren A. Determination of the tensile strength of the healing wound as a clinical test. *Acta Chir Scand* 1953. 105, 252-257.

31. Shuster S, Black M M, Mc Vitie, E. The influence of age and sex on skin thickness, skin collagen and density. *British Journal of Dermatology* 1975. 93, 639-643.

32. Sibbit W, Mills R, Bigler C, et al. Glucose inhibition of human fibroblast proliferation and response to growth factors is prevented by inhibitors of aldose reductase. *Mechanisms of Ageing and Development* 1989. 47, 265-279.

33. Stiller MJ, et al. A portable pulsed electromagnetic field (PEMF) device to enhance healing of recalcitrant venous ulcers: a double-blind, placebo-controlled clinical trial. *Br J Dermatol* 1992; 127:147-54.

34. Tepelidis NT. Wound healing in the elderly. *Clinic in Podiatric Medicine* 1991. 8[4], 817-826.

35. Uitto J. Connective tissue biochemistry of aging dermis: Age-related alterations in collagen and elastin. *Dermatologic Clinics* 1986. 4, 433-446.

36. Yamura H, Matsuzawa T. Decrease in capillary growth during aging. *Exp Gerontol* 1980. 15, 145-150.

REVIEW QUESTIONS

1.) Ageing results in changes to overall wound healing that creates a major problem for elders with:
   a. Pressure ulcers
   b. Venous stasis ulcers
   c. Skin tears
   d. All of the above

2.) Age associated changes in skin can be divided into sun-exposed and sun-protected changes. As a person ages between 20–80 years of age, the elastin content of the dermis in sun exposed areas increases while the elastin content of the dermis in sun protected areas:
   a. Has not been determined
   b. Remains the same
   c. Increases
   d. Decreases

3.) Which of the following is an age-related change that directly affects wound healing?
   a. Impaired glucose tolerance
   b. Slowed reaction time
   c. Impaired recall
   d. Decreased proliferation of fibroblasts

4.) Which of the following has shown to be of benefit in wound healing in older adults?
   a. Topical analgesics
   b. Topical platelet-derived growth factor
   c. Full-strength betadine solution
   d. Electromagnetic fields

5.) Which of the following is true of pressure ulcers in older adults?
   a. The incidence in homebound elders is 33%
   b. All pressure ulcers are preventable
   c. Nutrition has a limited role in healing pressure ulcers
   d. Prevention of pressure is a mainstay of treatment

Answers: 1d, 2d, 3d, 4d, 5d

NOTES

CHAPTER 25

Wound Care in Pediatric Patients

CHAPTER TWENTY-FIVE OVERVIEW

NOTES

Wound Care in Pediatric Patients

Melvin D. Smith

INTRODUCTION AND BACKGROUND

The overall care of pediatric patients has progressed to the point that they are no longer considered "little adults." In this respect, the care of wounds in the pediatric patient also must not be taken as care of adults in a little body. The author of this chapter is a pediatric surgeon who has taken care of patients in the pediatric age group since 1974. Many changes have occurred since that time and change continues to occur in the treatment of wounds of children, especially "problem" wounds.

This chapter will look at the care of wounds in the pediatric patient from the aspect of general principles that must always be considered and secondly, specific injuries that result in external wounds in the pediatric age group.

General principles that must be considered in all cases of wounds:

- Age of the patient at the time of injury
- Associated injuries are likely and/or probable
- Preexisting physical abnormalities, if any
- Preexisting metabolic/physiologic abnormalities, if any
- Characteristics of the agent causing the wound

GENERAL PRINCIPLES

Age of Patient at Time of Injury

Accidental injuries account for a major cause of debility in the pediatric age group between the ages of 1–16 years. It has been observed that over 700,000 patients present to the emergency rooms yearly in the United States from injuries sustained in various sporting activities. This number does not take into account injuries sustained in and about the proximity of the home. Combining all forms of injury, this number rises to over 2,000,000 children being hospitalized annually in the United States due to some form of trauma, more than 100,000 of which are permanently disabled.

The age of the patient is an important factor in discussing "trends" of accidental injuries and the resulting morbidities. An infant that is not yet ambulatory is less likely to be its own agent in contributing to an injury, but is more likely to be the recipient of another, older person causing the injury, either by accident or by purposeful abuse. A toddler that has recently mastered the skill of locomotion is, as we say in the hallways, "an accident waiting to happen." The newly found freedom of self assured ambulation, coupled with the desire to explore one's surroundings and a "no fear" factor added in, makes this age group prone to injury.

Thus enters now the spectrum of injuries including burns from hot liquids being pulled off the stove or table by the toddler onto himself or herself, pedestrian-motor vehicular accidents as the child chases into the street after a ball or pet animal, a fall into still-burning embers of a campfire, falls from heights such as from an unprotected second story (or higher) window or balcony.

As the age of the child increases, usually also does the awareness of the surroundings, but the fearlessness and "indestructible" attitude continue, making the pre-kinder and grade-school child subject to ongoing injuries mentioned above and new ones added to the list, such as fall from bicycles, injuries from organized contact sports, and bites from animals, especially dogs and snakes.

Unfortunately, also new in these recent years, we begin to see injuries afflicted by one's peer group, both on the school ground and in the neighborhood. Also, very unfortunately, in this school-age group the injuring agent, used by the peer group, has become more severe in its ability to cause bodily damage; it is not uncommon to hear on the local airways or read in the newspaper that a second or third grader or a middle-school student has shot or stabbed a fellow student.

As the pediatric age group extends into the teenage years, further injuries have become increasingly extensive as the teenager and the car become a serious vehicle for bodily harm as well as injuries sustained by "gang wars."

Lest the reader thinks that the author is too judgmental on teenage drivers, all one has to do is look up the statistics in any city vehicular accident report for any given week or month. The recurring statistic stands out: the driver is/was a male teenager. Because of this, many local county and state governing bodies are enacting ordinances to curtail teenage drivers by increasing the minimal age at which an unrestricted driving license can be issued, by restricting the number of passengers in the vehicle with the teenage driver, and by lowering the number for the alcohol breathalyzer, while raising the minimal age in which one can purchase alcohol.

Associated Injuries are Likely and/or Probable

As the physician is taking a phone report of any injured person being brought to the emergency room, not only must the care of the obvious, external injury be quickly considered, but also the possibility and/or probability of associated injuries has to be considered. Just as how the age of the person can place him or her into a rough, general category of what injuries might be received, so does the agent or mechanism of injury serve as a rough predictor of whether or not additional injuries may be associated and what they may be. Thus the patient who falls from a second story window or balcony might have similar associated injuries as a pedestrian-motor vehicle accident victim, with an obvious compound fracture of the femur or the obvious hemorrhagic discharge from the ear, but the other injuries not being readily obvious. On the other hand, neither of the above patients would be expected to have the same constellation of injuries as would be found in an assailant injury by stabbing or injuries sustained in a drive-by shooting. Saying it another way, penetrating injuries result in different, associated injuries than those of blunt trauma. Often, the associated, not-so-obvious injury may require more urgent attention than that of the obvious one. The physician at the receiving facility is always best prepared by considering the "worst-case scenario."

Preexisting Physical Abnormalities, if Any

Preexisting physical abnormalities seldom are directly responsible for the occurrence of injuries. Physical qualities, or lack thereof, that may play contributing factors are things such as poor eyesight resulting in misjudgment of position, extremity abnormalities that would affect dexterity, preexisting neuromuscular conditions that would affect inherent abilities, and leg-length discrepancies affecting ease of locomotion.

Preexisting Metabolic and/or Physiologic Abnormalities

Also during the reparative stages of care, the preexisting status of metabolic and/or physiological derangements play a major role in the ongoing care and eventual outcome of a wound sustained from any kind of injury, even purposefully fashioned ones as in an elective operation. The surgeon cannot afford to be so narrowly focused that metabolic or physiologic abnormalities are overlooked or not taken into account. The stabilization of these factors must occur simultaneously by the surgeon or specific consultative services must be rapidly utilized to participate in the initial and ongoing care, in efforts to maximize the desired and suitable outcome—a healed wound with minimal-to-no complications. In these regards, system reviews are as important as the history of the present illness (injury).

The concurrent knowledge of the presence of asthma, cystic fibrosis, and even an acute upper respiratory illness (URI) or acute pneumonia, all of which are extremely common in the pediatric age group, is of paramount importance. This knowledge is important not only for the immediate concern during an operation for repair, but also because of medications being taken may affect wound healing. This author has often lamented when a patient's medication list includes long-term steroids for asthma or cystic fibrosis, various antimetabolites for prevention of rejection of various organs that the injured patient may have received long before the problem currently at hand, or long-term antibiotic usage as occurs in patients with cystic fibrosis. The post renal transplant patient becomes "normal" for all intents and purposes and is therefore subject to any and all potential problems as noted in the discussion for age-related injuries. Nowadays, the post renal transplant patient is put in the mainstream of all activities, but the transplantation history is not hanging as a talisman around the patient's neck. The history must be sought after under Review-of-Systems interrogations. If luck would be on our side, the post transplant patient would have a wrist bracelet to identify the fact, but this author has seen many without this useful device.

The use of chronic medications such as steroids, antihypertensive medications, antibiotics, and antirejection medications has the potential and definite influence on fibroblastic and collagen synthesis, calcium and potassium metabolism, and the increased possibility of wound infection due to the immuno-compromised state and super-infection with selected-out antibiotic resistant organisms. Juvenile diabetes in the injured person can be especially challenging from the standpoint that, if the diabetes is not in exquisite control, any wound problems will be magnified. The poorly controlled juvenile diabetic is the same as an immuno-compromised child from the standpoint of infection.

Characteristics of the Agent Causing the Wound

The characteristics of the agent causing an injury is very closely related to the factors in the aforementioned paragraphs, in that, however the agent is categorized, there is a "general trend" of the agent to be with age. Also, as previously alluded to, the instrument of injury indicates the probability of associated injuries and thus, to a great extent, the eventual outcome, using this parameter alone. Again, independent of the agent of injury involved, the response to the injuring agent will vary, depending on the victim's premorbid condition. Thus, one can surmise that a previously healthy, middle-school age child or teenager who receives stab wounds to the abdomen and legs will have a predictably better outcome than would the pre-kinder or school-age child, with severe asthma or leukemia, who is hit by a fast moving vehicle.

IDENTIFICATION AND CARE OF SPECIFIC INJURIES RESULTING IN EXTERNAL WOUNDS

Moving Vehicular Accidents (MVA)

Among the most common of all accidents in the pediatric age group is the pedestrian-moving vehicular accident. The typical scenario is that of a three to six-year-old child running into the street after a ball, only to be struck down by an approaching vehicle. Usually the child suddenly emerges from behind a parked car and the driver of the approaching vehicle has no chance to avoid the collision. As you picture this in your mind, you see the child hit on the left side of the body (in the United States) with the resulting injuries: an open fracture of the leg with gravel imbedded into the soft tissues, a large, partially degloving injury to the right upper extremity, deep lacerations and abrasions to the chest and upper abdomen, ecchymosis around both eyes, hemorrhage coming from the right ear, an enlarging abdomen, and an overall motionless child with slow, shallow respirations. The Emergency Medical Services are called and arrive within minutes. The child is "scooped up," put into the van and rushed to the trauma center. Enroute, the child is intubated and appropriate intravenous fluids are started. In the emergency department, the services of the general surgeon, the neurosurgeon, and the orthopedist have been requested and they all assess the patient simultaneously. Operations by all three services are deemed urgently necessary. Minimal lab and x-ray studies are obtained while the child is being wheeled towards the operating sites: CBC, chemistry panel, type and cross-match, chest x-ray, cervical spine views, skull x-ray, and abdominal views. At operation, the following repairs are done after the initial resuscitation is secure: A subdural hematoma is evacuated and the depressed skull fracture is stabilized. A chest tube is inserted during the resuscitation period. The ruptured spleen is partially removed due to avulsion of the lower one third. The soft tissues are cleaned and debrided. The compound fracture is fixed with external devices because of the gross contamination of the wound. The skin is only partially approximated so as not to create the "closed compartment syndrome" of the lower extremity.

After the patient has recovered from the acute injuries of the head trauma, the thoracic and abdominal injuries, and the acute swelling of the leg injury, ongoing repair of the soft tissues become the main objective. Generally, the patient is returned to the operating room every other day for further debridement of ischemic tissue, if any, and a slow, but progressive, lessening of the separation of the skin edges until closure is complete. Skin grafting is needed for the degloving injury. The skin edges are approximated with minimally reactive sutures, such as nylon or prolene.

If a chronic or indolent infection should occur, such as osteomyelitis, a six-week course of intravenous antibiotics, culture specific (usually gram positive organisms), is administered via a central venous catheter, suitable for home-bound use. As an outpatient, the status of the healing process is evaluated at weekly intervals until the infection is eradicated.

In this severe type of skeletal and soft tissue injury, it rarely happens that a mixed infection of gram positive, gram negative, and synergistic microaerophilic organisms will produce a necrotizing fasciitis with rapidly advancing involvement of the extremity and adjacent abdomen. With this complication, the adjunctive use of hyperbaric oxygen therapy, along with ongoing debridement, offers the best chance of survival.

Falls

The commonality of falls from heights by children varies from community to community and is obviously more common in urban areas of high-rise, multifamily dwellings, such as apartments where the child has the opportunity to fall out of a window from two or more stories high. Falls from heights also occur from trees, embankments or cliff ledges, bridges, slides and jungle gyms on the school playground or city parks. This author had the occasion to chart review the care of 66 children, ages ranging from six months to 15 years, during a two-year period while in fellowship training during the nineteen seventies. This author personally cared for twelve of the 66 cases.

The mechanism of injury was, of course, that of a fast moving object (the child) suddenly impacting a resisting, non-displaceable force (the ground). The resulting injuries, to a large extent, varied with what body part impacted first. In the infants, the head was more frequently the most severely injured body part, while in the older child, the extremities took the brunt of the injuries, but often accompanied also by thoracic and/or abdominal involvement. The initial care required depended on the obvious injury, but, more often than not, included stabilization of the fracture of the radius (13 cases) or femur (nine cases) and protecting the cervical spine from further injury, until cleared. The progress in the emergency room always proceeded similar to that of the pedestrian-MVA, making sure all potential injuries were looked for and accounted for. In this series, the fractures sustained in falls from high places tended to be simple closed, but some were compound.

Compression of the fracture was also a common finding, as might be expected. These wounds tended not to be tattooed with dirt, as compared to the pedestrian-MVA cases, and thus primary closure of the skin following open reduction and internal fixation (ORIF) was carried out.

Burns

Few injuries or wounds can be as disfiguring or debilitating as a major burn of a child. Those burns that might seem minor or trivial in an adult might be greatly magnified in the child. The time-honored "Rule-of-Nines" does not apply in infants and small children, due to the proportional differences in the various body parts. The chart devised by Lund and Browder is the usual standard used by most burn centers that treat children with regularity. The main differences designated by this chart show the variation of the percentage of the body surface areas as the person ages from infancy to adulthood. From the Lund and Browder chart one sees that the infant's head is 19% of body surface, while the 15-year-old's head represents 9% and 7% in the adult. Likewise, the proximal extremities go in reverse: the thigh in the infant is 5.5% but enlarges to 9.5% in the adult.

The severity of a burn depends upon many variables, including the age of the patient, the location on the body of the burn, the surface area involved, the burning medium, the temperature of the burning medium, and the length of time of contact with the skin. Burns are further classified by the depth of involvement and referred to as being superficial partial thickness, deep partial thickness, full thickness, or char burn. Previous classifications used the terminology of first, second, and third degrees of burn depth. By way of examples, bad sunburn is a classic example of superficial partial thickness, characterized by erythema and possibly blistering, with excruciating pain and discomfort. Hot water or coffee spilled onto a two-year old will most likely yield a combination of both superficial and deep partial thickness burns. Agents such as burning gasoline, hot grease, burning clothes, or hot metal objects (stove tops) will produce, more times than not, a full thickness, leathery appearing, and painless burn.

The char burn is the most extensive regarding depth and is termed such because all tissues at the involved site are completely burned, including the skin, subcutaneous tissues, muscles, blood vessels and nerves, and bone. Such burns are characteristically seen with electrical burns such as a child touching a downed "hot" telegraph wire, or chewing on a "hot" electrical lamp cord. The survivor of a lightening strike will present with char burns.

The initial efforts in treating burn patients are mainly two-fold: 1) stop the ongoing injury or remove the burning agent and 2) support the patient with fluid resuscitation while minimizing ongoing losses. The efforts that immediately follow the initial care are designed to protect from infection as much as possible, restore ongoing fluid and electrolyte losses, control discomfort, and initiate steps for recovering the burned areas with autogenous skin.

The extent to which the foregoing is required varies with the body parts involved, the depth and extent of the body surface area involvement. It turns out that, although small in area by comparison, burns of the hands, feet, perineum, and face in children, stimulate as much, if not more, urgency than do burns of the chest and abdomen. This reasoning is due to the fact that resultant sequelae stand the chance of being more debilitating. A patient treated by this author will serve to illustrate the foregoing principles.

Case 1

A nine-year-old boy was helping his older brother clean the engine block of his car with gasoline. While the nine-year-old was looking on, a friend of the older brother came to the scene smoking a cigarette; the fumes from the gasoline ignited in a sudden fire resulting in a high intensity burn to the face, neck, and upper chest of the nine-year old boy (Figure 1A). The initial care consisted of intravenous fluids, immediate debridement, systemic antibiotics, topical silver sulfadiazine (Silvadine) cream on most of the burned areas and gentamycin solution around the eyes to lessen the chance of Silvadine contact conjunctivitis. Daily debridements were carried out as needed under the aid of conscious sedation medications (Figure 1B). At the time of this case, morphine and Valium were used, but now Fentanyl and Versed are more frequently used by this author at a rate of 1–2 micrograms per kilogram weight of the patient in combination with Versed at the rate of 0.1 mgs. per kilogram weight. Additional half doses are given as needed every 20–30 minutes. Within a matter of days, autogenous grafting was done. The graft was not meshed on the face, as is frequently done on other areas of the body, to discourage scar contracture and prevent the obvious "lattice-like" appearance of the meshed grafts. The patient was discharged to home at approximately two weeks post burn (Figures 1C and 1D).

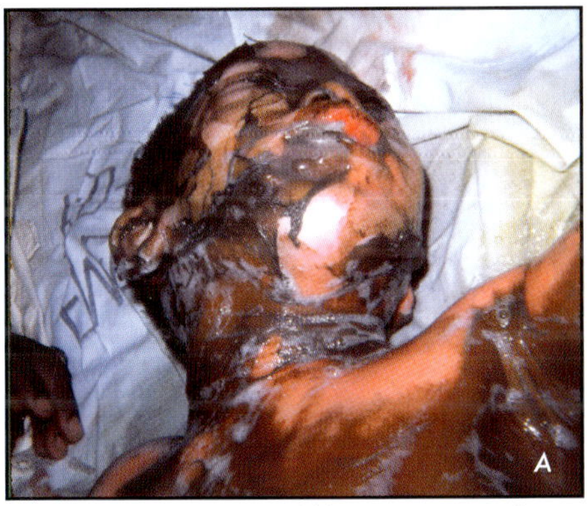

Figure 1A. Nine-year-old burn victim, with obvious varying burn depths depicted: blisters, erythematous areas, and white, leathery areas. Initial debridement is underway.

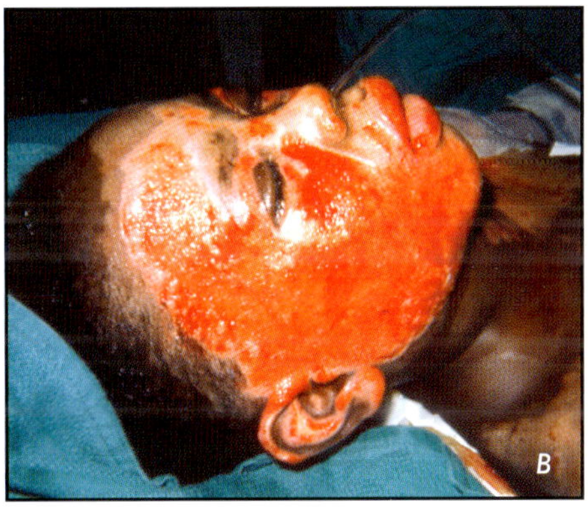

Figure 1B. Appearance of the bed of the facial burn after a debridemnt; approximately day number five.

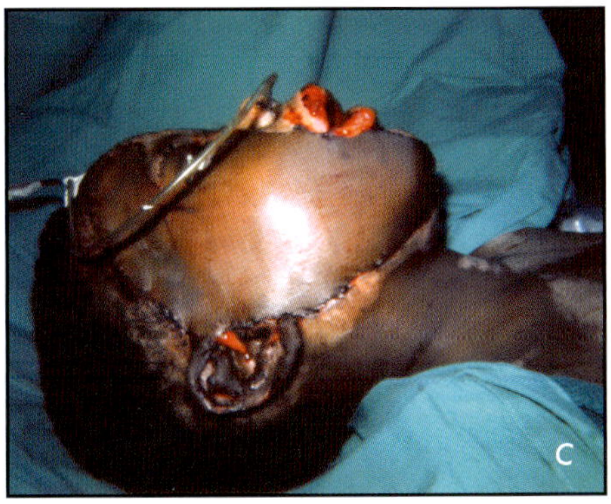

Figure 1C. Grafting completed; right side of the face shown here.

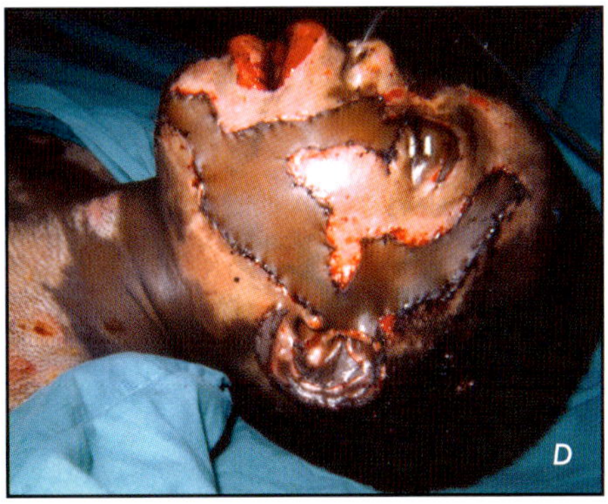

Figure 1D. Grafting completed; left side of the face shown here.

Bites

This author has seen problem wounds arising from bites from many different animals, varying from ants, spiders, dogs, snakes, lions, and even humans. We can watch the nightly news on television and learn of the severe wounds inflicted by Pit Bulls and Rottweilers occurring at an alarming frequency. During the height of the season of activity in Texas (April to October) the same can be said of rattlesnake bites, especially when inflicted on the infant or school age child. This discussion will not focus very much on dog bites; although they may be extensive, the care is straightforward and without controversy. Suffice it to say that the salient principles of treating the bites of dogs and other large animals, including humans, are thorough, extensive irrigation with copious amounts of saline, debridement of devitalized tissue, if present, and open drainage to deep puncture wounds, except on the face. Here, because of the rich vascular supply, most bites can be closed primarily.

Ant bites

Although it seldom makes the headlines, in the immunocompromised host, including diabetics, ant bites have produced very significant infections with deep subcutaneous abscesses. The first dilemma in the care of the juvenile diabetic, for example, is the question of did the infection cause the diabetes to be out of control or did the out-of-control diabetes allow the infection to progress to such a significant degree? It then takes the utmost cooperation between the endocrinologist and the surgeon to decide the proper timing of drainage and debridement of the extensive abscess (under general anesthesia, of course), while, at the same time, attempts to bring under control and stabilize the ketoacidosis with which the patient most likely presented. The following case illustrates how an otherwise insignificant insect bite can become a major event in the person with underlying metabolic problems.

Case 2

The patient was 17 years old at the time of this event. She had poorly controlled juvenile diabetes and had required approximately three admissions per year to treat ketoacidosis. On this admission, her blood sugar was 659 mg%, measured in the emergency room just prior to starting treatment. The gluteal lesion was already spontaneously draining minimally. There was a measured area of induration of approximately 6 cm. (Figure 2A). She was treated overnight by the endocrinologist with lowering of the blood sugar to 250–280 mg% at the time of operation. At operation a large cavity of purulent material was encountered (Figure 2B). Extensive debridement was carried out (Figure 2C) and copious irrigation with dilute Betadine (1% solution) was done (Figure 2D). The resultant wound now measured 9 cm. in greatest length (Figure 2E). The wound was packed initially with one-inch iodoform gauze (Figure 2F) and changed to saline soaked plain gauze the following day. She was discharged to home on daily saline irrigations and packing on the fourth hospital day, the diabetes under good control. Follow-up was scheduled with the surgeon at one week and the endocrinologist at two-week intervals.

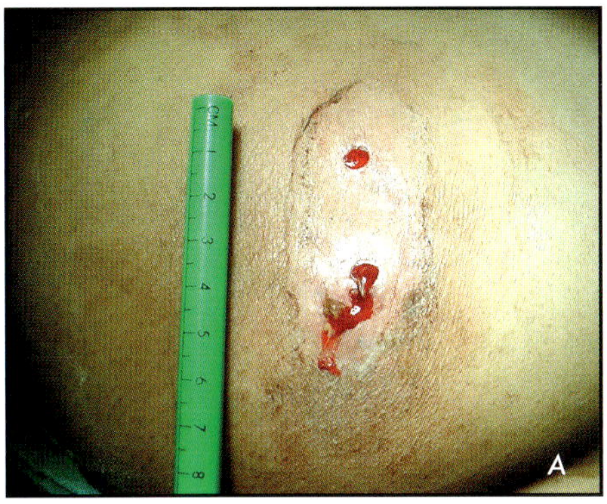

Figure 2A. Seventeen-year-old with juvenile diabetes presents with an already draining gluteal abscess. The area of induration was approximately 6 cm.

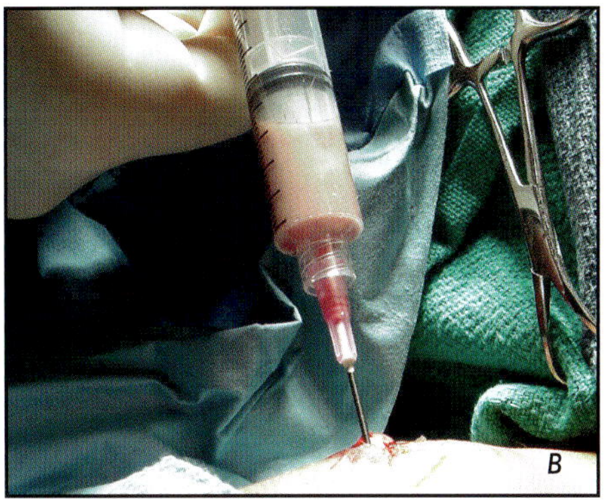

Figure 2B. Needle aspiration of the purulent fluid from the gluteal abscess. The fluid is gram strained and sent for culture and sensitivity.

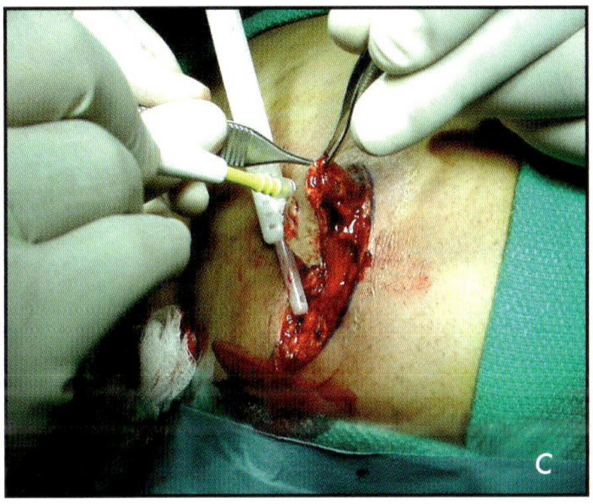

Figure 2C. Debridement of the gluteal abscess is underway. The area of induration was completely excised.

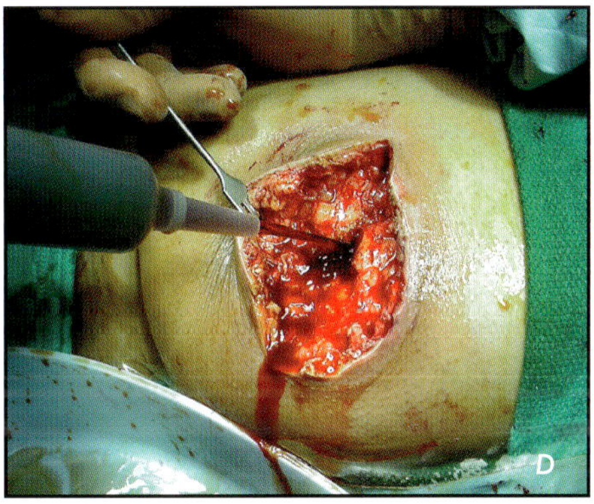

Figure 2D. Once debridement of all visible necrotic tissue is completed, the resulting wound is copiously irrigated with dilute Betadine solution.

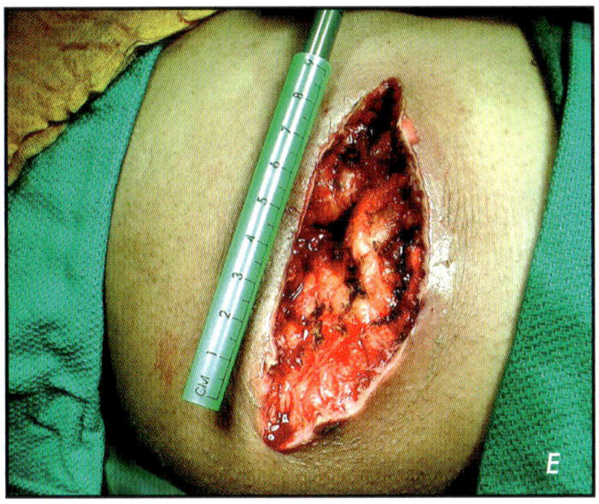

Figure 2E. The completed debridement and irrigated abscess cavity. Note that the wound is now 9 cm in greatest length. Hemostasis was secured using the electro-coagulation unit.

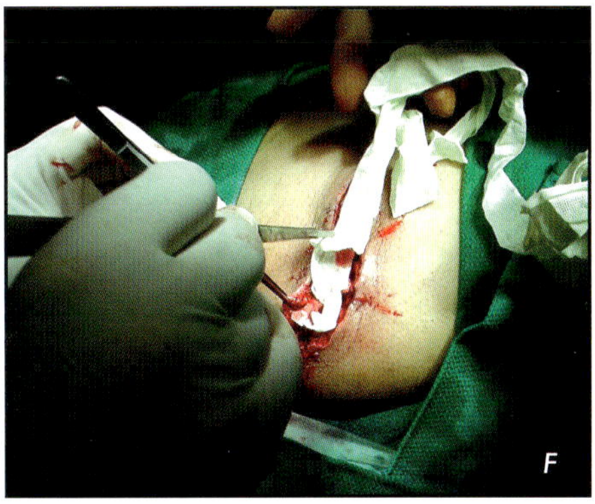

Figure 2F. Iodoform gauze packing is placed for further debridement and hemostasis for approximately 12 hours, then changed to saline-soaked plain gauze, to be changed once daily.

Snake bites

Those of us in the teaching profession of surgery always advocate that a snake bite in a small child portends a very bad scenario because the dosage of venom per body weight of the patient is important. The initial care by the person in the fields or the parent in the home is not to do cross cuts over the bites and attempt to suck out or squeeze out the venom. Tourniquets are not used in children for fear of compromising a potentially already compromised extremity. The initial care is directed at getting the child to the emergency care facility in a timely and calm manner. The patient should not run about, but is encouraged to be calm and still. If possible, the patient is carried from the scene of the bite to the vehicle, to be transported to the hospital. It is estimated that a time interval of bite-to-hospital of thirty minutes or less is optimal. Most snakebites that are inflicted on the proximal part of the extremity or trunk of the body are manageable most times by giving antivenin and supportive fluids. Careful monitoring of the extremity is required, looking for development of the compartment syndrome and monitoring for systemic signs of a developing coagulopathy. On the other hand, snakebite to the hands or fingers, wrist, foot or toes, or ankle will likely require, in addition to high dose antivenin, release of the skin and fascial compartments to save the extremity from ischemic necrosis due to rapidly developing edema in small, closed spaces.

Case 3

The accompanying series of pictures illustrate such a case in a four-year-old girl who was bitten near the wrist by a large rattlesnake while she was playing in her driveway. From the time of the bite to the appearance of the hand ischemia (Figure 3A) was only about 15 minutes. The width of the fang marks is obvious in the next photograph, indicating a very large snake (the fang puncture sites were excised in the operating room to evaluate the degree of tissue necrosis at the bite site) (Figure 3B). Over the next hour, as the antivenin was still underway, the hand was deemed to be in ischemic danger as measured by the parameters of loss of fine movement, pain on passive movement, loss of sensation, and decreasing Doppler signals. Operation was initiated at the conclusion of the administration of ten vials of antivenin (Figure 3C). The fasciotomies were required to include the hand and the entire lower arm (Figures 3C and 3D). Over several days, the skin edges were systematically drawn closer together (Figure 3E) until complete reapproximation could be carried out. Follow-up evaluation at two and five weeks later showed ongoing, good healing and good hand function (Figures 3F and 3G).

The underlying and mainstay treatment for snakebites is early use of multiple vials of antivenin in a continuous fashion until the prescribed dosage is completed. The need for fasciotomy is unusual, but it is not a zero percentage. The request from this author is that the care of snakebites not be the sole purview of the intensivist or hospitalist. Rather, the pediatric surgeon and/or the hand surgeon should be an early consultant in the care of the patient, so as to be "ready" for the potential need of a fasciotomy.

Adjunctive tests are also now available to aid in the clinical impression of the compartment, requiring operative intervention. In addition to the Doppler flow studies, direct measurement of the

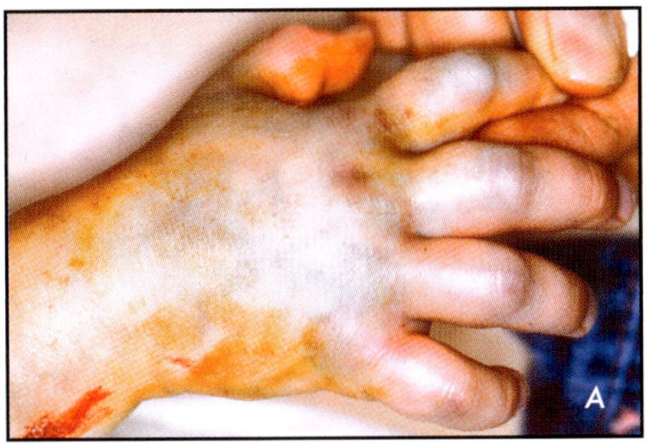

Figure 3A. Appearance of the right hand, in a 4-year-old patient, following a rattlesnake bite on the wrist approximately 15 minutes earlier. Note the marked edema and bluish discoloration.

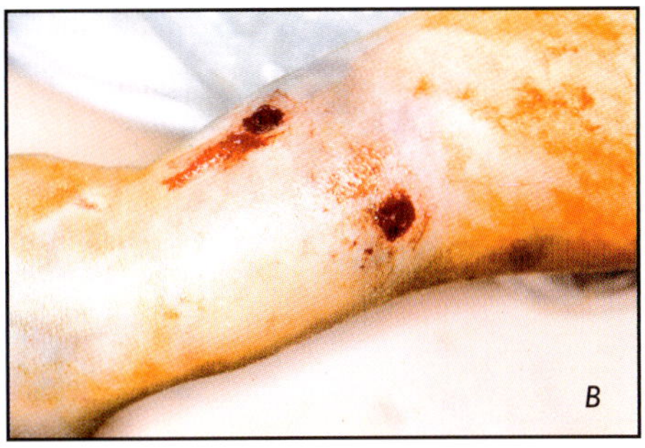

Figure 3B. The wide width of the fang puncture sites is pictured here. The puncture sites were excised in the operation room to evaluate the extent of tissue necrosis.

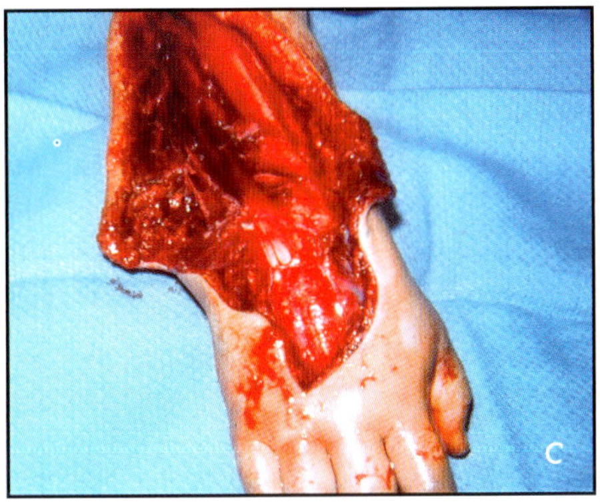

Figure 3C. Fasciotomy extended over the dorsum of the hand and subcutaneously into the fingers in this view.

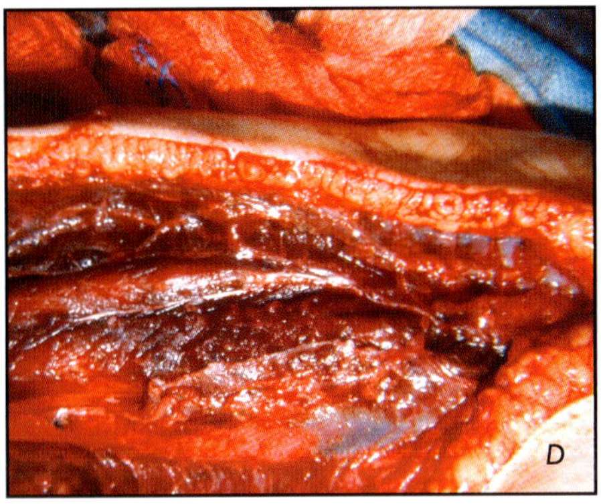

Figure 3D. Fasciotomy extending above the wrist into the arm. Note the discoloration of the deeper muscles.

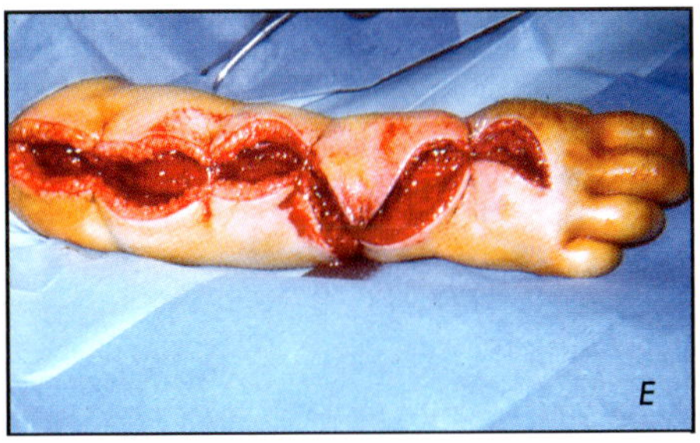

Figure 3E. The skin is loosely approximated at several, widely separated points. Although still discolored, all areas appear to be viable.

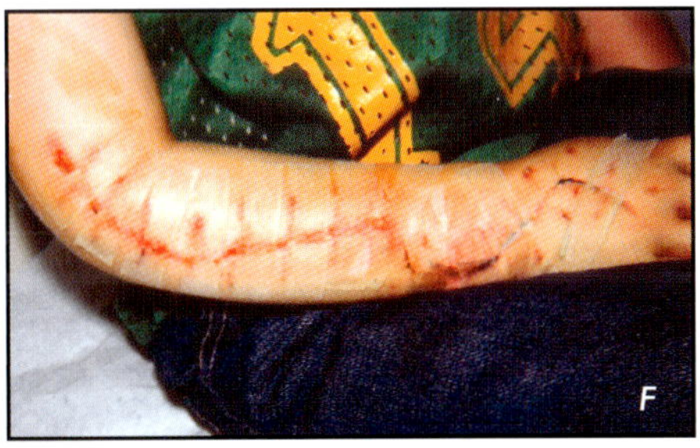

Figure 3F. Follow-up as outpatient from snake-bite on the wrist, requiring extensive fasciotomy. This is two weeks post-discharge.

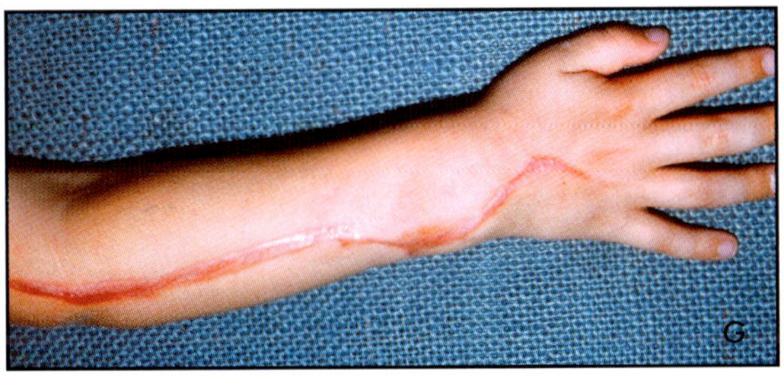

Figure 3G. Follow-up as outpatient from snakebite to the right wrist. The fasciotomy incision shows excellent healing at five weeks post-discharge.

compartment in question can be done with a needle attached to a pressure transducer. Pressures over 30 mm Hg are abnormal, while pressures of 20–30 mm Hg are considered marginal and pressures 20 mm Hg or less are normal, as long as one makes certain that the needle is patent in all the readings. A commercial device, made by Stryker, is available and has the advantage that the penetrating needle has a side opening to obviate tissue occlusion.

Spider bites

The need for a surgical undertaking for spider bites is in no way as frequent as for dog bites or even snakebites, but it occasionally occurs. In the case of brown recluse spider bites (Figure 4A), the teaching, just 10–15 years ago, was to excise the area that appeared necrotic and perform an immediate skin graft (Figure 4B). More recently therapy is directed at preventing a superficial infection and otherwise allowing the damaged tissue to regenerate as much as possible, prior to any escharotomy, hoping for a much smaller lesion to deal with. Thus, the mainstay of current treatment is local cleansing, antibiotics against staph and strep organisms and symptomatic pain management. There can be a systemic reaction to the brown recluse spider bite, producing red cell hemolysis, hemoglobinuria, and more severely, renal failure. As with the snakebites, the systemic symptoms are more likely to be seen in the small child, since the relative

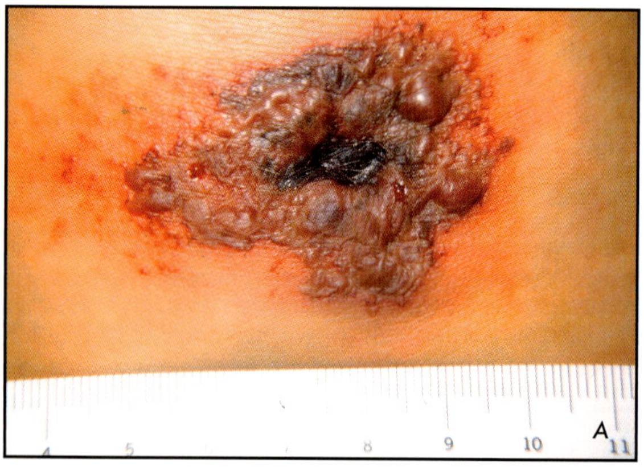

Figure 4A. Example of the lesion from a brown recluse spider bite. The distinctly necrotic (black) area measured approximately 15–77mm, while the area of bullous formation measures at least 50 mm, with lesser areas of patchy necrosis.

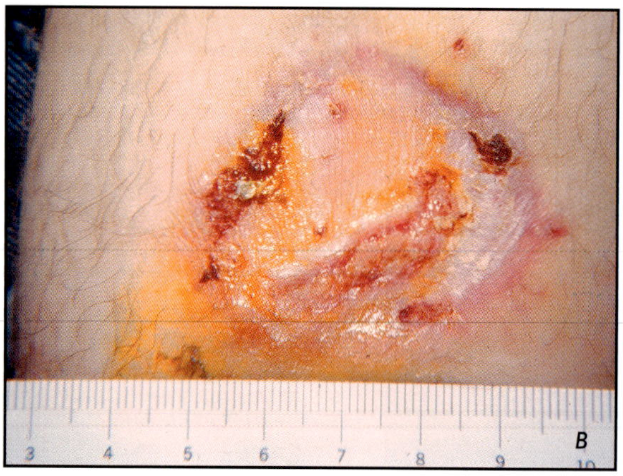

Figure 4B. Two weeks post immediate excision and skin grafting of a brown recluse spider bite. the STSG has had a very high percentage of "take."

dose of venom-to-patient is larger. The treatment for systemic reactions is plenty of hydration and otherwise supportive. More information about spider bites can be found in the chapter entitled "Necrotic Wounds Produced by Spider Bites" by CO Hagood and JR Wilson.

Internal Infections with Myocutaneous Extension

Wounds resulting from extensions of internal infections tend to be very indolent, debilitating, and test the skills of the surgeon as much as any other wounds produced by any other modality. Much to the chagrin of this author, he has had the opportunity to care for several of these wounds, produced both from diseases cared for by him as well as some inherited from others. Most prominent in this group of wounds are those derived from appendiceal abscesses, entero-cutaneous fistulae, especially with Crohn's Disease, and colo-cutaneous fistulae, associated with, and subsequent to, previous operative procedures.

Appendiceal abscess with a significant wound infection is by far the most common of those processes named above. The younger the child that develops appendicitis, the more likely there is to be a pre-operative peritonitis with abscesses in the so-called right colic gutter, interloop abscesses, and/or a pelvic abscess. Attempts at controlling the sepsis are begun with perioperative antibiotics to cover both aerobic and anaerobic organisms. The most common organisms involved include *Pseudomonas, Escherichia coli, Enterococcus, Streptococcus,* and *Bacteroides*. Double or triple antibiotic coverage is used, at the choice of the surgeon.

Appendectomy is now done either by the standard "open" method or via the laparoscopic approach. With persistent infection intra-abdominally, abdominal wall infection sometimes occurs with either method in the young, compromised host; it appears, however, to be less in those treated by the laparoscopic method. The treatment of the secondary infection continues to be that of establishing adequate drainage and wound debridement as well as internal drainage of abscesses. Especially if triple antibiotics were used initially, cultures are taken at the secondary procedure so that the antibiotics can be tailored as dictated by the sensitivities. The national rate of appendectomies is approximately 250,000 new cases yearly in the United States alone, with anywhere from 15–20 % of the cases having ruptures at the time of presentation. Over the past 32 years, this author has personally seen severe abdominal wall infections from appendicitis at the rate of approximately 3–4 per year per 100–120 appendectomies per year. Two of these abdominal wall infections progressed to involve a major portion of the abdomen towards the lower rib cage and umbilicus superiorly and inferiorly to the proximal thigh and all of the perineum, including the scrotum in a 15-year-old male and the labia in a two-year-old girl. The 15-year-old's infection proved to be necrotizing fasciitis clinically (and substantiated by gram stain of the exudates and a mixed flora of organisms from tissue biopsy. Frozen section of the same tissue specimen showed tissue necrosis and invading organisms). He required numerous debridements while receiving daily hyperbaric oxygen therapy (HBO2), initially twice a day for three days, then once daily for a total of a week. A diverting colostomy was required to divert the fecal stream because of the perineal involvement. He subsequently recovered from this devastating infection and was begun on reconstructive surgery of the perineum, scrotum, and staged closure of the abdominal wall.

The two-year-old defervesed with wide debridement daily and was not treated with HBO2 adjunctive therapy.

Case 4

This case clearly illustrates how other preexisting conditions might adversely affect the outcome of an otherwise seemingly "straightforward" operative procedure. This is the case of a 15-year-old female with chronic fecal incontinence due to spina bifida. To aid in controlling the incontinence, a tube cecostomy was fashioned so that antegrade enemas could be used to flush out the colon. The device worked well for only 3–4 days after which time she became distended and began to leak fecal material around the cecostomy tube. Subsequent studies showed intestinal strictures distal to the cecostomy tube as the cause of the leak complication. She had had two previous abdominal operations in the distant past. The abdominal wall developed severe erosion around the tube and progressed to the intertriginous areas on the right side. Multiple procedures were attempted to control the infection (Figure 5A). Large, retention sutures were also used due to the poor integrity of the edematous tissue. The system worked for 2–4 days, then broke down again. Figures 5B and C show the lack of good granulation tissue, although some is present. The close up view of Figure 5C shows the skin edges to be rolling inward, but minimal granulation tissue in the depths of the wound. Dressing changes were done four times daily, using multiple dilute solutions, including Dakin's solution because of the presence of *Pseudomonas* and other organisms. Also, Granulex (granulated growth hormone) was used for one month without noticeable change. After 9–10 weeks of wound "standstill" of non-healing, hyperbaric oxygen therapy was instituted with the idea to attempt stimulation of growth of granulation tissue. She only had two courses of HBO2 therapy because she was very aerophagic and developed

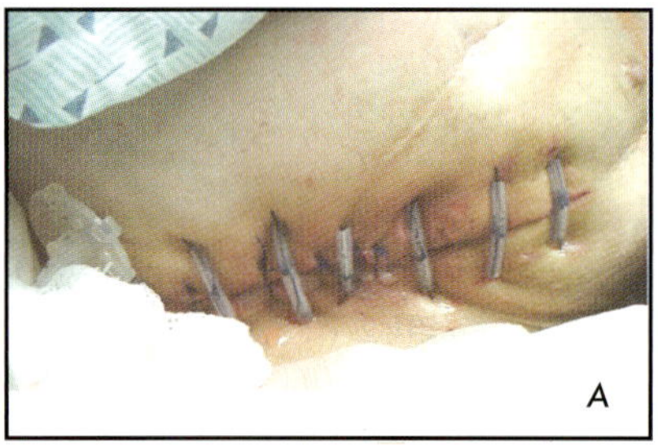

Figure 5A. One of the early attempts to control the wound breakdown in a patient with spina bifida.

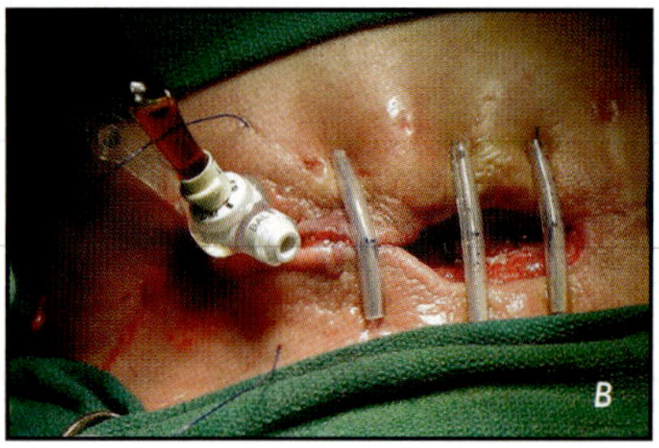

Figure 5B. This view depicts the wound breakdown and the ongoing attempts at control. The cecostomy tube is being irrigated with dilute Betadine (1% solution).

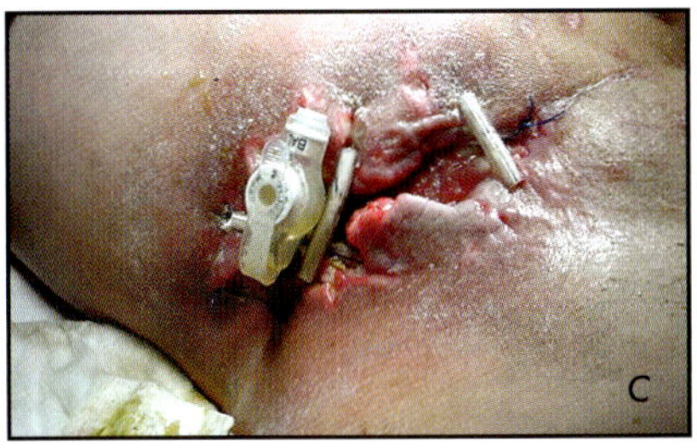

Figure 5C. A closer view to point out the lack of adequate granulation tissue to prevent ongoing fecal leakage.

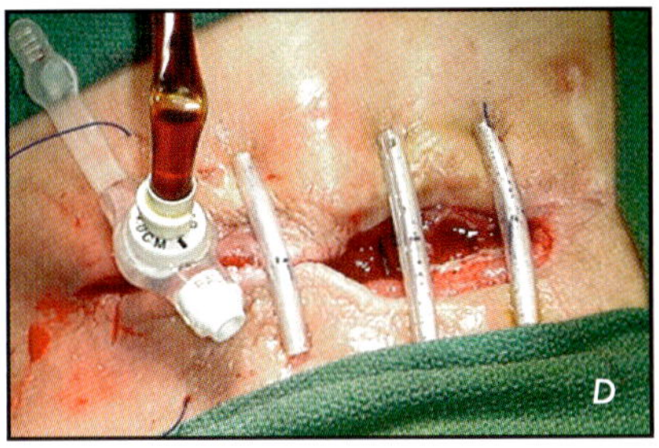

Figure 5D. After ten weeks of minimal progress, the wound appeared to be at a "standstill." Hyperbaric oxygen therapy was requested. Note the bile staining on the gauze pad at the patient's right.

massive intestinal distention on the two occasions. Figure 5D shows the appearance of the wound breakdown just at the start of the HBO2 therapy. The wound was able to be closed only after discontinuing the antegrade flushes, removing the cecostomy tube, and returning to the retrograde enemas per rectum. The wound finally stopped draining after another two months.

Major Postoperative Wound Infections

Wound infections in the post operative patient is a major cause of increased morbidity, prolonged hospital stay, and often times necessitates frequent return trips to the operating room for debridement due to the painful experience of debriding a given wound on the ward or in the treatment room. This is especially so in the childhood age group where adequate conscious sedation may require enough medication that it approaches general anesthetic levels. In most medical centers, most postoperative wound infections are managed by dressing changes at least once a day and sometimes as many as three times a day. Such routines expend a tremendous amount of time and energy on behalf of the patient, the nursing staff, and the treating surgeon. Further, if synthetic implants are involved, such as is common in orthopedic procedures, the problem is compounded. More often than not, the prosthetic device will require removal if successful treatment of the wound infection is to be obtained. This statement was the rule just a few years ago. Today, due to availability of new and exciting treatment modalities, it need not be the rule but rather, the exception. To be sure, sharp debridement of devitalized tissue is the primary initial mode of care, irrespective of the age of the patient. Adjunctive to sharp debridement, we have available for use in wound care several compounds for enzymatic debridement, substances to stimulate tissue growth, and the very exciting mechanical modality of negative pressure wound therapy (NPWT). One version of NPWT is the Vacuum Assisted Closure (VAC) device. Enzymatic debridement substances and progranulation substances currently are better known and understood than the VAC® system (Kinetic Concepts, Inc of San Antonio, Texas) especially in the pediatric age group, but that is rapidly changing. Reports of use of the VAC® of KCI system and its merits in adults are more numerous than its use in children, although a few reports are beginning to appear with more frequency since 2004. This portion of the chapter will discuss the use of NPWT in children, giving an example of a very major post operative complication in an eleven year old patient who had an orthopedic procedure.

Case 5

This 11-year-old male was born with spina bifida with the defect extending from mid thorax (T-7) to sacrum. He has been wheel chair bound all his life. Over time, he developed progressive kyphoscoliosis which resulted in a worsening of the ability to carry out his routine daily care with ease. To improve on this, he underwent correction of the kyphoscoliosis in the form of a procedure via a posterior spinal fusion with bone grafts and metal instrumentation. Twelve days postoperatively seropurulent drainage was expressible from the incision. The wound was opened and debrided by the primary surgeon, followed by referral to the wound care service for ongoing care.

After initial assessment by the wound care service, the skin and subcutaneous sutures were removed while the muscle sutures had been left in place. (Figure 6A) Because of persistent, intramuscular purulent drainage, the sutures in the muscle also required removal, exposing the metal hardware (Figure 6B). The open wound at the outset of therapy measured 17 cm long x 5.2 cm wide x 2.5 cm deep. Negative pressure wound therapy (VAC® of KCI, San Antonio, Texas) was applied at the initiation of care (Figure 6C). Specifically it was applied with the following details:

a. A polyurethane, highly porous sponge directly for the wound contact, cut to wound size and shape;
b. A plastic occlusive dressing;
c. Specially designed tubing attached to a graduated, vacuum pump;
d. Negative pressure is initiated at 100 mm Hg, continuous cycle;
e. Dressing changes and wound evaluations were done three times weekly (Monday, Wednesday, Friday);
f. Assessment consisted of evaluating overall appearance, volume changes of the wound, infection control, development of a healthy granulating bed, and migration of epithelium to the point of wound closure;
g. Changes of the degree of negative pressure were deemed necessary whenever a decrease in the rate of healing became apparent. This occurred on two occasions during the treatment period: at seven weeks and at 15 weeks after the start of NPWT therapy (Figures 6D and 6E). As can be seen in these two figures, the overall volume of the wound is considerably smaller and there is an excellent granulating bed, but some hardware is still exposed. The degree of negative suction was raised to -150 mm Hg (Figure 6D) and again to -175 mm Hg with a subsequent response of improved granulation tissue deposition and complete hardware coverage.

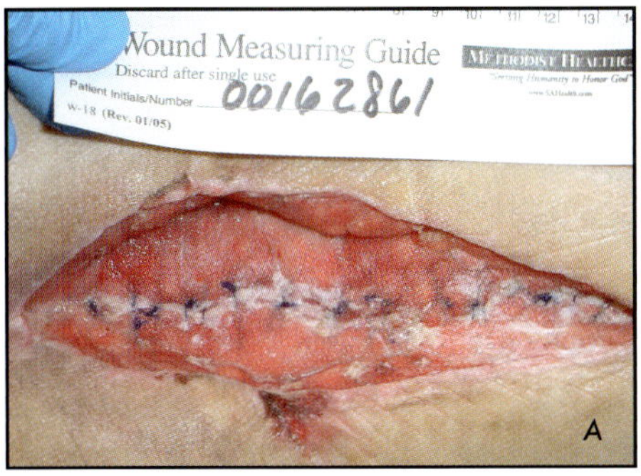

Figure 6A. Demonstrates initial view at start of treatment.

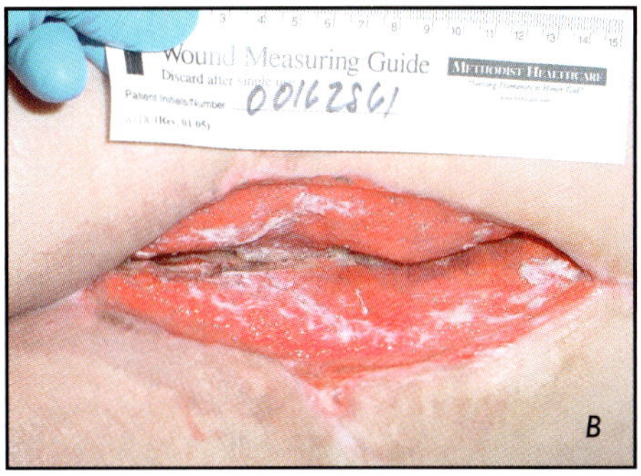

Figure 6B. Demonstrates view of ongoing treatment.

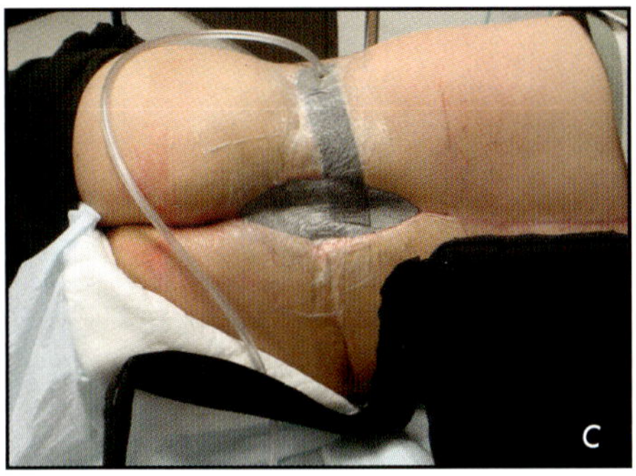

Figure 6C. Shows the Wound VAC in place.

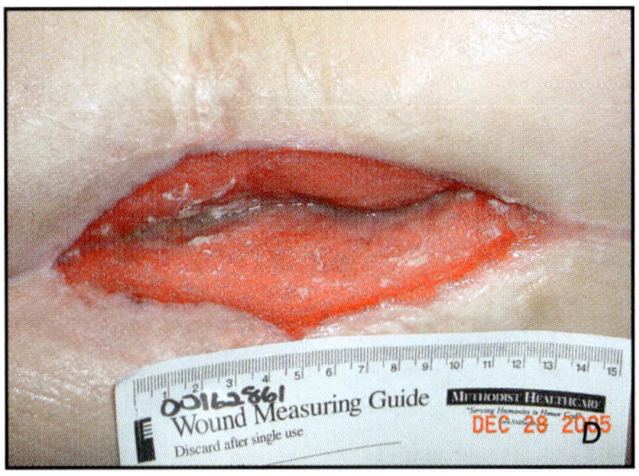

Figure 6D. Shows a much smaller wound is developing granulation tissue.

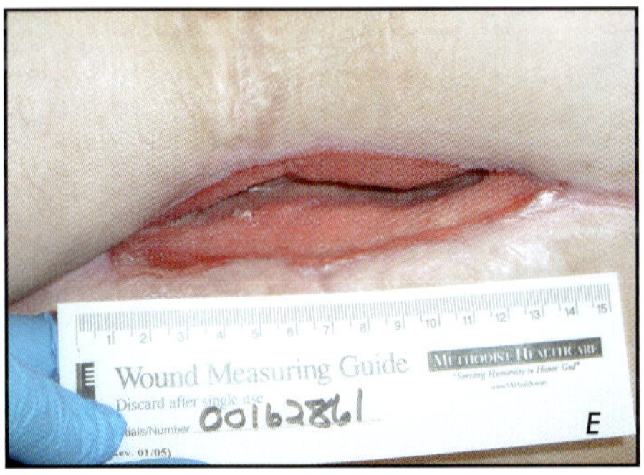

Figure 6E. This view shows an excellent response to therapy.

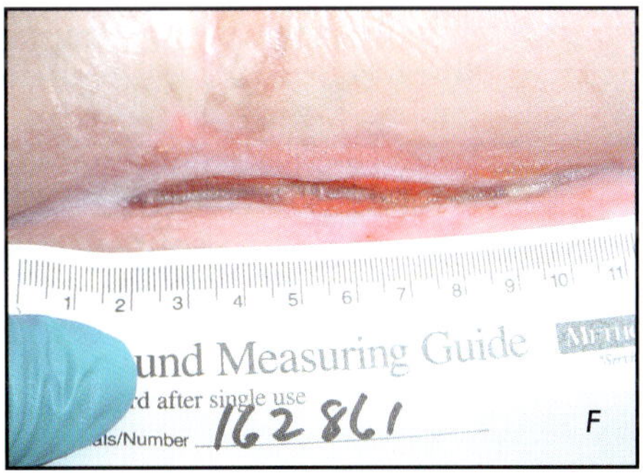

Figure 6F. The VAC was discontinued one week previously.

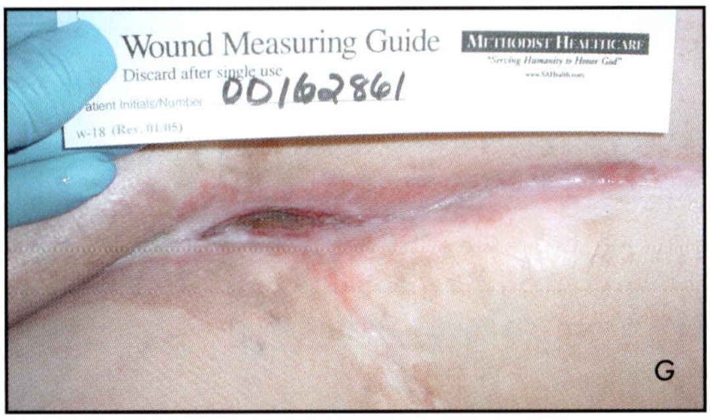

Figure 6G. Healing is virtually complete.

The overall impact of the use of the NPWT system allowed or provided three important features that most likely would have been impossible prior to its use in wound care:

1. Decrease in frequency of wound manipulation and decrease in the painful experience of dressing changes;
2. Ability to do the wound care of such large magnitudes without the need to be done in the operating suite;
3. The remarkable ability, in most cases, to "save" the hardware.

The last two Figures (6F and 6G) show the wound continuing to heal after discontinuation of the NPWT (which occurred one week prior to Figure 6F).

How to Make the Patients Comfortable

The following maneuvers/steps have been used by the author for the past 35 years of operation/caring for patients in the pediatric age group, ranging from six months to 16 years of age:

a. Establish initially a non-physical contact in a soft, non-threatening voice.
b. Discuss topics of interest to the patient, directly with the patient, disregarding the presence of the parent; acknowledge the parent, put him/her secondary.
c. Discuss play topics, school topics, favorite toy objects, etc.
d. Establish physical contact in a non-threatening manner; first "shake hands" with the parent, then shake hands with the patient; touch non-wounded areas of the body, clothing, etc; "listen" to the heart and lungs of the parent then let the patient "listen" to the heart and lungs of the parent. Finally, listen to the heart and lungs of the patient.
e. Lastly, look at/examine/treat the presenting wound.

For more information, see the chapter entitled "Comforting the Patient" by LL Soto and KM Sheffield.

SUMMARY

In summary, the reader should come to realize that to carry out optimal care of the wound in children, and, indeed, the whole child, it is paramount to have a good understanding that the child is not "just a little adult." Underscoring this dictum, the treating physician has to realize that the ever-changing child has ever-changing factors to contend with. These factors will: first, alter the child's response to an injury and, second, cause the physician to think "singularly" about the patient in hand and not "cookbook" treat the injury, as is often done in the adult situation.

Those influencing factors include, but are not limited to: age at time of injury, size of the patient, the high probability of associated injuries, preexisting physical abnormalities, and preexisting metabolic or physiologic conditions.

REFERENCES

1. Arensman RM, Fenner GC, Loe WA, et al. Care of traumatic wounds. *In Pediatric Trauma, Eichelberger(ed.)* St. Louis, MO: Mosby Year Book, 1993; 296–314.
2. Bergstein JM. Extremity compartment syndrome. In Cameron, JL (ed). *Current Surgical Therapy [7th ed]* St. Louis, Mosby, 2001;1140 - 1144.
3. Ein SH. Appendicitis. In Ashcraft KW, Murphy JP, Sharp RJ, (eds.): *Pediatric Surgery [3rd ed.]* Philadelphia, PA: WB Saunders, 2000; 571–579.
4. Fisher AC. Acute appendicitis. In Cameron JL (ed.). *Current Surgical Therapy [7th ed.]* St. Louis, MO: Mosby, 2001; 267-272.
5. Majeski J. Necrotizing infections of the skin and soft tissues. In Cameron JL (ed.). *Current Surgical Therapy [7th ed.]* St. Louis, MO: Mosby, 2001; 1246-1250.
6. McGill CW. Bites. In Ashcraft KW, Murphy, Sharp, Sigalet, Snyder (eds.): *Pediatric Surgery [3rd ed.]* Philadelphia, PA: WB Saunders, 2000; 153-158.
7. O'Neil JA. Burns. In Randolph JG, Ravitch MM, Welch KJ, Benson CD, Aberdeen E (eds.): *The Injured Child- Surgical Management* Chicago, IL: Year Book Medical Publishers, 1979; 303-329.
8. Patrick DA, Janik JE, et al. Increased CT scan utilization does not improve the diagnostic accuracy of appendicitis in children. *Journal Pediatric Surgery* 2003; 38: 659-662.
9. Pitts WJ. Snakebite. In Randolph JG, Ravitch MM et al (eds.) *The Injured Child- Surgical Management* Chicago, IL: Year Book Medical Publishers, 1979; 331-368.
10. Rause TM, Eichelberger MR. Trends in pediatric trauma management. In Filston, HC (ed.). *The Surgical Clinics of North America* Philadelphia, PA: WB Saunders,1992; 72: 1347-1364.
11. Silver GM, Gamelli RL. Burn wound management. In Cameron JL (ed.). *Current Surgical Therapy [7th ed.]* St. Louis, MO: Mosby, 2001; 1179–1185.
12. Smith MD, Burrington JD. Injuries in children sustained in free falls: an analysis of 66 cases. *The Journal of Trauma* Williams and Wilkins, 1975; 15: 987–991.
13. Vishal Saxena, S. M. Chao-Wei Hwang, Sui Huang, et-al. Vacuum-assisted closure: Microdeformation of wounds and cell proliferation. *Plastic and Reconstructive Surgery* 2004; 114: 1086-1096.
14. Butter A, Emran M, Al-Jazeri A, et al. Assisted closure for wound management in the pediatric population. *J Pediatric Surgery* 2006; 41:940-942.
15. Caniono DA, Ruth B, Teich S. Wound management with vacuum-assisted closure: Experience in 51 pediatric patients. *J Pediatric Surgery* 2005; 40:128-132.

REVIEW QUESTIONS

1.) General principles that must be considered in all children's wounds include all EXCEPT:
  a. Age of the patient at the time of injury
  b. Associated injuries are likely and/or probable
  c. Gender of the patient
  d. Preexisting metabolic/physiologic abnormalities, if any
  e. Characteristics of the agent causing the wound

2.) Wound care for a specific type of injury is the same regardless of the age of the patient.
  a. True
  b. False

3.) Motor vehicle accidents cause more injuries among infants than among teenagers.
  a. True
  b. False

4.) When treating bites of dogs and other large animals, including humans, the salient principles of treating the child include all of the following EXCEPT:
  a. Thorough, extensive irrigation with copious amounts of saline
  b. Debridement of devitalized tissue, if present
  c. Open drainage of all deep puncture wounds, including on the face.
  d. Closing primarily the puncture wounds on the face

5.) Wound infection in the post operative pediatric patient is a major cause of:
  a. Increased morbidity
  b. Prolonged hospital stay
  c. Frequent return trips to the operating room for debridement
  d. Medication doses for adequate conscious sedation that approaches general anesthetic levels
  e. All of the above

Answers 1c, 2b, 3b, 4c, 5e

CHAPTER 26

PREVENTION: THE SIXTH PHASE OF WOUND HEALING

CHAPTER TWENTY-SIX OVERVIEW

patient's problems, but should be considered the maestro in orchestrating the patient's need for specialty care. Obvious examples are referrals to vascular surgery, orthopedics, and endocrinology depending on the patient's underlying problems and complexity. This team approach is very important to the success of preventing wounds from occurring, but if the patient is sent to a specialist, the PCM needs to oversee the patient's overall care and be aware of the treatments prescribed by the various specialists.

Patients with diabetes may benefit from a referral to a podiatrist for routine foot care such as pressure point management at metatarsals, bunions, or heels, as well as for nail trimming and for problems with in-grown toenails. Foot deformities such as Charcot's foot or hammertoes may require surgical correction by a podiatrist or orthopedic surgeon to actually prevent limb threatening ulcers and infections. Close glucose control is also important in preventing wounds because minor scrapes or injuries will be less likely to become infected as when glucose levels are high. In brittle or hard to control diabetics, the patient may require the services of an endocrinologist and such technologies as an insulin pump.

Patients with hypertension or diabetes and signs of decreased lower extremity blood flow such as hair loss in the toes, feet, and lower leg may need early vascular evaluations by a vascular surgeon to determine if there are any significant blockages in the major arterial vessels. This can occur without classic signs of claudication. Monitoring foot pulses with Doppler readings and determining ankle-brachial indexes can track lower extremity vascular conditions. These can be done by the PCM or through referral to a wound care center or a vascular surgery clinic. Transcutaneous oxygen measurement is a non-invasive test that may indicate decreased oxygen tissue levels. This test is particularly important if any surgical procedures are anticipated. It helps determine the healing potential of the tissue and is useful after a vascular procedure to validate the tissue oxygenation.

Lower extremity vein harvest for cardiac bypass surgery or lower extremity arterial bypass surgeries will often result in venous and lymphatic return problems and an increase in the risk of venous stasis ulcers. If traditional compression is not effective, certain vascular surgery procedures may be of benefit. In severe cases, venous stasis ulcers are also associated with congestive heart failure and may require a cardiology consult to medically decrease the edema in concert with compression. If the patient is a candidate, vein harvesting may be prevented or postponed by endoarterial plaque removal procedures. This may increase arterial flow without compromising venous and lymphatic integrity and the associated edema problems.

PREVENTIVE MEASURES BY THE PRIMARY CARE MANAGER

In general, there are six main medical areas in wound prevention that need to be addressed by the PCM: obesity, lack of exercise, offloading, nutrition, skin care, and smoking. Education of the patient is a common thread within all of these areas. As with most medical treatments or health promotion efforts, the patient needs to be the one who accepts the responsibility for adhering to the recommendations. The use of support groups, family members, or community programs can often convert failure to success and the more opportunities to involve the patient, the better.

Obesity

Obesity has direct correlation with a number of areas that increase the risk of wound recurrence, particularly the lower extremity, sacral and buttock areas. The National Institutes of Health define obesity and overweight using a Body Mass Index (BMI), which is a calculation of a person's weight in kilograms divided by the square of their height in meters. An overweight adult is defined as one with a BMI between 25 and 29.9, while an obese adult has a BMI of 30 or higher. Comparing a BMI of 26 with a BMI of 21, the relative risks (RRs) of diabetes are about 8 for women and 4 for men. The corresponding RRs for congestive heart failure are 2 for women and 1.5 for men (2).

Regarding obesity, the first and most obvious effect is the pressure load expressed on the plantar surface or the foot. Although offloading of the healed wound area can be accomplished, the heavier an individual is, the more difficult it is to offload and the more pressure is exerted on compensatory tissues. This, in turn, increases the probability of recurrent or new wounds at these areas. Obesity is also associated with an increased risk of venous stasis disease and lymphedema of the lower extremities. Both of these conditions are more difficult to control in the obese patient and often lead to uncompensated edema in spite of traditional compression devices. This may lead to tissue breakdown with leakage areas that progress to blisters or open wounds.

Many patients with healed wounds are diabetic while others are at high risk of becoming diabetic. Obesity is closely associated with a precursor termed metabolic syndrome. The Third Report of the National Cholesterol Education Program (NCEP) Expert Panel provided a working definition of metabolic syndrome. Individuals with three or more of the following characteristics have the metabolic syndrome (4):

- Abdominal obesity: waist circumference >102 cm in men and >88 cm in women
- Hypertriglyceridemia: >150 mg/dl (1.69 mmol/L)
- Low high-density lipoprotein (HDL) cholesterol: <40 mg/dl (1.04 mmol/L) in men and <50 mg/dl (1.29 mmol/L) in women
- High blood pressure: >130/85 mm Hg
- High fasting glucose: >110 mg/dl (6.1 mmol/L)

Obesity is closely associated with cardiovascular disease. Peripheral vascular disease is often an important contributing factor to the development of lower extremity ulcers due to the low tissue oxygen levels. In addition, arterial bypass surgery wounds or wounds for vein harvest for cardiac bypass surgery are often seen in the wound care clinic due to delayed healing in many patients. Decreasing obesity empirically will decrease cardiovascular disease including peripheral vascular disease. The Look AHEAD (Action for Health in Diabetes) trial by the National Institute of Diabetes and Digestive and Kidney Diseases is studying over 5,000 obese patients with type 2 diabetes. Participants were randomly assigned to one of two interventions, the

TABLE 1. BODY MASS INDEX TABLE

	Normal						Overweight					Obese										Extreme Obesity														
BMI	19	20	21	22	23	24	25	26	27	28	29	30	31	32	33	34	35	36	37	38	39	40	41	42	43	44	45	46	47	48	49	50	51	52	53	54
Height (inches)	Body Weight (pounds)																																			
58	91	96	100	105	110	115	119	124	129	134	138	143	148	153	158	162	167	172	177	181	186	191	196	201	205	210	215	220	224	229	234	239	244	248	253	258
59	94	99	104	109	114	119	124	128	133	138	143	148	153	158	163	166	173	178	183	188	193	198	203	208	212	217	222	227	332	237	242	247	252	257	262	267
60	97	102	107	112	118	123	128	133	138	143	148	153	158	163	168	174	179	184	189	194	199	204	209	215	220	225	230	235	240	245	250	255	261	266	271	276
61	100	106	111	116	122	127	132	137	143	148	153	158	164	169	174	180	185	190	195	201	206	211	217	222	227	232	238	243	248	254	259	264	269	275	280	285
62	104	109	115	120	126	131	136	142	147	153	158	164	169	175	180	186	191	196	202	207	213	218	224	229	235	240	246	251	256	262	267	273	278	284	289	295
63	107	113	118	124	130	135	141	146	152	158	163	169	175	180	186	191	197	203	208	214	220	225	231	237	242	248	254	259	265	270	278	282	287	293	299	304
64	110	116	122	128	134	140	145	151	157	163	169	174	180	186	192	197	204	209	215	221	227	232	238	244	250	256	262	267	273	279	285	291	296	302	308	314
65	114	120	126	132	138	144	150	166	162	168	174	180	186	192	198	204	210	216	222	228	234	240	246	252	258	264	270	276	282	288	294	300	306	312	318	324
66	118	124	130	136	142	148	155	161	167	173	179	186	192	198	204	210	216	223	229	235	241	247	253	260	266	272	278	284	291	297	303	309	315	322	328	334
67	121	127	134	140	146	153	159	166	172	178	185	191	198	204	211	217	223	230	236	242	249	255	261	268	274	280	287	293	299	306	312	319	325	331	338	344
68	125	131	138	144	151	158	164	171	177	184	190	197	203	210	216	223	230	236	243	249	256	262	269	276	282	289	295	302	308	315	322	328	335	341	348	354
69	128	135	142	149	155	162	169	176	182	189	196	203	209	216	223	230	236	243	250	257	263	270	277	284	291	297	304	311	318	324	331	338	345	351	358	365
70	132	139	146	153	160	167	174	181	188	195	202	209	216	222	229	236	243	250	257	264	271	278	285	292	299	306	313	320	327	334	341	348	355	362	369	376
71	136	143	150	157	165	172	179	186	193	200	206	215	222	229	236	243	250	257	265	272	279	286	293	301	308	315	322	329	338	343	351	358	365	372	379	386
72	140	147	154	162	169	177	184	191	199	218	213	221	228	235	242	250	258	265	272	279	287	294	302	309	316	324	331	338	346	353	361	368	375	383	390	397
73	144	151	159	166	174	182	189	197	204	212	219	227	235	242	250	257	265	272	280	288	295	302	210	318	325	333	340	348	355	363	371	378	386	393	401	408
74	148	155	163	171	179	186	194	202	210	218	225	233	241	249	256	264	272	280	287	295	303	311	219	326	334	342	350	358	365	373	381	389	396	404	412	420
75	152	160	168	176	184	192	200	208	216	224	232	240	248	256	264	272	279	287	295	303	311	319	327	335	343	351	359	367	375	383	391	399	407	415	423	431
76	156	164	172	180	189	197	205	213	221	230	238	246	254	263	271	279	287	295	304	312	320	328	336	344	353	361	369	377	385	394	402	410	418	426	435	443

Lifestyle Intervention or Diabetes Support and Education, and will be followed for a total period of up to 11.5 years. The program began in 2004. The primary aim of Look AHEAD is to study the effects of the two interventions on major cardiovascular events that include: heart attack, stroke and cardiovascular-related death. Look AHEAD will also investigate the impact of the interventions on other cardiovascular disease-related outcomes, cardiovascular risk factors, and all-cause mortality. Additional outcomes include diabetes control and complications, fitness, general health, health-related quality of life and psychological outcomes. For the most current updates on findings, the reader is encouraged to access *www.niddk.nih.gov* and search "look ahead."

The Primary Care Manager needs to prescribe and encourage weight loss with the goal of converting the obese patient to an overweight one and the overweight patient to one with a BMI of less than 25. This is particularly true if the patient is already diabetic. Diet types have recently become controversial. Low carbohydrate diets have been criticized for adverse kidney effects. A recent review suggested that consumption of low-glycemic index (GI) foods/liquids was directly associated with reduction in subsequent hunger and increased satiety in most of the short-term feeding studies in humans (lasting for a single meal or a single day). In addition, voluntary energy intake increased after consumption of high-GI meals as compared with consumption of low-GI meals (5). The U.S. Department of Agriculture is currently studying various diets (*www.usda.gov*). A new food pyramid was rolled out in 2005 that personalizes food type and intake as well as considering exercise routines (*www.mypyramid.gov*). An example is at Figure 1.

Lack of Exercise

Regardless of what diet eventually is recommended by the PCM, exercise is an important component of any weight-control plan. Exercise is important in the overall prevention of wound recurrence from the standpoint of both weight control and cardiovascular conditioning. Even as a treatment modality for congestive heart failure, exercise has been shown to affect many peripheral changes, specifically abnormalities in the skeletal muscle, peripheral blood flow, and neurohormonal milieu, which improve with appropriate exercise regimes. Exercise also reduces the symptoms of exertional fatigue, improves quality of life, and increases survival. Patients with congestive heart failure are more likely to have edema in the lower extremities that increase the risk of stasis ulcers. If the PCM is not handling the care of the congestive heart patient, close coordination with the cardiologist would be necessary (6).

The National Institute of Diabetes and Digestive and Kidney Diseases' Diabetes Prevention Project (DPP), took 3,234 nondiabetic but overweight persons with impaired glucose tolerance (IGT) and randomly assigned them to placebo, metformin (850 mg twice daily), or a lifestyle modification program with the goals of at least a 7% weight loss and at least 150 minutes of physical activity per week. Diet and exercise that achieved a 5–7% weight loss reduced diabetes incidence by 58% in participants randomized to the study's lifestyle intervention group. Participants in this group exercised at moderate intensity, usually by walking an average of 30 minutes a day five days a week, and lowered their intake of fat and calories.

Lifestyle intervention worked equally well in men and women and in all the ethnic groups. It was most effective in people age 60 and older, who lowered the risk of developing diabetes by 71% (7).

Exercise of patients with healed wounds creates a problem regarding the healed area. For example, for wounds on the foot, the mechanical stress of exercise at the wound area needs to be addressed. This can be done by prescribing alternative exercises such as water workouts, stationary cycling (provided the wound is not at the pedal area or at an area where shear occurs from the shoe), or chair dancing. Stretching and using weights build flexibility and muscle tone. After a sufficient time of epithelialization, the patient can transition to limited weight bearing exercise. Exercise that challenges the wound area requires that the area be checked daily for stress points and the exercise duration must be short with gradual increase. As mentioned in the DPP study above, building up to 30 minutes of walking or similar exercise five times per week is the goal for weight loss, and suggests benefits for cardiovascular and diabetes control. An excellent resource for exercise for obese or diabetic patients is the National Institute of Diabetes and Digestive and Kidney Diseases web page (*www.niddk.nih.gov*) and its subsequent publications. Due to "fat city" lists by the news media, many communities such as San Antonio, TX now have official "fat to fit" programs in which the patient can be encouraged to participate.

Special attention must be given to the elderly and to those who have decreased mobility due to injury. These individuals are at risk for protein-energy malnutrition (PEM) which is discussed later in detail. It is

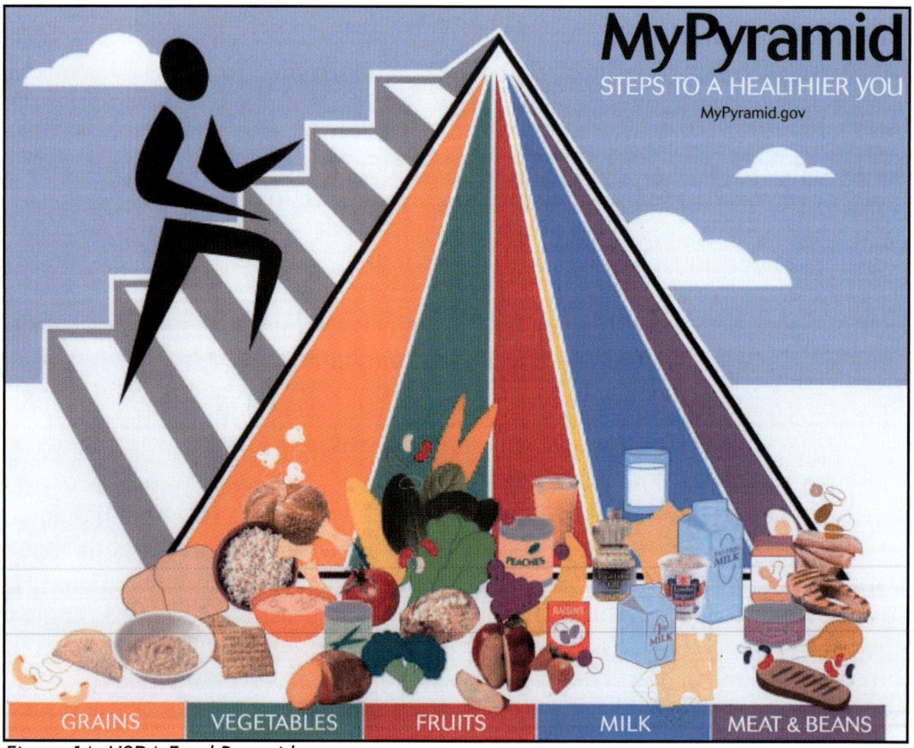

Figure 1A. USDA Food Pyramid.

Grains Make half you grain whole	Vegetables Vary you veggies	Fruits Focus on fruits	Milk Get your calcium-rich foods	Meat & Beans Go lean with protein
Eat at least 3 oz. of whole-grain cereals, breads, crackers, rice, or pasta everyday 1 oz. is about 1 slice of bread, about 1 cup of breakfast cereal, or 1.2 cup of cooked rice, cereal or past	Eat more dark-green veggies like broccoli, spinach, and other dark leafy greens Eat more orange vegatables like carrot and sweetpotatoes Eat more dry beans and peas like pinto beans, kidney beans, and lentils	Eat a variety of fruit Choose fresh, frozen, canned, or dried fruit Go easy on fruit juices	Go low-fat or fat-free when you choose milk, yogurt, and other milk products If you don't or can't consume milk, choose lactose-free products or other calcium sources such as fortified foods and beverages	Choose low-fat or lean meats and poultry Bake it, broil it, or grill it Vary your protein routine—choose more fish, beans, peas, nuts, and seeds
For a 2,000-calorie diet, you need the amounts below from each food group. To find the amounts that are right for you, go to MyPyramid.gov				
Eat 6 oz. every day	Eat 2.5 cups every day	Eat 2 cups every day	Get 3 cups every day; for kids aged 2 to 8, it's 2	Eat 5.5 oz. every day

Find your balance between food and physical activity

- Be sure to stay within your daily calorie needs.
- Be physically active for at least 30 minutes most days of the week.
- About 60 minutes a day of physical activity may be needed to prevent weight gain.
- For sustaining weight loss, at least 60 to 90 minutes a day of physical activity may be required.
- Children and teenagers should be physically active for 60 minutes every day, or most days.

Know the limits on fats, sugars, and salt (sodium)

- Make most of your fat sources from fish, nuts, and vegetable oils.
- Limit solid fats like butter, margarine, shortening, and lard, as well as foods that contain these.
- Check the Nutrition Facts label to keep saturated fats, *trans* fats, and sodium low.
- Choose food and beverages low in added sugars. Added sugars contribute calories with few, if any, nutrients.

Figure 1B. USDA Food Pyramid.

characterized by breakdown of body protein and can lead to muscle wasting. Resistance exercise should be considered for these patients and can be arranged by physical therapy staff or occupational therapy personnel, as well as the staff at some nursing homes or independent living facilities. By definition, resistance exercise is muscle movement against a resistance such as weights or elastic bands. In patients with PEM, resistance exercise diminishes the degree of protein loss and increases lean body mass, versus fat, particularly in the chronically ill population and the elderly. This, in turn, can decrease subsequent disability. Exercise of all muscle groups is important to maintain tone and relative strength. Exercising the large-muscle groups is especially crucial in reducing overall muscle loss and stimulates the body's anabolic drive (8).

Offloading

Offloading is crucial to both lower extremity and pressure point areas that have healed wounds or are at risk of forming wounds. Sumpio (9) found that after a heel ulcer heals, recurrence rates might be as high as 70% at three years. The mechanical goal of treatment after heel ulcer healing should be to reduce pressures so the cumulative load is below that at which tissue damage occurs (9). Oftentimes the clinician only thinks of the plantar surface or traditional pressure ulcer sites, but pressure can also be adversely applied to the sides of the foot from poor footwear or pathological deformities such as Charcot's foot or hammertoes. A compression dressing for venous stasis ulcers can cause enough pressure over the tibial area to retard wound healing or create new wounds. Supplemental padding on either side of the threatened area prior to the compression wrap will often take care of the problem.

For previous plantar metatarsal head ulcers, Birke et al. (10) demonstrated that adhesive backed quarter-inch-thick felt padding produced a 48% reduction over barefoot peak pressure at the previous wound area. The padding was fitted to the forefoot with a cutout over the previously ulcerated metatarsal area of interest. Pressure was further reduced when the padding was used in conjunction with a surgical shoe or wedged-sole surgical shoe (61% and 73% respectively). A short leg walker reduced pressure by 61%. The importance of such offloading techniques may require referral to a podiatrist, orthopedic surgeon, or orthotist. Simple shoe inserts with cutouts, non-medicated bunion rings, or toe separation pads may be all that are needed for small areas for offloading. Again, the patient must make routine daily checks of the threatened areas.

The Agency for Healthcare Research and Quality (AHRQ) Clinical Practice Guidelines of 1992 recommends offloading techniques and surfaces to prevent pressure ulcers. The guidelines should be one of the references used when the PCM has a patient who requires many hours in either a bed or in a wheelchair. Most of the fundamentals are widely used and will only be summarized here. The reader is urged to obtain a copy of the guidelines from the AHRQ.

Offloading the body surface at risk is the most critical aspect of prevention. The AHRQ recommends that bed-bound patients be turned at least every two hours and high risk patients be turned more frequently (11). A recent study that considered alternative turning schedules up to four hours when combined with Group 1 offloading surfaces and found it to be more effective than every two hours on a standard surface (12).

The AHRQ sponsored more recent studies regarding the effectiveness of Group 1 and Group 2 offloading surfaces in preventing pressure ulcers in at risk patients. Group 1 includes static overlays and mattress replacements primarily made of foam, air, water or gel. Group 2 includes alternating pressure mattresses, air mattress overlays and powered air flotation beds (low-air-loss therapy).

The results of the first study review demonstrated that "treatment with various support surfaces classified as Group 1 results in improved health outcomes for patients at risk of developing pressure ulcers. Preventing new pressure ulcers appears to be the main treatment effect associated with Group 1 support surfaces. Use of a standard surface (i.e., a standard hospital bed or standard operating table) is considered no treatment" (13).

The second study review concluded, "treatment with a Group 2 therapy is superior to no treatment in the prevention of pressure ulcers among patients who are at risk. It is plausible that extensive data are not available because any comparison between a Group 2 treatment and no treatment may be considered inappropriate, given that Group 1 treatments have been shown to be superior to no treatment in the prevention of pressure ulcers among patients who are at risk. The available evidence does not support the conclusion that treatment with alternating pressure therapy results in improved health outcomes as compared to treatment with a Group 1 pressure-reducing support surface" (14).

A more recent study review by the Cochrane Library showed a summary relative risk of 0.29 (95% CI: 0.19–0.43) favoring enhanced foam alternatives over standard mattresses. It also demonstrated similar results to the AHRQ study in that "comparison of alternating pressure devices with a variety of constant low-pressure devices (a water mattress, foam pad, static air mattress, and foam overlays) showed no significant difference in pressure ulcer development (15). Another important point regarding the use of any offloading surface is that it does not preclude or eliminate the need to turn the patient to further offload the area of concern. In wheelchair patients shifting of the weight from side to side every 15–20 minutes is recommended. Offloading cushions are beneficial in preventing wounds, but weight shifting is still necessary.

Patients that are admitted for surgery require attention for ulcer prevention during and after surgery. Baumgarten et al studied extrinsic factors associated with hospital-acquired pressure ulcers in at risk elderly patients who had hip fractures. These included longer wait before surgery, intensive care stay, longer surgical procedure, and general anesthesia (16). In addition, the heels of patients are often times forgotten and are at particular risk in diabetics or patients with low blood flow. From 1997–2000, the incidence of hospital-acquired heel ulcers has increased from 19% to 30% (17). Offloading by turning, placing pillows under the calves, or providing multipodal boots prevent heel contact with the mattress surface and prevent subsequent heel ulcers.

Shear and friction are other factors that produce pressure ulcers. The standard recommendation is to avoid inclining the head of the bed by greater than 30% to decrease the probability of shear injuries in the reclined bed patient.

The risk of friction injury is reduced by careful movement techniques, such as the use of sheets or assistance devices to slide the patient without direct contact with the underlying material. In addition, morbidly obese patients will benefit from bariatric beds and chairs that aid the movement of the obese patient by staff or family members.

Nutrition

Proper nutrition, particularly in elderly and diabetic patients is often overlooked. Malnutrition, including obesity as mentioned above, is a critical factor in healing wounds, preventing recurrences, and preventing new wounds. Total calorie intake is often too low in the elderly, but too high in the diabetic. Calorie levels should be sufficient to maintain the body's ability to heal any scrapes or lacerations, but low enough to allow one to two pounds of weight loss per week in the obese patient.

Nutrition should also take into consideration adequate vitamins and minerals. The most important are reviewed here with details discussed in the chapter entitled "Nutrition and Hydration" by Aimee Dennis Wauters (18). Vitamin C (ascorbic acid) has the primary function of collagen production, which forms the basis for connective tissue in bones, teeth, and cartilage. It also plays an important role in wound healing, immunity, and the nervous system, and acts as a water-soluble antioxidant. This is particularly important in wound prevention. Clinical signs of vitamin C deficiency includes purplish blotches or lightly traumatized areas and extreme transparency of the skin in the upper extremities. The primary role of vitamin E is to act as an antioxidant by being incorporated into the lipid portion of cell membranes and other molecules. There, it protects these structures from oxidative damage and prevents the propagation of lipid peroxidation. Vitamin E has been shown to have protective effects against cancer, heart disease, and complications of diabetes. It also protects the skin from photodamage and improves skin texture. A linoleic acid mixture of essential fatty acids, vitamin A, and vitamin E applied over the body inclusive of all potential wound sites for a mean of 21 days demonstrated a protective effect for the development of pressure ulcers (19).

Carotenoids act as a source of vitamin A in the diet and have important antioxidant actions. Conversion of carotenoids to vitamin A requires protein, thyroid hormone, zinc, and vitamin C. Deficiencies in vitamin A will clinically manifest as waxy perifollicular hyperkeratosis with nonpigmented areas that are dry and rough, anorexia, apathy, and increased susceptibilty to infections.

Selenium is the most important antioxidant mineral. It is essential for the function of the antioxidant enzyme glutathione peroxidase and it is also important for healthy immune and cardiovascular systems (20, 21).

Zinc is important in establishing a strong immune system at the cellular level and increases the number of T-lymphocytes. But it also is essential in tissue growth that continues during the remodeling phase. The ability to absorb zinc decreases with age. A deficiency in zinc will be evident clinically by seborrhea like dryness and redness of the nasolabial folds and eyebrows and white flecks in the fingernails.

Water intake is critical to optimize metabolism, keep skin turger intact, and maintain proper electrolyte balance. Indeed, dehydration is the most common cause of fluid and electrolyte disturbances and is particularly critical in the elderly. There are many different methodologies to determine proper hydration and one must also take into consideration losses from disease or medications, the patient's living environment (heat and humidity, air conditioning versus none) and activity levels, especially if performed out of doors. Daily fluid intake can be calculated as 25–30 ml per kg body weight or 1–1.5 ml per calorie consumed. Also, a minimum of 1500 ml per day is generally recommended. In Simmons' study, prompted fluid intake was found to improve hydration status, and giving individuals their beverage of choice works best, especially for cognitively intact people (22).

Protein levels should be checked in elderly patients and in those who had difficulty in healing their wound in spite of good vascular supply and glucose control. This would also include albumin and pre-albumin levels. For the prevention of pressure ulcers, the AHRQ recommends 30–35 calories per kg of ideal weight per day including 1.25–1.5 grams of protein per kg per day.

Indeed, Protein-Energy Malnutrition (PEM) is being recognized as a detrimental condition that leads to new wounds due to loss of skin integrity. PEM occurs when the intake of energy and protein is inadequate to meet the body's needs. It is frequently associated with significant involuntary weight loss. Involuntary weight loss has a number of definition parameters and can be defined as 5% loss of body weight in 30 days, 7% loss in three months, or 10% loss in six months and should be based on the patient's weight prior to any unintended loss. This is particularly common when a patient becomes immobile for a variety of reasons, but usually due to injury. During the weight loss period, there is the loss of body protein usually monitored as lean body mass (LBM). In the protein deficient patient, a wound heals by assimilating the amino acids from muscle and other stores. This deficit needs to be replaced. When the LBM is less than 15% of usual for the patient, the body becomes at risk for developing wounds. With a loss of LBM exceeding 20% of total, spontaneous wounds can develop due to the thinning of skin from lost collagen. A decrease in LBM approaching 25% is manifested by profound weakness, infections, and further development of new wounds or breakdown of prior healed wounds. An LBM loss greater than 25% leads to life threatening infections and a high mortality rate. Reduction of the LBM causes a depletion of glutamine, antioxidants, and micronutrients.

Confirming PEM is usually done by measuring serum albumin, total protein and serum transferrin. A serum albumin level less than 3.5 g/dl indicates low protein storage levels and less than 2.5 g/dl indicates seriously deficient protein stores. Total protein levels below 6.6 g/dl are considered low, but the total protein levels have the longest lag time and will be the last indicator to change in PEM. Pre-albumin and serum transferrin offer a more acute and accurate snapshot of protein stores. Prealbumin levels less than 18 mg/dl are considered low. Transferrin levels below 200 mg/dl are of concern with values less than 100 mg/dl indicating severe PEM. Lymphocyte cell count will also be decreased with protein-energy malnutrition with counts less than 800 in severe cases.

Reversing PEM, especially when severe, requires both macro and micronutrients. Generally, a target protein amount of 1.5 g/kg/day will be sufficient to satisfy protein requirements. The body will usually not be able to process more than 2.0 grams of protein per kilogram per day. Target carbohydrate amounts are 7–8 grams per kilogram per day with an emphasis on complex carbohydrates, if possible. The total number of calories should be 30–35 cal/kg/day. Vitamins, particularly A and C, and minerals (zinc, copper, and manganese) are required to correct PEM. Although the doses of micronutrients are not well defined, a dose 5–10 times the recommended daily allowance is usually suggested until the PEM is corrected. Although enteral or nasogastric tube feeding is preferred, the parenteral route may become necessary if enteral feeding does not adequately meet the requirements discussed above.

Optimum nutrition and resistance exercise is essential to increase anabolism. The addition of an anabolic agent can markedly accelerate restoration of lean body mass and favor consumed protein to building lean body mass instead of being used as an energy source. Anabolic steroids include human growth hormone, testosterone, and oxandrolone. The FDA approved oral oxandrolone for restoration of weight loss after severe trauma, major surgical procedures, or infections with a recommendation up to 20 mg per day. Contraindications include tumors that have androgenic receptors such as prostate or male breast cancer and hypercalcemia. Side effects include rare or mild hepatotoxicity and potential androgenic effects such as hirsutism, hypersexualism, and mood changes although also rare. Maintaining body weight and protein (muscle mass) is an essential aspect of the wound prevention management plan (23).

Skin Care

Skin care is very important in preventing wounds whether it be in the diabetic, venous stasis, bedridden, or paralytic patient. Patients first need to be educated on inspecting their skin for breaks, abrasions, redness or swelling. This is especially important for areas prone to pressure whether it be from bedding, chair surface, or orthotic devices. It is critical for patients compromised neurologically and who have difficulty feeling pain or temperature to focus on those body areas affected. In addition, they need to be taught to identify objects and equipment they use which may cause injury. Hot water from a faucet or a hot cup from a microwave may not be felt, causing catastrophic burns. A patient with foot neuropathy, who goes barefoot, courts trauma from stubbed toes, splinters, and needles, all of which can lead to lower extremity infection and amputations. If patients cannot physically inspect themselves because of mobility or blindness, then family members or caregivers need to be educated. If a suspected area or an open wound is found, the patient should be instructed to see the PCM as early as possible. The patient should gently clean the area with an antibiotic liquid soap and apply an antibiotic ointment or cream to the area.

Dry skin is often a problem of the venous stasis or diabetic patient. This sometimes leads to eczema that is uncomfortable causing itching. When the patient scratches the area, open sores may develop if the skin is broken especially in patients with venous stasis disease.

Topical corticosteroid ointment or antipuritic such as 5% doxepin may be used for short periods of time until the underlying problem is relieved. Remember that steroid creams can cause skin atrophy and thinning if it is used for more than two weeks (24).

In addition, the skin needs to be moisturized on a routine basis to counteract the dryness. Poore et al. suggest applying equal parts of white soft paraffin and liquid paraffin or other simple emollient (25). Commercial lotions often work well and the less expensive, non-prescription ones should be considered. One needs to remember that many of the lotions contain lanolin and may cause dermatitis for a patient who is allergic to wool and can actually add to the problem. Petroleum products may also cause sensitization.

The opposite problem is found in bedridden patients, wheelchair bound patients, and obese patients. That is the problem of wet or macerated skin. This is often associated with urine or fecal contamination in the incontinent patient and is a considerable concern in preventing sacral or buttock wounds. Vigilant patient hygiene or nursing care is critical in keeping the area clean and the fecal and urine milieu from breaking down the skin. Skin barrier creams or lotions can be used after sufficient cleaning has been accomplished. This may be as simple as applying zinc oxide ointment, A + D ointment, or more commercial skin barrier products. Liquid bandages that form a waterproof seal on the skin may also be beneficial. In the obese patient skin folds are prone to moisture related breakdown. These areas should be cleaned and dried. A hair blower on the "no heat" setting can be used after towel drying for added benefit. To reduce friction, the area can then be powdered with antifungal powder (if at risk for candida) or a light application of cornstarch.

Smoking

The effects of smoking include vasoconstriction due to the powerful nicotinic effect and carbon monoxide, cyanide, and other detrimental chemicals. Chronic smokers will also develop pulmonary problems such as COPD or emphysema and hypertension which in turn can lead to peripheral vascular disease and cardiac disease. All of these play a part in reducing tissue oxygen levels. Krupsi (26) investigated changes in the microvasculature of skin exposed to cigarette smoke, which include which include chronic reduced blood flow to the skin. When the tissue is traumatized, there is less capability to respond and thus a greater risk of developing a serious wound or infection.

The obvious solution is for the Primary Care Manager to have the patient stop smoking, which is something easier said than done. The patient must be ready and motivated to quit. The PCM needs to discourage the patient from smoking with every visit, regardless of the patient's reason for coming. Once the patient has contemplated stopping, then the PCM can offer various methods alone or in combination that the patient can use in the attempt to stop. This may include nicotine withdrawal programs, vitamin supplements, or antidepressants, behavioral modification, or even hypnosis. Training classes offered by community health programs, military health promotion offices, or service organizations are often beneficial from a group support standpoint. Regression should be expected by the PCM and considered a setback, not a failure, in the patient's attempt to stop. It is important for the PCM to continue supporting the patient's efforts to stop smoking.

ROUTINE PREVENTIVE MEASURES

Other routine measures may be taken by the PCM for monitoring and patient education. For diabetic patients, tight blood glucose control is associated with a decrease in foot ulcers. Patients should be encouraged to bring their blood glucose monitor during their appointment to review the historical measurements since the last visit. A glucose A1c will also give a picture as to how well the patients are controlling their glucose levels over time. Good glycemic control will slow down the development of diabetic complications including neuropathy. Inspection of the feet by the PCM or staff will allow intervention if suspect areas are found. A nylon monofilament test allows a method of early determination for the loss of peripheral sensation and identifies patients at risk for ulceration.

For the venous stasis patient, the main focus of patient education should be on compression, compression, and compression. The use of compression socks or hose will alter the lifestyle of patients. They need to be put on the first thing in the morning, before fixing breakfast or reading the morning newspaper. Otherwise, walking around the home will allow dependent edema to begin and when the compression system is put on, it will already be behind functionally. The patients need to be encouraged to wear the compression even during the summer although they will be uncomfortable in the heat. New materials are being developed that breath easier and the PCM is encouraged to keep abreast of the changes. The patient should try to bathe at night, so the compression system can be taken off, the patient can bathe, and then go to bed with the legs at least level. Elevation, however, needs to be balanced with arterial supply. A transcutaneous oxygen measurement ($TcpO_2$) may demonstrate significant decrease in tissue oxygen levels with leg elevation (usually 30°) due to underlying peripheral vascular disease. Hence, too much elevation may decrease the edema in the leg, but produce overall hypoxic tissue in the lower extremity. Although higher compression (40 mm Hg) support systems have shown the best results in preventing recurrence in venous stasis ulcers, they also have the least compliance due to discomfort and difficulty in donning and doffing the system. The PCM needs to work with the patient to achieve a mutual agreement as to what the patient will wear on a routine basis with the realization that a recurrence can occur and may result in aggressive treatment later.

SUMMARY

Due to the rising cost of treating wounds and patient discomfort, morbidity, and even mortality associated with them, preventing wounds from occurring is a goal for any medical provider to strive for. The proverb, "an ounce of prevention is worth a pound of cure" has never been more apropos.

REFERENCES

1. Hunt TK, Goodson WH. Wound healing in current surgical diagnosis and treatment. Norwalk, Conn: *Lange* 1988; 86-98.
2. Willett WC, Dietz WH, Colditz GA. Guidelines for healthy weight. *N Engl J Med* 1999;341:427.
3. Hu FB. Overweight and obesity in women: health risks and consequences. *Journal of Women's Health* 2003; 12(2): 163-172.
4. Executive Summary of The Third Report of The National Cholesterol Education Program (NCEP) Expert Panel on Detection, Evaluation, and Treatment of High Blood Cholesterol in Adults (Adult Treatment Panel III). *JAMA* 2001; 285:2486.
5. Roberts SB. High-glycemic index foods, hunger, and obesity: Is there a connection? *Nutr Rev* 2000; 58:163.
6. Monchamp T, Frishman WH. Exercise as a treatment modality for congestive heart failure. *Heart Dis* 2002 Mar-Apr; 4(2):110-6
7. NIDDK: Clinical Research: Look AHEAD action in health in diabetes. *http://www.niddk.nih.gov/patient/SHOW/lookahead.htm*
8. Evans W. Exercise, nutrition and aging. *J Nutr* 1992; 122:796-861.
9. Sumpio BE. Foot ulcers. *N Engl J Med* 2000; 343(11):787-92.
10. Birke JA, Fred B, Krieger LA, et al. The effectiveness of an accommodative dressing in off-loading pressure over areas of previous metatarsal head ulceration. *Wounds* 15:33-39, 2003.
11. Panel for the Prediction and Prevention of Pressure Ulcers in Adults. Pressure ulcers in adults, prediction and prevention. Clinical practice guideline, number 3. Rockville MD: US Department of Health and Human Services, 1992.
12. Defloor T. Less frequent turning intervals and yet less pressure ulcers. *Tijdschrift voor Gerontologie en Geriatrie* 2001; 32:174-177.
13. Special Report: Pressure-reducing support surfaces in the prevention and treatment of pressure ulcers: Group 1 Technologies; TEC Assessor, Technology Evaluation Center, Blue Cross and Blue Shield Association, Chicago, Illinois, *Agency for Health Care Policy and Research (AHCPR)* March 1998.
14. Special Report: Pressure-reducing support surfaces in the prevention and treatment of pressure ulcers: Group 2 Technologies; Marymargaret Sharp-Pucci, Ed.D., M.P.H., TEC Assessor, Technology Evaluation Center, Blue Cross and Blue Shield Association, Chicago, Illinois, *Agency for Health Care Policy and Research (AHCPR)* June 1998.
15. Cullum N, Deeks J, Sheldon TA, et al. Summary RR 0.84, 95% CI: 0.57-1.23. Beds, mattresses and cushions for pressure sore prevention and treatment. *In: The Cochrane Library*, Issue 4, 2000. Oxford: Update Software.
16. Buamgarten M, Margois D, Berlin J, et al. Risk factors for pressure ulcers among elderly hip fracture patients, *Wound Repair Regen* 2003; 11(2):96-103.
17. Donnelly J. Hospital-acquired heel ulcers: A common but neglected problem. *J Wound Care* 2001;10(4):131-4
18. Dennis Wauters A. Nutrition and hydration. In: PJ Sheffield, CE Fife, APS Smith, (eds.) *Wound Care Practice.* Flagstaff, AZ: Best Publishing Company, 2004, pp 471-502.
19. Declair V. The usefulness of topical application of essential fatty acids (EFA) to prevent pressure ulcers. *Ostomy Wound Manage* 1997 Jun; 43(5):48-52, 54 ISSN: 0889-5899
20. Burke KE. Few vitamins effectively prevent or reverse skin damage. New York, Medscape Wire, Feb 28, 2002. *www.medscape.com/viewarticle/429171.*
21. McDermott JH. Antioxidant Nutrients: Curent dietary recommendations and research update. *J Am Pharm Assoc* 2000; 40(6):785-799.

22. Simmons SF, Alessi C, Schnelle JF. An intervention to increase fluid intake in nursing home residents: prompting and preference compliance. *J Am Geriatr So* 2001; 49:926-933.

23. Demling RH, and DeSanti L. Protein-energy malnutrition, and the nonhealing cutaneous wound Updated May 22, 2002, Medscape Portals, Inc.

24. Demling RH, DeSanti L. Topical doxepin significantly decreases itching and erythema in the healed burn wound. *Wounds* 14(9): 334-339, 2002. © 2002 Health Management Publications, Inc.

25. Poore S, Cameron J, Cherry G. Venous leg ulcer recurrence: prevention and healing, *J Wound Care* Vol 11 No 5 May 2002.

26. Krupsi WC. The peripheral vascular consequences of smoking. *Ann Vasc Surg* 1991; 5:291-304.

REVIEW QUESTIONS

1.) Which of the following statements about the Primary Care Manager (PCM) is FALSE?
   a. The PCM is crucial to preventing wound recurrence.
   b. The PCM sees the patient on a routine basis.
   c. The PCM is always a wound care specialist.
   d. Ideally, the PCM actively treats all of the patient's problems, but should be considered the maestro in orchestrating the patient's need for specialty care.
   e. The PCM needs to oversee the patient's overall care and be aware of the treatments prescribed by the various specialists.

2.) All of the following are important medical areas the primary care manager needs to address in the prevention of wounds except:
   a. Weight control
   b. Offloading
   c. Nutrition
   d. Antibiotics
   e. Smoking

3.) Pressure point areas that are at risk of forming wounds can be caused by:
   a. Walking on the plantar surface
   b. Poor footwear on the side of the foot
   c. Pathological deformities such as Charcot's foot or hammertoes
   d. Compression dressing for venous stasis ulcers
   e. Any of the above

4.) An overweight adult is defined as one with a Body Mass Index between:
   a. 15 and 19.5
   b. 20 and 24.9
   c. 25 and 29.9
   d. 30 and 34.9

5.) For the prevention of pressure ulcers, the AHRQ recommends:
   a. 30–35 calories per kg of ideal weight per day
   b. 1.25–1.5 grams of protein per kg per day.
   c. Both a and b
   d. Neither a or b

Answers: 1c, 2d, 3e, 4c, 5c

NOTES

Section 4
Pain, Infection, & Adjunctive Therapies

CHAPTER 27

NUTRITION AND HYDRATION

CHAPTER TWENTY-SEVEN OVERVIEW

Nutrition and Hydration

Aimee Dennis-Wauters

INTRODUCTION

Wound healing remains a challenge for medical professionals in both inpatient and outpatient settings. While provision of appropriate nutrition has long been recognized for its importance in preventing and healing wounds, it continues to be a predicament. Unintentional weight loss and protein-energy malnutrition are the most frequently observed nutritional deficits that lead to the development of chronic or non-healing wounds. However, one must not overlook potential deficiencies of micronutrients or trace minerals.

Malnutrition is a complex process involving much more than a decline in nutritional intake. Diseases, injuries, and other factors can dramatically effect the regulation of metabolism, resulting in an internal imbalance that sets the stage for the development of malnutrition and the development of or difficulty of healing a wound. We will examine populations at risk for wound development as well as protein-energy malnutrition, factors contributing to the development of malnutrition, its resultant risk for the development of wounds, macro and micronutrients to be considered for optimum healing, and the effects of appropriate hydration.

MALNUTRITION

Protein-Energy Malnutrition (PEM)

Protein-energy of malnutrition represents a wide variety of metabolic issues—energy and protein deficiency occurring simultaneously, in addition to probable micronutrient deficiency. Increased total protein turnover in conjunction with protein deficiency can result in metabolic crises and rapid loss of lean body mass. Decreased calorie intake, combined with increased calorie needs due to metabolic stress can further contribute to unintentional weight loss.

Protein-energy malnutrition develops slowly. This is largely due to adaptive mechanisms of metabolism that occur during prolonged fasting and starvation. Many individuals develop PEM because they are metabolically starving, not literally starving. While they may be eating regularly, needs may not be met as a result of concomitant hypermetabolism and catabolism. It is in the context of metabolism that the word starvation will be used.

During early starvation, gluconeogenesis will be the primary source of energy. Glucagon, cortisol, and catecholamine levels will be increased and insulin and other anabolic hormones such as growth hormone will be decreased. Muscle will begin to breakdown, releasing amino acids to drive gluconeogenic processes. Amino acids enter the citric acid cycle (Krebs or TCA) and are converted into acetyl-CoA. Acetyl-CoA is then converted into pyruvate to drive gluconeogenesis. The amino acids luecine and lysine are strictly ketogenic and therefore will not be used for glucose formation, but will be converted into ketone bodies. The ketone bodies acetone, acetoacetate, and β-hydroxybutyrate are used by the brain, heart, and skeletal muscle as an energy source in order to spare glucose for other tissues. As a result of protein catabolism, urinary nitrogen losses will increase.

As starvation progresses, protein will need to be conserved for essential functions, such as the formation of antibodies, enzymes, and hemoglobin, as well as wound healing. Gluconeogenic processes will decline, and lipolysis will begin. Free fatty acids will be converted into acetyl-CoA in the liver, contributing to the formation of ketone bodies. As long as there are fat stores available to drive the production of ketone bodies, protein will continue to be spared. When fat stores are depleted, protein stores will become the primary source of energy. If starvation is not ended, body protein will be rapidly depleted, resulting in multiple organ failure and ultimately death.

As described above, during starvation lean body mass (LBM) will decline. Various complications are associated with the amount of lean body mass lost. If approximately 10% of LBM is lost, immune function will be impaired, resulting in increased risk of infection. At this point, free fatty acids have become the primary energy source, allowing spared protein to be allocated to wound healing. A loss of more than 15% LBM further increases the risk for infection and slows the rate of wound healing. A loss of 25% LBM results in extreme weakness, further risk of infection, and a lack of healing. As loss of LBM progresses, spared protein is less available for wound healing as restoring LBM becomes the priority. Additionally, when malnutrition becomes this severe there is also a risk that new wounds will form as a result of collagen losses and a thinning of the skin.

Protein-energy malnutrition is not always the result of poor dietary intake. Often there will be a condition or acute illness that hastens the development of PEM. In the case of a wound, often PEM is caused by infection of the wound site. Presence of a chronic disease such as diabetes, cardiovascular disease, or COPD increases risk for the development of PEM. In such cases, it will be necessary to treat the precipitating cause of malnutrition in addition to treating the PEM.

Populations Nutritionally at Risk for Wound Complication

The elderly

While all people are at risk for the development of a wound, there are certain subsets of the population particularly at risk for a non-healing wound. One such group is the elderly. Many of those living in long-term care facilities develop pressure ulcers. It has been reported that 3–5% of hospitalized elderly and as many as 45% of elderly in long-term care facilities will develop pressure ulcers. Coincidentally, a separate study confirmed that 4% of community-dwelling elderly, 50% of acute-care hospitalized elderly, and 30–40% of elderly in long-term care facilities suffer from protein-energy malnutrition.

Changes in body composition increase the risk among the elderly for wound development. As humans age, it has long been observed that there is a decline in lean body mass, and an increase in percentage of total body fat. A redistribution of body fat is also noted. It seems that in the elderly, presence of internal body fat increases while the presence of subcutaneous body fat decreases. At the same time, elasticity of the skin declines and the skin becomes thinner. This loss of muscle, combined with decreased subcutaneous fat cushioning and changes in the skin increase the risk for skin tears and subsequent wound development.

Observed commonly among, but not limited to the elderly are the issues of dentition and dysphagia. Aging can cause a decline in dental health and can result in the loss of teeth. If teeth are lost or a source of pain when eating or chewing, dietary intake will most likely decrease, increasing patient risk for the development of malnutrition. Protein intake should be a foremost consideration in these patients. Meats are the primary source for dietary protein. However, meats are among the more difficult foods to chew, and therefore, one of the first foods patients tend to avoid.

A common solution to endentulism in patients is the provision of dentures. However, if they do not fit properly or are found to be uncomfortable, poor compliance is likely and will result in similar risk for malnutrition. Dysphagia will produce a similar result. The inability to swallow will result in a number of problems, from a decline in fluid intake leading to dehydration to a total decline in calorie intake, resulting in the development of some degree of malnutrition.

Macro and microvascular disease

The presence of vascular disease will play a significant role in effecting the rate of healing in a wound. While having a disease such as diabetes, cardiovascular disease, or chronic obstructive pulmonary disease may not predispose one to wound development, vascular diseases can significantly delay wound healing due to consequential endothelial dysfunction. Endothelial dysfunction results in the inability of oxygen, macronutrients (carbohydrate, protein, fat), and micronutrients (vitamins, minerals, trace elements) to effectively penetrate the endothelial layer. The result is inadequate oxygen and nutrient supply to the wound site, causing delayed healing and increased risk for infection. Other risk factors for endothelial dysfunction include hypertension, hypercholesterolemia, obesity, and smoking.

The three major categories of macrovascular disease are coronary artery disease, cerebral vascular disease, and peripheral vascular disease. Diabetes mellitus is highly associated with all three of these, and numerous studies of diabetic populations confirm the benefits of dietary changes in decreasing macrovascular disease risk. The Diabetes Control and Complications Trial (DCCT) found that participants undergoing intensive blood glucose control, including dietary restriction, were at significantly lower risk for the development of hyperchloesterolemia, thereby decreasing risk for all macrovascular diseases. The United Kingdom Prospective Diabetes Study (UKPDS) found that a reduction in blood pressure would reduce risk for development of macrovascular complication such as stroke, and microvascular complications such as retinopathy. In a study of elderly Framingham subjects, weight reduction, glucose, lipid, and blood pressure control, as well as smoking cessation were found to decrease risk of macrovascular disease. All except the latter of these have dietary implications both in the prevention and treatment of wounds.

Feeding Problems

Functional loss

While the complications associated with chronic disease are largely uncontrollable for patients and healthcare providers, there are a number of factors contributing to poor nutritional status that can be controlled. Among these are functional losses of the patient, such as inability to self-feed or prepare meals. Inability to self-feed is a commonly observed problem following a cerebrovascular accident. Loss of motor skills will impair one's ability to self-feed. Simply picking up a fork or spoon and bringing it to the mouth become monumental tasks. Often, it will require great energy, patience, and concentration on behalf of the patient, resulting in frustration and a feeling of helplessness. This may result in a refusal to eat. More commonly, the result is inadequate food intake, and the consequential development of malnutrition. Appropriate physical and occupational therapies are necessary to prevent depression and help the patient regain basic skills and self-confidence.

The inability to prepare meals can be manifested in a variety of ways. For the individual with a lower extremity ulcer, such as a diabetic, standing to prepare meals becomes an almost impossible task. This person may not even be able to walk to the kitchen and find foods to prepare. It is common among the elderly, especially widowers that live alone, to not have the ability to prepare meals. The person may not know how to cook, or simply does not see the purpose in cooking a meal for just one person. Assistance from a home health care provider or public program that provides meals to the ill or elderly can help decrease the occurrence of malnutrition in these situations.

Psychosocial issues become a dominant consideration in these situations. Lack of access to food due to financial hardship or lack of transportation to purchase groceries can be of concern. Assessment of mental status should not be overlooked, as depression often results in nutrient deficiency. In most cultures, eating is very often a social activity. Those who live alone or who are disabled due to a disease or accident may not see the "joy" in eating a meal for the purpose of survival. Inadequate intake in such situations is not uncommon. Assistance from family, church, or community organizations is often available to provide assistance with transportation or financial issues. Counseling is helpful not only in the presence of depression, but for many patients as it provides the patient an outlet to communicate regularly with another person.

Dietary restrictions

Patients who are unable to eat solid foods or have difficulty with self-feeding are frequently placed on special diets, such as pureed foods or liquid diets. Pureed food diets have a very low acceptance rate. The texture is unpleasing and often makes the adult feel helpless as pureed foods can be likened to baby foods. Additionally, the taste can be rather unpleasant. Many would rather go hungry than eat pureed foods. Such diets should be ordered only as a last resort when all other nutritional possibilities have been exhausted.

Other dietary restrictions can also result in poor intake. It is not uncommon to observe a patient in either an acute care or long-term care environment with multiple dietary restrictions, such as "low fat, low cholesterol," "low sodium," or even "bland." To many, these diets are just that—bland. They lack the taste and flavor to which the patient may be accustomed. While the clinician means well, such restrictions can compromise nutritional status. If intake of an individual declines so dramatically that it places the person at risk for or causes malnutrition, dietary restrictions should be reconsidered. It would be preferential to have a patient eat some "inappropriate" foods than to develop malnutrition. Remember, foods are only nutritious if they are eaten.

Assessment of Nutritional Status

There are various parameters to consider in the assessment of nutritional status. As different deficiencies manifest in different ways over differing amounts of time, diagnosis of nutritional deficiency is not always straightforward. When assessing nutritional status, it is always helpful to remember the ABC's of nutrition assessment (Table 1). All of these factors should be considered so as to determine the type and degree of nutrient deficiency and level of malnutrition.

TABLE 1. ABC'S OF NUTRITION ASSESSMENT

Anthropometrics	Height, Weight, Skinfold thickness, Circumference measurements (i.e., waist-to-hip ratio, mid-upper arm)
Biochemical Indices	Albumin, pre-albumin, transferrin, total lymphocyte count, glucose, minerals (Na, K, P, Ca, Mg), BUN, creatinine, WBC count, hemoglobin, hematocrit
Clinical Signs	Skin: pale, dry/scaly, facial swelling Hair: thinning, lack of shine, change of texture Eyes: sunken, Bitot's spots, scleral yellowing, xerosis (corneal and conjunctival), redness of eyelids Mouth: angular cheilosis, color of tongue, atrophy or hypertrophy of filiform papillae, missing teeth, dental caries, bleeding gums
Dietary Intake	Calorie counts, plate waste assessment, food-frequency questionnaire, intake recall

Anthropometrics

Anthropometry involves measurement of the human body in various fashions, such as height, weight, or arm circumferences. In a state of illness, a decline in body weight can often be attributed to a decline in nutritional status. Measurements of circumference in various areas of the body can provide a great deal of information on nutritional status, such as presence and amount of muscle wasting and decline in subcutaneous fat. Or conversely, the amount of muscle generated and subcutaneous fat deposited. However, this information is most useful if baseline data have been obtained. Additionally, if measurements are not repeated with the same equipment or performed by the same person, results may not be as useful for comparison.

Biochemical indices of nutrition deficiency

Biochemical indices are perhaps the best early indicator of changing nutritional status, particularly when considering those particles for which the half-life is short. For example, a nutritional deficit of protein will appear in a pre-albumin screening earlier than in an examination of albumin, and both of these exams will detect a potential problem before physical signs of wasting are apparent. Hydration status is an important factor to consider when blood is being inspected. Dehydration will increase the concentration of particles in the blood, which can lead to a "false high" in a laboratory test. Similarly, urine concentration will increase and yield irrelevant results.

Clinical signs

Clinical signs of deficiency are physical symptoms of deficiency. In many instances, presentation of a clinical sign yields an easy diagnosis. One could not easily attribute the magenta tongue of riboflavin deficiency or the deteriorating scurvy gums of vitamin C deficiency to another cause. Other deficiencies, such as protein wasting, are not so easily elucidated. Physical changes, such as dry eyes, can also occur out of sight of the clinician, so it is important to thoroughly question the patient about physical changes he or she may be experiencing.

Dietary intake and nutrition deficiency

Interviewing the patient and assessing intake from day-to-day can best obtain changes in dietary intake. A food frequency questionnaire (FFQ) is convenient as the individual can answer questions at his own pace and does not require the presence of a clinician. A FFQ can reveal a variety of details—avoidance of or aversion to certain foods, likes or dislikes of specific foods, and changes in intake, such as a decrease in meat intake because of recent difficulty chewing. It has been confirmed that such methods can provide reasonable accuracy, especially when an interview with the patient is conducted. Assessing plate waste provides us with a reasonable estimate of calories and amounts of nutrients consumed. In an outpatient setting, a food diary kept by the patient or a 24-hour recall will perform a similar function. While some research shows these methods to be inaccurate, numerous studies have concluded to the contrary.

THE MACRONUTRIENTS

Macronutrients are those nutrients needed by the human body in the greatest quantities. They are carbohydrate, protein, fat or lipid, and water. All are necessary for human function and survival, and deletion of any of these nutrients over time will lead to malnutrition of varying degree.

Determining Energy Requirements

The macronutrients, particularly carbohydrate and fat, are the energy source for the human body. In states of severe stress, protein too can be utilized as a form of energy. A wound imparts metabolic stress. In the presence of stress, energy requirements are greater, not only due to ongoing catabolism, but to fight infection as well as heal the wound.

Needs can be directly measured or calculated. Measurements are best obtained through indirect calorimetry. This can be expensive and results are not easily obtained. Calculation however, allows for a quick estimation of needs and despite controversy, has been proven to be effective. Most calculations are aimed at determining the basal metabolic rate (BMR).

The basal metabolic rate is predicted using one of a series of equations, and accounts for the amount of energy needed to maintain vital functions when one is completely at rest and fasting. A popular formula for determining the BMR is the Harris-Benedict equation (Table 2). It considers the height, weight, and age of an individual, multiplied by a series of constants. Different equations exist for males and females. Once the BMR is calculated, it can then be multiplied by any one of a number of stress factors (Table 3), in addition to an activity factor (Table 4) to estimate the amount of energy being consumed in a 24-hour period. In a healthy individual, a stress factor of 1.0 is used. A sample calculation of calorie needs is at Figure 1.

The efficacy of predictive equations such as the Harris-Benedict equation in assessing needs of individuals of low or high body weight has been questioned. Arguments state that predictive equations will overestimate needs in obese populations and underestimate needs in underweight populations. Recent studies have found the Harris-Benedict equation to be an effective tool in these cases.

A study of critically ill obese individuals compared estimated needs to those measured using indirect calorimetry. The Harris-Benedict equation was

TABLE 2. HARRIS—BENEDICT EQUATION

Females:
BMR (kcal) = 655 + (9.6 x wt in kg) + (1.8 x ht in cm) – (4.7 x age in yr)
BMR (kJ) = 2741 + (40 x wt in kg) + (7.7 x ht in cm) – (28.4 x age in yr)
Males:
BMR (kcal) = 66 + (13.7 x wt in kg) + (5 x ht in cm) – (6.8 x age in yr)
BMR (kJ) = 278 + (57.5 x wt in kg) + (7.7 x ht in cm) – (19.6 x age in yr)

TABLE 3. STRESS FACTORS

Maintenance	1.0
Infection:	
Minor	1.2
Moderate	1.4
Severe	1.6
Burns:	
40% BSA	1.5
100% BSA	2.0
Surgery:	
Minor	1.1
Major	1.2
Trauma	1.5
Fracture	1.3

Bedridden 75-year-old female with infected pressure sore, weight: 105 lbs.; height: 61in	
	105 ÷ 2.2 = 47.7 kg; 61 x 2.54 = 154.9 cm
BMR (kcal)	= 655 + (9.6 x wt in kg) + (1.8 x ht in cm) – (4.7 x age in yr)
	= 655 + (9.6 x 47.7) + (1.8 x 154.9) – (4.7 x 75)
	= 655 + 457.9 + 278.8 – 352.5
	= 1039 Calories
BMR x activity factor x stress factor	
	= 1039 x 1.0 x 1.4 = 1455 Calories
This woman requires 1455 Calories/day to maintain weight and heal the wound.	

Figure 1. Sample calculation of calorie needs.

found to overestimate needs when actual body weight was used, however, it reasonably predicted needs when an adjusted body weight was considered. Another study of critically ill patients found the Harris-Benedict equation multiplied by an appropriate stress factor to be accurate for determining needs in short-term nutrition support situations.

Energy needs can also be calculated using empirical formulas. It has been established that in a healthy individual, the BMR will be approximately 25 Calories per kilogram (kcal/kg). As many as 30–35 kcal/kg should be allotted to the stressed patient. A study of severely underweight patients (mean weight was 40.9 ± 5.1 kg) compared measurements of indirect calorimetry to the empirical measurement. While 25 kcal/kg was found to underestimate needs, 30–32 kcal/kg was suggested based on data provided by indirect calorimetry. As indirect calorimetry is not commonly available to the clinician, predictive equations can provide a reasonable estimate of calories required for maintenance and healing.

Assessment of the body mass index (BMI) can also provide information about nutritional status. The BMI is calculated by dividing weight in kilograms by height in meters^2. BMI is usually considered in determining degree of obesity. However,

TABLE 4. ACTIVITY FACTORS

Sedentary: Bedridden, no activity Ambulatory, no exercise	 1.0 1.2
Light Activity: Light exercise/sports 1–3 x week	 1.3
Moderate Activity: Moderate exercise/sports 3–5 x week	 1.5
High Activity: Hard exercise/sports 6–7 x week	 1.7
Extreme Activity: Strenuous exercise/sports daily, physical labor, twice daily training	 1.9

A 65-year-old male with non-healing wound,
weight: 110 lbs.; height: 65 in.

$120 \div 2.2 = 50$ kg $\rightarrow 65 \times 2.54 = 165.1$ cm

$165.1 \div 100 = 1.65$ m

$(1.65\text{m})^2 = 2.73\ \text{m}^2$

$50\ \text{kg} \div 2.73\ \text{m}^2 = 18.3$

Body mass index is 18.3, indicating mild nutritional deficiency.

Figure 2. Calculating the BMI.

TABLE 5. CLASSIFICATION OF NUTRITIONAL STATUS USING THE BMI

Normal	≥18.5
Mild Deficiency	17.0–18.4
Moderate Deficiency	16.0–16.9
Severe Deficiency	<16.0

it can also be used to determine severity of malnutrition. As body weight decreases, so will the BMI, just as it increases in the presence of obesity. BMI is simple to use, as it does not take into consideration age, sex, or body frame size. Table 5 details categories of the BMI and Figure 2 shows how to calculate a BMI.

Protein

Protein serves the human body a variety of ways. It is essential for the building and maintenance of muscle tissue, as well as the internal organs, hair, nails, blood, and more pertinent to wounds, skin. Protein is required for the development of collagen, a primary structural component within the cell. It is a necessary precursor to and/or component of many hormones, enzymes, and antibodies. If necessary, it can serve as a source of energy.

Proteins are composed of differing combinations of amino acids. While over 300 amino acids are known to exist in nature, 22 of these have been identified as necessary for growth and development of the human. They are assigned into one of two categories: essential and non-essential. In general terms, these descriptors can be misleading, as all of these are required for human health. Nutritionally, these designations are accurate. The essential amino acids are termed as such because they are only available to humans through dietary consumption. They cannot be synthesized endogenously. The non-essential amino acids can be endogenously synthesized from the essential amino acids as well as from products and intermediates of transamination and deamination. Therefore, they are not nutritionally essential. Some non-essential amino acids can be considered "conditionally essential" or "semi-essential." For example, in children and during phases of rapid tissue repair, histadine becomes essential. Arginine is also sometimes needed in greater quantities than can be endogenously produced. While the non-essential amino

TABLE 6. ESSENTIAL AND NON-ESSENTIAL AMINO ACIDS

Essential Amino Acids		Non-Essential Amino Acids	
Isoleucine	Phenylalanine	Alanine	Glutamine
Leucine	Threonine	Arginine*	Glycine
Lysine	Tryptophan	Asparagine	Histadine*
Methionine	Valine	Aspartate	Proline
		Cysteine	Serine
		Glutamate	Tyrosine

* Indicates conditionally essential amino acids.

acids can be endogenously produced, often times this process is dependant on the presence of essential amino acids. The essential and non-essential amino acids are listed in Table 6.

Functions of protein

While proteins serve numerous functions within the human body, here we will limit our discussion to protein function in terms of wound healing. Plasma proteins can be placed into one of three categories: fibrinogen, albumin, and globulins. Fibrinogen is required for clot formation at the wound site, and albumin is a necessary transport protein. Antibodies are protein immunoglobulins that are vital in the prevention of infection of the wound site. Additionally, protein is the precursor to enzymes throughout the body.

Albumin is the major transport protein within the bloodstream. It is synthesized in the liver and signifies about 25% of total hepatic protein synthesis. Albumin constitutes approximately 60% of all serum protein, 40% of it is found in the plasma and about 60% of it is found in the extracellular space. It binds and transports various nutrients, such as copper, zinc, and calcium, in addition to free fatty acids, some steroid hormones, the amino acid tryptophan, and bilirubin. Albumin has a significant pharmacological function as the transport protein for a variety of drugs such as penicillin and aspirin.

Fibrinogen is also a plasma protein and will be converted by thrombin into fibrin in the presence of calcium ions. Fibrin is one of the first proteins to arrive at the site of the wound to induce blood clotting. The staggered pattern of fibrin at the wound forms a fibrin mesh, allowing red blood cells, platelets, and other factors to aggregate at the site and form a blood clot. While protein intake will impact the amount of fibrinogen available to aid wound healing, vitamin K is necessary for the conversion of prothrombin to thrombin.

Perhaps one of the most important protein products in the healing of a wound is collagen. Collagen is found in the extracellular matrix of tissues and represents approximately 25–30% of mammalian protein. While 19 different types of collagen have been identified in humans, some of these are found only in small amounts. Type I collagen is the more predominant form, comprising about 80% of total collagen in skin, the other 20% being type III. All types of collagen are indispensable in influencing the physical properties of tissue.

Collagen is present in all phases of wound healing—the inflammatory phase, epithelialization (or re-epithelialization), and fibroplasia. Immediately following development of a wound, the inflammatory response is initiated. Fibroblasts will be attracted to the wound by cytokines, and will begin to produce collagen. In this process, oxygen is used by the amino acids proline and lysine to synthesize the collagen chain. Angiogenesis will occur, and fibroblasts will continue to proliferate at the wound site. Collagen will continue to be synthesized during the process of epithelialization, and during fibroplasia, the final phase of wound healing, collagen will be the primary component of scar tissue.

The amount of collagen synthesized is dependant on the availability of nutrients and oxygen. Nutrients required for protein synthesis include vitamin A, vitamin C, amino acids, particularly proline and lysine, iron, copper, and zinc. If there is poor perfusion, as occurs when there is endothelial dysfunction, availability of these nutrients, even when the diet is adequate, will be compromised.

Biochemical indicators of protein status

In the initial phases of protein-energy malnutrition hepatic albumin synthesis will begin to decline. Within only a few days, albumin stores will shift from extravascular to intravascular spaces in an attempt to maintain serum albumin levels. Additionally, the adaptive mechanisms of starvation will contribute to the stability of serum albumin by slowing the rate of albumin breakdown. Albumin levels will not decline significantly until severe protein depletion occurs and adaptive mechanisms can no longer continue. As malnutrition progresses, albumin levels will further decline. Table 7 illustrates the severity of protein deficiency based on albumin status.

TABLE 7. SERUM ALBUMIN LEVELS

Normal	3.5–5.0 g/dL
Mild Deficiency	2.8–3.4 g/dL
Moderate Deficiency	2.1–2.7 g/dL
Severe Deficiency	< 2.1 g/dL

While serum albumin levels provide accurate information regarding protein status, it has a half-life of 15–20 days. Considering that albumin levels do not decline in the initial phases of protein-energy malnutrition, and its rather long half-life, albumin is not always the best indicator of nutritional status. An individual may be experiencing protein-energy malnutrition, but until the deficiency becomes somewhat advanced a serum albumin level will not provide the clinician with much data regarding protein status.

Examination of a transferrin level however, will provide more accurate information. Transferrin has a half-life of only 8–10 days. This allows the clinician to diagnose and treat the malnutrition at a much earlier stage than with an albumin level. Examination of transferrin levels will also provide information about iron status. As it is an iron transport protein, if serum levels of transferrin decline, so will serum levels of iron. Total lymphocyte count (TLC) will decrease in protein-energy malnutrition; therefore it too can be used as an indicator of protein status in

TABLE 8. PARAMETERS OF TRANSFERRIN AND TOTAL LYMPHOCYTE COUNT

	Transferrin	Total Lymphocyte Count
Normal	> 200 mg/dL	> 2000 per µL
Mild Deficiency	150–200 mg/dL	1200–2000 per µL
Moderate Deficiency	100–149 mg/dL	800–1199 per µL
Severe Deficiency	< 100 mg/dL	< 800 per µL

addition to providing information regarding immune response. As TLC declines, protein deficiency becomes more severe. At the same time, immune response will decline, meaning that in addition to impaired wound healing as a result of protein deficiency, the risk of infection is also increased. Table 8 details the severity of protein deficiency based on transferrin and total lymphocyte count.

Examination of a pre-albumin level would allow for an even quicker diagnosis of protein-energy malnutrition. With a half-life of only two days, a pre-albumin will provide the clinician with "up to the minute" information about protein status. A pre-albumin level is therefore the preferred biochemical indicator of protein status. For indicators of pre-albumin status see Smith's 'Pre-albumin Rule of Fives' in the chapter entitled, "Etiology of the Problem Wound." For in-depth discussion of biochemistry of wound healing, see the chapter by Chin and associates entitled, "Biochemistry of Wound Healing in Wound Care Practice."

Biochemical parameters such as albumin, transferrin, and pre-albumin are not only indicators of protein status in terms of assessing degree of malnutrition, but may also be useful in determining potential delays in the rate of healing. Numerous studies have been conducted to assess if biochemical indices related to nutrition can be used to determine potential delays in the rate of wound healing. In a study of the composition of wound fluid, protein and albumin levels were found to be higher in exudates collected from healing wounds versus non-healing wounds. Similar results were found in a study of patients undergoing knee disarticulation and the rate of healing with the use of a flap. Of seven patients that experienced major dehiscence of the wound, six were found to have serum albumin levels of less than 30 mmol/L.

Other studies have found that while albumin may not correlate with delayed healing, other biochemical parameters may be worth examining. In a study of delayed wound healing after total hip arthroplasty, the researchers concluded that only pre-operative transferrin levels were of value in predicting development of delayed healing. Still another study concluded that only a pre-operative total lymphocyte count would be useful in determining delays in healing. According to this study, complications are three times more likely to occur if the lymphocyte count is less than 1500 cells/mm^3.

Combinations of parameters have also been found to be of use in determining the potential for problems with healing. A study examining the relationship between nutritional status and wound complication concluded that serum albumin and transferrin levels are useful in predicting the potential development of a complication. Patients with serum albumin levels of

Individual weighing 150 lbs. with non-healing foot ulcer, requiring 1.5 g of protein per kg body weight:

1. Convert pounds into kilograms
   150 lbs ÷ 2.2 = 68.2 kg
2. Multiply kilograms body weight by protein requirement to obtain protein needs
   68.2 kg x 1.5 g = 102.3 g protein required per day to meet needs
3. Convert to Protein Servings
   7 g protein = 1 oz of meat
   →102.3 g ÷ 7 = 14.6 or 15 oz protein needed per day

Figure 3. Determining protein requirements.

greater than 3.0 g/dL and/or transferrin levels of greater than 150 mg/dL were less likely to suffer complicated wound healing. While research is contradictory as to which parameters, if any, are most useful in predicting the potential for delayed wound healing, it is reasonable to assume that a normal biochemical profile will be more favorable in terms of the rate of healing.

Determining protein requirements

As previously stated, in the presence of a wound, it is appropriate to provide 30 kcal/kg to meet increased energy needs. Protein provides four calories per gram of protein consumed. A healthy individual requires only 0.6 g of protein/kg of body weight to maintain muscle mass, build new muscle tissue, and contribute to other protein-dependant structures. The average American consumes between 0.8–1.0 g of protein per day, more than the necessary amount. In a catabolic state, such as that of a wound, protein needs will be increased. Protein is now not only required to maintain essential functions, but also to replace protein lost in catabolic processes as well as to heal the wound. When treating a wound 1.5 g of protein/kg of body weight is recommended. Figure 3 illustrates how to determine protein requirements.

Dietary sources of protein

The most significant dietary source of protein is meat. Meat is not just beef, but is a term that can be used to categorize beef, chicken, fish, pork, cheeses, and eggs. Leaner meats are lower in calories than higher fat meats. Keeping in mind that calorie needs are increased in the presence of a wound, the idea of feeding higher fat meats in order to provide more calories per protein serving is appealing. However, higher fat meats are higher in calories because of their high fat content. These fat calories will come primarily from saturated fats, which increase the risk for the development of heart disease. Feeding extra fat is sometimes necessary to meet increased calorie needs, but it is best to provide these calories in the form of monounsaturated fats (see Dietary Sources of Fat in this chapter). Leaner meats will be the best protein source by virtue of their lower fat content.

Protein quality should also be considered when choosing a protein. A protein is more complete when it contains a variety of amino acids. The most perfect proteins will contain all of the essential amino acids. Protein quality considers the proportion of specific amino acids present in foods versus the proportion of amino acids needed for good nutrition. The closer the

TABLE 9. SOURCES OF DIETARY PROTEIN

Milk: whole, 2%, 1%, skim (skim and 1% are lowest in fat & cholesterol)
Eggs: whole eggs, egg whites, egg substitute (egg yolks are high in cholesterol)
Very Lean & Lean Meats: skinless chicken or turkey; fresh fish or shellfish, fish canned in water; low-fat or fat-free cheeses, cottage cheese; select or choice grades of lean beef, especially loin, flank, or round, ≥ 90% lean ground beef; loin pork chops, Canadian bacon, ≥ 95% lean luncheon/sandwich meats
Legumes: all varieties of beans

Remember: Milk and eggs are the standards against which all other proteins are graded.

proportion of amino acids in a food to the standard, the higher the protein will be in quality. Such proteins are said to have a high biological value, meaning they will provide more nutrition and be more available in metabolic processes. Egg and milk are high quality proteins and are the standard against which all other proteins are compared. Meats are considered to be high quality protein. Plant sources of protein will be of varying quality. Many plant sources of protein will be rich in some amino acids, but lacking others. For example, beans contain a variety of amino acids but often lack methionine, and corn, while high in some amino acids, is deficient in tryptophan. In a normal varied diet, the deficiencies of essential amino acids in some foods are made up for in other foods. When the diet is lacking in reference proteins such as milk, a greater amount of protein must be consumed in order to meet amino acid needs. In a healthy individual this usually does not pose a problem. However, in a patient with malnutrition for whom intake may be low, this can be difficult to achieve. Supplements can be used if needed, and will be discussed shortly. Table 9 contains a list of sources of dietary proteins.

Carbohydrate

Carbohydrate is the macronutrient responsible for the provision of energy. The majority of dietary carbohydrate consists of polysaccharides, such as starch, cellulose, and glycogen. Disaccharides, such as lactose and sucrose are also consumed in the diet. The endpoint of carbohydrate digestion is conversion of saccharide chains into the monosaccharides, galactose, fructose, and glucose. Virtually all dietary carbohydrate is eventually converted into glucose to provide energy to numerous tissues or to be stored as glycogen.

During digestion, starch breakdown begins in the mouth with salivary amylase. This process continues until salivary amylase is inactivated by the low pH of HCl in the stomach. In the small intestine, pancreatic amylase will further digest starches into maltose. The microvilli of the wall of the small intestine secrete the disaccharidases lactase, maltase, and sucrase into the microvillar spaces and break disaccharides into monosaccharides. Glucose and galactose are then absorbed by active transport while fructose is absorbed by facilitated diffusion. Glucose, fructose, and galactose are absorbed into the bloodstream via the portal vein. Most galactose and fructose that enters the liver will be converted into glucose.

Functions of carbohydrate

The primary function of carbohydrate is to provide energy in the form of glucose to tissues where it can be utilized to drive cellular processes, thereby sparing body protein. Nearly all carbohydrate is converted into glucose to be used as an energy source. Glucose is the preferred energy source of the brain, heart, and skeletal muscle.

In the fed state, the pancreas will release insulin into the bloodstream in the presence of glucose. Insulin will stimulate cellular uptake of glucose via glucose transporters. GLUT-1 is not dependant on insulin and is primarily responsible for glucose uptake in the brain. GLUT-4 is an insulin dependant transporter responsible for the transport of glucose to the heart, skeletal muscle, and adipose tissue. Glucose then enters glycolysis and the citric acid cycle to drive the generation of ATP. Excess glucose will be converted into glycogen in the liver. As serum glucose levels decline, so will insulin levels. Conversely, as insulin declines glucagon levels will rise and gluconeogenesis may be initiated in the liver. In a healthy individual, these counter-regulatory hormones work to keep blood glucose levels stable. Diabetes Mellitus is the hallmark example of what happens when this regulation disappears.

The high blood sugars that result from diabetes can be attributed to any number of causes that will not be discussed here. What will be discussed is hyperglycemia in type 1 diabetes. The hyperglycemia of type 1 diabetes sets off a chain of events not dissimilar to what takes place in starvation. Despite the availability of glucose in the blood, a lack of or inability to use insulin will prevent its uptake by the tissues. Gluconeogenesis will begin, further raising glucose levels. Meanwhile, tissues such as skeletal muscle are still in need of an energy source, and when glucose is unavailable, protein will become the primary source of energy until ketone bodies are available so that body protein can be spared. In type 1 diabetes the result will be diabetic ketoacidosis. In a non-diabetic, over time, the result is protein-energy malnutrition.

It is well documented that hyperglycemia will impair wound healing. While proper medical treatment and medication are critical to the treatment of diabetes, dietary changes are equally important. Since the primary source of glucose is carbohydrate foods, by eating the appropriate foods in the appropriate amounts, better glycemic control can be achieved. The Diabetes Control and Complications Trial (DCCT) found that intensive treatment resulted in better glycemic control, and diet was one of the components of intensive treatment. The United Kingdom Prospective Study (UKPDS) found that complications of type 2 diabetes would be reduced if glucose control were obtained. Dietary interventions were also a strategy in this study. The earlier in the disease course that control was obtained, the lower the risk for complications. The UKPDS showed that in early stages of type 2 diabetes, diet alone would be enough to achieve appropriate glycemic control. Many individuals with non-healing diabetic wounds can improve glycemic control by making simple diet changes with the help of a registered dietitian. See the chapter by Reasner entitled, "Glycemic Control in the Patient with Diabetes."

Determining carbohydrate requirements

Carbohydrate, like protein, provides four calories per gram of carbohydrate consumed. Recommendations of the American Dietetic Association, the American Diabetes Association, and the American Heart

In Figure 1, using the BMR multiplied by activity and stress factors, it was estimated that 1455 Calories are needed per day.

1. Determine 50–60% of Calories to come from carbohydrate

   1455 x .5 = 727.5, 1455 x .6 = 873

   → 728–873 kcal should come from carbohydrate

2. Determine grams of carbohydrate needed

   728 ÷ 4 = 182, 873 ÷ 4 = 218

   → 182–218 g of carbohydrate are needed per day

3. Convert to carbohydrate servings

   15 g carbohydrate = 1 carbohydrate serving

   → 182 ÷ 15 = 12, 218 ÷ 15 = 14.5

So, 12–15 carbohydrate servings are needed per day.

Figure 4. Determining carbohydrate requirements.

Association currently state that 50–60% of calories consumed should come from carbohydrate, preferably high fiber carbohydrate. Carbohydrate calorie needs can easily be calculated once total energy needs have been determined as previously discussed. Carbohydrate needs are determined in Figure 4.

In type 2 diabetes, hyperglycemia is frequently accompanied by obesity and insulin resistance. While it is reasonable to assume that eating less carbohydrate (40% of calories versus 50–60%) will result in better blood sugar control, there lacks evidence in the form of a large, controlled trial to support such recommendations. However, small studies have found lower carbohydrate diets to be beneficial in diabetic populations. One study compared the benefits of a low-carbohydrate versus a low-fat diet in obesity. Carbohydrate consumption in the low-carbohydrate consumption group averaged around 40% of calories at both baseline and after six months. The low-fat group consumed approximately 50% of calories from carbohydrate at both baseline and after six months. The investigators found that the low-carbohydrate diet group had improved triglyceride levels and improved insulin sensitivity after adjusting for weight loss. With interest in low-carbohydrate diets ever growing, it is likely that more research will be conducted in the near future evaluating the efficacy of lower carbohydrate diets.

Dietary sources of carbohydrate

Starch foods are the primary source of carbohydrate. Starch is a general name for a group of foods that includes, but is not limited to bread, rice, beans, pasta, cereal, potatoes, corn, and peas. Fruits of all types and fruit juices are carbohydrates, as are milk and yogurt. Natural sugars such as sugar,

TABLE 10. CARBOHYDRATE CHOICES

Starch	Fruit	Milk
1/2 c of one of the following: • potatoes, corn, peas • pasta, rice, beans • hot cereals one slice of bread	one small piece, such as: apple, orange, peach, pear, plum, apricot one large piece, such as: grapefruit, mango, banana	1 cup 1% or skim milk 1 cup light yogurt

brown sugar, honey, syrup, and molasses are also carbohydrates, as are foods made with these sugars, such as candies, cookies, cakes, and pies. Table 10 provides examples of the carbohydrate choices and appropriate portion sizes.

As with proteins, not all carbohydrates are created equal. While all carbohydrates are sources of glucose, some carbohydrates are also sources of fiber. What has long been called "roughage," fiber is found exclusively in plant-based foods and is the portion of the plant that cannot be digested by non-microbial enzymes in the digestive tract. It is categorized as a carbohydrate, but does not breakdown into glucose. Therefore, it will not raise blood glucose levels.

There are two types of dietary fiber: soluble and insoluble. Each type of fiber functions differently. Soluble fiber can be partially broken down by bacterial enzymes in the large intestine while insoluble fiber cannot. It has long been accepted that fiber can prevent or relieve constipation. Fiber has also been shown to help decrease the risk for colon and intestinal cancers. The exact mechanism for this has not been identified, but hypotheses include increased bulk of the stool to dilute potentially cancerous substances in the feces, increased transit time in the gut resulting in decreased exposure to carcinogens, and changes in the metabolism of bile acids and increases of possibly beneficial products of bacterial fermentation.

Until recently, other benefits of fiber have been largely unknown. Consumption of high fiber diet can result in improved lipid levels, improvements in blood pressure, better glycemic control, and improved appetite control. However, for a long time it has been unclear if these benefits are the result of consumption of fiber itself or simply the result of the lower-fat, more nutritious diet that fiber imparts. This is still thought to be the reason fiber helps prevent coronary heart disease. In the case of cholesterol, while studies have shown that certain types of fiber do help improve lipid levels, these changes are usually modest. Blood glucose improvements are also modest; fiber consumption does not need to be greater in diabetics than in the rest of the population. The bulk that fiber creates in the stomach produces a feeling of fullness, helping control appetite and increase satiety. Therefore, it is not clear if substances in fiber are responsible for producing weight loss or if it is merely the result of bulkiness in the gut. It is also important to note that in order for fiber to be effective, fluid must also be consumed regularly. Otherwise, high fiber with little fluid actually causes constipation or even bowel obstruction.

TABLE 11. FIBER FOODS

Whole Grains	Legume	Vegtables	Fresh Fruit
oatmeal/oat bran bran flakes brown rice whole wheat bread whole wheat pasta	beans such as: kidney, lentil, pinto, black-eyed peas, grean peas potatoes, sweat potatoes, corn	spinach & greens broccoli carrots cauliflower green beans	apples (with peels) oranges pears (with peels) grapes prunes

Note: Fruits and vegetables have more fiber if eaten with their peels.

The Dietary Guidelines for Americans recommend a daily intake of 20–35 grams of fiber per day. Aerage intake for an American adult is about half of that amount. The highest fiber foods available in the diet are whole grains, vegetables, fresh fruits, and legumes. Table 11 provides a list of examples of foods that contain fiber.

Fat

Fats or lipids in the diet provide the body with an energy source in addition to carbohydrates. Most dietary fats are in the form of glycerides, or acylglycerols. 95–98% of fats consumed are in the form of triglyceride. Ingested triglyceride will travel through the stomach to the duodenum where glyceride digestion really begins. As fat enters the duodenum, this signals the release of cholecystokinin. Cholecystokinin causes contraction of the gallbladder, forcing bile into the duodenum. The phospholipids and bile acids present in bile will emulsify fats into droplets in a water medium. After emulsification, pancreatic lipase then enters the duodenum and cleaves fatty acids in positions 1 and 3 from the triglyceride backbone. This yields a monoglyceride and two free fatty acids. Fatty acids less than ten carbons in length (short chain fatty acids) are absorbed directly into the portal vein. Many of these free fatty acids are synthesized into triglyceride in the liver to be used by tissues for energy. The brain and red bloods cells will not accept this form of lipid as an energy source.

Free fatty acids containing ten or more carbon molecules (medium and long chain fatty acids) will form micelles, and intestinal cells will take up the micelle contents. Once in the intestinal cell, micelle contents are re-packaged into triglycerides. These triglycerides will form chylomicrons. Chylomicrons carrying dietary triglycerides and cholesterol leave the intestinal cells through the lymph system and enter into circulation via the thorasic duct.

Chylomicrons carry dietary triglyceride through the bloodstream, and very low-density lipoproteins (VLDL) carry triglyceride synthesized in the liver. Lipoprotein lipase (LPL) will hydrolyze these molecules in the capillaries. The triglyceride products are then absorbed by muscle to be utilized as an energy source. The destination of the newly freed fatty acids is determined largely by the rate constant (Km) of lipoprotein lipase in different tissues. The Km of LPL in the heart is relatively low. The Km of LPL in adipose tissue is ten times that of the heart. Km will be influenced by the counter-regulatory hormones. Glucose and insulin are positive effectors of LPL in adipose and negative effectors of LPL in heart and skeletal muscle. Conversely, glucagon is a positive effector on adipose tissue, and a negative effector of heart and skeletal muscle. Trigylcerides are only stored in adipose tissue as a last resort when other tissues cannot use them as an energy source.

Functions of fat

The primary function of fat is as an energy source for body tissues, primarily the heart and skeletal muscle. This is best demonstrated in dire situations such as protein-energy malnutrition. Fat also acts as an energy storage reserve in the form of triglyceride in adipose tissue. Fat serves to cushion the organs and provides padding between the skin and bones. It is also vital to the structure and permeability of cell membranes. Without dietary fats, fat-soluble substances such as the fat-soluble vitamins would not be able to be absorbed into cells.

Fat is the most concentrated source of calories available in the diet. Fats provide nine calories per gram of fat consumed as opposed to only four calories per gram in carbohydrates and protein, more than double the amount of energy. Because of their energy density, fats are an efficient way to provide calories in small quantities of food. In protein-energy malnutrition or other forms of starvation, it would seem reasonable to increase dietary fat intake to meet calorie needs. However, excess consumption of fat is not without disadvantages.

Recently much attention has been given to both omega fatty acids and medium chain triglycerides as a therapy for reducing lipid levels, particularly cholesterol. Consumption of a diet high in omega-3 and omega-6 fatty acids will improve the lipid profile. These fats have also been investigated for other benefits, such as in wound healing. One study examined the effects of structured lipid emulsions (medium and long chain triglycerides) on protein sparing. It was found that rats receiving a chemically structured lipid formula had greater nitrogen balance and higher serum albumin levels than rats receiving a physically structured mixture of triglycerides, indicating that chemically mixed triglycerides could be beneficial to injured patients. A more recent study found similar results, concluding that omega-3 fatty acids in combination with a protein and vitamin rich diet would improve nitrogen balance in hypermetabolic patients suffering from thermal injury. Numerous other studies have found that omega fatty acids, particularly omega-3, improve immunity after injury. Additional studies point to the anti-inflammatory effects of omega-3 fatty acids that may improve the rate of wound healing. Despite studies like these, there is also literature reporting that no benefit is observed when omega-3 fatty acid is supplemented. However, it is more widely accepted that these fatty acids improve immunity and the anti-inflammatory response, indicating that they can be beneficial to wound healing. Caution must be exercised in supplementation of fats as overfeeding of fat can lead to increased lipid levels, increased adiposity, and fatty liver. Indeed, if fats are over-consumed, regardless of the source, the result will likely be impaired wound healing due to improper immune response resulting in increased susceptibility to infection.

Determining fat requirements

As previously stated, fats provide nine calories per gram, making them the most calorie dense macronutrient. According to the guidelines of the National

In Figure 1, using the BMR multiplied by activity and stress factors, it was estimated that 1455 Calories are needed per day.

1. Determine 25–35% of Calories to come from fat

    1455 x .25 = 364, 1455 x .35 = 509

    → 364–509 kcal should come from fat

2. Determine grams of fat needed

    364 ÷ 9 = 40.4, 509 ÷ 9 = 56.6

    → 40–57 g of fat are needed per day

Providing 50 grams of fat per day will assure that needs are met.

Figure 5. Determining fat requirements.

TABLE 12. RECOMMENDED FAT INTAKE FOR THE TLC DIET

Nutrient	Recommendation
Total fat	25–35% of total daily calories
Saturated fat	> 7% of total daily calories
Polyunsaturated fat	≤ 10% of total daily calories
Monounsaturated fat	≤ 20% of total daily calories

(NCEP ATP III)

Cholesterol Education Program (NCEP) Adult Treatment Panel III (ATP III) fats should provide 25–35% of calories for those on the diet for therapeutic lifestyle changes (TLC) designed to lower LDL levels. The newest NCEP guidelines correlate with the 2000 Dietary Guidelines for Americans. Once total daily needs have been calculated, requirements for fat can be determined as seen in Figure 5.

The NCEP ATP III guidelines for fat intake are listed in Table 12. The same dietary guidelines can be applied to the individual with a non-healing wound.

Dietary sources of fat

Fat usually enters the diet in one of three forms-—monounsaturated fat, polyunsaturated fat, or saturated fat. Saturated fat has long been associated with increased risk of cardiovascular complications such as atherosclerosis and arteriosclerosis. Consumption of a diet high in saturated fat will lead to increased serum cholesterol and LDL levels. Monounsaturated fats have been documented to be beneficial on lipid levels. Particular attention has been focused on omega fatty acids in this area. Consumption of monounsaturated fats in place of saturated fats will lead to improvements in cholesterol and LDL levels, thereby reducing cardiovascular risk. Polyunsaturated fats will improve LDL levels but are also associated with a decline in HDL levels. They should be consumed in moderation. Table 13 details dietary sources of the different fats.

TABLE 13. SOURCES OF DIETARY FAT

Monounsaturated Fats	Polyunsaturated Fats	Saturated Fats
• Oils such as: canola, olive, peanut • Nuts such as: peanuts, pecans, cashews • Natural peanut butter • avocadoes	• vegetable oils such as: soybean, corn, sunflower, safflower oils • mayonnaise • tub margarines • salad dressings	• butter & stick margarine • lard shortening • fried foods • high fat meats such as: hot dogs, sausages, bacon, bologna, salami

Since fats are very dense in calories, it takes only a very small serving to provide a good deal of calories. One fat serving will provide five grams of fat and 45 calories. Table 14 lists examples of fat serving sizes. As other foods in the diet such as meats and milk will contain fat, it is important to monitor use of added fats so as not to exceed recommendations.

TABLE 14. FAT CHOICES

1 teaspoon of:	cooking oil, margarine, mayonnaise
1 tablespoon of:	salad dressing, nuts, peanut butter, low-fat mayonnaise or low-fat margarine
2 tablespoons of:	avocado, low-fat salad dressing

Supplementation of macronutrients

In an individual suffering from protein-energy malnutrition or with increased nutrient needs, it is often difficult to meet needs using foods alone. Often the quantities of food required to meet needs are more than an individual can or is willing to consume, especially if appetite is poor or feeding problems are present. In the presence of diarrhea or emesis, excess intake will worsen the condition. In such cases, dietary supplements are helpful in meeting needs.

There are a variety of supplements available for providing extra nutrition to individuals with non-healing wounds. These supplements include powders, ready-to-drink liquids, and enteral products. There are so many in fact, that choosing a product can become overwhelming. Always try to choose a product most suited to your patients' needs at the lowest possible cost. More importantly, choose a product that the patient is willing to take. Remember, foods are only nutritious if they are eaten, and the patient will be far more likely to accept the supplement if his/her opinion is given consideration when the product is selected. If choosing a supplement is confusing or if you are not quite sure what to do, consult with a registered dietitian. Nutritional supplements are constantly changing, and the dietitian will be the best source for current information. Additionally, the dietitian is often the best-suited person to interview the patient for his concerns, review his nutritional needs, and choose the supplement.

In an acute or long-term care setting, use the facility formulary as a guideline when choosing a supplement. Selecting a product from the formulary helps to assure product availability. This also helps to reduce potential costs for the patient. In an ambulatory setting, determine what sort of supplementation the individual is agreeable to, and just as in acute-care settings, be sure it is a product the patient can purchase easily and at a minimum cost. It is always best to consider an oral supplement as opposed to an enteral or parenteral product. If self-feeding is possible, it is always the best option, if not, choose an enteral product. Many of the ready-to-drink formulas are available for purchase in regular grocery stores and pharmacies at substantially lower cost than some of the "designer" supplements. Parenteral nutrition should be considered a final option, and used for as few days as possible. If the gut works, use it.

Protein supplements are often needed in wound care due to protein-energy malnutrition and catabolism. There are a number of "high protein" ready-to-drink products available; some even have increased amounts of fiber or calories. These products too are easily purchased at grocery stores and pharmacies. There are isotonic and elemental formulas with increased amounts of protein for enteral use and even products specifically for hypermetabolic patients. Another alternative for protein supplementation is protein powder. These products can usually be mixed into hot beverages or foods. They do not alter food taste and are virtually undetectable in foods when used correctly. Powders are very helpful in diabetic patients needing more protein. There are currently no ready-to-drink, high protein supplements available for diabetics. A simple solution is to provide a ready-to-drink diabetic supplement with protein powder added to it. One company also makes an amino acid supplement in both powder and liquid forms so that it can be used as needed.

Particular attention has been focused on amino acid supplementation in recent years, especially the use of glutamine and arginine. Glutamine is a non-essential amino acid synthesized in the liver from the nitrogenous waste product ammonia. It plays a critical role in preserving nitrogen balance, protein synthesis, cellular structure, and metabolism. Various components of glutamine are used to drive cellular reactions. For example, glutamine donates an amide group that can be used in the synthesis of asparagine, glucosamine, and NAD+. Another function of glutamine is as a source of energy for cellular respiration. Because glutamine can be utilized in so many processes, in catabolic states skeletal muscle stores of glutamine may be rapidly utilized, resulting in decreased protein synthesis. However, supplementation will result in sparing of muscle proteins and increased muscle protein synthesis. One study in rats concluded that protein synthesis correlated with glutamine concentration in the muscles. A study conducted on amino acid supplementation and collagen deposition found that collagen synthesis was enhanced in healthy elderly volunteers supplemented with a formula that included glutamine. Therefore, benefits of glutamine supplementation may be even greater in a stressed individual.

Arginine is also a non-essential amino acid that is involved in protein synthesis and serves as an intermediate in the urea cycle. One of the products of arginine metabolism is nitric oxide, which is necessary for collagen accumulation and angiogenesis. Arginine is a substrate for proline synthesis, so it is indirectly involved in collagen synthesis. Arginine is also known to enhance immunity, although the mechanism by which this occurs is unknown. In the same study of glutamine supplementation carried out in healthy, elderly volunteers, arginine supplementation proved to be equally as beneficial as glutamine. Another study found that arginine supplementation in breast cancer patients stimulated lymphocyte and killer cell activity. It is reasonable to conclude that supplementation with glutamine and arginine could decrease the risk of developing malnutrition and enhance wound healing.

There are some products available to increase dietary fat intake. As discussed previously, research has shown that excessive fat intake can delay wound healing. However, in severe malnutrition, extra calories may be beneficial. Increasing fat intake not only provides more fat but also more calories. Remember that fats contain more than double the calories per gram of carbohydrate or protein. Most fat in supplements is in the form of medium-chain triglyceride (MCT). These smaller triglyceride chains are more easily digested and have become the popular choice for supplementation. There is an MCT product available for use as a beverage or enterally. MCT is also available as a liquid or oil that can be added to other supplements. Another available product is a lipid supplement of polyunsaturated fats, the goal of which is to provide linoleic acid, an omega-3 fatty acid, to assist wound healing. As discussed, increased intake of omega-3 fats in place of other fats can improve immunity.

Most products will contain about one calorie per milliliter of product. For individuals with increased calorie needs, there are also products containing 1.5 or 2 calories per milliliter. Some of the ready-to-drink products are called "Plus." The "plus" in such products is added calories. The extra calories in these sorts of products are almost exclusively provided in the form of carbohydrate. Powdered carbohydrate supplements are also available and can be added to hot foods and beverages, much like the powdered protein supplements. Whatever type of supplement is needed, be sure to research available products and consult with the patient for the best outcome.

THE MICRONUTRIENTS

Micronutrients are those nutrients that are needed in small amounts. They include the fat-soluble vitamins D, E, A, and K, and the water-soluble vitamins C and the B family. While these nutrients may be needed only in small quantities, they are essential to human health. Each nutrient is responsible for performing different functions that contribute to metabolism and maintenance.

Water-Soluble Vitamins

The water-soluble vitamins are vitamin C (also known as ascorbic acid) and the entire B family. The B vitamins include thiamin (B1), riboflavin (B2), pyridoxine (B6), folic acid (B9), cyanocobalamin (B12), niacin, pantothenic acid, and biotin. Water-soluble vitamins must be obtained from the diet and excessive quantities are usually excreted in the urine. Because of this, toxicities of the water-soluble vitamins are rare. For the same reason, deficiencies can develop rather quickly.

The B vitamins

Most of the B vitamins function as cofactors in enzymatic reactions, making them critical to regulation of metabolism. There have been no reported benefits of B vitamins specific to wound healing. Table 15 lists the B vitamins and their various physiological functions.

Vitamin C

Vitamin C, also known as ascorbic acid, serves a variety of functions, a number of which are critical to the wound healing process. Vitamin C stimulates the inflammatory response and improves resistance to infection by increasing white blood cell activity. Additionally, vitamin C drives collagen synthesis, and stimulates the formation of scar tissue. As stated in the amino acids discussion, collagen synthesis is dependant on the hydroxylation of proline and lysine. Ascorbic acid is necessary in this process. As collagen is needed in all phases of wound healing, vitamin C deficiency can create a significant delay in the healing process.

Scurvy is the well-documented deficiency disease of vitamin C. It can appear after about 60 days, but as late as 3–4 months after deficiency is initiated. Scurvy is characterized by bleeding, receding gums, loose teeth, swollen joints, blotches on the skin, and muscle weakness. Another known deficiency symptom is

TABLE 15. THE B VITAMINS

Thiamin (vitamin B1)	• Activated in brain by thiamin diphosphotransferase • Coenzyme thiamin diphosphate transfers activated aldehydes - Oxidative decarboxylation of α-ketoacids (example: α-ketogluterate →succinyl CoA) - Transketolase reactions (example: pentose phosphate pathway) • Deficiency disease is Beriberi- causes peripheral neuropathy, weakness, anorexia, edema, cardiac, neurological, muscular degeneration • Dietary Sources: grains, wheat germ, pork, liver, fortified cereal, enriched rice
Riboflavin (vitamin B2)	• Active forms are flavin mononucleotide (FMN) & flavin adenine dinucleotide (FAD) • Coenzyme of flavoprotein enzymes - Glycerol-3-phosphate dehydrogenase (in glycolysis) - Succinate dehydrogenase (citric acid cycle) - Acyl-CoA dehydrogenase (b oxidation of fats) - Dihydrolipoyl dehydrogenase (oxidative decarboxylation of pyruvate→acetyl CoA) - Oxidation of NADH in mitochondrial respiratory chain • Generalized deficiency symptoms include: magenta tongue, glossitis, cheilosis, angular stomatitis, edema • Dietary Sources: milk, liver, kidney, meats
Pyridoxine (vitamin B6)	• Coenzyme in amino acid metabolism - Transamination, decarboxylation, threonine aldolase activity - Glycogenolysis (glycogen→glucose-1-phosphate) - Conversion of tryptophan→niacin - Heme formation • Deficiency is rare; symptoms include: seborrheic dermatitis, cheilosis, stomatitis, glossitis • Dietary Sources: meat, wheat, corn, yeast, pork, liver
Folic Acid (vitamin B9)	• Active form is tetrahydrofolate • Carries activated single carbon units • Coenzyme in formation of heme, nucleic acids • Deficiency is megaloblastic anemia • Supplement with 400 mg daily if deficient and for women of child-bearing age to prevent neural tube defects • Dietary Sources: fortified cereals, orange juice
Cyanocobalamin (vitamin B12)	• Coenzyme in various reactions: - Deoxyadenosylcobalamin (methymalonyl CoA→Succinyl CoA) - Methylcobalamin (homocysteine→methionine) (methyltetrahydrofolate→tetrahydrofolate) • Absorption requires intrinsic factor • Deficiency is anemia: 1. Pernicious anemia- macrocytic, megaloblastic anemia due to lack of intrinsic factor 2. Megaloblastic anemia-characterized by large, immature red blood cells in the bone marrow 3. Lack of Methylcobalamin causes -"Folate Trap" (inability to convert methyltetrahydrofolate) - Methionine deficiency (inability to convert homocyteine), homocyteinuria • Dietary Sources: animal proteins such as meat, liver, milk
Niacin	• Active forms are nicotinamide adenine dinucleotide (NAD+), nicotinamide adenine dinucleotide phosphate (NADP+) • NAD+, NADP+ are coenzymes in oxidoreductase reactions - Converts pyruvate→acetyl CoA - Various reactions of citric acid cycle • Deficiency disease is Pellegra- characterized by diarrhea, dermatitis, delerium, death • Toxicity causes flushing of skin due to histamine release, excess can cause liver damage • Dietary sources: protein rich foods- meat, milk; enriched breads, cereals, pastas
Pantothenic Acid	• Active forms are coenzyme A (CoA), acyl carrier protein (ACP) • No known deficiency in humans • Dietary sources: most all foods- grains, legumes, animal protein products (meat, milk)
Biotin	• Coenzyme of carboxylase reactions • Synthesis or oxidation of fatty acids • Deamination & removal of NH2 from amino acids • Deficiency is rare, consumption of raw eggs can cause deficiency- avidin protein binds biotin (avidin denaturated by cooking egg whites) • Dietary Sources: most foods, especially egg yolk, soybeans, yeast

impaired wound healing. Impaired healing associated with vitamin C deficiency is well documented. Provision of adequate vitamin C to deficient individuals will improve healing, but it is unlikely that supplementation in the absence of deficiency will increase the rate of healing. However, one study concluded that provision of calcium ascorbate supplemented with vitamin C resulted in increased formation of mineralized nodules and collagenous proteins in vitro, indicating that supplementation may be beneficial.

Iron absorption is enhanced by vitamin C. Therefore, iron deficiency can develop secondary to vitamin C deficiency. Vitamin C is also involved in the degradation of tyrosine and the resultant synthesis of epinephrine, and bile acid formation. Vitamin C also functions as an antioxidant, reducing oxidized tocopherol in cell membranes and inhibiting the formation of nitrosamines (see Vitamin E). Due to its antioxidant properties, supplementation of vitamin C might be considered by the clinician for wound healing. However, due to its water-solubility, excessive amounts will be excreted in the urine, and little evidence exists to support supplementation of vitamin C in wound therapy.

While toxicity is rare, chronic excessive intake of vitamin C may contribute to the development of nephrolithiasis. Vitamin C is metabolized into oxalate, which along with calcium can cause kidney stones. Good dietary sources include oranges, strawberries, spinach, and broccoli.

Table 16 lists the recommended dietary allowances for the water-soluable vitamins.

TABLE 16. RECOMMENDED DIETARY ALLOWANCES FOR WATER-SOLUBLE VITAMINS

	Recommended Dietary Allowances*		
	Males	Females	Pregnancy
Thiamin (B1)	1.2 mg/d	1.1 mg/d	1.4 mg/d
Riboflavin (B2)	1.3 mg/d	1.1 mg/d	1.4 mg/d
Pyridoxine (B6)†	1.3 mg/d	1.3 mg/d	1.9 mg/d
Folic Acid (B9)	400 μg/d	400 μg/d	600 μg/d
Cyanocobalamin (B12)	2.4 μg/d	2.4 μg/d	2.6 μg/d
Niacin	16 mg/d	14 mg/d	18 mg/d
Pantothenic Acid	5 mg/d	5 mg/d	6 mg/d
Biotin	30 μg/d	30 μg/d	30 μg/d
Vitamin C	90 mg/d	75 mg/d	85 mg/d

* Recommended Dietary Allowances listed are for ages 19–70+ in both sexes.
† Values listed are for ages 19–50 in both sexes. In age 50+, the RDA for males is 1.7 mg/d and 1.5 mg/d for females.

Fat-Soluble Vitamins

The fat-soluble vitamins include D, E, A, and K. They cannot be synthesized by the body, and therefore must be obtained through the diet. Once they have been ingested, the fat-soluble vitamins can be stored in adipose tissue. As a result of this, deficiency diseases of the fat-soluble vitamins are rare, but do exist. Deficiencies are most likely to effect individuals lacking adequate fat stores, such as is observed in protein-energy malnutrition or other conditions of starvation. Recommended Dietary Allowances can be found in Table 17.

TABLE 17. RECOMMENDED DIETARY ALLOWANCES FOR FAT-SOLUBLE VITAMINS

	Recommended Dietary Allowances*		
	Males	Females	Pregnancy
Vitamin D†	5 μg/d	5 μg/d	5 μg/d
Vitamin E	15 mg/d	15 mg/d	15 mg/d
Vitamin K	120 μg/d	90 μg/d	90 μg/d
Vitamin A	900 μg/d	700 μg/d	770 μg/d

* Recommended Dietary Allowances listed are for ages 19–70+ in both sexes.

† Values listed are for ages 19–50 and 70+ in both sexes. In age 50–70, the RDA is 10 μg/d for both sexes.

Vitamin D

Vitamin D_3 is formed by sunlight from 7-dehydrocholesterol. Vitamin D_3 is then hydroxylated in the liver into its active form, 25-hydroxyvitamin D_3. For the remainder of this discussion, 25-hydroxyvitamin D_3 will be referred to as vitamin D. Vitamin D has little direct involvement in wound healing, but it is involved in other important functions. Some of its functions, sources, and toxicities are listed here:

- Enhances active transport of calcium across the gut by stimulating calbindin, the calcium binding protein of the brush border
- It is a component of calcitonin, which along with PTH regulates mobilization and deposition of calcium and phosphorous in the bones and teeth
- In the kidney, vitamin D increases renal tubular reabsorption of calcium and phosphorous
- Under hypocalcemic conditions, vitamin D acts to restore plasma calcium by enhancing enteric calcium absorption & renal retention, and mobilizing calcium from the bone
- Dietary sources include egg yolks, fortified milk, and fish liver oils; the best source is sunlight
- Rare deficiency disease is Rickets (in children) or Osteomalacia (in adults)
- Toxicity results in elevated serum calcium and phosphorous levels, leading to calcification of soft tissues

Vitamin E

Vitamin E is also known as tocopherol. The most active form, D-α-tocopherol has the greatest biologic activity and is the most desirable dietary form of vitamin E. The primary function of vitamin E is as an antioxidant. The antioxidant properties of vitamin E make it indirectly important in the wound healing process. Vitamin E maintains cell membrane integrity by preventing peroxidation of polyunsaturated fatty acids contained in the membrane phospholipids. The antioxidant functions of vitamin E are effective at high oxygen concentrations. Vitamin E tends to be found in tissues exposed to the greatest O_2 partial pressure, such as erythrocyte membrane and the retina of the eye. For the same reason, it is reasonable that supplementation of vitamin E would be beneficial in hyperbaric oxygen therapy of wounds. By fighting oxidative damage, vitamin E can also be effective in reducing risk for infection. One report indicates that in the days following wound development, non-enzymatic antioxidants, vitamin E, and glutathione are decreased, and by the 14th day post-wounding, only glutathione levels will completely recover. All substances recover following healing. The non-enzymatic antioxidants studied included superoxide dismutase, glutathione peroxidase, and glutathione-S-transferase. Glutathione peroxidase and superoxide dismutase are both vitamin E derived enzymes. Therefore, supplementation during wound treatment will be beneficial to the healing process. Appropriate vitamin E supplementation is 400 IU per day of vitamin E as D-a-tocopherol. The deficiency disease of vitamin E is hemolytic anemia, and dietary sources include green leafy vegetables and whole grains.

Vitamin K

Vitamin K is found in primarily plant-based foods in the form phylloquinone, or vitamin K1. Vitamin K2, also known as menaquinone-7, is the form of vitamin K synthesized by bacteria in the intestine. Dietary vitamin K is absorbed in the ileum, and vitamin K synthesized by bacteria is absorbed in the colon. Vitamin K is important to wound healing in the time immediately following wounding. Vitamin K is necessary for the formation of the clot factors II, VII, IX, and X. Prothrombin (clot factor II) will combine with the other clot factors to produce thrombin. Thrombin and fibrinogen form fibrin, resulting in a blood clot.

Deficiency of vitamin K is rare due to endogenous bacterial synthesis. However, deficiency can be caused by chronic antibiotic therapy (friendly bacteria are killed), fat malabsorption, and liver disease. Deficiency of vitamin K needs to be treated aggressively and immediately to prevent potentially lethal hemorrhage. Dietary sources include green leafy vegetables, broccoli, and liver.

Vitamin A

Vitamin A or retinal is derived from the provitamin b-carotene and similar structures called carotenoids. Vitamin A is critical to vision. Retinal, a form of vitamin A is a component of the visual pigment rhodopsin, which is essential to photoreception. Retinal participates in glycoprotein synthesis, promoting the growth and differentiation of tissues. Vitamin A contributes to immune function and like vitamin E, has antioxidant properties, particularly at higher partial pressures of O_2. Vitamin A supplementation is beneficial in individuals undergoing glucocorticoid therapy. The anti-inflammatory effects of glucocorticoids impair wound healing, and vitamin A supplementation can lessen these effects. One rat study showed that vitamin A supplementation improved wound healing despite persistent hyperglycemia, indicating potential for supplementation in diabetic patients. Another rat study showed that treatment with polyprenoid, a vitamin A compound, stimulated collagen deposition and neo-vascularization in burn treatment.

Deficiency disease of vitamin A will result in visual disturbances and ultimately blindness. Night-blindness, which develops earlier in deficiency, can be reversed with supplementation. Deficiency of vitamin A is the leading cause of blindness in under-developed countries. This form of blindness is known as xeropthalmia. Xeropthalmia involves atrophy of the periocular glands, hyper keratosis of the conjunctiva, and softening of the cornea, the endpoint of which is irreversible blindness. Strides are being made to correct this problem. One solution is the development of a functional food known as golden rice, a b-carotene enriched rice. Toxicity occurs if the capacity of retinal binding protein for vitamin A is exceeded and cells are exposed to free retinal. This can happen if vitamin A is over-consumed or over-supplemented. Symptoms of toxicity are dry lips, scaling or peeling of the skin, headache, nausea, vomiting, diarrhea, and hair loss.

THE MINERALS AND TRACE ELEMENTS

The minerals include calcium, magnesium, sodium, potassium, phosphorous, and chloride. Minerals are essential for fluid balance and enzymatic activity. Proper balance of all the minerals is indirectly essential to wound healing. The trace elements include minerals needed in small amounts, such as zinc, copper, and iron. Even though only a "trace" of these minerals is present in the human body, that small amount is necessary for proper function and critical to wound healing. As these three trace minerals are all directly involved in the healing process, they will be the focus of discussion. Table 18 lists the recommended dietary allowances for the trace minerals.

TABLE 18. RECOMMENDED DIETARY ALLOWANCES OF TRACE MINERALS

	Recommended Dietary Allowances*		
	Males	Females	Pregnancy
Iron	8 mg/d	18 mg/d†	27 mg/d
Zinc	11 mg/d	8 mg/d	11 mg/d
Copper	900 μg/d	900 μg/d	900 μg/d

* Recommended Dietary Allowances listed are for ages 19–70+ in both sexes.
† Values listed are for females of ages 19–50. In ages 50–70+, the RDA is 8mg/d.

Iron

The primary function of iron is as a constituent of heme enzymes, such as hemoglobin and in cytochromes of the electron transport chain. It is responsible for respiratory transport of oxygen and carbon dioxide. Iron is also necessary for the oxidation of pyruvate. Iron is involved in the wound healing process. Iron is a cofactor in the hydroxylation of proline and lysine during collagen synthesis.

Deficiency of iron results in decreased hemoglobin and hematocrit levels. This will cause a decrease in red blood cell proliferation at the wound site. However, this lack of hemoglobin at the wound site should not impair healing, as long as there is adequate profusion of the wound site. Iron deficiency can also decrease circulating T lymphocytes and natural killer cells, which will impair immunity.

Excessive iron consumption can result in infection. Bacteria require iron for growth and proliferation. Over-consumption will allow for bacterial proliferation. Dietary sources include lean meats, shellfish, dried beans, dried fruits, fortified breads & cereals, and dark green leafy vegetables.

Zinc

Zinc serves a variety of functions in the body. Zinc is involved in the synthesis and degradation of carbohydrate, protein, and fat, as well as DNA & RNA. It supports immunity in that it is necessary for the formation of T lymphocytes. It is a cofactor in approximately 100 enzymes such as lactate dehydrogenase, alkaline phosphatase, and carbonic anhydrase.

Because of its activity as a cofactor and in immune processes, zinc deficiency can result in impaired wound healing. Zinc deficiency leads to decreased epithelialization and fibroblast proliferation at the wound site. Studies have shown that zinc supplementation in zinc deficient individuals results in improved healing. However, routine supplementation of zinc in individuals not suffering from deficiency will not improve the rate of healing.

Deficiency is very common in the elderly, one of the populations at increased risk for the development of malnutrition. One survey concluded that both zinc and copper intake were low in elderly populations and this was associated with age, low income, and lower education level. Deficiency of zinc is usually due to inadequate consumption of zinc containing foods, such as meats and milk. Intake of meats tends to decline with age, often due to functional losses previously discussed. Another side effect of zinc deficiency is altered taste acuity, which in itself will lead to decreased food intake. Zinc deficiency is difficult to diagnose, as there are currently no biochemical markers of zinc deficiency. Serum zinc levels may be inaccurate due to other factors. Some medications will decrease serum zinc levels despite adequate stores, and hypoalbuminemia will also cause low serum readings of zinc, as albumin is the zinc transport protein. If deficiency is suspected, zinc supplementation is indicated in low amounts. The current recommendation is 15–25 mg per day. Toxicity of zinc is very rare.

Copper

The primary function of copper is as a component of enzymes such as cytochrome-C oxidase, superoxide dismutase, and lysl oxidase. While all enzymes are essential, lysl oxidase is of particular interest here as it is the enzyme required for collagen synthesis and formation of collagen cross-linkages. Inadequate copper will impair the formation of collagen, delaying wound healing.

Copper is bound to ceruloplasmin and transported by albumin. Protein deficiency can result in secondary copper deficiency due to lack of transport.

Copper deficiency diseases include hypochromic, microcytic anemia and Menke's disease (a genetic disorder of intestinal malabsorption). Deficiency of copper can also decrease iron absorption, cause demineralization of bone, failure of erythropoeisis, neutrapenia, and leukopenia. Deficiency is observed in populations at risk for malnutrition as discussed above. Copper toxicity is rare but occurs in the genetically inherited disorder Wilson's disease. Dietary sources include meats, legumes (beans, peas, lentils), whole grains, and nuts.

HYDRATION

Provision of adequate water is necessary to maintain skin turgor and prevent tissue breakdown. The consequences of dehydration will all have a negative impact on the wound healing process. Dehydration results in low blood pressure and body temperature, which will affect blood flow and oxygenation to the wound site. Dehydration will result in impaired nutrient transport and absorption, and rapid pulse. Another consequence of dehydration is inaccuracy of biochemical indices. If serum or urinary laboratory parameters are examined during dehydration, values will be erroneously high, or "false highs." In such a case, low levels of nutrients will appear to be normal. This could delay diagnosis of conditions such as hypoalbuminemia and anemia.

There are several recommendations for daily fluid needs. A good guideline is 30 milliliters per kilogram of body weight. One set of guidelines for wound care states that 35 mL should be provided for every kilogram of body weight for individuals ages 18–55, and ≥30mL with a minimum of 1500 mL per day in individuals older than 55, unless renal or cardiac disease does not permit it. These guidelines likely are accounting for fluids lost from the wound itself and through diarrhea, emesis, fever, or increased perspiration. Another guideline states that 1 mL should be provided per calorie consumed, however, this may not always be enough. It is important to examine input/output records if they are available.

Fluids can be provided in forms other than as drinking water. Table 19 lists appropriate fluid choices.

TABLE 19. APPROPRIATE FLUID CHOICES

• Water • Decaffeinated tea (best if without sugar) • Caffeine-free diet sodas • Sugar-free flavored drinks	• Ice chips • Broth • Sugar-free Popsicles

SUMMARY

Here are some key points to remember when assessing nutrition and hydration status in wound care:

- Protein-energy malnutrition can set-in quickly with few initial physical symptoms and will not result in severe weight loss until it is very advanced.
- Keep in mind populations at risk—the elderly, those with macro or microvascular disease or a functional loss—and use the ABC's of Nutrition Assessment to detect risk of malnutrition.
- Protein is found in the body as albumin, fibrinogen, or globulin, all of which are essential to wound healing. Albumin acts primarily as a transport protein, fibrinogen forms the clot allowing collagen synthesis to occur, and globulins produce infection-fighting antibodies.
- Biochemical indices of protein status include albumin, transferrin, total lymphocyte count, and pre-albumin.
- Carbohydrate functions primarily as an energy source. Glucose is the endpoint for virtually all ingested carbohydrate.
- Hyperglycemia delays wound healing, therefore, glycemic control is vital to healing the wound. This will require dietary changes in individuals with diabetes.
- Starches, fruit, and milk are the primary sources of carbohydrate in the diet. It is best to consume higher fiber carbohydrates.
- Fat functions as an additional energy source for the body, serves as insulation and padding under the skin for organs and bones, and contributes to integrity of cell membranes.
- Monounsaturated fats are the best dietary fat choice. Polyunsaturated fats should be consumed in smaller quantities, and saturated fats should be avoided. Servings are very small due to calorie density.
- There are a large variety of supplements available to meet an individual's specific needs. Be sure the patient is agreeable to supplementation and the product selected—this will assure the best compliance of consumption.
- The water-soluble vitamins include vitamin C and the B family. They function in wound care in immunity, inflammatory responses, and collagen synthesis.
- The fat-soluble vitamins include D, E, A, and K. They function in wound healing, in clotting, and have antioxidant properties.
- The trace elements iron, zinc, and copper are only needed in very small amounts by the body, but these elements are critical in the wound healing process.
- Maintaining adequate hydration will assist healing and decrease the risk of developing of additional wounds.

REFERENCES

1. Adler AI, Stratton IM, Neil HA, et al. Association of systolic blood pressure with macrovascular and microvascular complications of type 2 diabetes (UKPDS 36): prospective observational study. *BMJ* Aug 2000; 321: 412-9.
2. Ahmad A, Duerksen DR, Munroe S, et al. An evaluation of resting energy expenditure in hospitalized, severely underweight patients. *Nutrition* May 1999; 15: 384-8.
3. Aida T, Murata J, Asano G, et al. Effects of polyprenoic acid on thermal injury. *Br J Exp Pathol* Jun 1987; 68: 351-8.
4. Ayala A, Chaudry, IH. Dietary n-3 polyunsaturated fatty acid modulation of immune cell function before or after trauma. *Nutrition* Jan 1995; 11: 1-11.
5. Blaylock, B. Pressure ulcers: a review. *Dermatol Nurs* Oct 1990; 2: 278-82.
6. Bowker JH, San Giovanni TP, Pinzur MS. North American experience with knee disarticulation with use of a posterior myofasciocutaneous flap. Healing rate and functional results in seventy-seven patients. *J Bone Surg Am* Nov 2002; 82-A: 1571-4.
7. Constans T, Alix E, Dardaine V. Protein-energy malnutrition. Diagnostic methods and epidemiology. *Presse Med* Dec 2000; 29: 2171-6.
8. Cutts ME, Dowdy RP, Ellersjeck MR, Edes TE. Predicting energy needs in ventilator-dependent critically ill patients: effect of adjusting weight for edema or adiposity. *Am J Clin Nutr* Nov 1997; 66: 1250-6.
9. Demling RH, DiSanti L. Protein-Energy Malnutrition, and the Honhealing Cutaneous Wound. *http://www.medscape.com/viewprogram/714_pnt*
10. Food and Nutrition Information Center. *http://www.nal.usda.gov/fnic/etext/000105.html*
11. Gherini S, Vaughn BK, Lombardi Jr. AV, et al. Delayed wound healing and nutritional deficiencies after total hip arthroplasty. *Clin Orthop* Aug 1993; 293: 188-95.
12. Griffiths A, Russell L, Breslin M, et al. A comparison of two methods of dietary assessment in peritoneal dialysis patients. J Ren Nutr, Jan 1999; 9: 26-31.
13. James TJ, Hughes MA, Cherry GW, et al. Simple biochemical markers to assess chronic wounds. *Wound Repair Regen* Jul 2000; 8: 264-9.
14. Jeschke MG, Herndon DN, Ebener C, et al. Nutritional intervention high in vitamins, protein, amino acids, and omega3 fatty acids improves protein metabolism during the hypermetabolic state after thermal injury. *Arch Surg* Nov 2001; 136: 1301-6.
15. MacDonald A, Hildebrandt L. Comparison of formulaic equations to determine energy expenditure in the critically ill patient. *Nutrition* Mar 2003; 19: 233-9.
16. MacLennan PA, Brown RA, Rennie MJ. A positive relationship between protein synthetic rate and intracellular glutamine concentration in perfused rat skeletal muscle. *FEBS Lett* May 1987; 215: 187-91.
17. Mahan L, Escott-Stump S. Krause's Food, Nutrition, & Diet Therapy, 9th ed. Philadelphia, PA: W.B Saunders Co. 1996.
18. Marin LA, Salido JA, Lopez A, et al. Perioperative nutritional evaluation as a prognostic tool for wound healing. *Acta Orthop Scand* Jan 2002; 73: 2-5.
19. Mead Johnson Nutritionals. The Role of Nutrition in Wound Healing. MJ Publication No. MB 183. Evansville, IN: 2001.
20. Mok KT, Maiz A, Yamazaki K, et al. Structured medium-chain and long-chain triglyceride emulsions are superior to physical mixtures in sparing body protein in the burned rat. *Metabolism* Oct 1984; 33: 910-5.
21. Morgan KJ, Johnson SR, Rizek RL, et al. Collection of food intake data: an evaluation of methods. *J Am Diet Assoc* Jul 1987; 87: 888-96.
22. Murray RK, Granner DK, Mayes PA, et al. Harper's Biochemistry, 25th ed. Appleton & Lange. 2000.

23. Nichols PJ, Porter C, Hammond L, et al. Food intake may be determined by plate waste in a retirement living center. *J Am Diet Assoc* Aug 2002; 102: 1142-4.

24. Park KG, Heys SD, Blessing K, et al. Stimulation of human breast cancers by dietary L-arginine. *Clin Sci (Lond)* Apr 1992; 82: 413-7.

25. Samaha FF, Igbal N, Seshadri P, et al. A low-carbohydrate as compared with a low-fat diet in severe obesity. *N Engl J Med* May 2003; 348: 2074-81.

26. Schroder H, Covas MI, Marrugat J, et al. Use of a three-day estimated food record, a 72-hour recall and a food-frequency questionnaire for dietary assessment in a Mediterranean Spanish population. *Clin Nutr* Oct 2001; 20: 429-37.

27. Shils ME, Olson JA, Shine M, et al. Modern Nutrition in Heath and Disease, 9th ed. Baltimore, MD: Williams & Wilkins. 1999.

28. Shukla A, Rasik AM, Patnaik GK. Depletion of reduced glutathione, ascorbic acid, vitamin E and antioxidant defense enzymes in a healing cutaneous wound. *Free Radic Res* Feb 1997; 26: 93-101.

29. Singh R, Gopalan S, Sibal A. Immunonutrition. *Indian J Pediatr* May 2002; 69: 417- 9.

30. Smith APS. Etiology of the Problem Wound. In PJ Sheffield, CE Fife, APS Smith (eds.). Wound Care Practice. Flagstaff, AZ: Best Publishing Company, 2004: pp 3-48.

31. Tashiro T, Yamamori H, Takagi K, et al. n-3 versus n-6 polyunsaturated fatty acids in critical illness. *Nutrition* Jun 1998; 14: 551-3.

32. Williams JZ, Abumrad N, Barbul A. Effect of a specialized amino acid mixture on human collagen deposition. *Ann Surg* Sep 2002; 236: 369-74; discussion 374-5.

33. Wilson PW, Kannel WB. Obesity, diabetes, and risk of cardiovascular disease in the elderly. *Am J Geriatr Cardiol* Mar 2002; 11: 119-23,125.

REVIEW QUESTIONS

1.) During starvation, the rate of wound healing slows when there is a loss of lean body mass (LBM) of more than:
   a. 5%
   b. 10%
   c. 15%
   d. 25%

2.) The primary reason for protein-energy malnutrition among seniors is:
   a. They tend to avoid eating meat
   b. There is an increase in percentage of total body fat
   c. Internal body fat increases while subcutaneous body fat decreases
   d. There is a decline in fluid intake

3.) Which of the following statements about nutrition is FALSE?
   a. Pureed food diets have a very high acceptance rate
   b. A nutritional deficit of protein will appear in a pre-albumin screening earlier than in an examination of albumin
   c. A vitamin C deficiency can be detected by examining the gums for deteriorating scurvy
   d. Foods are only nutritious if they are eaten

4.) The major transport protein within the bloodstream is:
   a. Albumin
   b. Fibrinogen
   c. Globulin
   d. Thrombin

5.) The preferred biochemical indicator of protein status is:
   a. Albumin level
   b. Transferrin level
   c. Pre-albumin level
   d. Vitamin K level

Answers: 1c, 2a, 3a, 4a, 5c.

CHAPTER 28

Glycemic Control in the Patient with Diabetes

CHAPTER TWENTY-EIGHT OVERVIEW

NOTES

Glycemic Control in the Patient with Diabetes

Charles A. Reasner

INTRODUCTION

Patients with diabetes are at increased risk of developing both microvascular (retinopathy, nephropathy, and neuropathy) and macrovascular complications (heart attacks, stroke, and peripheral vascular disease). Diabetes is the leading cause of blindness, renal disease, and lower extremity amputations in the United States. Heart attacks and stroke occur two to four times more frequently in persons with diabetes than in those without the disease. Macrovascular complications are caused by components of the insulin resistance syndrome commonly seen in diabetics including hypertension, dyslipidemia, obesity, and enhanced clotting. The major risk factor for microvascular complications in the diabetic patient is hyperglycemia. The evidence that tight control of the blood glucose can reduce or prevent microvascular complications is outlined below.

GLYCEMIC CONTROL AND COMPLICATIONS

The Diabetes Control and Complications Trial (DCCT) compared conventional insulin therapy with intensive insulin treatment in patients with type 1 diabetes mellitus. Lowering the hemoglobin A_{1c} (A_{1c}) from 9% in the conventional treatment group to 7% in the intensively treated patients resulted in a 50% reduction in the development or progression of retinopathy, nephropathy or neuropathy. No glycemic threshold for the prevention of long-term microvascular complications was observed in the DCCT. Similarly, intensive insulin verse conventional insulin therapy in Japanese patients with type 2 diabetes resulted in lowering of blood glucose and improvements in retinopathy, nephropathy, and neuropathy comparable to those observed in the DCCT.

The United Kingdom Prospective Diabetes Study (UKPDS) evaluated conventional therapy (mainly diet and exercise) versus intensive therapy with oral antidiabetic agents or insulin in newly diagnosed type 2 diabetic patients. After a dietary run-in period of three months, 3867 patients with newly diagnosed type 2 diabetes were randomly assigned to intensive therapy with a sulfonylurea or insulin (n = 2729) or to conventional diet therapy (n = 1138).

In the intensive group, the aim was to achieve a fasting plasma glucose level less than 6 mmol/L (108 mg/dL). In the sulfonylurea group, patients were switched to insulin therapy or metformin was added if they did not achieve the target blood sugar with sulfonylurea therapy alone. The treatment target in the conventional diet treatment group was a fasting plasma glucose level less than 15 mmol/L (270 mg/dL) without symptoms. If the fasting plasma glucose level exceeded 15 mmol/L (270 mg/dL) or symptoms occurred, patients were randomly assigned to receive therapy with a sulfonylurea or insulin. During the 11 year follow-up period a 1% difference in A_{1c} values was seen between the intensive versus the conventional treatment groups (7.0% verse 8.0%; P = 0.009). This modest difference in blood glucose resulted in a 25% reduction in combined microvascular end points (eye, kidney, and nerve). No difference in macrovascular end points between the two groups was observed. In addition to the main randomization described above, 342 overweight patients were randomly assigned to intensive treatment with metformin and were compared with 411 overweight diabetic patients receiving conventional diet therapy and with 951 overweight diabetic patients receiving intensive therapy with sulfonylureas or insulin. Each of the drug-treated groups of patients achieved similar glycemic control with an A_{1c} value of 0.6 percentage points lower than the conventionally treated patients (7.4% compared with 8.0%; P = 0.002) (Figure 1). There was a 25% reduction in microvascular endpoints seen in drug treated patients. Only patients treated with metformin showed a reduction in macrovascular complications with a 36% reduction (P = 0.021) for death from any cause, a 42% reduction in diabetes-related death (P = 0.11), a 39% lower risk (P = 0.010) for myocardial infarction, and a 41% lower risk (P = 0.032) for stroke compared with patients who received conventional treatment. The risk reduction for any diabetes-related end point (P = 0.003) and death from any cause (P = 0.021) in the metformin group was significantly greater than that in the group assigned to intensive therapy with insulin or sulfonylureas (Figure 2).

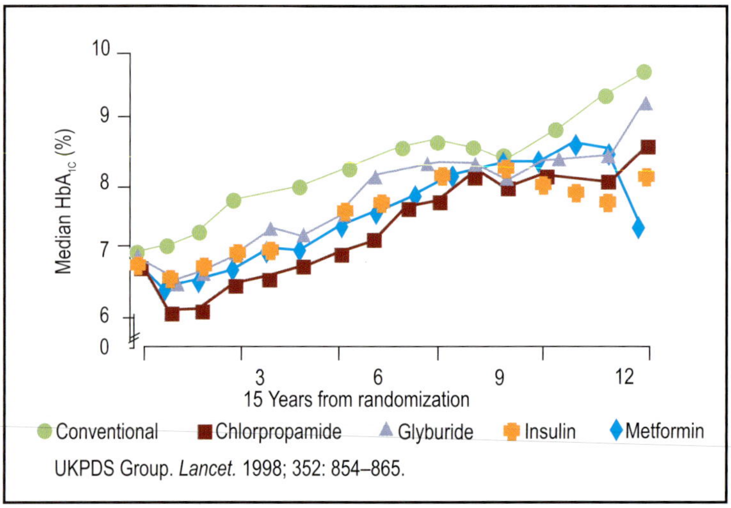

Figure 1. UKPDS: Effects of treatment on HbA_{1C}.

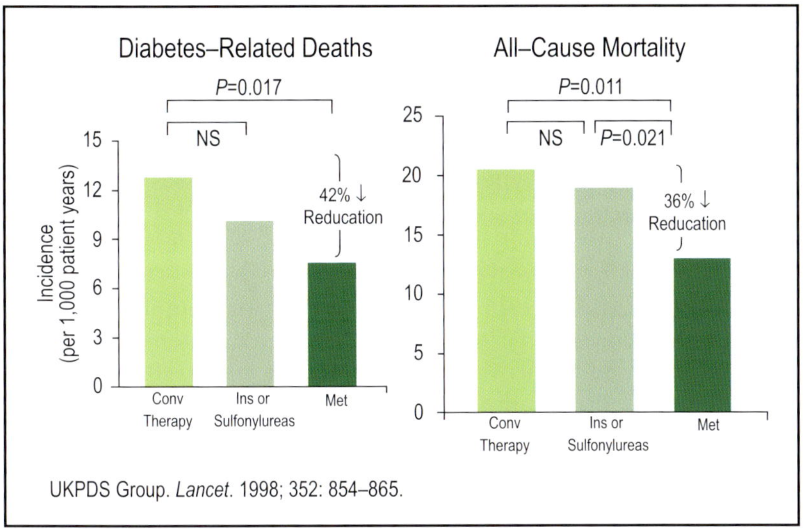

Figure 2. Metformin improves survival in type 2 diabetes.

The UKPDS showed that type 2 diabetes mellitus is a progressive disorder (Figure 1). After an initial and similar decrease in the HbA_{1c} value with metformin, sulfonylureas, or insulin, the rate of increase in HbA_{1c} value was identical to that in the group treated with diet therapy. Measurement of serum insulin levels showed an unrelenting annual 6% reduction in insulin levels in all treatment groups. Therefore, glycemic control requires constant adjustment of the therapeutic regimen.

In summary, the results of the UKPDS show that 1) the development of microvascular complications was similarly reduced in patients with type 2 diabetes treated with sulfonylureas, insulin, or metformin; 2) in patients with type 2 diabetes assigned to intensive therapy with sulfonylureas or insulin, the incidence of macrovascular complications was not increased compared with the group assigned to conventional therapy; 3) a decrease in macrovascular complications was seen only in patients with type 2 diabetes assigned to intensive therapy with metformin; and 4) diabetes is a progressive disease due to an inexorable decline in beta cell function. Thus, the findings of the UKPDS are consistent with those of the DCCT and extend the benefit of tight glycemic control to type 2 patients treated with either oral agents or insulin.

THERAPEUTIC GOALS

The American Diabetes Association (ADA) recommends use of hemoglobin A_{1c} (A_{1c}) determinations to monitor glycemic control in known diabetic patients. The A_{1c} level reflects the mean blood glucose levels over a three month period and correlates with the microvascular complications of diabetes. The ADA recommends maintaining an A_{1c} level $< 7\%$ while the European Diabetes Association and the American College of Endocrinology set the standard below 6.5%. In the individual patient it seems most prudent to try to achieve glucose levels as close to normal as possible without causing medically significant hypoglycemia.

GLUCOSE METABOLISM (FIGURE 3)

Approximately 85% of glucose production in the fasting state occurs in the liver. The majority of glucose metabolism in the fasting state takes place in the brain and splanchnic tissues which are not dependent on insulin. After we eat, the increase in plasma glucose stimulates insulin release from the pancreatic beta cells. The resultant hyperinsulinemia 1) suppresses hepatic glucose production and 2) stimulates glucose uptake by peripheral tissues. The vast majority of glucose in the fed state is taken up by muscle with only a small amount metabolized by adipocytes.

Although fat tissue is responsible for only a small amount of total body glucose disposal, it plays a very important role in the maintenance of total body glucose homeostasis. Small increments in the plasma insulin concentration exert a potent antilipolytic effect, leading to a marked reduction in the plasma free fatty acid (FFA) level. The decline in plasma FFA concentration results in increased glucose uptake in muscle and reduces hepatic glucose production. Thus, a decrease in the plasma FFA concentration lowers plasma glucose by both decreasing its production and enhancing the uptake in muscle.

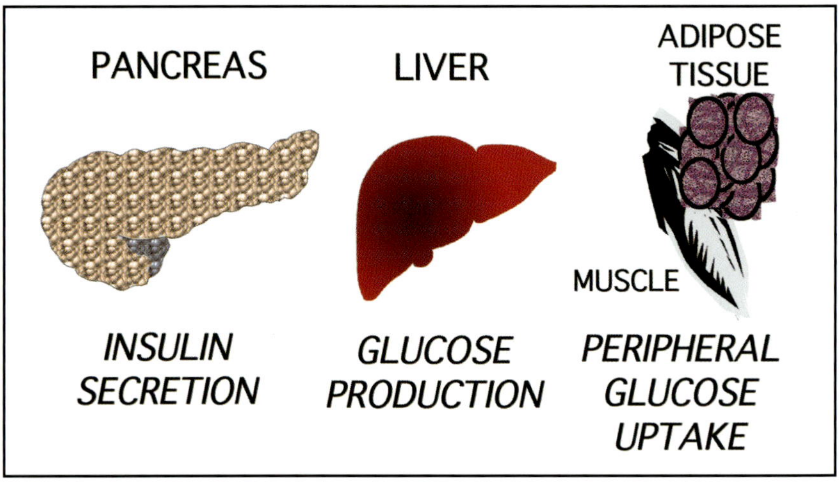

Figure 3. Role of tissues involved in glucose metabolism.

GLUCOSE METABOLISM IN TYPE 2 DIABETES MELLITUS

Type 2 diabetic individuals are characterized by: 1) defects in insulin secretion; and 2) insulin resistance involving muscle, liver, and the adipocyte. Insulin resistance is the first defect.

Insulin Resistance

During the night the liver of nondiabetic individuals produce glucose at the rate of ~2.0 mg•kg-1•min-1. This glucose production is essential to meet the needs of the brain and other neural tissues which accounts for ~50–60% of glucose disposal during the fasting state and this uptake is insulin independent. In type 2 diabetic subjects with fasting hyperglycemia (140–200 mg/dL, 7.8–11.1 mmol/L), basal hepatic glucose production is increased by

25% (~0.5 mg/kg•min). Consequently, during the overnight sleeping hours the liver of a 80 kg diabetic individual with modest fasting hyperglycemia adds an additional 35 g of glucose to the systemic circulation. This increase in overnight hepatic glucose production is the cause of fasting hyperglycemia.

After a meal, insulin is secreted into the portal vein and carried to the liver, where it suppresses hepatic glucose output. If the liver is resistant to insulin and continues to produce glucose, there will be two inputs of glucose into the body, one from the liver and another from the gastrointestinal tract. Thus insulin resistance at the liver may contribute to both fasting and postprandial hyperglycemia.

In the fed state, muscle is the major site of glucose disposal accounting for about 80% of total body glucose uptake. In diabetic patients glucose uptake into muscle is reduced by approximately 50% compared to nondiabetic controls. In addition, the onset of glucose uptake into the muscle is delayed about 40 minutes compared to nondiabetic individuals.

In summary, insulin resistance involving both muscle and liver are characteristic features of the glucose intolerance in type 2 diabetic individuals. In the basal state, the liver represents a major site of insulin resistance, and this is reflected by overproduction of glucose. This accelerated rate of hepatic glucose output is the primary determinant of the elevated fasting plasma glucose concentration in type 2 diabetic individuals. In the fed state, both decreased muscle glucose uptake and impaired suppression of hepatic glucose production contribute to the insulin resistance.

Impaired Insulin Secretion

The pancreas in people with a normal-functioning beta cell is able to adjust its secretion of insulin to maintain normal levels of blood glucose. Diabetes develops when the pancreas can no longer make enough insulin to overcome the insulin resistance. DeFronzo et al. measured the fasting plasma insulin concentration and performed oral glucose tolerance tests in 77 normal-

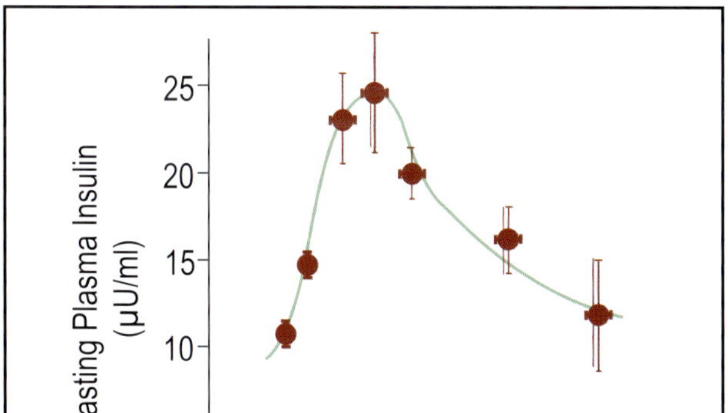

Figure 4. Relationship between rise in fasting plasma glucose and fall in fasting plasma insulin.

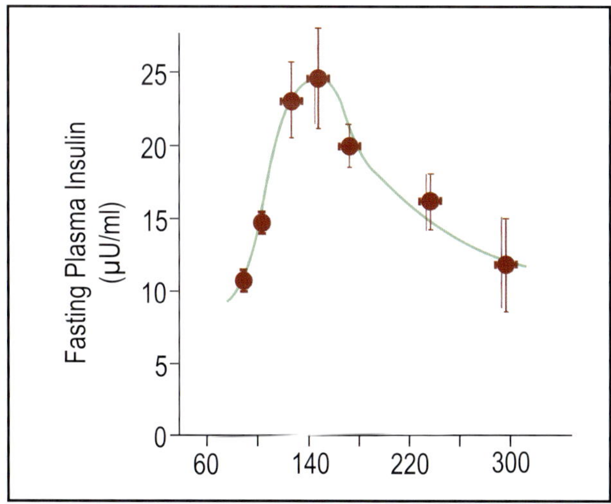

weight type 2 diabetic patients and over 100 lean subjects with normal or impaired glucose tolerance (Figure 4). The relationship in diabetic patients between the fasting plasma glucose concentration and the fasting plasma insulin concentration resembles an inverted U or horseshoe. As the fasting plasma glucose concentration rises from 80–140 mg/dL, the fasting plasma insulin concentration increases progressively, peaking at a value that is 2–2.5 fold greater than in normal weight, nondiabetic controls. When the fasting plasma glucose concentration exceeds 140 mg/dL, the beta cell has been unable to maintain its elevated rate of insulin secretion and the fasting insulin concentration declines precipitously. This decrease in fasting insulin leads to an increase in hepatic glucose production which results in an elevated fasting plasma glucose concentration.

A type 2 diabetic patient with a fasting plasma glucose concentration of 150–160 mg/dL secretes an amount of insulin that is similar to that in a healthy nondiabetic individual. However, a "normal" amount of insulin in absolute terms in the presence of this degree of hyperglycemia is markedly abnormal. When the fasting glucose exceeds 200–220 mg/dL, the plasma insulin response to a glucose challenge is markedly blunted.

Role of Obesity in Insulin Resistance

A similar degree of insulin resistance is seen in obese nondiabetic and lean type 2 diabetic individuals. The insulin resistance in obese individuals is caused by an increase in visceral fat. Since visceral fat is resistant to the antilipolytic action of insulin, visceral adiposity leads to an elevation in plasma free fatty acid levels which, as mentioned earlier, lead to the development of muscle/hepatic insulin resistance and impaired insulin secretion. Interestingly, normal-weight diabetic subjects manifest marked glucose intolerance, whereas the obese nondiabetic individuals have normal plasma glucose. This difference is explained by the plasma insulin response to a glucose challenge. Obese nondiabetic individuals secrete more than twice as much insulin as lean diabetic controls and compensate for the insulin resistance. In contrast, normal-weight diabetic subjects are unable to augment the secretion of insulin sufficiently to compensate for the insulin resistance.

Treatment

In developing a treatment strategy for patients with type 2 diabetes, it must be remembered that glucose intolerance occurs as part of a complex metabolic syndrome that includes dyslipidemia, hypertension, obesity, and clotting abnormalities. Each of these abnormalities increases the risk of macrovascular complications which will be responsible for the death of 75% of all patients with diabetes. Therefore, weight loss, exercise and appropriate treatment of lipid abnormalities and hypertension is essential.

Oral antihyperglycemic agents

Figure 5 lists the site of action of the classes of oral agents approved for use in the United States. Each of these drugs targets a single metabolic defect present in patients with type 2 diabetes. It is not surprising that most patients will require at least two and often three drugs to achieve target levels of A_{1c}.

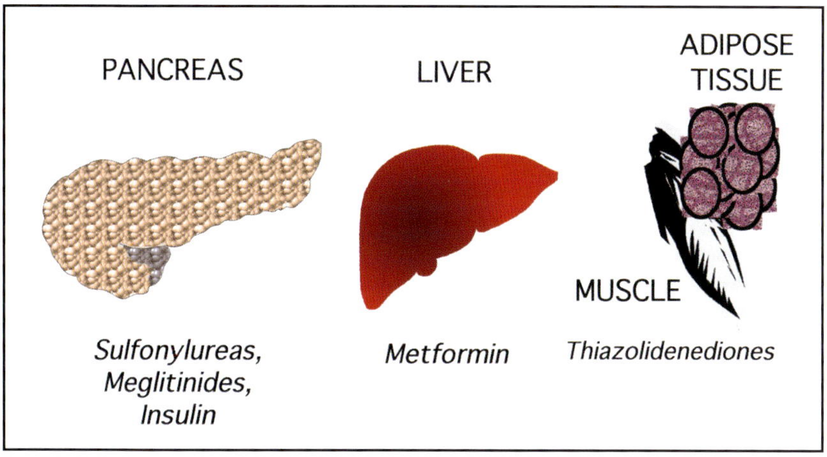

Figure 5. Site action of oral agents.

Sulfonylureas

Sulfonylureas primary mechanism of action is enhancement of insulin secretion. They initiate their action by binding to a specific sulfonylurea receptor on pancreatic [beta]-cells which causes translocation of secretory granules to the cell surface and extrusion of insulin into the portal vein. Insulin delivered to the liver suppresses hepatic glucose production to control fasting glucose. In the fed state, the elevated insulin level improves muscle glucose uptake resulting in improved postprandial glucose levels. In patients with baseline A_{1c} values around 10, sulfonylurea therapy will reduce levels by 1.5–2.0%. Clinical experience suggests that all sulfonylureas when given in maximally effective doses will achieve similar reductions in A_{1c} levels.

The major adverse effects of sulfonylurea therapy is hypoglycemia and weight gain. Both of these adverse effects may be less with the long-acting glipizide preparation. Three clinical trials showed little or no weight gain with this preparation. When dosing these agents it is important to recognize that most of the efficacy of these agents is actually seen at the starting dose. Increasing the dose beyond half of the FDA approved maximal dose results in little, if any, improvement in glycemic control.

Metformin

Metformin is the only biguanide approved for use in the United States. Metformin enhances the sensitivity of hepatic tissues to insulin through mechanisms that are still not completely understood. The reduction in A_{1c} value of 1.5–2.0% in poorly controlled patients with diabetes is comparable to that seen with sulfonylureas. Metformin therapy is effective in combination therapy with a sulfonylurea. In 423 sulfonylurea-treated patients with a fasting plasma glucose level of 250 mg/dL the addition of metformin decreased the fasting plasma glucose level by 63 mg/dL and the HbA_{1c} value by 1.7%. Thus, the hypoglycemic action of metformin and the sulfonylureas are completely additive.

In addition to lowering blood glucose, metformin decreases plasma triglyceride and low-density lipoprotein (LDL) cholesterol levels by 10% to 15%.

Most studies show modest weight loss—2 to 3 kg—during the first six months of treatment. The beneficial effects on plasma lipids combined with weight loss likely contribute to the reduction in macrovascular complications seen with metformin therapy.

This author initiates metformin therapy with one 500 mg tablet given with the largest meal to minimize gastrointestinal side effects. The dosage should be increased by 500 mg/d every 1–2 weeks until a dose of 2000 mg/d (two tablets with breakfast and supper) is reached. The slow titration schedule allows the patient's gastrointestinal system to adjust to the medication. Unlike sulfonylureas, little therapeutic benefit is seen at the starting dose and the author attempts to maximize the dose of metformin in all patients. Because metformin is an insulin-sensitizer, hypoglycemia does not occur when the drug is used as monotherapy.

Gastrointestinal side effects, including nausea, abdominal discomfort and diarrhea occur in over 30% of patients. These side effects can be minimized by the slow titration described above. If symptoms occur during titration, one should return to the previous metformin dose at which no symptoms were encountered and wait at least two weeks before increasing the dose. The most severe side-effect, lactic acidosis, had been reported to occur with a frequency of three per 100,000 patient-years. Lactic acidosis is rare in the absence of other serious medical disorders, including renal insufficiency or severe tissue hypoperfusion seen in cardiogenic or septic shock. Therefore, metformin should not be given to an individual with significant renal insufficiency (serum creatinine >1.5 mg/dL in men or > 1.4 mg/dL in a woman) or in individuals with uncompensated congestive heart failure. Impaired renal function is the most important contraindication to metformin use because the drug is excreted through the kidneys. In elderly patients with reduced muscle mass, the serum creatinine concentration may underestimate the glomerular filtration rate, and the creatinine clearance should be determined. If the creatinine clearance is less than 65 ml/min metformin should not be given.

Thiazolidenediones

Two thiazolidenediones (TZDs) are presently in use in the United States, pioglitazone (Actos) and rosiglitazone (Avandia). These agents enhance insulin sensitivity in the peripheral tissues. Thiazolidenediones bind to an intranuclear receptor called the peroxisome proliferator activated receptor [gamma], leading to increased glucose transporter expression. In addition the TZDs stimulate the conversion of undifferentiated subcutaneous mesenchymal cells to fat cells. These newly produced fat cells are metabolically more active than older adipocytes and actively take up plasma glucose and circulating free fatty acids. These cells also are able to accept fat stored in intraabdominal and splanchnic tissues leading to a shift of fat from the intraabdominal, hepatic and muscle tissue to these newly formed subcutaneous adipocytes. Intraabdominal fat produces cytokines which are released into the portal circulation and increase insulin resistance. Shifting fat from the intraabdominal to the subcutaneous site improves insulin sensitivity.

The thiazolidenediones are most effective in lowering blood glucose in individuals who are making significant amounts of insulin and who have peripheral insulin resistance. Conversely, thin individuals who make little insulin show only modest reductions in glucose in response to thiazolidenedione treatment. The mean reduction in A_{1c} is approximately 1.5% but the individual variation is quite large.

Thiazolidenediones consistently increase HDL cholesterol levels by 10–20%. In addition, pioglitazone significantly lowers triglycerides and has little effect on LDL-cholesterol. Rosiglitazone has little effect on triglycerides and may raise LDL-cholesterol levels by 5–10%. One of the most intriguing effects of the TZDs is their ability to preserve beta cell function. The TRIPOD study evaluated the ability of troglitazone to prevent the development of diabetes in 199 women with a history of gestational diabetes. The rate of development of diabetes in the placebo arm of the study was approximately 12% per year compared to about 5% in the treatment group. Dr. Buchannan was able to demonstrate total preservation of beta cell function over a five year period in women who had near normal beta cell function at baseline and initially responded to the drug. The baseline ability to secrete insulin was intact even eight months after the drug had been discontinued.

Weight gain may be significant in some patients given a TZD. As noted above, one of the mechanisms of action of the thiazolidenediones is to increase subcutaneous fat cell number. Therefore, patients given TZDs should be advised to strictly adhere to their diet and exercise regimens to avoid a significant increase in weight. Lower extremity edema and exacerbation of underlying congestive heart failure may be seen with the TZDs. This is likely the result of the increase in plasma volume seen with the TZDs (similar to the effect of calcium channel blockers) as well as an enhancement of the effect of insulin on the kidney to resorb sodium. Edema is most likely to be seen in patients with underlying cardiovascular disease who are taking insulin. The weight gain and edema seen with the TZDs are dose related.

This author starts patients with no contraindications to TZD treatment on 30 mg/d of pioglitazone or 4 mg/d of rosiglitazone. If the patients are not at their target A_{1c} after three months of therapy the dosage can be increased to the maximal dose of 45 mg/d of pioglitazone or 4mg b.i.d. of rosiglitazone. The recommended starting dosages of pioglitazone and rosiglitazone are 15 mg once daily and 2 mg once daily, respectively in patients who are elderly, on insulin, or have underlying cardiovascular disease.

Because troglitazone, the first TZD introduced to the market, was associated with idiosyncratic liver failure, it is recommended that patients should have their liver function tests monitored q two months while they are taking TZDs. Patients with baseline transaminase levels more than two fold the upper limit of normal should not be given TZD therapy. The incidence of elevated liver enzyme levels in diabetic patients treated with pioglitazone and rosiglitazone are 0.25% and 0.2%, respectively (data on file with FDA). These incidences of abnormal liver enzyme levels were similar to those in patients who received placebo.

Alpha-glucosidase inhibitors

Acarbose (Precose) and miglitol (Glyset) competitively inhibit the ability of enzymes (maltase, isomaltase, sucrase, and glucoamylase) in the small intestinal brush border to break down oligosaccharides and disaccharides into monosaccharides. By delaying digestion of carbohydrates, it shifts their absorption to more distal parts of the small intestine and colon increasing the time the beta-cell has to augment insulin secretion after a meal.

Clinical trials have shown that the hypoglycemic potency of acarbose is less than that of sulfonylureas, metformin, and the TZDs. As monotherapy, acarbose decreases A_{1c} value by 0.7%–1.0%. Plasma lipids and body weight do not change significantly with these agents.

The glucosidase inhibitors should be initiated at the lowest dose pill given once a day with the smallest meal to minimize gastrointestinal side effects. Patients are advised to take their pill with the first bite of food because the drug must be present in the small bowel with food to be effective. The dose of the medication can be increased weekly until the patient is taking medication with each meal.

Gastrointestinal side effects, including bloating, abdominal discomfort, diarrhea, and flatulence, occur in most patients treated with alpha glucosidase inhibitors but these effects tend to diminish with continued drug use. Initiation of therapy with a low dose and slow titration helps to minimize these adverse effects. These agents are contraindicated in patients with inflammatory bowel disease. If hypoglycemia occurs when alpha glucosidase inhibitors are being used, patients should be instructed to ingest pure glucose to avoid delay in absorption of more complex carbohydrates.

Meglitinides

The meglitinides available in the United States are Repaglinide (Prandin) and Nateglinide (Starlix). These drugs are short acting insulin secretagogues given before each meal. These drugs bind to a site close to the sulfonylurea receptor and the insulin stimulatory effect is not additive to sulfonylureas. When used as monotherapy repaglinide decreases A_{1c} values 1.5%. Nateglinide is shorter acting and reduces A_{1c} levels approximately 1.0%. These agents have no significant effect on plasma lipid levels. Most patients treated with these drugs gain little or no weight.

The main advantage of these agents is a lower risk of hypoglycemia than the longer-acting sulfonylureas. Because of the short half-life, nocturnal hypoglycemia is significantly decreased. However, the need to administer the drugs before each meal and their relatively high cost has limited their use.

INJECTABLE AGENTS

Incretin

The term incretin describes the physiologic observation that glucose given orally is associated with a greater increase of insulin than the same amount of glucose administered intravenously. This suggests that a gastrointestinal hormone, stimulated by a local increase in glucose, results in an increase in insulin secretion. We now know that there are several incretin hormones but only two, glucagons-like peptide 1 (GLP-1) and glucose-dependent insulinotropic polypeptide (GIP) are responsible for over 90% of the increase in insulin secretion. The first agent to be released in this family of antidiabetic agents is Exenatide (Byetta), a GLP-1 analogue.

GLP-1 is secreted by L-cells in the intestine in response to an increase in glucose. An increase GLP-1 leads to: 1) an increase in insulin secretion, 2) a decrease in glucagons secretion, 3) an increase in time of gastric emptying, and 4) an increase in satiety. These actions of GLP-1 all lead to a reduction in postprandial glucose elevation. GLP-1 levels decline progressively as individuals progress from impaired glucose tolerance to diabetes and continuous intravenous infusion of GLP-1 normalizes glucose in diabetic patients.

Exenatide was discovered in the saliva of a Gila monster. Administration of Exenatide to diabetic individuals results in a dose dependent lowering of the plasma glucose due to an increase in insulin secretion and a decrease in plasma glucagon. Exenatide is approved by the Food and Drug Administration to be used with metformin and/or sulfonylureas. When added to patients on these agents there was a decrease in A_{1c} of 1% at the five microgram twice daily dose and 1.5% at the ten microgram twice daily dose. In these trials, 83% of the Exenatide-treated patients lost weight. Weight loss varied significantly with those in the lowest quartile of weight loss gaining approximately 2 kg while patients in the highest quartile lost an average of 12 kg. As expected, greater weight loss was associated with beneficial effects of serum triglycerides and HDL-cholesterol.

Insulins

All insulin preparations available in the United States are human insulin. They differ mainly in their onset and duration of action. Short acting insulins are given prandially to limit glucose elevations associated with eating. Long acting insulin preparations are used to control hepatic glucose output.

COMBINATION THERAPY WITH ORAL AGENTS

Patients with diabetes have three major defects in glucose metabolism: 1) insulin resistance in peripheral tissues (muscle and fat), 2) insulin resistance at the liver, and 3) decreased insulin secretion. It should not be surprising that mainstays of oral antidiabetic therapy, i.e. TZDs, metformin, and the sulfonylureas target these three defects. Since all these defects are present in an individual patient it follows that most individuals will require combination therapy with two or three drugs to achieve tight glycemic control. Recently, pharmaceutical companies have manufactured tablets containing the most commonly used drug combinations: Metaglip (metformin plus glipizide), Glucovance (metformin and glyburide), and Avandamet (metformin and Avandia). The recent addition of Exenatide, which increases insulin secretion and is associated with weight loss, make it an attractive option for overweight diabetic patients.

Strategy

The author believes the clinician should make every effort to prescribe a treatment regimen that has a high likelihood of having the patient achieve their A_{1c} goal. It is easy to see how a patient can get discouraged if they follow a diet and exercise program faithfully for several months and still are far from reaching their A_{1c} goal. In my opinion it is much more motivating to be able to reduce the number of medications you have prescribed for your patient as you observe them losing weight and achieving their target glucose levels. If you understand that each of the individual agents will lower the A_{1c} 1.5–2.0% and your A_{1c} goal is < 7% it follows that monotherapy has a reasonable chance of success if the A_{1c} is < 8.5%. In these individuals one should initiate therapy with an insulin sensitizer. As monotherapy, these agents have no risk of hypoglycemia so the patients do not have to worry about this unpleasant and potentially dangerous condition. Metformin has the major advantage of reducing cardiovascular complications of diabetes and is the only oral antidiabetic agent associated with weight loss. The TZDs are the most potent insulin sensitizers and hold the most promise of preserving beta cell function. Many physicians are initiating treatment with both metformin and a TZD reasoning insulin resistance is the major defect in diabetes and is present in both the periphery and the liver. There is the hope that metformin use may ameliorate some of the weight gain seen with the TZDs. In the author's practice, Exenatide is added to sensitizers to increase insulin recreation and facilitate weight loss.

In patients with an A_{1c} greater than 10%, the author usually initiates therapy with sensitizers and Exenatide. These individuals have insulin resistance and an absolute reduction in insulin secretory capacity. If the patient does not reach their A_{1c} goal after three months of continuous therapy, another oral agent should be added or insulin should be given.

Combination Therapy with Bedtime Insulin Plus Oral Agents

The effectiveness of bedtime insulin therapy in patients with type 2 diabetes in whom acceptable glycemic control does not occur with combination therapy described above is well documented. In such patients, the elevated fasting plasma glucose level is caused by incomplete suppression of basal hepatic glucose. Although the medications are still working, they are not producing the desired hypoglycemic effect. Bedtime insulin takes advantage of the differential sensitivity of hepatic compared with peripheral tissues to insulin. Relatively low doses of insulin effectively suppress hepatic glucose production and have a much smaller effect on stimulating muscle glucose uptake. By giving a modest dose of long-acting insulin at bedtime, the elevated basal rate of hepatic glucose production can be reduced to normal, and the likelihood of hypoglycemia will decrease because muscle glucose uptake is only minimally stimulated.

It is important to continue insulin sensitizers such as metformin and a TZD when insulin therapy is initiated. Patients who no longer make adequate amounts of insulin remain insulin resistant. Moreover, tight control of blood glucose cannot be achieved with insulin therapy alone in a type 2 diabetic. Because these patients are resistant to insulin, insulin doses exceeding 100 units per day are often required to control the blood glucose. These doses cause weight gain which increases insulin resistance.

The author initiates insulin therapy with ten units of long-acting insulin given at bedtime. The patient is instructed to increase the dose of insulin by one or two units daily until the fasting glucose is less than 120 mg/dL. In patients who have significant postprandial hyperglycemia, short-acting insulin preparations are administered before meals.

REFERENCES

Pathogenesis

1. Rubin RJ, Altman WM, Mendelson DN. Health care expenditures for people with diabetes mellitus, 1992. *J Clin Endocrinol Metab* 1994;78:809A-809F.
2. DeFronzo RA. Pathogenesis of type 2 diabetes: metabolic and molecular implications for identifying diabetes genes. *Diabetes Rev* 1997;5:177-269.
3. Groop LC, Bonadonna RC, Del Prato S, et al. Glucose and free fatty acid metabolism in non-insulin-dependent diabetes mellitus. Evidence for multiple sites of insulin resistance. *J Clin Invest* 1989;84:205-213.
4. Mitrakou A, Kelley D, Veneman T, et al. Contribution of abnormal muscle and liver glucose metabolism to postprandial hyperglycemia in NIDDM. *Diabetes* 1990;39:1381-1390.
5. Polonsky KS. Lilly Lecture 1994. The [beta]-cell in diabetes: from molecular genetics to clinical research. *Diabetes* 1995;44:705-717.
6. Saad MF, Knowler WC, Pettitt DJ, et al. Sequential changes in serum insulin concentration during development of non-insulin-dependent diabetes. *Lancet* 1989;1:1356-1359.
7. DeFronzo RA. Lilly Lecture 1987. The triumvirate: beta-cell, muscle, liver. A collusion responsible for NIDDM. *Diabetes* 1988;37:667-687.

Complications

8. The effect of intensive treatment of diabetes on the development and progression of long-term complications in insulin-dependent diabetes mellitus. The Diabetes Control and Complications Trial Research Group. *N Engl J Med* 1993;329:977-986.
9. The absence of a glycemic threshold for the development of long-term complications: the perspective of the Diabetes Control and Complications Trial. *Diabetes* 1996;45:1289-1298.
10. Intensive blood-glucose control with sulphonylureas or insulin compared with conventional treatment and risk of complications in patients with type 2 diabetes (UKPDS 33). UK Prospective Diabetes Study Group. *Lancet* 1998;352:837-853.
11. Effect of intensive blood-glucose control with metformin on complications in overweight patients with type 2 diabetes (UKPDS 34). UK Prospective Diabetes Study. *Lancet* 1998;352:854-865.
12. Ohkubo Y, Kishikawa H, Araki E, et al. Intensive insulin therapy prevents the progression of diabetic microvascular complications in Japanese patients with non-insulin-dependent diabetes mellitus: a randomized prospective 6-year study. *Diabetes Res Clin Pract* 1995;28:103-117.

Therapeutic Goals

13. Standards of medical care for patients with diabetes mellitus. American Diabetes Association. *Diabetes Care* 2003;26(Suppl 1):S33-50.
14. Pyorala K, Pedersen TR, Kjekshus J, et al. Cholesterol lowering with simvastatin improves prognosis of diabetic patients with coronary heart disease. A subgroup analysis of the Scandinavian Simvastatin Survival Study (4S) Group. *Diabetes Care* 1997;20:614-620.
15. Tight blood pressure control and risk of macrovascular and microvascular complications In type 2 diabetes: UKPDS 38. UK Prospective Diabetes Study. *BMJ* 1998;317:703-713.
16. Kelley DE. Effects of weight loss on glucose homeostasis in NIDDM. *Diabetes Rev* 1995;3:366-377.
17. Schneider SH, Morgado A. Effects of fitness and physical training on carbohydrate metabolism and associated cardiovascular risk factors in patients with diabetes. *Diabetes Rev* 1995;3:378-407.

Oral Agents

18. United Kingdom Prospective Diabetes Study 24: a 6-year, randomized, controlled trial comparing sulfonylurea, insulin, and metformin therapy in patients with newly diagnosed type 2 diabetes that could not be controlled with diet therapy. United Kingdom Prospective Diabetes Study Group. *Ann Intern Med* 1998;128:165-175.

19. DeFronzo, RA. Pharmacologic Therapy for Type 2 Diabetes Mellitus. *Ann Intern Med* 1999;131:281-303.

20. Lebovitz HE. Stepwise and combination drug therapy for the treatment of NIDDM. *Diabetes Care* 1994;17:1542-1544.

21. UKPDS 28: a randomized trial of efficacy of early addition of metformin in sulfonylurea-treated type 2 diabetes. U.K. Prospective Diabetes Study Group. *Diabetes Care* 1998;21:87-92.

22. Simonson DC, Kourides IA, Feinglos M, et al. Efficacy, safety, and dose-response characteristics of glipizide gastrointestinal therapeutic system on glycemic control and insulin secretion in NIDDM. Results of two multicenter, randomized, placebo-controlled clinical trials. The Glipizide Gastrointestinal Therapeutic System Study Group. *Diabetes Care* 1997;20:597-606.

23. Groop LC. Sulfonylureas in NIDDM. *Diabetes Care* 1992;15:737-754.

24. Lebovitz HE, Melander A. Sulfonylureas: basic aspects and clinical uses. In: Alberti KG, Zimmet P, DeFronzo RA, eds. *International Textbook of Diabetes Mellitus* 2d ed. New York: J Wiley; 1997:817-840.

25. Bailey CJ, Turner RC. Metformin. *N Engl J Med* 1996;334:574-579.

26. DeFronzo RA, Goodman AM. Efficacy of metformin in patients with non-insulin-dependent diabetes mellitus. The Multicenter Metformin Study Group. *N Engl J Med* 1995;333:541-549.

27. DeFronzo RA, Barzilai N, Simonson DC. Mechanism of metformin action in obese and lean noninsulin-dependent diabetic subjects. *J Clin Endocrinol Metab* 1991;73:1294-1301.

28. Stumvoll N, Nurjhan N, Perriello G, et al. Metabolic effects of metformin in non-insulin-dependent diabetes mellitus. *N Engl J Med* 1995;333:550-554.

29. Cusi K, DeFronzo RA. Metformin: a review of its metabolic effects. *Diabetes Rev* 1998;6:89-131.

30. Johansen K. Efficacy of metformin in the treatment of NIDDM. Meta-analysis. *Diabetes Care* 1999;22:33-37.

31. Reaven GM, Johnston P, Hollenbeck CB, et al. Combined metformin-sulfonylurea treatment of patients with noninsulin-dependent diabetes in fair to poor glycemic control. *J Clin Endocrinol Metab* 1992;74:1020-1026.

32. Lebovitz HE. A new oral therapy for diabetes management: alpha-glucosidase inhibition with acarbose. *Clinical Diabetes* 1995;13:99-103.

33. Chiasson JL, Josse RG, Hunt JA, et al. The efficacy of acarbose in the treatment of patients with non-insulin-dependent diabetes mellitus. A multicenter controlled clinical trial. *Ann Intern Med* 1994;121:928-935.

34. Saltiel AR, Olefsky JM. Thiazolidenediones in the treatment of insulin resistance and type II diabetes. *Diabetes* 1996;45:1661-1669.

35. Maggs DG, Buchanan TA, Burant CF, et al. Metabolic effects of troglitazone monotherapy in type 2 diabetes mellitus. A randomized, double-blind, placebo-controlled trial. *Ann Intern Med* 1998;128:176-185.

36. Nolan JJ, Ludvik B, Beerdsen P, et al. Improvement in glucose tolerance and insulin resistance in obese subjects treated with troglitazone. *N Engl J Med* 1994;331:1188-1193.

37. Horton ES, Whitehouse F, Ghazzi MN, et al. Troglitazone in combination with sulfonylurea restores glycemic control in patients with type 2 diabetes. The Troglitazone Study Group. *Diabetes Care* 1998;21:1462-1469.

38. Schwartz S, Raskin P, Fonesca V, et al. Effect of troglitazone in insulin-treated patients with type II diabetes mellitus. Troglitazone and Exogenous Insulin Study Group. *N Engl J Med* 1998;13:861-866.

39. Marbury T, Huang WC, Strange P, et al. Repaglinide versus glyburide: a one-year comparison trial. *Diabetes Res Clin Pract* 1999;43:155-166.

40. Inzucchi SE, Maggs DG, Spollett GR, et al. Efficacy and metabolic effects of metformin and troglitazone in type II diabetes mellitus. *N Engl J Med* 1998;338:867-872.

41. Buchanan TA, Xiang AH, Peters RK, et al. Preservation of pancreatic ß-cell function and prevention of type 2 diabetes by pharmacological treatment of insulin resistance in high-risk Hispanic women. *Diabetes* 2002; 51:2796-803.

Insulin Therapy

42. Yki-Jarvinen H, Ryysy L, Nikkila K, et al. Comparison of bedtime insulin regimens in patients with type 2 diabetes mellitus. A randomized, controlled trial. *Ann Intern Med* 1999;130:389-396.

43. Bergenstal R, Johnson M, Whipple D, et al. Advantages of adding metformin to multiple dose insulin therapy in type 2 diabetes. *Diabetes* 1998;7(Suppl 1):A89.

44. Riddle MC. Evening insulin strategy. *Diabetes Care* 1990;13:676-686.

45. La Barre J, Still EU. Studies of the physiology of secretin: III. Further studies on the effects of secretin on the blood sugar. *Am J Physiol* 1930; 91:649-653.

46. Nauck M, Stöckmann F, Ebert R, et al. Reduced incretin effect in type 2 (non-insulin-dependent) diabetes. *Diabetologia* 1986: 29:46-52.

47. Drucker DJ. Development of glucagon-like peptide-1-based pharmaceuticals as therapeutic agents for the treatment of diabetes. *Curr Pharm Des* 2001; 7:1399-1412.

48. Drucker DJ. Glucagon-like peptides: Regulators of cell proliferation, differentiation, and apoptosis. *Mol Endocrinol* 2003; 17:161-171.

49. Toft-Nielsen M-B, Damholt MB, Madsbad S, et al. Determinants of the impaired secretion of glucagon-like peptide-1 in type 2 diabetic patients. *J Clin Endocrinol Metab* 2001; 86:3717-3723.

50. Rachman J, Barrow BA, Levy JC, Turner RC. Near-normalization of diurnal glucose concentrations by continuous administration of glucagon-like peptide-1 (GLP-1) in subjects with NIDDM. *Diabetologia* 1997; 40:205-211.

51. Kolterman OG, Buse JB, Fineman MS, et al. Synthetic Exendin-4 (Exenatide) significantly reduces postprandial and fasting plasma glucose in subjects with type 2 diabetes. *J Clin Endocrinol Metab* 2003; 88:3082-3089.

52. DeFronzo RA, Ratner RE, Han J, et al. Effects of Exenatide (Exendin-4_ on glycemic control and weight over 30 weeks in metformin-treated patients with type 2 diabetes. *Diabetes Care* 2005; 28:1092-1100.

53. Buse JB, Henry RR, Han J Kim DD Fineman MS, Baron AD, for the Exenatide-113 Clinic Study Group. Effects of Exenatide (Exendin-4) on glycemic control over 30 weeks in sulfonylurea-treated patients with type 2 diabetes. *Diabetes Care* 2004; 27-2628-2635.

54. Kendall DM, Riddle MC, Rosenstock J, et al. Effect of Exenatide (Exendin-4) on glycemic control over 30 weeks in patients with type 2 diabetes treated with metformin and a sulfonylurea. *Diabetes Care* 2005; 28:1083-1092.

REVIEW QUESTIONS

1.) Metabolic defects in patients with type 2 diabetes include:
- a. Insulin resistance in muscle
- b. Hepatic insulin resistance
- c. Decreased insulin secretion
- d. Elevation of free fatty acids
- e. All of the above

2.) Which antidiabetic agents are associated with weight loss?
- a. Insulin
- b. Metformin
- c. Exenatide
- d. TZDs
- e. Sulfonylureas
- f. b and c
- g. a, d, and e

3.) Physiologic effects of "incretins" include:
- a. Increased insulin secretion
- b. Decreased glucagon secretion
- c. Increased satiety
- d. Delayed gastric emptying
- e. All of the above

Answers: 1e, 2f, 3e

CHAPTER 29

BIO-FILM BASED WOUND CARE

CHAPTER TWENTY-NINE OVERVIEW

NOTES

Bio-film Based Wound Care

Randall D. Wolcott

INTRODUCTION

A good clinical model should be able to explain what we see in the daily care of patients. A wound bio-film model has shown an exciting power for explaining even the most frustrating elements of delayed wound healing. It is important for all wound care providers to firmly grasp the wound bio-film concept, its importance in delayed wound healing, and how it differs from a planktonic bacterial concept.

The most widely held concept of what is happening on the surface of a chronic wound is the contamination-infection continuum (Figure 1). This concept holds that bacteria randomly land on the surface of the wound in relatively small numbers (contamination). Then, feeding on necrotic tissue and nutrient-rich exudate, the bacteria grow on the surface of the wound (colonization). If the bacteria become more aggressive, invading the host boundary (critical colonization) or if they spread deeper into the tissue causing a

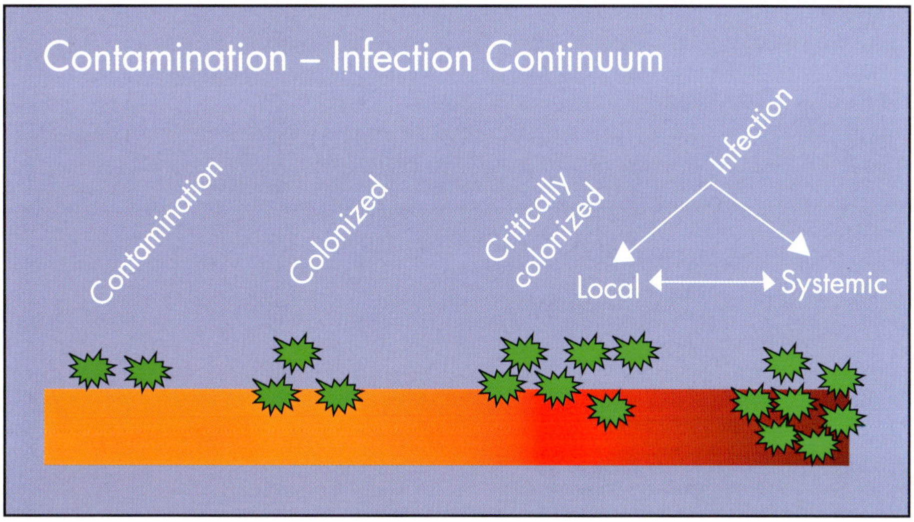

Figure 1. The contamination-infection continuum is possible, but is not scientifically valid for bacteria on the surface of the wound. This is, at best, only a minor pathway of how bacteria survive on the surface of the wound and is insignificant in wound healing.

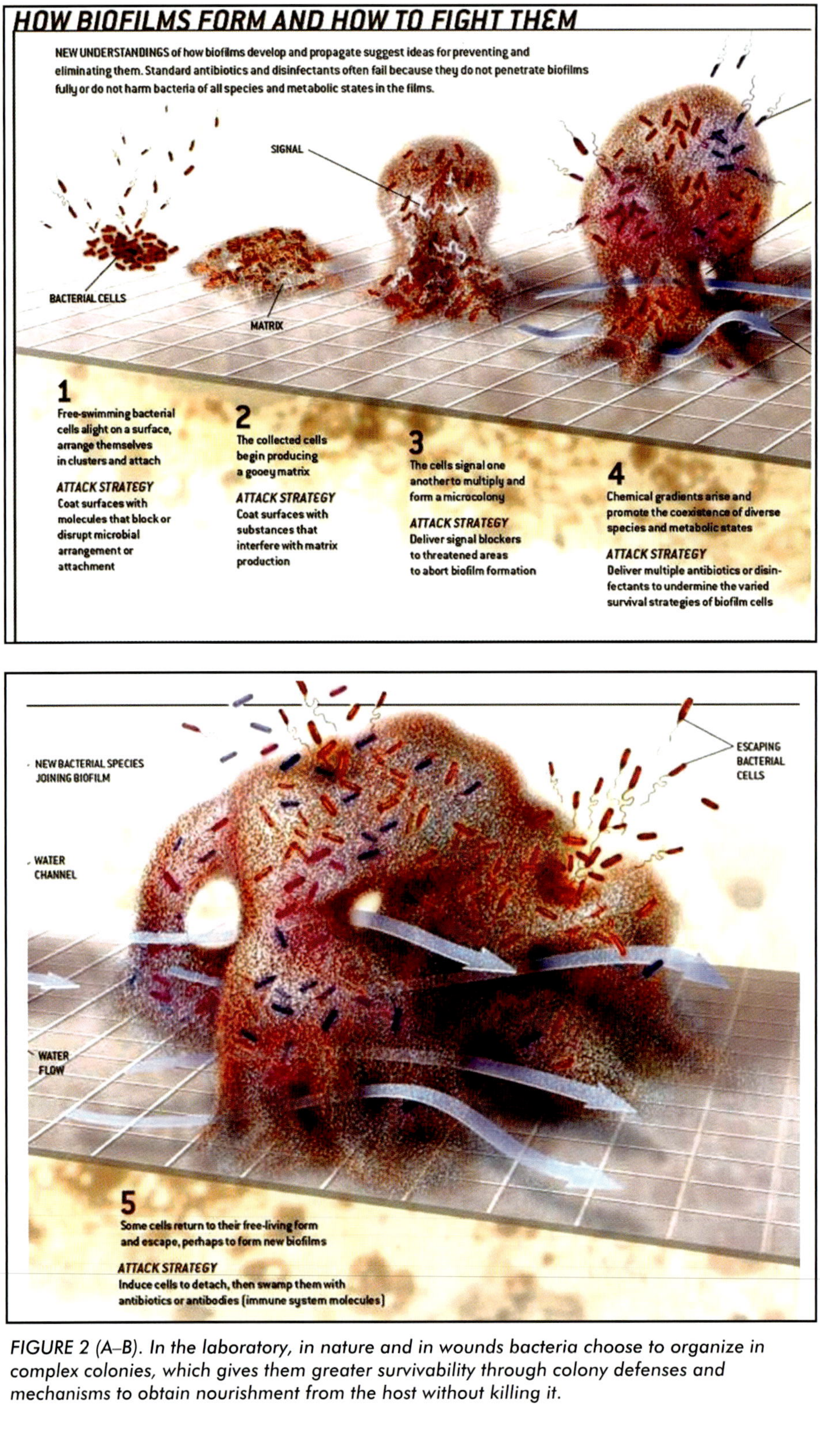

FIGURE 2 (A–B). In the laboratory, in nature and in wounds bacteria choose to organize in complex colonies, which gives them greater survivability through colony defenses and mechanisms to obtain nourishment from the host without killing it.

broader inflammatory host response (infection), then the bacteria may become detrimental to wound healing. The only trouble with this scenario is it just doesn't apply to chronic wounds. The contamination-infection continuum is a planktonic concept, which is only a very minor pathway of how bacteria behave on the surface of a wound, and is not an acceptable model for chronic wounds.

The way bacteria behave on a wound—the dominant pathway—is to form a dense organized colony, which has multiple defensive strategies to ensure bacterial survival (Figure 2). This colony organization of bacteria on the surface of a wound is called wound bio-film.

In the wound bio-film model a single planktonic bacterium randomly lands on a freshly exposed wound surface. The tissue exposed in the wound bed has no protection against bacterial attachment. The bacterium twitches to prepare the surface, irreversibly attaches and starts secreting an extracellular slime that protects the bacterium and its progeny. When enough bacteria are present (quorum) in the slime, chemical signals become concentrated enough to upregulate the bio-film pathways. This concentrated chemical signal, called quorum sensing, allows the bio-film to form a complex colony structure, which confers multiple defenses that protect each bacteria in the colony. The colony is most successful if the wound stays open; therefore, bio-films have developed a number of different strategies to prevent wound closure. It is bio-films' defenses, their ability to adapt to selective stresses and their need to keep the wound open that make knowledge of bio-film so important to the wound care provider.

The awesome power of molecular techniques and advanced imaging has not been fully utilized in studying chronic wounds. There have been extremely few microscopic studies (2–3) of the chronic wound over the last two decades. This totally neglects the rapid advances in imaging including confocal, transmission electron microscopy and scanning electron microscopy. The little work that has been reported leads to the conclusion that bacteria must not be acting as single cell individuals but rather as a colony. Many times these conclusions must be made tangentially from studies where the primary focus was not on bacterial phenotype. For example, Diegelmann et al. in a wound bed photomicrograph (Figure 3) showing excess neutrophils in the wound bed of a decubitus ulcer serendipitously captured a colony of bacteria on the surface most consistent with bio-film. Wound bio-film in the photomicrograph best explains the excessive neutrophils documented in the study (1).

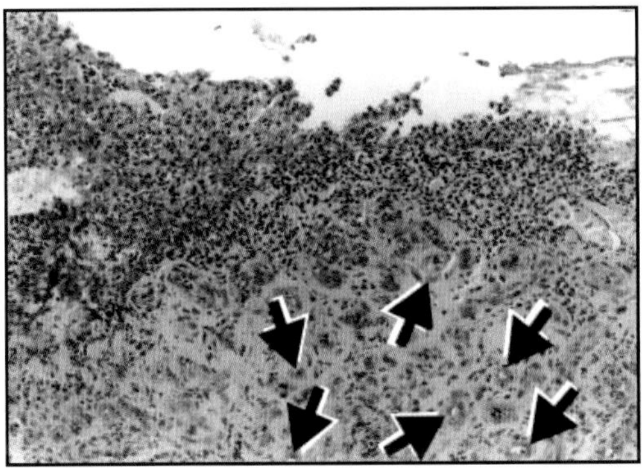

Figure 3. This photomicrograph was produced to demonstrate the excessive neutrophils present in a decubitus ulcer. Fortunately, the cause for the excess neutrophils was inadvertently captured in the frame. The bacteria on the surface show architecture most consistent with bio-film.

Over the last few years, several articles have appeared linking bio-film to chronic wounds (2, 3). Bio-film, such as the plaque on our teeth, is defined as "a microbially derived sessile community characterized by cells that are irreversibly attached to a substratum or interface or to each other, are embedded in a matrix of extracellular polymeric substances (EPS) that they have produced, and exhibit altered phenotype with respect to growth rate and gene transcription" (4). Donlan's and Costerton's excellent review of bio-

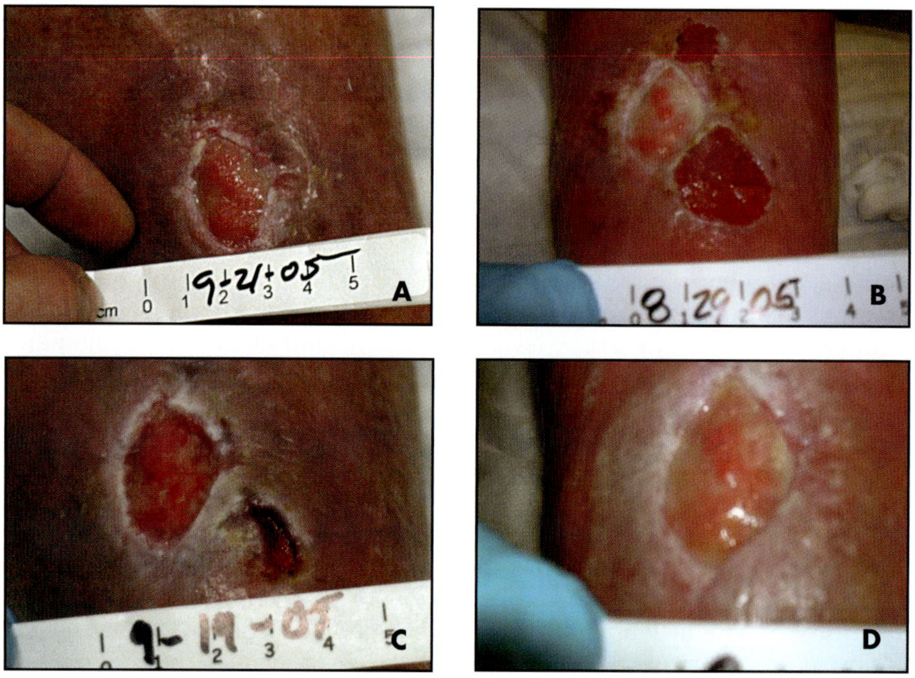

Figure 4 (A–D). This series of photographs captures the development of a full thickness acute wound in the same region as a chronic wound. The acute wound heals in three weeks and the chronic wound does not. The difference may be bio-film.

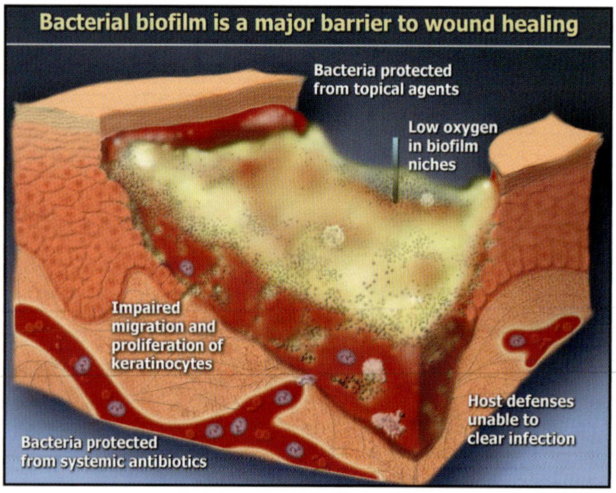

Figure 5. Wound bio-film is the best model for the behavior of chronic wounds.

TABLE 1. OBSERVATIONS IN CHRONIC WOUNDS EXPLAINED BY BIO-FILM CONCEPT VERSUS PLANKTONIC CONCEPT

Observation	Planktonic Concept	bio-film Concept
In vitro	Planktonic bacterium (seed) express proteins and structures for motility and attachment (flagella, fimbria). Its function is to spread the colony to a different location	Bio-film (vegetation) is a complex colony of bacteria that can express different proteins (phenotype) to fulfill different roles to help the community survive. Bio-film is stationary, protecting its location with multiple defenses
In vivo	Planktonic bacteria are susceptible to antibiotics, biocides and the immune system	Bio-films are resistant to antibiotics and biocides. Once bio-film is established it cannot be eradicated by the immune system
Acute wounds heal in 2–4 weeks; chronic wounds in the same area heal in 4–6 months	Acute wounds have intact defenses and clear planktonic bacteria not allowing bio-film formation	Random planktonic bacteria evade host defenses and set up bio-film. Bio-film possesses defenses against host immune system and strategies to keep the wound open
Antibiotics not effective in chronic wounds but work in acute wounds	Sensitive planktonic bacteria show a rapid 4- to 5-log reduction	Sensitive bio-film phenotype bacteria show only a grudging 1- to 2-log reduction at 50 to 1000 times planktonic doses and quick adaptation
Biocides not effective in chronic wounds	Nonspecific biocides eradicate planktonic bacteria	Nonspecific biocides eradicate host healing cells and host defenses doing little damage to the bio-film
Drying the wound (open to air, heat lamp, etc.) is ineffective in chronic wounds	Planktonic bacteria are very sensitive to environment	Bio-films are very resistant to drying and other environmental changes
Closing a traumatic wound after 4 to 12 hours leads to increased dehiscence	Planktonic phenotypes dominate the surface early on (1–2 hours) and are sensitive to biocides and amenable to closure	Bio-films form in 3–8 hours and are resistant to surgical scrubs. Closure of the wound puts two surfaces in contact with the bio-film and leads to dehiscence
Increased surgical site infections in patients with chronic wounds	Surgical preps and prophylactic antibiotics are highly effective against planktonic bacteria	Chronic wounds shed bio-film fragments continuously. These fragments have all the defenses of bio-film and are resistant to surgical preps and prophylactic antibiotics
Wet to dry dressings are detrimental to chronic wounds	Planktonic bacteria quickly (six hours) seeds gauze and forms bio-film on gauze	Detachment fragments foul the gauze dressing forming bio-film that produces fragments, toxins, etc., that are detrimental to the wound
Autograft or Allograft failure on wounds	Planktonic cells are easily cleared by neutrophils, antibodies and common wound bed preparations	Laying unprotected cells over bio-film just adds a second surface and a food source leading to the rapid deterioration of the graft with increased exudate, inflammation and odor
Negative wound cultures	Most clinical bacteria in planktonic phenotype are easily cultured	Wounds have bacteria on their surface yet culture negative when only bio-film phenotype is present (i.e., viable but not culturable)
Wounds "stuck" in chronic inflammatory state	Planktonic bacteria are easily cleared by host inflammatory response and try to avoid causing inflammation	Bio-films are impervious to the host inflammatory response and can even feed off the exudate produced by inflammation. Bio-films try to cause inflammation
Corticosteroids known to slow the host healing response help in healing some chronic wounds	Steroids decrease the host immune response making planktonic infections worse	Steroids rob bio-films of nutrition by decreasing the host inflammatory response
No blood clot formation on chronic wound	Planktonic bacteria are overwhelmed by host defenses post injury and clot will form on surface of the wound	Bio-films prevent clot formation on the surface of a wound post debridement by direct competition and increased proteolytic environment

film seems relevant to chronic wounds since wounds possess many of the clinical characteristics of the other bio-film based infections summarized in their article. The article also reveals many attributes of bio-film, which elucidates why chronic wounds are stuck in the chronic inflammatory phase and fail to heal.

The contamination-infection model is a planktonic bacterial concept and does not help us in the management of clinical wounds. A bio-film model clarifies why wounds are resistant to antibiotics, nonspecific biocides, debridement, etc. Bio-films may also shed light on why acute wounds (without significant bio-film) heal quickly while chronic wounds (with bio-film) in the same area of the acute wound fail to heal (Figure 4). The difference may be the presence of bio-film.

This chapter will attempt to make a scientific and clinically relevant connection between chronic wounds and bio-film. The major premise throughout is that bio-film, a polymicrobial, organized colony of bacteria, is a major barrier to wound healing (Figure 5). Evidence will be produced showing that bio-film is present in chronic wounds yet insignificant in acute wounds. However, the presence of bio-film does not necessarily establish its role in impaired wound healing. It is the remarkable improvement in wound healing produced by wound care specifically targeting bio-film (bio-film based wound care) that is the most compelling argument for bio-film's pivotal role in delayed wound healing.

BIO-FILM

Bio-films are shown in the fossil record to have been present since near the beginning of life, and are ubiquitous in nature(5). It seems bio-film is the preferred way bacteria choose to live in nature (6). Bio-films also constitute the majority of bacteria in pathogenic ecosystems (7). Bio-films are organized colonies of multiple combined species of bacteria that are found throughout nature; in streams, water systems, food processing, petroleum, and anywhere bacteria are present. If there is an available surface, bacteria will work very hard to form a bio-film because it gives them much better survivability.

The formation of a differentiated multicellular community gives bio-films defenses against biocides, antibiotics, UV light, bacteriophages, immune responses, and many environmental stresses (4). Bio-film, as an organized colony, allows bacteria to survive all these assaults that would easily kill the single cell (planktonic form) bacteria.

Microscopically a mature bio-film is 60–200 microns thick, possesses an irregular (variegated) surface, and has a rubbery or gelatinous texture. The mature bio-film grown in a flow state has been described as having pillars that attach to the surface with enlarged tops often called "mushrooms." This arrangement allows for water channels and the flow of nutrients throughout the bio-film. Nutrients penetrate inside the bio-film though diffusion. The arrangement of water channels, mushrooms and pillars seems to be directed by cell-cell communication of the different bacteria within the bio-film. Bio-films are true multicellular organisms with well-differentiated bacteria pursuing different functions throughout the structure to provide for success of the entire colony.

The life cycle of a bio-film begins when a planktonic bacterium (seed) bumps into a surface with its fimbria, pili, and/or flagella. These structures allow the bacterium to have a true sense of touch. Attachment is a very complex process that produces significant changes within the individual bacterium. The exact signal for attachment is unknown, but the individual bacterium will move (twitch) along the surface until it is satisfied (reversible attachment), and then will attach itself solidly to the surface (irreversible attachment). Once attachment is complete, the bacteria divide until a critical density (microcolony) of bacteria is reached. At that point, quorum-sensing molecules, when in high enough concentrations, will upregulate genes that produce the bio-film phenotype (maturation) (5). The focus of the bacteria at this stage is no longer for survival of itself, but for survival of the colony (Figure 2).

To date there are still many undefined variables in the differentiation of bacteria to form the bio-film. There is no single bio-film phenotype, since each cell expresses different proteins to fulfill its role in the community. Sauer et al., using RNA microarray, have shown that over 30 operons are changed two-fold or greater in bio-film versus planktonic cells (8). Also her group showed that 50% of the detectable proteome (800 proteins) had six-fold or greater change (9). Multiple other groups that have evaluated bio-film using microarray techniques also see a high percentage of change in the genes expressed and the proteins produced (10–12). However, there is no strong correlation between the genes or the proteins identified for the bio-film phenotype in the different labs. Bio-film phenotype is highly variable.

Early in the differentiation process a small group of bacteria (microcolony) envelope themselves in a gooey substance. This substance has been given many names including exopolysaccharide, extracellular polysaccharide matrix, glycocalix, extracellular matrix and bio-film matrix, but is formally known as extracellular polymeric substance (EPS). The EPS comprises approximately 85% of the bio-film volume with the individual bacteria making up only about 15% of the mature bio-film (4).

The bio-film extracellular matrix is composed of polysaccharide strands, proteins and DNA (13). DNA, cations and side chains of the polymers allow the EPS to cross link much like the knots on a fishing net to provide the structural support of the EPS (14). The EPS composition is not only dependent upon the bacterial species involved, but also on nutritional substrates and environmental conditions. There are even posttranslational modification mechanisms by the bacteria outside the cell. For example, Staphylococcus using icaB covalently bound to the outside of the cell can deacetylate the polysaccharide chains of the EPS, changing the properties of the EPS post transcription (15). This allows a mature bio-film to adapt to attacks and changes in the environment. Therefore, the macroscopic characteristics of bio-film (that is the sliminess, friability, etc.) vary widely.

An important property of the bio-film matrix is protection against the host immune system. EPS has been shown to completely inhibit macrophage activity (16) as well as antibodies (17). In *S. aureus* the major EPS component is polysaccharide intercellular adhesin (PIA). When PIA is absent, polymorphonuclear white blood cells and macrophages can clear the bacterial cells from the bio-film (18).

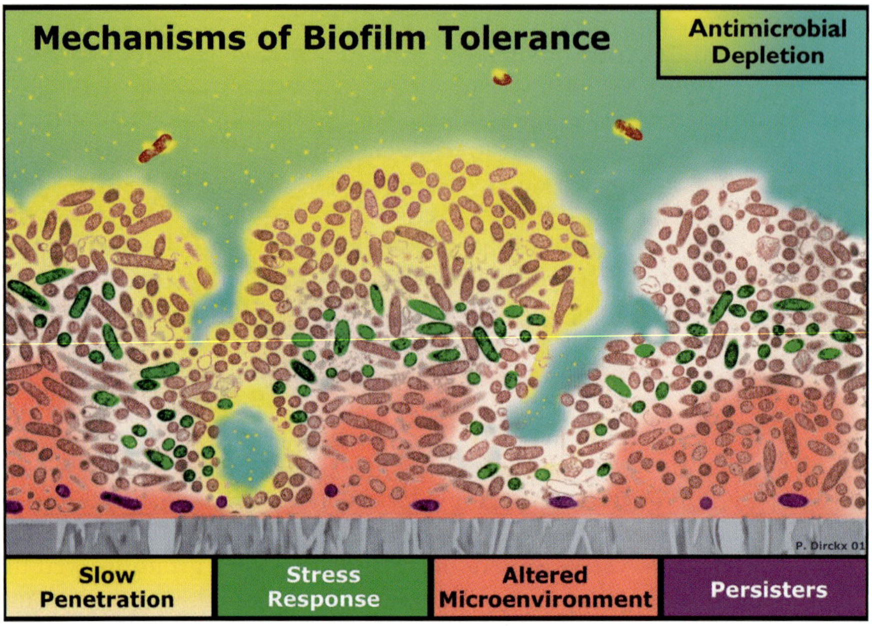

Figure 6. This illustration of bio-film demonstrates the three regions of the bio-film with bacteria in each region having a different bio-film phenotype. This leads to the colony defenses, which protect bio-film from biocides, antibiotics and immune responses.

Stewart has demonstrated that most antibiotics can penetrate the EPS (19), yet the EPS material does contribute to bio-film's antibiotic resistance. It has been shown that beta lactamase can accumulate in the bio-film matrix faster than beta lactam antibiotics can diffuse through the EPS material (20, 21). Also, extracellular polymeric substance is usually positively charged and will adhere aminoglycosides, sequestering this antibiotic away from bacterial cells (22). Properties of the EPS of coag negative staph have been shown to inhibit glycopeptide antibiotics (23, 24).

The EPS material of bio-films provides the necessary structure and function for many of the defenses of bio-film. The bio-film matrix is important for inhibition of host defenses, resistance to antibiotics and resistance to biocides. These are key characteristics of bio-film, which are used to define its presence, setting it apart from planktonic bacteria.

After attachment and production of early EPS material, the planktonic bacteria phenotype quickly changes. This means that each bacterium produces a large number of new proteins not found in its free-floating state. Bio-film bacteria have only a 30 to 50% protein homology in the outer membrane proteins when compared to their genetically identical planktonic counterpart (8, 9). This change in the bacteria is just like the change of a caterpillar into a butterfly. They are genetically identical but structurally and functionally they are vastly different.

The organizational structure of bio-film is critical to its defenses and, therefore, its survival. The three most important layers into which the bacteria will differentiate are the outer edge (which interfaces with the environment), the mid portion of the bio-film, and the metabolically inactive base attached to the surface (Figure 6).

The environmental edge of the bio-film is composed of metabolically active bacterial cells imbedded in the bio-film matrix. All along the surface of the bio-film the bacteria of the environmental edge are in the process of developing small pods, which change back into planktonic cells and are being dispersed out into the environment. This has been termed "seeding dispersal" (25). This appears to be a reproductive mechanism. Also, this portion of the bio-film is constantly shedding large fragments out into the environment, which again is felt to be reproductive but may also provide a defense much like our skin, which constantly sheds.

Another major function of the environmental edge is defensive, and that is to prevent penetration of toxic substances into the bio-film. This has been termed "reaction defusion interaction." When bio-film was treated with high doses of hydrogen peroxide, a microelectrode deep inside the bio-film registered no sign of penetration of the peroxide for over 50 minutes (26). The environmental edge cells catalyzed (reaction) the hydrogen peroxide even after they were dead. The reaction at the environmental edge limits diffusion into the bio-film. This gives bio-film the property of being very resistant to hydrogen peroxide as well as other reactive substances.

In another biocide experiment, glutaraldehyde was tested against *P. aeruginosa* bio-film. Glutaraldehyde showed little or no penetration into the bio-film up to 200 minutes, and it was only at 800 minutes that there was a 3-log killing of the bacteria in the bio-film. On the other hand, the planktonic form of the *P. aeruginosa* from the same strain showed a 3-log killing in just a few minutes (27). With prolonged exposure to monochloromine, bio-film resists penetration and produces a neutralizer (28). Resistance to the penetration and, therefore, the killing by commonly used biocides such a glutaraldehyde, bleach, hydrogen peroxide, acetic acid and others is a very important defense and is often used to define the presence of bio-film.

Bacteria that differentiate into the mid portion phenotype in the bio-film have a different function. These bacteria remain metabolically active, but they are geared to produce protective responses, which are not well understood. Two-D gel experiments show that the mid portion of the bio-film will produce different, yet uncharacterized proteins in a very rapid fashion when the bio-film is subjected to stress. When antibiotics are applied, this region usually has subinhibitory concentrations of these antibiotics (29). This finding plus high cell density with mobile genetic material (30) may allow for the horizontal transfer of resistance in this region. It is unclear what benefit the other protein production confers on the bio-film, but this will probably be found to be very clever defenses.

A better characterized defense is the altered microenvironment in the base of the bio-film. The bacteria, which differentiate in the basilar region of the bio-film where it is attached to a surface, show no metabolic activity. These individual bacteria, whether due to cell-cell signaling, metabolic byproducts, the extremely low oxygen tension in the region, or yet undetermined factors, have shut down all their DNA synthesis, protein synthesis and other cell functions. This may lead to the production of cells that are viable but not culturable (31).

Detachment fragments are "packets" of bacterial cells enveloped in extracellular polymeric substance. Detachment fragments may result from preprogrammed sloughing by the bio-film or from physical forces such as irrigation or debridement. Detachment fragments vary in size from just a few bacterial cells up to a thousand individual bacteria (32). Because of the presence of the EPS material and the metabolic inactivity in the center of the fragment, these detachment fragments have many of the defenses of mature bio-film.

The pre-programmed sloughing of detachment fragments has been thought to be a reproductive mechanism. Because of the defenses that detachment fragments retain, this may make them more successful in reproducing the bio-film. A mature bio-film has the ability to replace its entire mass in approximately 24 hours through the sloughing of detachment fragments (32). This means the entire area of a chronic wound may be reproduced and shed each day. These detachment fragments are shed into the environment and, in the case of a chronic wound, have the ability to "seed" the skin of the host. Because of the intact bio-film defenses of slow penetration, stress response and metabolic inactivity, these detachment fragments are resistant to biocides and antibiotics. This means they are resistant to many surgical preps and prophylactic antibiotics. Detachment fragments can explain why patients with chronic wounds tend to get more surgical site infections than patients who do not have chronic wounds.

Bio-film's most fearsome defense is its ability to reconstitute itself from these detachment fragments and other bio-film residual after disruption. Like a phoenix rising up from the ashes, bio-film can reconstitute its fragments, quickly reestablish its defenses and rise up off the surface. This one property of bio-film bestows upon it, its incredible survivability.

It is bacteria's ability to differentiate into these three different layers, produce EPS material, and reconstitute itself from fragments that has given bio-film its overwhelming success. Of current interest are the mechanisms bio-films possess at the molecular level to commandeer host systems as well as defending against host responses. Bio-films have been able to remain successful over an enormous time period without having to change their structure, function or defenses. They truly are a formidable foe.

MOLECULAR HEALING

Studies have shown that the wound bed of all chronic wounds, regardless of etiology, have excessive presence of neutrophils (1), massive overexpression of active MMP 8 and elevated proinflammatory cytokines (33). Also, the hostile proteolytic environment leads to decreases in cytokines, especially growth factors, degraded receptors on the cell membrane and decreased tissue inhibitors of metalloproteases (34). There is universal acceptance, based on multiple studies, that all chronic wounds are stuck in a chronic inflammatory state. This suggests a common element in every chronic wound. When molecular healing agents such as proinflammatory cytokines, matrix metalloproteases (MMP), tissue inhibitors of metalloprotease (TIMP), etc., are evaluated in chronic wounds, regardless of the etiology and regardless of age, gender, or any other patient factor, they all show a similar biochemistry.

Chronic wounds show a marked increase in proinflammatory cytokines such as interleukin 1, tumor necrosing factor alpha, and gamma interferon.

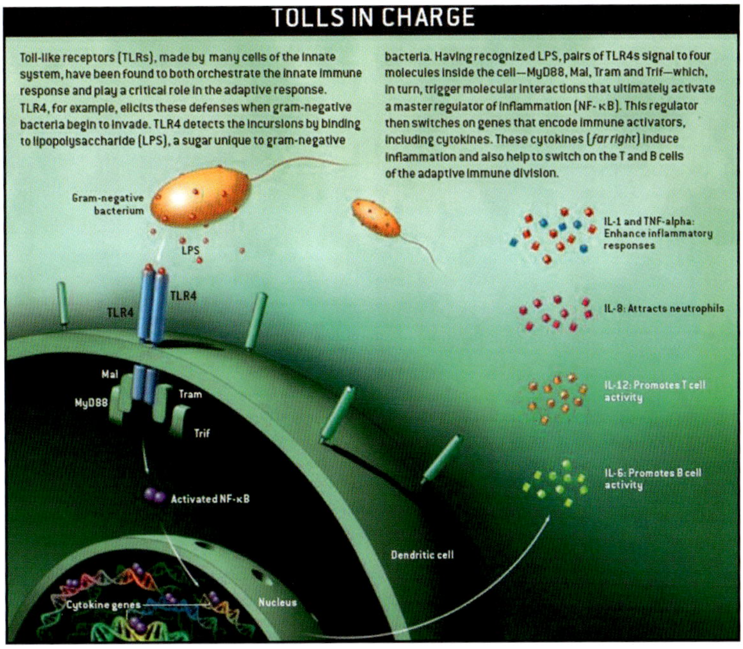

Figure 7. Toll-like receptors of the innate immune system may be the link between wound bio-film and the chronic inflammatory state of chronic wounds.

Matrix metalloproteases (MMP) are upregulated up to 30-fold (35). Also, certain patterns such as increases in matrix metalloprotease 8 (neutrophil-derived) and matrix metalloproteases 2 and 9 (macrophage-derived) are usually present (35). Of the four tissue inhibitors of metalloproteases, tissue inhibitor of metalloprotease 1 (TIMP-1) seems to have the most importance. TIMP-1 is down regulated in chronic wounds, producing a hallmark feature of chronic wounds, which is a very high ratio of MMPs to TIMP-1. The other findings in the chronic wound environment seem to be secondary to the above phenomena. There is a significant decrease in growth factors and cytokines in general due to proteolytic degradation, and there is a reduction in functional receptors on the somatic cells making up the wound bed resulting in their senescence (34).

The presence of the proinflammatory cytokines is interesting and may be explained as a response to foreign agents (Figure 7). The innate immune system is designed to be vigilant and reactive to foreign insults, especially bacteria. Toll-like receptor 4 is very sensitive to LPS material. When LPS material stimulates this receptor, it results in response yielding proinflammatory cytokines (interleukin 1, tumor necrosing factor alpha and gamma interferon). These are chemotactic and inductive biochemicals, which cause the stimulation of the immune system leading to mobilization of cellular and humoral immunity (36). A factor in the ongoing overproduction of proinflammatory cytokines may be explained by the effect of bio-film on the innate immune system.

The most active component of cellular immunity is neutrophils. These are the wolves of the host cellular defenses, running in packs and swarming the invader.

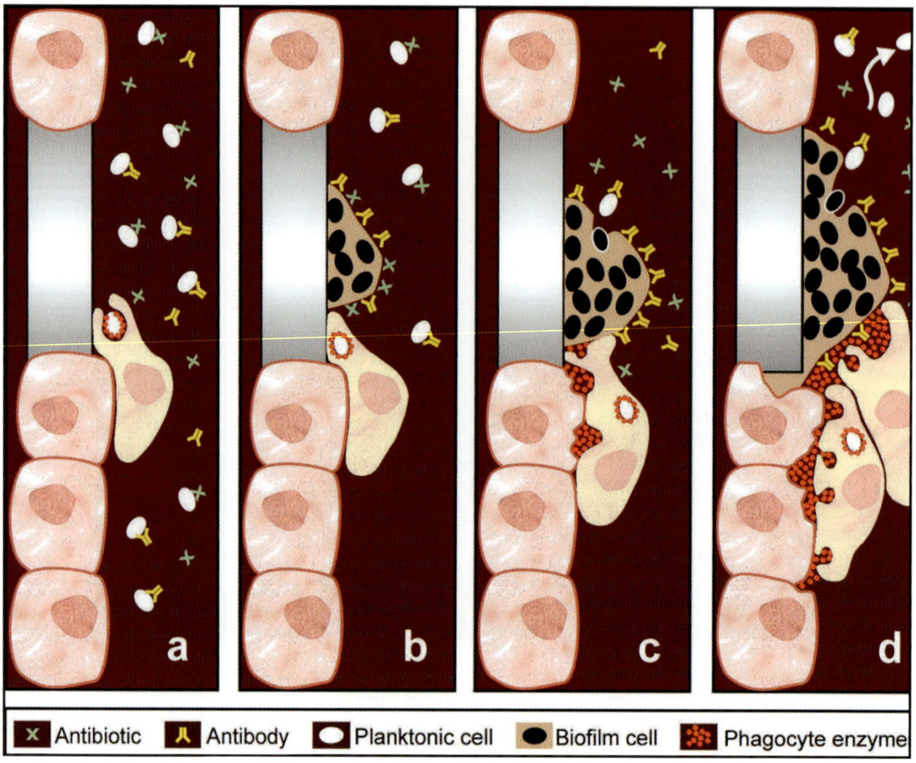

Figure 8. This illustration by Peg Dirks represents the behavior of bacteria on the surface of the lung in cystic fibrosis. It also gives insight into the behavior of bacteria in a wound.
(A) The planktonic bacterium randomly contacts the open surface of a wound. The exposed tissue has no defenses to prevent attachment and the planktonic bacterium quickly attaches.
(B) The individual bacterium quickly divides and creates a small microcolony, which excretes EPS to wall itself off from host defenses and to adhere itself tightly to its substrate. The bacteria begin producing new proteins (differentiation) immediately after attachment.
(C) Once a critical density of bacteria is present, enough signaling molecules will accumulate (quorum sensing), which allows the bacteria to rise up off the surface and differentiate into a complete complex community known as bio-film.
(D) The mature bio-film is impervious to host defenses (white blood cells, antibodies, etc.) and actually uses host mechanisms to cause collateral damage and grow the wound.

It is the ability of the neutrophils to clear the invading bacteria that prevents infection. In chronic wounds it is felt that it is the over recruitment of neutrophils which may play a significant role in the pathophysiology of chronic wounds (37, 38). Armstrong et al. report, "…it can be postulated with some confidence that neutrophil derived MMP 8 is the predominant collagenase present in normal human wounds and that overexpression and activation of this collagenase may be involved in the pathogenesis of nonhealing chronic ulcers (33)." Neutrophils not only express MMP 8 but also other enzymes, which can cause collateral damage such as elastase, myeloperoxidase, and many others (34). It has been shown in cystic fibrosis and may be true in chronic wounds that the overexpression of phagocytic enzymes by the host may cause collateral damage to the host and actual benefit to the bacterial bio-film.

The similar biochemistry in every chronic wound points to a "common cause." Also, the prolonged "chronic inflammatory state" suggests a persistent agent. Bio-film firmly entrenched on the surface of the wound impervious to host defenses is a likely candidate for the common cause of the chronic inflammatory state of chronic wounds.

BIO-FILMS AND CHRONIC WOUNDS

Drs. Bill Costerton and Phil Stewart unintentionally but eloquently demonstrated the connection between bio-film and chronic wounds in a 1999 article in Science (39). In this article on cystic fibrosis, there is an illustration of bio-film in the lung, which is an amazingly accurate conceptualization of what may be taking place in chronic wounds (Figure 8).

The illustration in that article shows that a planktonic bacterium adheres to an exposed susceptible surface. The planktonic bacterium evades host defenses such as antibodies and white blood cells. It is able to form a microcolony with a small amount of EPS and quickly begins differentiating into its different functional components. The bio-film grows, which incites an inflammatory reaction from the host that does collateral damage, which enlarges the wound.

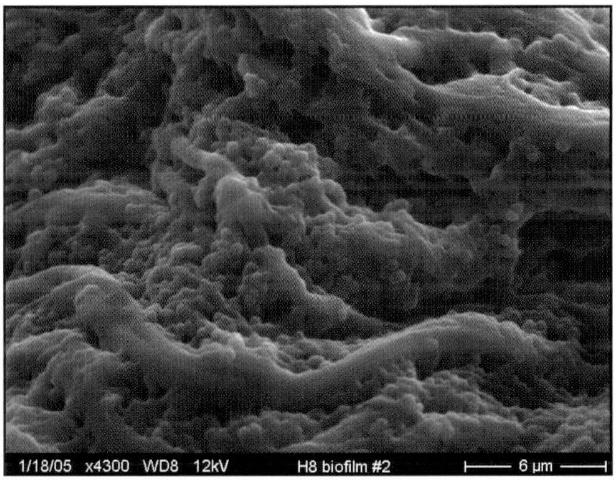

Figure 9. This is scanning electron micrograph of bio-film coating the surface of a venous leg ulcer. Because of the moister environment of a venous leg ulcer the bio-film is thick and very dense. The ECM of the wound bed cannot be seen.

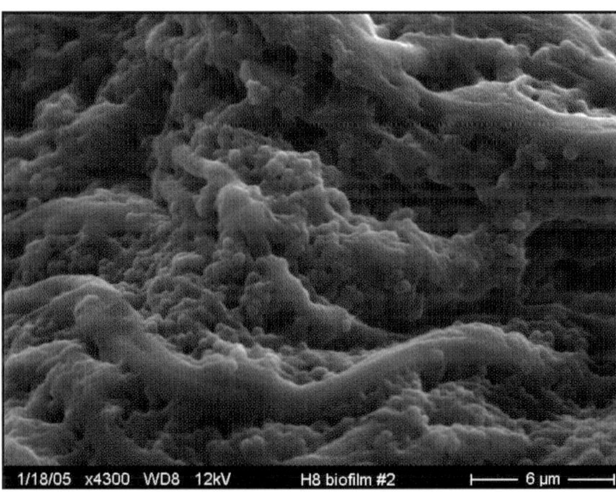

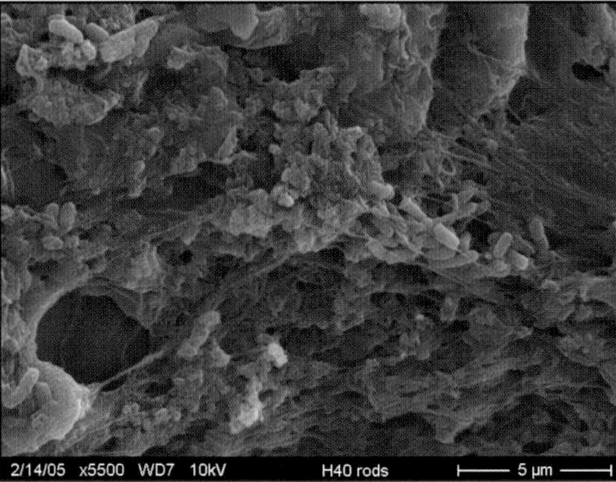

Figure 10. This bio-film present on a diabetic foot ulcer is much thinner and is patchy. The ECM of the wound bed can be easily seen. This is staph aureus, which has the ability to commandeer fibrinogen and form fibrin strands to adhere it more tightly to the surface and protect from host attacks and/or environmental changes in the wound bed.

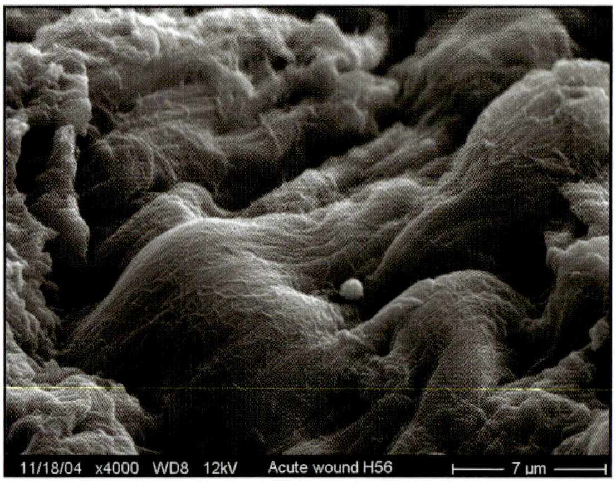

Figure 11. Acute wound electron micrograph showing clean extracellular matrix material and one lone bacterium.

Bio-film is common in our daily lives and is implicated in 60-80% of human infectious diseases (40). We can see it as plaque on our teeth or as slime on a pond rock. So if it is present on chronic wounds, why haven't we recognized it and what does it look like?

In the literature, slough is commonly referred to as dead host tissue with some proteinaceous exudate, white blood cells and bacteria (41). Slough is a frequent target of sharp debridement yet in the majority of wounds it reaccumulates by the next week. The slough is removed week after week and yet the wound does not get deeper. Where does the new layer of "dead tissue" come from each week? Slough acts more like a living organism growing on the surface of the wound. Indeed slough is a well-differentiated polymicrobial multicellular organism growing on the surface of chronic wounds. Slough is bio-film.

Slough found on chronic wounds has many of the physical characteristics of bio-film grown in a laboratory. But can slough really be bio-film? And if it is bio-film, is it really keeping the wound open?

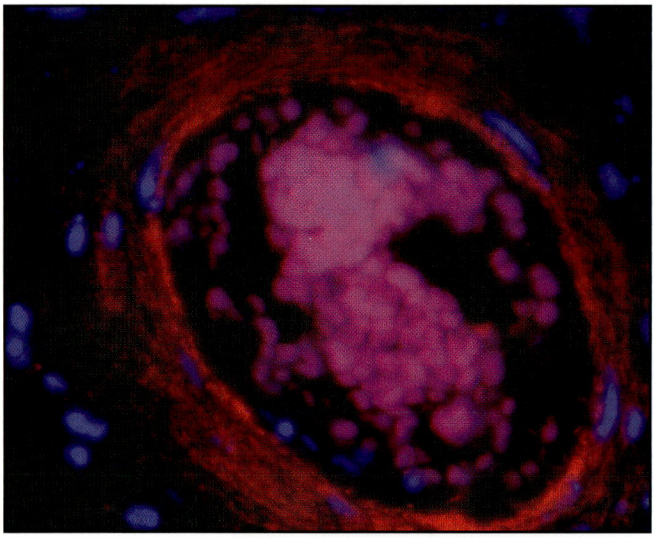

Figure 12. A dense population of Pseudomonas aeruginosa cells can be seen organized around a capillary in this mouse model of a burn-inection. The P. aeruginosa cells are stained red using fluorescent in situ hybridization (FISH). Eukaryotic nuclei are stained blue, and red blood cells are stained pink. Image courtesy of Kendra Rumbaugh, Ph.D.

James et al. pursued microscopic evaluation of acute and chronic wounds. The gram stains of the chronic wounds suggested that there were multiple species of bacteria present on each wound. Also, bacteria tend to penetrate deeply into intact tissue with capillaries present, and there was quite a bit of amorphous material surrounding the bacteria consistent with bio-film (42).

Using scanning electromicroscopy there appeared to be organized bio-film with extracellular polymeric substance adhered around colony bacteria in up to 70% of the chronic wounds (42). One of the problems with scanning electromicroscopy of chronic wounds is that the preparation of the samples distorts the bio-film matrix. Also, scanning electromicroscopy looks at a very small area of the total wound bed and frequently may have only been looking at degraded material, which was too difficult to define. These difficulties may have lead to an underreporting of bio-film in chronic wounds (Figures 9 and 10).

The same methodology was used to evaluate 16 acute wounds (Figure 11). Only one of the 16 wounds was found to have any bio-film (42). Most of these wounds were in the same limb and even in the same area as a chronic wound that was present. Yet each one healed quickly in two to three weeks, whereas the chronic wound in the same area was still open two to three months later.

This difference in healing between acute and chronic wounds is indirect evidence that bio-film may be an essential barrier to healing. It seems that two wounds having the same host defenses and the same host healing properties available to them should heal the same. Yet the acute wounds without bio-film healed while the chronic wounds with bio-film did not. Bio-film must be the barrier to healing.

Rumbaugh et al. using green fluorescent PAO1 (*P. aeruginosa*) have

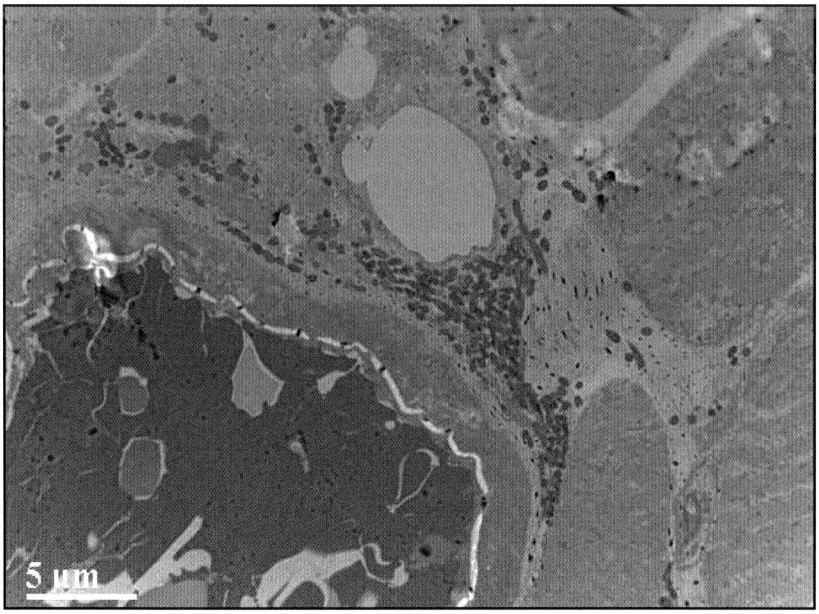

Figure 13. This high-pressure fast freeze transmission electron micrograph demonstrates a capillary with bio-film tightly adhered to a capillary basement membrane using the capillary for structural support and for nutrition.

determined some very interesting early bio-film behavior in a burn mouse model (43). Bio-film was shown to form within three hours in the adipose tissue. Using confocal microscopy the bio-film was observed to penetrate deeply (1–2 millimeters) through the adipose tissue in tubular "green rivers" of epifluorescence encompassing capillaries and venules (Figures 12 and 13). Rumbaugh et al. have termed this "perivascular cuffing" by the bio-film. Of interest is that planktonic PAO1 develop bio-film early (three hours) in the mouse host and preferentially spreads along the vascular system in adipose tissue (43).

These findings correlate with our microscopic studies of the human wound bed that showed bio-film penetration deeper than expected. Bio-films may use the capillary and venular walls as the preferred surface to spread, which raises some interesting possibilities. Since the bio-film is impervious to the host defenses, proximity to the vasculature would not be detrimental. Also it may be that bio-film feeds more off the transudate from the vasculature system than necrotic tissue. Bio-film, through direct contact, production of counterfeit signaling molecules, or stimulation of host inflammatory pathways, may control transudate production for its own nourishment.

These studies demonstrate that bio-films are prevalent on chronic wounds, and that bio-film does not appear to play a significant role on the surfaces of acute wounds. Also it is clear that wound bio-films contain multiple species of bacteria. Bio-film forms quickly in an impaired host and penetrates into the surface of the wound possibly using vascular structures as a surface. Although these studies show that these polymicrobial bio-films are prevalent on chronic wounds, it still needs to be shown how wound bio-film plays a significant role in producing wound healing impairment.

TREATING WOUNDS AS IF BIO-FILM IS THE CAUSE

Is the bio-film on the surface of chronic wounds just filling a niche that is open, or are the bacteria intentionally keeping the wound from healing? The direct evidence and exact mechanisms of how bio-film impairs wound healing still needs to be worked out, but until then there is clinical evidence that bio-film is a major barrier in nonhealing wounds. If suppression of bio-film through multiple simultaneous strategies enables wounds to heal better, then there is good indirect evidence that bio-film is producing impaired wound healing.

Medicine is behind when it comes to management of bio-films. Although the majority of human infectious diseases are bio-film based and many nosocomial reservoirs of resistant bacteria are bio-film problems, medicine has been slow to respond to the concept of bio-film. Antibacterial bio-film agents have long histories in industry such as manufacturing, food preparation, food packaging, meatpacking, dairy, dentistry and the petroleum industry. The literature concerning bio-film in these industries has volumes of information on agents that are effective against bio-films. Many of these industrial agents used to control bio-film hold promise in medicine.

Lactoferrin

Lactoferrin is used for many purposes. Meat packing plants use it to treat the surfaces of meat to prevent bio-film formation. Lactoferrin has also been a popular nutritional supplement for a number of decades, which may have contributed to a lack of rigorous study of this very powerful component of the innate immune system. Copious amounts of lactoferrin are in human external secretions, such as tears, saliva, mucous, milk, etc. Since lactoferrin is a main component of the innate immune system and ubiquitous in surface secretions, it seems logical that lactoferrin would play a significant role in antimicrobial surface protection of the host. Exactly what roles it plays and how it plays those roles is just now coming to light.

Singh and coworkers demonstrated that lactoferrin prevents free-floating (planktonic) *P. aeruginosa* from attaching to a surface. If the attachment is prevented, then bio-film formation is prevented. It seems that as a planktonic bacterium adheres to a surface in the presence of lactoferrin, the movement of the individual bacterium (referred to as twitching) is increased. If twitching is increased for the parent cell and all its progeny, they fail to group into microcolonies, which is the first step in expressing bio-film behavior. In Singh's study, *P. aeruginosa* cultures without lactoferrin demonstrated thick bio-film formation. When lactoferrin was added, the planktonic bacteria were able to divide but not attach, so no bio-film structures were identified (44). Lactoferrin worked purely in preventing the attachment of planktonic bacteria, thus preventing bio-film formation.

To determine if lactoferrin is effective in managing wounds, the author's group conducted an eight-week prospective randomized controlled study of 50 patients. Twenty-five patients with a total of 37 wounds were randomly placed in the lactoferrin gel treatment group while the control group was randomly assigned 25 patients with 30 wounds receiving the same gel without lactoferrin. The study demonstrated that patients receiving lactoferrin gel had a higher percentage of wounds with complete healing in the eight weeks. Overall lactoferrin was an effective agent for improvement in the healing of chronic wounds (Wolcott, RD, unpublished *www.woundcarecenter.net*).

Xylitol

Xylitol, as well as other sugar alcohols such as sorbitol, have an absence of reducing carbonyl groups, which exerts a negative effect on the formation of extracellular polymeric substance. Xylitol has been documented to bind to the outer membrane of pathogenic organisms such as strep mutans and makes the outer structures of these organisms less effective. The most common finding is that there is a lower ability of pathogenic organisms to adhere to epithelial cell surfaces and other host structure surfaces. Recent scanning electron microscopy of *Streptococcus pneumoniae* treated with xylitol showed marked cell wall changes (45).

Xylitol has shown clinical efficacy in use to prevent bio-film-based diseases of dental plaque, otitis media and sinusitis. Katsuyama et al. showed that use of Xylitol along with farnesol synergistically inhibited *S. aureus* bio-film formation on the epidermis, which produces the symptoms of atopic dermatitis (46, 47). Using volunteers with normal microflora and patients with atopic dermatitis, which cultured *S. aureus*, xylitol and farnesol inhibited bio-film formation. In their study using scanning electron microscopy, xylitol inhibited the formation of glycocalyces (EPS) in *S. aureus* through unknown pathways (46).

QUORUM SENSING INHIBITORS

An exciting area in antibacterial bio-film agents is in the specific signaling agents that can control the language of bio-films. The original name given to these signaling agents was quorum-sensing molecules because it required a critical density of individual bacteria (quorum) to trigger bio-film gene expression. In other words, a certain number of these molecules needed to be present to cause upregulation or downregulation of operons and regulons, which controls a suite of genes responsible for bio-film formation. It was clear from the beginning that if this communication language could be understood, certain behaviors could be blocked, thus subverting the impenetrable defenses of bio-film.

Many gram-positive bacteria such as *S. aureus* produce RNA-III Activating Peptide (RAP). Once enough of RAP accumulates around its receptor called Target of RNA-III Activating Peptide (TRAP), that receptor is upregulated. Phosphorylation of TRAP, in turn, upregulates the agr regulon. The agr regulon is responsible for production of RNA-III, but also contains a number of other genes responsible for bio-film behavior. RNA-III works to upregulate the production of toxins such as hemolysin, enterotoxin B, and other virulence factors. These virulence factors can be considered the offensive weapons of *S. aureus*. Other upregulated genes produce defensive mechanisms such as the extracellular polymeric substance, phenotype changes (differentiation) and the other bio-film factors. Therefore, it was hoped that by blocking the stimulation of the agr regulon, *S. aureus* would show less bio-film behavior, and not cause the tissue destruction that is so often seen with the *S. aureus* (48).

RNA-III Inhibitory Peptide (RIP). A seven amino acid peptide that blocks TRAP was discovered. Because it inhibited the effects of RAP, it was given the name RNA-III Inhibitory Peptide (RIP). RNA-III Inhibitory Peptide is a gram-positive quorum sensing inhibitor. RIP blocks RAP and, therefore, the upregulation of the agr regulon. RIP, a true quorum sensing inhibitor, only blocks bio-film behavior, but it does not kill planktonic bacteria (49).

Animal studies using mice with infected metal devices showed that mice treated with RIP were able to clear their bio-films with antibiotics whereas mice not treated with RIP were not able to clear the bio-film from the metal devices (50). This is a very exciting step towards specific, well-understood agents for use in clinical wound care.

BIOCIDES

Nonspecific Biocides

Nonspecific biocides are common in chronic wound care management but need to be carefully reexamined. What makes a biocide nonspecific is its ability to attack any organic material, bacterial or host. Therefore, agents such as acetic acid, carbolic acid, bleach, alcohol, Mercurochrome, Betadine and many other agents can attack bacteria, but also attack and do harm to the host.

Studies over the last two decades have shown that all these non-specific biocides impair the healing process in chronic wounds. Bio-film is the best explanation for this. In thc laboratory, full-strength bleach placed on a bio-film for up to 60 minutes only kills about one-half the bacteria making up the bio-film (51). Whereas just **60 seconds** of 5% bleach (Dakin's solution) will kill 100 percent of all host cells and denature important proteins such as antibodies, growth factors, etc. The bio-film that is only partially damaged quickly repairs itself while it takes much longer for the host (especially the impaired host) to regenerate the cell lines it needs for healing. Nonspecific biocides do more damage to the host than to the bio-film; therefore, they should be avoided.

Silver Compounds

More specific agents against bacteria that spare host cells and proteins have been developed and are gaining wider use in wound care. Probably none is more popular than silver compounds.

Silver appears to work through inhibiting cell respiration, cell membrane disruption and denaturing of nucleic acids. It is probable that these multiple pathways contribute to the lack of resistance seen with silver use. In vivo, much higher concentrations of silver are necessary to achieve antimicrobial effects. In biologic fluids, 12.5 to 25 parts per million of silver atoms are needed to be bacteriocidal. Acticoat™ (trademark of Smith and Nephew) has been shown to obtain these levels and, interestingly, is proving some efficacy against mature bio-film.

Multiple Concurrent Strategies

However, using only one selective pressure will be quickly overcome by bio-film adaptation because of the law of large numbers. Bio-films have high density of bacteria (10–8th/cm^2) with a protective coating. Through normal spontaneous mutation rates (1/10–6th), stress response, posttranslational modification and bacterial synergies, the bacteria present will quickly adapt to any single attack. This has led Fux et al. to postulate that a combined strategy will be necessary to clear bio-film (30).

The use of lactoferrin, xylitol, quorum sensing inhibitors, antibiotics, and specific biocides is not mutually exclusive. Synergies using multiple concurrent strategies are scientifically possible. So it seems reasonable that combinations of these agents should allow us to be more successful in managing bio-film.

DEBRIDEMENT

Debridement of the wound is the central point around which all the other elements of wound care must revolve. The physical removal of bio-film gives the best chance at healing. "Industry currently relies on mechanical cleansing and oxidative biocides; the former removes bio-film and the latter gradually dissolves the bio-film matrix material and eventually kills the sessile cells" (4). In every industry sector and in our daily lives, when we deal with bio-film, removal is the primary goal.

Steed et al. reported that extensive frequent debridement was a positive independent variable in the healing of diabetic foot wounds. Steed concluded, "Debridement is a vital adjunct to the care of patients with chronic diabetic foot ulcers" (52). Unfortunately there have been few important studies looking at wound debridement since that time (41).

Recently Steed revisited wound debridements stating, "Despite the fact that most physicians, and certainly all surgeons, know what debridement is, there is no universal agreement on how to debride, when to debride, or how much tissue to take. Similarly, although it is widely recognized that debridement is a key element to wound healing, there are few randomized controlled studies showing the benefit of debridement". Steed went on to say, "Although every surgeon can attest to the benefit of debridement, the literature does not elaborate on it" (53). This does not put wound debridement on a very strong scientific foundation. However, bio-film based wound care may provide some insight into the questions that Steed poses as to when, how often, and how much to debride.

There is universal acceptance that devitalized tissue produces no positive effect on wound healing. Therefore, sharp removal of devitalized tissue seems to accelerate wound healing by removal of a food source for bacteria as well as relieving the host of the burden of autolytically removing dead material. Also sharp debridement exposes a new wound bed, which has not been subjected to the excess proteolytic environment of the chronic wound, stuck in the chronic inflammatory phase. This exposes new cells that aren't senescent, cells that aren't stripped of their receptors and cells that are better perfused. Yet in the context of wound bio-film, frequent debridement accomplishes much more than this.

Sibbald et al. showed that the removal of "bioburden" from the wound has significant important benefits for wound bed preparation and, therefore, for wound healing (54). How much more important is removal when the bioburden is not a random group of individual bacteria but an organized bio-film? Removing wound bio-film may be the most important factor of wound debridement.

Science can provide insight into the frequency of debridement. Steed's group showed that patients debrided frequently had a significantly higher healing rate than those debrided less often (52). Also, experiments suggest bio-film reconstitutes itself within ten hours and is a young functional bio-film within 24 to 48 hours (55). Also, dental plaque will form a climax, mature bio-film community 50–100 microns thick within just one week if left undisturbed (56). Other bio-film experiments suggest that moisture, types of bacteria, host factors, nutrient source, etc., all impact the time it takes for bio-film to reestablish itself on the surface of a wound.

Our personal experience can also give us some guidance on the frequency of wound debridements. We see from our personal experience that we manage bio-film at different frequencies based on their environments. In a very moist environment such as our mouth, we remove the bio-film by brushing twice a day. In the intermittently wet environment of a shower we scrub two times a week and in the drier environment with intermittent use such as the trash can lid we manage the surface once a week. The moister the environment, the greater the food source and the greater the bacterial seeding, the more frequent is the need to debride.

Frequent removal of bio-film from surfaces is the mainstay for preventing damage by bio-film. The frequent removal of bio-film reduces toxins, proteases, excessive neutrophils, and the molecules that bio-film produces to commandeer host systems. Also the physical disruption of EPS material exposes parts of the bio-film to the treating agents such as specific biocides, anti-bio-film agents and host defenses. It has also been shown that young bio-films are less resistant to antibiotics and biocides and that resistance increases with maturity of the bio-film (4, 57). Therefore, frequent debridement keeps bio-films suppressed and more sensitive to wound care treatments. Two guiding principles for debridement have emerged out of this experiential and scientific knowledge base. These debridement recommendations will still require scientific validation.

The first principle of bio-film based wound care is shaping the wound to favor the host over the bio-film. Surfaces favor bio-film; therefore, tunnels, undermining, tracks, redundant folds in the wound bed or any condition that causes two wound surfaces to touch, favor the bio-film (4, 5, 30). So it is important through sharp debridement to open tracks, tunnels, undermining, etc., and shape the surface of the wound (saucerize). Hopefully, over the first few debridements the wound bed architecture can be changed to favor the host. Then as the wound heals, it is still very important to assess the shape of the wound each visit.

The second principle of debridement in bio-film based wound care is to frequently remove the slough (bio-film) from the surface of the wound. We have learned from dental plaque that brushing twice a day is better than once a day for the prevention of cavities (58). We have learned from science that we have a better chance at suppressing a young bio-film than a more mature bio-film. We have learned from industry that frequent removal of bio-film from a surface reduces the destruction that it does to that surface. And from our personal experience we realize there are a number of variables that impact bio-film and dictate when it needs to be removed.

In the final analysis the clinician will have to decide the timing of the surface management of bio-film based on the appearance of the wound. Generally a chronic wound will require sharp debridement every one to two weeks to manage wound bio-film. An important factor to consider is the environment of the wound. For example, venous leg ulcers tend to drain edema fluid as well as exudate from inflamed capillaries, making them a moister environment. In impaired hosts, bio-film tends to be faster growing. In limbs with critical limb ischemia, bio-films may not grow as fast, but even the small amount that bio-film does grow may have a large impact on the marginal tissue. This may contribute to the dying back often seen in ischemic wounds. These wounds may require more than once a week debridement.

The goal of debridement in bio-film-based wound care is to develop a wound bed free of any necrotic material, which is granular, red in appearance, and ready for proactive wound care treatment such as tissue engineered skin or growth factors.

ANTIBIOTICS

In a bio-film system of wound management, antibiotics are an adjunct to therapy. Antibiotics are just one piece of the overall program. Bio-film must be removed frequently and then multiple strategies are engaged to keep it suppressed. Using high dose antibiotics for longer periods (30–60 days) in a coordinated system of multiple strategies, which achieves wound healing

in a reasonable time (20 weeks) may decrease overall antibiotic exposure.

But using antibiotics as a single strategy, without regard to the dose or duration, is not appropriate.

The use of antibiotics in terms of dose and duration is controversial in many bio-film-based human infections. Yet Fux et al. state, "Successful treatment in these cases (bio-film infections) depends on long-term, high dose antibiotic therapies and the removal of any foreign body material" (30). This statement is widely accepted for bio-film disease and supported by the emerging science.

Several bio-film-based diseases can be used to give guidance for antibiotic regimens for treatment of chronic wounds. In treating native value endocarditis it has been demonstrated that antibiotics are more successful when used at ten times the minimal bacteriocidal concentration for the entire course of treatment (59) and that longer durations are better (60). Osteomyelitis, prostatitis and other bio-film diseases tend also to be treated with high doses of antibiotics for long durations, usually exceeding one month. The need for this long and strong approach to antibiotics for bio-film diseases is based on bio-film's inherent resistance to antibiotics.

Identifying bacteria and their antibiotic sensitivity is predicated on the time-honored methods for determining antibiotic sensitivities. These antibiotic sensitivity tests always use planktonic bacteria in exponential growth phase to determine minimal inhibitory concentration and minimal bacteriocidal concentration (30). Bio-films, causing greater than 60% of human infections (7), are fundamentally different from planktonic bacteria and are highly resistant to antibiotics and biocides. This suggests that classical culturing and antibiotic sensitivity tests are not sufficient for bio-film diseases.

Denaturing Gradient Gel Electrophoresis (DGGE) has demonstrated in venous leg ulcers (61) and in all wound etiologies (62) that the bacteria within the bio-films of wounds are much more diverse than what is cultured. This is explained by the finding that much of the bacterial cell population is dormant yet still alive, and difficult to culture (31). These bacteria are exceedingly resistant to antibiotics, yet if they can be isolated and grown on fresh medium in planktonic conditions, they can regain their antibiotic sensitivity (21). These findings have led to the concept of "viable but not culturable."

Many experiments have demonstrated that the superficial layers of bio-film are susceptible to high, prolonged doses of antibiotics for reasons noted above. These high levels are 50 to 1000 times higher than required to kill planktonic cells. This has produced a "top to bottom" killing pattern for antibiotics in in vitro bio-films (21, 22). However, it may be that instead of producing cell death, these antibiotics may only damage the cell, allowing it to protect deeper layers (30). This or other adaptive mechanisms like it must be true or we could just kill the bio-film a layer at a time by prolonged use of antibiotics. This strategy does not work at all with bio-film.

Bio-films adapt. Bio-films have been shown to change their susceptibility to antibiotics after a 2- to 3-log killing. Bio-films first lose their surface layers, and then the pattern of antibiotic killing becomes patchy, and then ineffective (63–65). It is clear that antibiotics alone cannot eradicate a bio-film, neither in the lab nor in the patient.

The management of wound bio-film, with a goal of producing a wound bed with suppressed bio-film, will necessarily include multiple concurrent strategies.

Antibiotics used based on current sensitivity techniques in high doses for durations longer than 4 weeks are appropriate only when combined with other strategies and if clinical progression is evident. Antibiotics, when combined with frequent debridement, anti bio-film agents (lactoferrin, xylitol, etc.), specific biocides, and anti bio-film dressings are clinically important in obtaining a self-sustaining wound bed. Once a healthy wound bed is obtained that can respond to proactive wound healing agents, antibiotics can still play a role in bio-film suppression. The concept is not eradication of the bio-film but rather suppression until the wound is healed and the reservoir is closed.

ADVANCED TECHNOLOGIES

The advanced technologies being brought to bear on chronic wound care are awe-inspiring. But all the advanced technologies need to be evaluated in the context of bio-film. For example, the tissue-engineered product, Apligraf®, uses living human cells including fibroblasts and keratinocytes. These cells are proactive agents in stimulating healing pathways within the chronic wound to achieve faster complete wound healing. However, in the presence of bio-film deeply embedded in the surface of the wound, these cells may become counterproductive.

To place the nutrient rich bilayer of Apligraf® on a wound that is still heavily laden with bio-film provides a surface and a food source for the bio-film to use. The naked keratinocytes and fibroblasts that are exposed are no match for the organized multicellular organism on which it is laid. This creates quick degradation of the graft, increased exudate, odor and erythema along with a deterioration of the wound. Clearly some wounds have excessive bioburden, but even wounds with 100% granulating tissue and little or no visible slough can possess bio-film, which will ambush the graft that is applied.

It is important with graft material to provide some sort of protection for the cells that are being applied to the wound bed. Using anti-bio-film agents such as xylitol and lactoferrin can keep bio-films suppressed and prevent bio-film from harming the cells. Also, antibiotics systemically and sometimes topically can protect the graft and allow it to be much more effective in increasing wound healing. Additionally, selective biocides such as silver have proven to be a very good adjunct in protecting the tissue engineered grafts from the ravages of bio-film.

Other advanced technologies include small peptide or protein cytokines. Platelet derived growth factor, PDGF (REGRANEX Gel) is commercially available. It has had limited success even in its initial clinical studies, not because it is not a potent growth factor but because of the hostile proteolytic wound bed environment. The proteolytic enzymes and excessive neutrophils produced by the wound bed in response to the bio-film also destroy the exogenously applied PDGF.

Therefore, when these protein cytokines are brought into the clinical setting, their effects have been disappointing. Eming et al. state, "However the outcome of the clinical studies, up to now demonstrates that an important often underestimated aspect of the growth factor wound healing paradigm is the effective delivery of these polypeptides to the wound site. However, the wound site is often a relatively hostile environment. Consequently, it is possible that a great deal of growth factor activity is either lost by binding to other molecules in the extracellular space or by being subjected to degradative action of exogenous enzymes released by inflammatory and mesenchymal cells during the course of wound repair and remodeling" (66). The presence of wound bio-film causing recruitment of excessive numbers of active neutrophils, along with excess proteolytic enzymes, seems to be the single most important barrier to the efficacy of exogenously applied peptides.

Once wound bio-film is adequately suppressed and host-healing barriers are adequately addressed, then exogenously applied cytokines can be and are successful. Early work involving frequent debridement of wounds conducted by Steed et al. showed that a properly prepared wound was responsive to exogenously applied platelet derived growth factor (52). Recent clinical experience suggests that use of bio-film suppression agents along with debridement produces enough anti-proteolytic effect on the wound to allow exogenous peptides to be successful.

CONCLUSION

A planktonic concept of the bacteria present on the surface of a chronic wound is no longer viable. Microscopic studies show that bio-film is present on chronic wounds yet does not seem to be prominent on the surface of acute wounds. Bio-film is able to neutralize our host defenses and commandeer host systems, and possesses an impressive array of defenses and virulence factors. Clinically we see a significant difference in the healing behavior between chronic and acute wounds. Also, suppression of bio-film using multiple simultaneous strategies including debridement, anti-bio-film agents, specific biocides, antibiotics and advanced technologies improves wound healing. This suggests bio-film plays an important role in delayed wound healing.

REFERENCE

1. Diegelmann RF. Excessive neutrophils characterize chronic pressure ulcers. *Wound Repair Regen* 2003 Nov;11(6):490-5.
2. Mertz PM. Cutaneous Bio-films: Friend or Foe? *Wounds: A Compendium of Clinical Research and Practice* 2003 May;15(5):1-9.
3. Percival SL, Bowler Philip G. *Bio-films and Their Potential Role in Wound Healing. Wounds* 2004 Jul;16(7):234-40.
4. Donlan RM, Costerton JW. Bio-films: survival mechanisms of clinically relevant microorganisms. *Clin Microbiol Rev* 2002 Apr;15(2):167-93.
5. Stoodley P, Sauer K, Davies DG, Costerton JW. Bio-films as complex differentiated communities. *Annual Review of Microbiology* 2002;56(1):187-209.
6. Costerton JW, Lewandowski Z, Caldwell DE, Korber DR, Lappin-Scott HM. Microbial bio-films. *Annu Rev Microbiol* 1995;49:711-45.
7. Costerton JW, Stewart PS, Greenberg EP. Bacterial bio-films: a common cause of persistent infections. *Science* 1999 May 21;284(5418):1318-22.
8. Sauer K, Camper AK. Characterization of phenotypic changes in Pseudomonas putida in response to surface-associated growth. *J Bacteriol* 2001;183:6579.
9. Sauer K, Camper AK, Ehrlich GD, Costerton JW, Davies DG. Pseudomonas aeruginosa displays multiple phenotypes during development as a bio-film. *J Bacteriol* 2002;184:1140.
10. Brozel VS, Cloete TEE, Strydom GM. A method for the study of de novo protein synthesis in Pseudomonas aeruginosa after attachment. *Biofouling* 1995;8:195.
11. Whiteley M, Bangera MG, Bumgarner RE, Parsek MR, Teitzel GM, Lory S, et al. Gene expression in Pseudomonas aeruginosa bio-films. *Nature* 2001 Oct 25;413(6858):860-4.
12. Prigent-Combaret C, Vidal O, Dorel C, Lejeune P. Abiotic surface sensing and bio-film-dependent regulation of gene expression in Escherichia coli. *Journal of Bacteriology* 1999;181(19):5993-6002.
13. Whitchurch CB, Tolker-Nielsen T, Ragas PC, Mattick JS. Extracellular DNA required for bacterial bio-film formation. *Science* 2002 Feb 22;295(5559):1487.
14. Stewart PS. Matrix mysteries hold keys to controlling bio-films. Web 2006 February 15Available from: URL: *http://www.bio-filmsonline.com/cgi-bin/bio-filmsonline/00345.html*
15. Vuong C, Kocianova S, Voyich JM, Yao Y, Fischer ER, DeLeo FR, et al. A crucial role for exopolysaccharide modification in bacterial bio-film formation, immune evasion, and virulence. *J Biol Chem* 2004 Dec 24;279(52):54881-6.
16. Shiau AL, Wu CL. The inhibitory effect of Staphylococcus epidermidis slime on the phagocytosis of murine peritoneal macrophages is interferon-independent. *Microbiol Immunol* 1998;42(1):33-40.
17. Meluleni GJ, Grout M, Evans DJ, Pier GB. Mucoid Pseudomonas aeruginosa growing in a bio-film in vitro are killed by opsonic antibodies to the mucoid exopolysaccharide capsule but not by antibodies produced during chronic lung infection in cystic fibrosis patients. *J Immunol* 1995 Aug 15;155(4):2029-38.
18. Vuong C, Voyich JM, Fischer ER, Braughton KR, Whitney AR, DeLeo FR, et al. Polysaccharide intercellular adhesin (PIA) protects Staphylococcus epidermidis against major components of the human innate immune system. *Cellular Microbiology* 2004 Mar;6(3):269-75.
19. Stewart PS. Theoretical aspects of antibiotic diffusion into microbial bio-films. *Antimicrob Agents Chemother* 1996 Nov;40(11):2517-22.
20. Bagge N, Hentzer M, Andersen JB, Ciofu O, Givskov M, Hoiby N. Dynamics and spatial distribution of beta-lactamase expression in Pseudomonas aeruginosa bio-films. *Antimicrob Agents Chemother* 2004 Apr;48(4):1168-74.

21. Anderl JN, Zahller J, Roe F, Stewart PS. Role of nutrient limitation and stationary-phase existence in Klebsiella pneumoniae bio-film resistance to ampicillin and ciprofloxacin. *Antimicrobial Agents And Chemotherapy* 2003 Apr;47(4):1251-6.

22. Walters MC, III, Roe F, Bugnicourt A, Franklin MJ, Stewart PS. Contributions of antibiotic penetration, oxygen limitation, and low metabolic activity to tolerance of Pseudomonas aeruginosa bio-films to ciprofloxacin and tobramycin. *Antimicrob Agents Chemother* 2003 Jan;47(1):317-23.

23. Konig C, Schwank S, Blaser J. Factors compromising antibiotic activity against bio-films of Staphylococcus epidermidis. *European Journal Of Clinical Microbiology & Infectious Diseases: Official Publication Of The European Society Of Clinical Microbiology* 2001 Jan;20(1):20-6.

24. Souli M, Giamarellou H. Effects of slime produced by clinical isolates of coagulase-negative staphylococci on activities of Various antimicrobial agents. *Antimicrobial Agents And Chemotherapy* 1998;42(4):939-41.

25. Purevdorj-Gage B, Costerton WJ, Stoodley P. Phenotypic differentiation and seeding dispersal in non-mucoid and mucoid Pseudomonas aeruginosa bio-films. *Microbiology* 2005 May;151(Pt 5):1569-76.

26. Stewart PS, Roe F, Rayner J, Elkins JG, Lewandowski Z, Ochsner UA, et al. Effect of catalase on hydrogen peroxide penetration into Pseudomonas aeruginosa bio-films. *Applied and Environmental Microbiology* 2000;66(2):836-8.

27. Stewart PS, Grab L, Diemer JA. Analysis of biocide transport limitation in an artificial bio-film system. *J Appl Microbiol* 1998 Sep;85(3):495-500.

28. Sanderson SS, Stewart PS. Evidence of Bacterial Adaption to Monochloramine in Pseudomonas aeruginosa Bio-films and Evaluation of biocide Action Model. *Biotechnol Bioeng* 1987.

29. Rachid S, Ohlsen K, Witte W, Hacker J, Ziebuhr W. Effect of subinhibitory antibiotic concentrations on polysaccharide intercellular adhesin expression in bio-film-forming Staphylococcus epidermidis. *Antimicrobial Agents And Chemotherapy* 2000 Dec;44(12):3357-63.

30. Fux CA, Costerton JW, Stewart PS, Stoodley P. Survival strategies of infectious bio-films. *Trends in Microbiology* 2005 Jan;13(1):34-40.

31. Rayner MG, Zhang Y, Gorry MC, Chen Y, Post JC, Ehrlich GD. Evidence of bacterial metabolic activity in culture-negative otitis media with effusion. *Journal of the American Medical Association* 1998;279(4):296-9.

32. Stoodley P, Wilson S, Hall-Stoodley L, Boyle JD, Lappin-Scott HM, Costerton JW. Growth and detachment of cell clusters from mature mixed species bio-films. *Appl Environ Microbiol* 2001;67:5608.

33. Armstrong DG, Jude EB. The role of matrix metalloproteinases in wound healing. *J Am Podiatr Med Assoc* 2002 Jan;92(1):12-8.

34. Yager DR, Nwomeh BC. The proteolytic environment of chronic wounds. *Wound Repair Regen* 1999 Nov;7(6):433-41.

35. Trengove NJ, Stacey MC, MacAuley S, Bennett N, Gibson J, Burslem F, et al. Analysis of the acute and chronic wound environments: the role of proteases and their inhibitors. *Wound Repair Regen* 1999 Nov;7(6):442-52.

36. O'Neill LA. Immunity's early-warning system. *Sci Am* 2005 Jan;292(1):24-31.

37. Yager DR, Chen SM, Ward SI, Olutoye OO, Diegelmann RF, Cohen IK. Ability of chronic wound fluids to degrade peptide growth factors is associated with increased levels of elastase activiy and diminished leves of proteinase inhibitors. *Wound Repair Regen* 1997.

38. Nwomeh BC, Yager DR, Cohen IK. Physiology of the chronic wound. *Clin Plast Surg* 1998 Jul;25(3):341-56.

39. Costerton JW, Stewart PS, Greenberg EP. Bacterial bio-films: a common cause of persistent infections. *Science* 1999 May 21;284(5418):1318-22.

40. Costerton JW, Cheng KJ, Geesey GG, Ladd TI, Nickel JC, Dasgupta M, et al. Bacterial bio-films in nature and disease. *Annu Rev Microbiol* 1987;41:435-64.

41. Williams D, Enoch S, Miller D, Harris K, Price P, Harding KG. Effect of sharp debridement using curette on recalcitrant nonhealing venous leg ulcers: a concurrently controlled, prospective cohort study. *Wound Repair Regen* 2005 Mar;13(2):131-7.

42. James G, Swogger E, Secor P, Pulcini E, Costerton B, Wolcott R. *Examination of Wounds for the Presence of Bio-film and Analysis of the Bacterial Community Structure.* 2006. Ref Type: Personal Communication

43. Rumbaugh K, Oliver J, Hastert M, Griswold J, Hamood A, Schaber J. Pseudomonas aeruginosa forms *Bio-films in Acute Infection Independently of Cell-to-Cell Signaling*. 2006. Ref Type: Personal Communication

44. Singh PK, Parsek MR, Greenberg EP, Welsh MJ. A component of innate immunity prevents bacterial bio-film development. *Nature* 2002 May 30;417(6888):552-5.

45. Tapiainen T, Sormunen R, Kaijalainen T, Kontiokari T, Ikaheimo I, Uhari M. Ultrastructure of Streptococcus pneumoniae after exposure to xylitol. *J Antimicrob Chemother* 2004 Jul;54(1):225-8.

46. Katsuyama M, Ichikawa H, Ogawa S, Ikezawa Z. A novel method to control the balance of skin microflora. Part 1. Attack on bio-film of Staphylococcus aureus without antibiotics. *J Dermatol Sci* 2005 Jun;38(3):197-205.

47. Katsuyama M, Kobayashi Y, Ichikawa H, Mizuno A, Miyachi Y, Matsunaga K, et al. A novel method to control the balance of skin microflora Part 2. A study to assess the effect of a cream containing farnesol and xylitol on atopic dry skin. *J Dermatol Sci* 2005 Jun;38(3):207-13.

48. Giacometti A, Cirioni O, Gov Y, Ghiselli R, Del Prete MS, Mocchegiani F, et al. RNA III inhibiting peptide inhibits in vivo bio-film formation by drug-resistant Staphylococcus aureus. *Antimicrob Agents Chemother* 2003 Jun;47(6):1979-83.

49. Balaban N, Stoodley P, Fux CA, Wilson S, Costerton JW, Dell'Acqua G. Prevention of staphylococcal bio-film-associated infections by the quorum sensing inhibitor RIP. *Clin Orthop Relat Res* 2005 Aug;(437):48-54.

50. Giacometti A, Cirioni O, Ghiselli R, Dell'Acqua G, Orlando F, D'Amato G, et al. RNAIII-inhibiting peptide improves efficacy of clinically used antibiotics in a murine model of staphylococcal sepsis. *Peptides* 2005 Feb;26(2):169-75.

51. Costerton JW, Stewart PS. Battling bio-films. *Sci Am* 2001 Jul;285(1):74-81.

52. Steed DL, Donohoe D, Webster MW, Lindsley L. Effect of extensive debridement and treatment on the healing of diabetic foot ulcers. Diabetic Ulcer Study Group. *J Am Coll Surg* 1996 Jul;183(1):61-4.

53. Steed DL. Debridement. *Am J Surg* 2004 May;187(5A):71S-4S.

54. Sibbald RG, Williamson D, Orsted HL, Campbell K, Keast D, Krasner D, et al. Preparing the wound bed—debridement, bacterial balance, and moisture balance. *Ostomy Wound Manage* 2000 Nov;46(11):14-8, 30.

55. Harrison-Balestra C, Cazzaniga AL, Davis SC, Mertz PM. A wound-isolated Pseudomonas aeruginosa grows a bio-film in vitro within 10 hours and is visualized by light microscopy. *Dermatol Surg* 2003 Jun;29(6):631-5.

56. Lamont RJ, Jenkinson HF. Life below the gum line: pathogenic mechanisms of Porphyromonas gingivalis. *Microbiol Mol Biol Rev* 1998 Dec;62(4):1244-63.

57. Nickel JC, Ruseska I, Wright JB, Costerton JW. Tobramycin resistance of Pseudomonas aeruginosa cells growing as a bio-film on urinary catheter material. *Antimicrob Agents Chemother* 1985 Apr;27(4):619-24.

58. Quirynen M, Bollen CM, Vandekerckhove BN, Dekeyser C, Papaioannou W, Eyssen H. Full- vs. partial-mouth disinfection in the treatment of periodontal infections: short-term clinical and microbiological observations. *J Dent Res* 1995 Aug;74(8):1459-67.

59. Joly V, Pangon B, Vallois JM, Abel L, Brion N, Bure A, et al. Value of antibiotic levels in serum and cardiac vegetations for predicting antibacterial effect of ceftriaxone in experimental Escherichia coli endocarditis. *Antimicrob Agents Chemother* 1987 Oct;31(10):1632-9.

60. Sandoe JA, Kerr KG, Reynolds GW, Jain S. Staphylococcus capitis endocarditis: two cases and review of the literature. *Heart* 1999 Sep;82(3):e1.

61. Davies CE, Hill KE, Wilson MJ, Stephens P, Hill CM, Harding KG, et al. Use of 16S ribosomal DNA PCR and denaturing gradient gel electrophoresis for analysis of the microfloras of healing and nonhealing chronic venous leg ulcers. *J Clin Microbiol* 2004 Aug;42(8):3549-57.

62. James G, Secor P, Wolcott R. Use of Denaturing Gradient Gel Electrophoresis for Evaluation of Chronic Wounds. 2006. Ref Type: Personal Communication

63. Danese PN, Pratt LA, Kolter R. Exopolysaccharide production is required for development of Escherichia coli K-12 bio-film architecture. *Journal of Bacteriology* 2000;182(12):3593-6.

64. Huang CT, Yu FP, McFeters GA, Stewart PS. Nonuniform spatial patterns of respiratory activity within bio-films during disinfection. *Appl Environ Microbiol* 1995 Jun;61(6):2252-6.

65. Mason DJ, Power EG, Talsania H, Phillips I, Gant VA. Antibacterial action of ciprofloxacin. *Antimicrob Agents Chemother* 1995 Dec;39(12):2752-8.

66. Eming SA, Smola H, Krieg T. Treatment of chronic wounds: state of the art and future concepts. *Cells Tissues Organs* 2002;172(2):105-17.

REVIEW QUESTIONS

1.) Planktonic phenotype bacteria differ from genetically identical bio-film phenotype bacteria in that:
   a. Planktonic bacteria are attached to a surface
   b. Planktonic bacteria differentiate into multiple phenotypes to enable colony survival
   c. Planktonic bacteria possess colony defenses
   d. Planktonic bacteria are individual and free floating

2.) Bio-film phenotype bacteria on the surface of the wound are:
   a. Very sensitive to antibiotics
   b. Very sensitive to biocides (hydrogen peroxide, Dakin's solution, Betadine)
   c. Not detrimental to wound healing
   d. Very resistant to antibiotics

3.) Bio-films are difficult to culture by routine culture methods because:
   a. They are too slippery to get in the culture tube
   b. The bio-film phenotype cells are viable but not culturable
   c. It is impossible to get bio-film off the surface so it can be cultured
   d. Bio-films culture just as easily as planktonic bacteria

4). An acute wound that occurs in the same area as a chronic wound usually will heal in 2–3 weeks while the chronic wound remains open. The reason for this is:
   a. Good wound care by the wound care provider
   b. Acute wounds know how to get healing agents from the blood better than chronic wounds
   c. Acute wounds do not have much bio-film and chronic wounds have a lot of bio-film on their surface
   d. Acute wounds are better looking and, therefore, deserve to heal faster

5.) The developmental phases of bio-films are:
   a. Twitching, attachment, microcolony formation, maturation
   b. Twitching, maturation, attachment, microcolony formation
   c. Attachment, twitching, maturation, microcolony formation
   d. Attachment, twitching, microcolony formation, maturation

6.) Debridement to remove bio-film (slough) from the chronic wound bed should be done:
   a. As often as the clinician thinks is necessary, even if it is two or three times in one week
   b. Every two weeks
   c. Every three weeks
   d. Every month

Answers: 1a, 2d, 3b, 4c, 5a, 6a

NOTES

CHAPTER 30

Skin, Skin Structure, and Muscle Infections

CHAPTER THIRTY OVERVIEW

NOTES

SKIN, SKIN STRUCTURE, AND MUSCLE INFECTIONS

Jack L. Le Frock, Jon T. Mader

INTRODUCTION

Skin and soft tissue (subcutaneous tissue, fascia, skeletal muscle) infections account for a lot of visits to physicians and emergency rooms, as well as prolong the stay of postoperative patients. Many of these infections are superficial and are treated with oral antibiotics and local care. However, others such as, group A beta hemolytic streptococcal gangrene, necrotizing cellulitis, and clostridial myonecrosis are life threatening and require immediate medical and surgical care.

Many of these syndromes are similar in nature and have common or overlapping signs and symptoms leading to confusion in classification, diagnosis and management. Some people classify the syndromes as clostridial and nonclostridial syndromes. Others classify them based on anatomical location, (skin, fascia, muscle, etc.).

This chapter does not follow any specific classification, but discusses the most common syndromes. This chapter will cover the following topics: cellulitis, diabetic foot, phycomycotic gangrenous cellulitis, clostridial cellulitis, non-clostridial anaerobic cellulitis, synergistic necrotizing cellulitis, progressive bacterial synergistic gangrene, necrotizing fasciitis, myositis, pyomyositis, anaerobic streptococcal myositis, streptococcal myositis, clostridial myonecrosis (gas gangrene), and infected vascular gangrene. The differential diagnoses of some necrotizing infections of the skin and subcutaneous tissues are summarized in Table 1.

CELLULITIS

Cellulitis is an acute spreading infection of the skin which may extend to involve the subcutaneous tissues as well. Cellulitis may be caused by Group A streptococcus, *Staphylococcus aureus*, gram-negative bacteria (*Serratia, Proteus, Aeromonas hydrophila, Vibrio supp., Pseudomonas aeruginosa*), Mycobacterium, and fungi.

A history of previous trauma (laceration, puncture wound) or an underlying skin lesion (ulcer, furuncle) predisposes one to the development of a cellulitis. Several days after the inciting trauma, the signs of celsus (rubor, calor, dolor, tumor) will develop.

TABLE 1. DIFFERENTIAL DIAGNOSIS OF NECROTIZING INFECTIONS OF SKIN & SUBCUTANEOUS TISSUES

	Necrotizing fasciitis, strepto-coccal	Necrotizing fasciitis, mixed	Synergistic necrotizing cellulitis	Infected vascular gangrene	Progressive bacterial synergistic gangrene	Clostridial cellulitis	Non clostridial anaerobic cellulitis
Pain	Moderate to severe	Moderate to severe	Severe; marked tenderness	Variable	Moderate	Mild	Mild
Tissue gas	Absent	May be present	Crepitus in 25% of cases	Often present	May be present	Extensive	Extensive
Odor to exudate	Little	Foul	Foul	Foul	±Foul	Sometimes Foul	Foul
Skin changes	Variable amounts of erythema, anesthesia and gangrene with extensive undermining	Variable amounts of erythema, anesthesia and gangrene with extensive undermining	Patchy secondary necrosis of skin and subsutaneous tissues	Discolored often black	Shaggy ulcer with gangrenous margin and erythe-matous periphery	Minimal discoloration	Minimal discoloration
Systemic toxicity	Prominent	Prominent	Marked	Nil or minimal	Nil or minimal	Minimal	Moderate
Progression	Rapid	Rapid	Rapid once infection established	Slow	Slow	May be rapid	May be rapid
Predis-posing factors	Local trauma	Diabetes mellitus, abdominal surgery; perirectal infection	Diabetes mellitus, cardiorenal disease Obesity, perirectal abscess	Diabetes mellitus peripheral arterial insufficiency	Surgery, draining sinus	Local trauma or surgery	Diabetes mellitus, pre-existing localized infection
Muscle involvement	0	0	++	Dead	0	0	0

Malaise, fever, and chills develop. The area which is involved may be extensive and unlike erysipelas the borders are not sharply demarcated and the area involved is not elevated. Regional lymphadenopathy is common, local abscesses may occur, areas of overlying skin may undergo necrosis, with super infection with gram-negative bacilli and bacteremia can occur.

Cellulitis should be taken seriously because of its propensity to spread via the lymphatics and blood stream. In older patients it may be complicated by thrombophlebitis.

A special form of cellulitis occurs in patients whose saphenous veins have been removed for coronary artery bypass surgery. Systemic symptoms such as chills, high fever, and toxicity occurs. Marked erythema, edema, and tenderness extend along the course of the saphenous venectomy. The portal of entry is often an associated area of tinea pedis. To date non-group A B-hemolytic streptococci (groups C G B) have been isolated from skin or blood.

Group A streptococci and *S. aureus* are responsible for the overwhelming majority of cases of cellulitis, but other organisms may be involved occasionally.

Cellulitis due to group A streptococci may occur as a postoperative wound infection. Although uncommon today it can occur very quickly manifesting itself within 6–48 hours of surgery. Rare cases of pneumococcal cellulitis acquired through the bacteremic route have been reported. This type of cellulitis can bear a striking resemblance to streptococcal erysipelas.

Erysipelas is a characteristic form of cellulitis which affects the superficial epidermis, producing marked swelling. It occurs in all ages in patients with predisposing medical or post surgical conditions, such as skin ulcers or eczematous lesions, chronic fungal infections, local trauma, and venous or lymphatic compromise are present in many patients who develop erysipelas. Beta-hemolytic streptococci, primarily group A, cause the vast majority of cases of erysipelas.

Erysipelas skin lesion has a raised border which is sharply demarcated from normal skin. This allows it to be differentiated from other types of cellulitis which are flat or macular. The affected skin is painful, edematous, intensely erythematous and indurated. When it occurs on the face, a classic butterfly rash develops.

There are only a few conditions that can mimic erysipelas. Herpes zoster of the trigeminal nerve may be confused with erysipelas of the face. One also has to consider contact dermatitis, giant urticaria and inflammatory carcinoma of the breast in the differential diagnosis. Penicillin is the treatment of choice in acute therapy. Choose penicillin G (2 million units q 4 hrs IV) for parenteral therapy for hospitalized patients, and penicillin VK (500 mg PID oral) for non hospitalized patients. Use erythromycin 500 mg QID IV or oral for patients with a penicillin allergy.

A variety of unusual pathogens may invade the skin of immunocompromised patients after some local, often minor laceration or abrasion. Such pathogens include fungi (paecilomyces, Penicillium, Trichosporon, Fusarium, alternaria), and even algae (Prototheca wickerhamm).

The lesions are usually ulcerative or nodular. In immunocompromised or granulocytopenic patients, a variety or bacteria (*Serratia*, *Proteus*, and other *Enterobacteriaceae*), and fungi (*Cryptococcus neoformans*) may produce a cellulitis. *Legionella sp*. has on an occasion produced cellulitis.

Pseudomonas aeruginosa bacteremia is often accompanied by metastatic gangrenous lesions, particularly in the immunocompromised host. The characteristic lesion produced is ecthyma gangrenosum. *Aeromonas hydrophila*, Serratia *marcescens*, *S. aureus* and *Aspergillus sp*. can occasionally cause ecthyma.

Aeromonas hydrophila has been reported to cause crepitant cellulitis and myonecrosis. Patients give a history of penetrating trauma either in a fresh water environment or associated with fishing in the Gulf of Mexico. The onset is rapid and may resemble clostridial myonecrosis. Gas production is not prominent and bacteremia is frequently present. Massive surgical debridement and occasional amputation may be required for control of the infection. Antibiotic therapy is based on susceptibility testing.

Cellulitis, bullous lesions, or necrotic ulcers may complicate infection of a traumatic wound sustained in salt water or exposed to drippings from raw seafood produced by *Vibrio sp*. (primarily *V. vulnificus*). This organism can result in bacteremia and progress to necrosis, requiring extensive surgical debridement and antibiotics.

Another presentation is a primary septicemia due to *V. vulnificus* may follow entry of the organism through the gastrointestinal tract (i.e., consumption of raw oysters). Cellulitis with hemorrhagic skin bullae often rapidly follows the bacteremia. People at increased risk are those with alcoholic cirrhosis, hemochromatosis, and thalassemia.

Rapidly growing mycobacteria (*Mycobacterium fortuitum* and *Mycobacterium chelone*) can cause localized cutaneous infection, often involving the foot and lower extremities. *M. marinum* may produce a nodular lymphangitis extending from the original focus. Most patients give a history or a penetrating injury with soil or water contamination at the site of infection. The cellulitis is localized and abscess formation occurs. Discharge from the abscess is watery, not purulent. In the absence of abscess formation, nodular reddish appearing lesions are common.

The diagnosis is usually made on histologic examination of biopsy specimens, which show acid fast bacilli (AFB). Smears from the watery discharge may on occasion also reveal the presence of AFB. Cultures usually turn positive in 4–10 days. *M. fortuitum* and *M. chelone* are resistant to standard anti-tuberculous drugs (i.e., isoniazid, rifampin).

Agents such as amikacin, cefoxitin, erythromycin and doxycycline are often required for therapy. See Table 2 for presumptive treatment of cellulitis.

TABLE 2. TREATMENT OF CELLULITIS

Type	Etiology	Primary Antibiotic	Penicillin Allergy or Alternative Therapy
Mild Cellulitis	*Streptococcal*	Ceftriaxion 1 gram IV Q24 hrs or Pen VK 500 mg po TID Dicloxacillin 500 mg po TID	Erthromycin 500 mg po TID Azithromycin 250 mg po QID
	Staphylococcal	Cephalexin 500 mg po QID	Clindamycin 150–300 mg po TID Linezoilid 600 mg po BID
Serious Cellulitis	<u>Gram Positive</u> *Streptococcal*	Nafcillin 1–2 grams IV Q6 hrs or Cefotaxime 1–2 grams IV 28 hrs	Vancomycin 15 mg/kg IV Q12 hrs or Clindamycin 900 mg IV Q8 hrs
	Staphylococcal	Vancomycin (for resistant strains)	
	<u>Gram Negative</u> *Aeromonas hydrophilia*	Aminoglycoside (Tabramycin/gentamicin IV 1.5 mg/kg Q8 hrs or Cefotaxime 2 grams IV Q8 hrs	Ciprofloxacin 400 mg IV Q12 hrs Levofloxacin 500 mg IV Q12 hrs Trimethoprim Sulfa methoxazole 160/800 mg TMP–SMX BID
	Vibrio vulnificus	Aminoglycoside 1–5 mg/kg Q8 hrs IV+ Cefotaxime 2 grams Q8 hrs IV Ceftazidime 2 grams Q8 hrs IV	Ciproflaxacin 400 mg IV Q12 hrs or Doxycycline 100 mg IV Q24 hrs
	Legionella	Clarithromycin 500 mg Q12hrs po Azithromycin 500 mg IV Q24 hrs for 2 days then 250 mg po Qday	Doxycycline 100 mg IV Q12 hrs
	Atypical mycobacterium *Mycobacterium marinum* *M. Fortuitum*	Rifampin 600 mg 1 day & Ethambutol 15 mg/kg 1 day TMP–SMX BID Ciprofloxacin 500 mg po BID TM12–SMX 100/800 mg po BID	Doxycycline 100mg po BID Clarithromycin 500mg po BID Azithromycin 250mg po Qday

Dosage: Q—every, PO—perfered orally, BID—two times per day, TID—three times per day, Q10—four times per day.

Using aspirates from the advancing edge of cellulitis, skin biopsy, and blood cultures, only gives isolates in 25% of patients. Positive cultures can be obtained from 30% of closed lesions of cellulitis by use of a fine needle aspiration technique. In view of the overall limited yield of pathogens on aspiration of areas of cellulitis, it is reasonable to employ this method when unusual pathogens are suspected or in immunocompromised hosts.

Diseases sometimes confused with cellulitis include acute dermatitis, such as that due to contact with an allergen; gout, with marked cutaneous inflammation extending beyond the joint involved; and herpes zoster. Acute lipodermatosclerosis, a panniculitis that occurs predominantly in obese women with lower extremity venous insufficient, causes painful, erythematous, tender, warm indurated, and sometimes scaly areas in the medial leg that resemble cellulitis.

Emerging antibiotic resistance among *S. aureus* (methicillin resistance) and *S. pyogenes* (erythromycin resistance) have become a big problem because these organisms are common causes of a variety of skin and soft tissue infections. Empirical antimicrobials must include agents with activity against resistant strains. Minor infections may be empirically treated with semi-synthetic penicillin, first or second generation oral cephalosporins, macrolides, or clindamycin. Fifty percent of *S. aureus* (MRSA) strains have inducible or constitutive clindamycin resistance. Most community acquired MRSA strains are susceptible to trimethoprim-sulfamethoxazale and tetracycline.

DIABETIC FOOT

Diabetic patients frequently develop foot ulcers, cellulitis, soft tissue necrosis, and osteomyelitis with a draining sinus or distal gangrene. This is discussed in the chapter by Khan, Derksen and Steinberg entitled, "Diabetic Foot Wounds."

PHYCOMYCOTIC GANGRENOUS CELLULITIS

The phycomycetes are a class of fungi that belong to the order Mucorales which includes Rhizopus, Absidia, and Mucor. Infections caused by these fungi are also called "mucormycosis." Infections by Phycomycetes can produce various manifestations, including sinusitis, rhino cerebral involvement, pneumonitis, and disseminated disease. Phycomycotic infections generally occur in immunocompromised patients (e.g., acute leukemia, lymphoma, diabetes mellitus or burn patients). It also has been described in patients in whom adhesive tape contaminated with *Rhizopus sp.* was applied over open wounds. Local factors (open fracture sites, ileostomy stomas, fistulous tracts) also play a predisposing role in this type of infection. The infection may exhibit an indolent course with minimal fever and slowly enlarging black ulcer, or it may follow a rapidly progressive febrile course. The cutaneous lesions usually produce necrosis, ulceration, and eschar formation. The eschar is usually black and may be misleading because fungi stain poorly. Furthermore, the smear may be contaminated with surface bacteria. The diagnosis is best established by performing histologic examination of biopsy specimens. Broad branching and nonseptate hyphae are visualized.

Management consists of aggressive surgical excision and intravenous amphotericin B, especially if multi focal lesions occur or the cellulitis is progressive.

CLOSTRIDIAL CELLULITIS

Clostridial cellulitis is a necrotizing infection of devitalized subcutaneous tissue produced by *Clostridium sp.* usually *Cl. Perfringens* and less commonly *Cl. Septicum.* Deep fascia is not appreciably involved. The organisms are introduced into the subcutaneous tissue through either a traumatic wound, or at surgery with bowel flora. Localized infections in the perineum, abdominal wall, buttocks, and lower extremities may also become contaminated with *Clostridium sp.* and serve as the source of entry into subcutaneous tissues. The presence of foreign debris and necrotic tissue in the depths of a wound provides a suitable environment for clostridial proliferation.

The clinical features consist mainly of local signs and symptoms with very little systemic toxicity. The relative mildness of the process helps differentiate it from Clostridial myonecrosis toxicity. The onset may be gradual, but progression can be fairly rapid. Local pain is minimal; however, there is extensive gas production with frank crepitus and swelling. A dark, serous malodorous exudate is usually present.

Diagnosis is easily established by the examination of a Gram-stained smear of the drainage showing thick Gram-positive bacilli. Soft tissue x-ray reveals abundant gas.

Surgical exploration is mandatory in order to determine the extent of involvement and to distinguish clostridial cellulitis from myonecrosis. The involved tissues must be laid open to expose the underlying muscles, which are normal in appearance.

Management includes surgically removing all necrotic tissue and allowing the wound to remain wide open. Antibacterial therapy consists of high dose (16–20 million units/day) intravenously administered penicillin.

NON-CLOSTRIDIAL ANAEROBIC CELLULITIS

This infection is similar to clostridial cellulitis except that it is caused by a variety of non-spore forming anaerobic bacteria including *Bacteroides sp.*, *Peptostreptococcus*, and *Peptococci* either alone or in combination with facultative bacteria (*Enterobacteriaceae*, *Streptococci*, *S. aureus*). Cultures frequently reveal more than one bacterial agent. Diabetes mellitus and pre-existing localized infection are the major predisposing factors.

The onset may be either gradual or acute. The involved area is edematous, and a dark frequently foul smelling, purulent exudate is usually present. Local pain is mild, but systemic toxicity may be moderate. Tissue gas formation is extensive and crepitation may extend beyond the infected areas.

Diagnosis is established by examining the Gram-stained smears of wound exudate. Surgical exploration is required. With similar findings as those seen in clostridial cellulitis, debridement of all necrotic tissue should be performed.

Initial therapy should be directed against anaerobes and *Enterobacteriaceae*. A combination of clindamycin, timentin or tazobactam plus aminoglycoside, ciprofloxacin or aztreonam is good initial therapy. Therapy may be modified according to the susceptibility of the organism(s) isolated.

SYNERGISTIC NECROTIZING CELLULITIS

Synergistic necrotizing cellulitis is a variant of necrotizing fasciitis, one in which there is prominent involvement of skin and muscle as well as of subcutaneous tissue and fascia. This was first described in 1972 by Stone and Martin. Predisposing factors include diabetes mellitus, obesity, advanced age, and cardiorenal disease. Most infections are located on the lower extremities or near the perineum.

The infection is usually polymicrobial involving a mixture of anaerobes (*Pepto-Streptococcus sp.*, *Bacteroides sp.*, and facultative bacteria (*Klebsiella*, *Enterobacter*, *E. coli*, *Proteus*). Bacteroides sp. has been reported as the major pathogen on occasion.

The onset is acute, local pain occurs in the affected area, and systemic toxemia occurs. The lesion manifests with small skin ulcers surrounded by circumscribed areas of gangrene and draining foul-smelling, reddish brown exudate. The areas involved are edematous, painful, and exquisitely tender. Tissue gas is noted in about a quarter of the patients and blood cultures are positive in approximately half of the patients.

Therapy consists of surgical debridement (amputation if necessary), antimicrobial therapy, and management of diabetic ketoacidosis, if present. Initial surgery involves incision and drainage, but radical debridement is often necessary because of extensive involvement of deep fascia and muscle antibiotic therapy. Antibiotic therapy should cover anaerobes as well as gram-positive and gram-negative aerobes. The prognosis is poor. Forty-eight (76%) of 63 patients described by Stone and Martin died.

PROGRESSIVE BACTERIAL SYNERGISTIC GANGRENE

This was first described by Brewer and Meleney in 1926. This lesion usually follows infection of an abdominal operative wound site, where wire sutures have been used. Sometimes it develops slowly around an ileostomy or colostomy site or in proximity to a chronic ulceration on an extremity.

Initially, the wound becomes red, swollen and tender. Within the next few days the wound margins develop an indurated appearance. The central area is purplish in color, surrounded by a 1–10 cm zone of erythema. As the lesion progresses, the central portion of the purplish area becomes necrotic, the color changing to a dirty gray brown or yellow green with a type suede leather appearance. As the lesion enlarges, the inner margin of the gangrenous zone becomes undermined and melts away. Eventually the center of the lesion becomes a granulating ulcer which is encircled by a gangrenous margin. Surrounding the latter is a violaceous zone which fades into an outer pink edematous area. The major system is the extraordinary pain and tenderness of the lesion. Untreated, the process extends slowly ultimately producing large ulcerations.

This differs from necrotizing fasciitis in that it is a more slowly progressing lesion affecting the total thickness of skin, but not involving deep fascia. A related lesion, Meleney's ulcer, is essentially bacterial synergistic gangrene with the additional feature of burrowing necrosis tracts through tissue planes emerging at distant skin sites.

Microaerophilic or anaerobic streptococci can be recovered from aspirates of the advancing margin of the lesion, and *S. aureus* (or occasionally *Proteus* or other Gram-negative bacilli) are present in the ulcerated area. In experimental animals, this lesion can only be produced by the bacterial combination and not by the individual bacteria.

Therapy consists of prompt surgical excision in addition to the appropriate antimicrobial agents. The choice of antibiotics is guided initially by the gram stained smears and later the results of the culture of the exudate. On occasion excision of the lesion is required to cure progressive bacterial synergistic gangrene. Hyperbaric oxygen has been used successfully as adjunctive therapy.

NECROTIZING FASCIITIS

Necrotizing fasciitis is a deep seated infection of the subcutaneous tissue that is rapidly progressive with severe systemic toxicity and 40% mortality. In 1921, Meleney first described this syndrome and called it hemolytic streptococcal gangrene. This disease can lead to progressive destruction of fascia and fat, but may spare the skin itself. This is caused by Group A streptococci, either alone or in combination with other species, *S. aureus* most commonly.

The older reports of necrotizing fasciitis differ from current reports of cases associated with streptococcal toxic shock syndrome (TSS). Recent cases have mainly been seen in young healthy individuals who have no underlying disease, but have sustained minor trauma to an extremity. Most earlier cases reported older people who have significant underlying diseases. Meleney's cases (from China) were probably among young healthy persons who sustained minor trauma, but had only 20% mortality prior to antibiotics versus 20–60% mortality today with Streptococcal TSS in lieu of antibiotics. Most of Meleney's patients did not have shock, organ failure, or require amputation. In contrast, today we see severe systemic toxicity and high morbidity in spite of the use of antibiotics, dialysis, intravenous fluids, ventilators, and improved surgical techniques. A question arises as to whether the increased mortality rate in streptococcal necrotizing fasciitis is due to the emergence of more virulent streptococci.

The other type of necrotizing fasciitis is produced by at least one anaerobic species (*Bacteroides*, *Peptostreptococcus sp.*) that is isolated in combination with one or more facultative anaerobic species such as *Streptococci* (non Gr A). Members of the *Enterobacteriaceae* only anaerobes are very rare.

The sine qua non of necrotizing fasciitis is the rapid spread of necrosis along fascial planes, with subsequent undermining and necrosis of overlying skin. It is most often an acute process, but can occasionally follow a subacute course. It can affect any part of the body, but most commonly involves the extremities, particularly the legs. Other sites may include the abdominal wall, perianal and groin areas, and postoperative wounds. The portal of entry is usually a site of trauma, either burn, laceration, abrasion, or insect bite, but it can be seen in the post surgical setting as well, particularly after laparotomy performed in the presence of peritoneal soiling such as with intestinal perforation.

Predisposition exists in compromised hosts such as diabetes mellitus, alcoholism, parenteral drug abuse, and obesity.

Clinical presentations can be acute, with sudden onset of pain and swelling, with or without chills and fever. Within 24 hours considerable phlegmon may be present, with accompanying erythema and cellulitis. The affected area initially is erythematous, swollen, without sharp margins, hot shiny exquisitely tender and painful. Lymphangitis and lymphadenitis are infrequent. The process progresses rapidly over several days, with sequential skin color changes, from red purple to patches of blue gray. Within 3–5 days of onset, skin breakdown with bullae and frank cutaneous gangrene occurs. By this time, the involved area is no longer tender, but has become anaesthetic secondary to thrombosis of small blood vessels and destruction of superficial nerves located in the necrotic undermined subcutaneous tissues. Development of anesthesia may antedate the appearance of skin necrosis, and may provide a clue that the process is necrotizing fasciitis and not a simple cellulitis. Subcutaneous gas is often present in the polymicrobial form of necrotizing fasciitis, particularly in patients with diabetes mellitus. Systemic toxicity is prominent, and the temperature is elevated in the 39–41°C (102–105°F) range.

Extensive undermining of the skin and subcutaneous tissue occur, and is classically demonstrated when a surgical clamp or even the surgeon's finger will pass along a fascial plane, which is normally tight and resists such probing. Subcutaneous crepitation may be noted on occasion, but x-ray examination reveals tissue gas in the majority of cases. Bacteremia is common especially with *S. pyogenes* and metastatic foci of infection may be seen. Hypocalcemia may occur and is most likely related to extensive fat necrosis.

DIAGNOSIS

The early recognition of tissue necrosis is by far the most important step in the effective treatment of necrotizing fasciitis. Outcomes are clearly affected by early diagnosis and treatment. It should be suspected clinically when the typical findings especially cutaneous anesthesia is present. The findings on gram stained smears of the exudate and consideration of the role of anaerobes in the infectious process can guide initial antibiotic therapy. However, prompt surgical intervention is of paramount importance. On incision, the diagnosis is confirmed by the findings of extensive undermining of skin by necrotic superficial fascia and subcutaneous tissue as evidenced by the easy passage of a blunt instrument along the fascial plane.

If shock and multiple organ failure occurs early in the course of illness (the first 24–36 hours) streptococcal toxic shock syndrome (TSS) should be suspected. This is caused by Group A Streptococcal (GAS) strains of M protein serotypes 1, 3, 6, 12, and 28. M proteins inhibit phagocytosis of streptococci by polymorphonuclear leukocytes, which may enhance the virulence of GAS strains. The production of streptococcal exotoxins type A and B (found in most severe infections) and M protein fragments act as superantigens, interacting with the major histocompatibility complex class II antigens. This interaction causes a substantial release of cytokines responsible for the dramatic shock and multiple organ failure (respiratory, liver, renal).

Gas in soft tissue whether found by radiograph, physical exam, or computed tomography is an ominous sign and should alert the physician to a significant underlying infection. Gas in the soft tissue is more commonly associated with nonclostridial infections. Some clinicians advocate the use of MRI/CT Scan for early diagnosis treatment of necrotizing fasciitis.

Therapy for necrotizing fasciitis is the following: resuscitation and stabilization, appropriate antibiotics, aggressive surgical debridement, and adjunctive hyperbaric oxygen therapy. Empiric therapy should begin immediately with broad spectrum coverage such as: Ampicillin-sulbactam, Ticarcillin-clavulanate, Piperacillin-Tazobactam or a combination of Clindamycin or any of the above with an aminoglycoside aztreonam or a fluoroquinolone.

Surgically multiple linear incisions should be made through the skin and subcutaneous tissues going beyond the area of involvement until normal fascia is found. Necrotic fat and fascia should be excised and the wound should be left open. Debridement may be considered adequate when the subcutaneous tissue can no longer be separated from the underlying fascial planes by finger or probe dissection. Repeated debridement may be necessary. Secondary closure and/or skin grafting is usually required after the infection is cured.

In general, HBO2 has been reported to be beneficial. Gozal and coworkers, using combined HBO2, radical surgery and antibiotics, reduced the mortality rate from the expected 38–12.5%. Other series also noted beneficial effects of HBO2.

Patient risk is increased in association with age greater than 50, pre-existing disease, underlying vascular disease, truncal involvement, poor nutrition, and, most especially, delayed diagnosis.

FOURNIER'S GANGRENE

Fournier's gangrene is a form of necrotizing fasciitis that initially affects the male genitalia. Its differentiation from necrotizing fasciitis is only by anatomical location. Microbiology, diagnosis, and treatment are very similar.

CLOSTRIDIAL MYONECROSIS (GAS GANGRENE)

Gas gangrene represents a true medical emergency. It is a destructive infectious process of muscle associated with local crepitance and systemic signs of toxemia, which are caused by the anaerobic, gas forming bacilli of the clostridium genus. It occurs in the setting of muscle injury and contamination (with the spores of *C. perfringens* or other clostridial species), such as accidental trauma, penetrating injuries, (gunshot wounds, frost bite) wounds associated with biliary tract or bowel surgery, as a complication of thermal burns, and in the setting of arterial insufficiency. The onset is usually acute with pain occuring early at the site of injury. The pain rapidly increases in intensity and is accompanied by acute systemic toxemia. Tachycardia, hypotension and shock follow, giving the patient a moribund appearance. Hypothermia, when present, indicates a poor prognosis.

Locally, the skin may initially be tense and blanched as a result of edema. Crepitus is often present, although not a prominent feature of gas gangrene. Gas is seen on x-ray films of soft tissue. A dark, serosanguinous discharge is often present which contains many organisms with a paucity of polymorphonuclear leukocytes. Rapid tissue necrosis occurs and is caused by clostridial toxins.

These toxins produced by the bacteria directly kill the muscle and adjacent tissue. In addition, these toxins cause vascular stasis, ischemia and inhibit neutrophil emigration. As a result, there is very little local neutrophil response. Nine of the 20 different clostridial exotoxins have been identified which are implicated in the local and systemic changes in gas gangrene; alpha-toxin, theta-toxin, kappa-toxin, mu-toxin, nu-toxin, fibrinolysin, neuraminidase, "circulating factor," and "bursting factor." The most prevalent is the oxygen-stable lecithinase-C (alpha-toxin), which is hemolytic, tissue necrotizing and lethal. Stevens and coworkers described the lethal effects and cardiovascular effects of purified alpha and theta toxins from *Clostridial perfringens*.

The involved muscles undergo degeneration and acquire a reddish purple hue. They become friable, lose their contractility, and fail to bleed when cut with a surgical knife. Gram stained material usually reveals large gram positive bacilli, but no spores are seen.

The clinical features should arouse suspicion early in the course of the disease, so that it can be recognized and early aggressive surgical debridement can be done. The definite diagnosis is based on the appearance of the muscle on direct visualized by surgical exposure. Gas in the wound is a late finding and by the time crepitans is noted, the patient may be near death. The mortality rate is 60% and is highest in cases affecting the abdominal wall and lowest in cases affecting the extremities.

Successful treatment depends on early recognition, antibiotics, debridement of all devitalized and infected tissues and hyperbaric oxygen which can reduce tissue loss and mortality. High dose intravenous penicillin is the antibiotic of choice. Major clinical studies indicate that the lowest morbidity and mortality are achieved with initial conservative surgery and rapid initiation of HBO2. Results decline progressively when HBO2 therapy is delayed. Early aggressive surgery and delayed HBO2 treatment lead to a significantly higher mortality and morbidity than when HBO2 is administered promptly. The work of Brummelkamp and Boerema and later updated by Bakker totaling 409 cases, showed a mortality of 11.7%, and HBO2 therapy reduced the amputation rate to 18% versus 50–55% following primary surgery. The advantages of early HBO2 therapy are that:

1. It is life saving since it requires less heroic surgery in a very ill patient and it rapidly stops the production of alpha-toxin.
2. It prevents major amputation or excisions prematurely (except opening of wounds). It clarifies the demarcation in 24–30 hours, so there is a clear distinction between dead and living tissue. These things lead to a decrease in number and extent of amputations.

INFECTED VASCULAR GANGRENE

Infection frequently complicates the distal gangrene seen with peripheral vascular insufficiency. It usually manifests by the development of a putrid odor and accumulation of gas in the gangrenous tissue. Pain and systemic toxicity are usually minimal, but can become prominent especially if cellulitis spreads to viable tissues. These infections are usually polymicrobial involving anaerobes and aerobes. Anaerobic bacteria appear to be of major significance, as evidenced by frequent crepitus and foul smell.

It is important to differentiate gangrene and infection in a cold or warm foot. In the former, gangrene is primary and amputation is usually required. In the latter, infection may be primary and although debridement and appropriate antibiotics are required, amputation may be avoided.

Table 1 summarizes as well as gives the differential diagnosis of necrotizing infections of skin and subcutaneous tissues. Table 2 summarizes the presumptive treatment for cellulitis. Table 3 summarizes the empiric therapy of necrotizing soft tissue infections.

MYOSITIS

Myositis is an uncommon infection of skeletal muscle. Bacteria can invade muscle either from contiguous sites of infection (skin and subcutaneous abscesses, penetrating wounds, decubitus ulcers, osteomyelitis), or by hematogenous spread from a distant focus. One may see myositis presenting as different clinical patterns such as pyomyositis, gas gangrene, non-clostridial (crepitant) myositis, infected vascular gangrene, Aeromonas hydrophila myonecrosis and psoas abscess.

TABLE 3. EMPIRIC THERAPY OF NECROTIZING SOFT TISSUE INFECTIONS

Syndrome	Treatment	Penicillin Allergy
Type 1 Polymicrobial necrotizing fasciitis Mixed aerobes and anaerobes	Piperacillin/tazobactum, 3.375 g IV Q6 hrs or Imipenem 500 mg IV Q6 hrs	Vancomycin 15 mg/kg Q12 hrs Plus ciprofloxan, 400 mg IV Q12 hrs and metronidazole, 500 mg IV Q6 hrs
Type 2 Streptococcal necrotizing fasciitis	Penicillin G 4 million U IV Q4 hrs and clindamycin 900 mg IV Q8 hrs	Clindamycin, 900 mg IV Q8 hrs
Progressive bacterial synergistic gangrene Microaerophilic Streptococci and S. aureus	Piperacillin/tazobactram, 3.375 g IV Q6 hrs or Ampicillin-sulbactam 1.5–3.0 g IV Q6-8 hrs	Clindamycin, 900 mg IV Q8 hrs plus Ciprofloxacin, 400 mg IV Q12 hrs or Vancomycin,15 mg/kg IV Q12 hrs plus Ciprofloxacin 400 mg IV Q12 hrs
Clostridial Myonecrosis (gas gangrene)	Penicillin G, 4 million U IV Q4 hrs plus Clindamycin, 900 mg IV Q8 hrs	Metronidazole, 500 mg IV Q6 hrs
Clostridial anaerobic cellulitis *C perfringens*	Penicillin G, 4 million U IV Q4 hrs	Metronidazole, 500 mg IV Q6 hrs or Clindamycin 900 mg IV Q8 hrs
Non Clostridial Anaerobic Cellulitis mixed aerobes and anaerobes	Piperacillin/Tazobactam 3.375 g IV Q6 hrs or Imipenem 500 mg IV Q6 hrs Meropenem 1g IV Q8 hrs Ertapenem 1g IV Q24 hrs	Vancomycin 15 mg/kg IV Q12 hrs plus Ciprofloxacin 400 mg IV Q12 hrs plus Metronidazole 500 mg IV Q6 hrs

PYOMYOSITIS

Pyomyositis is an acute bacterial infection of skeletal muscle usually due to *S. aureus*. The accumulation of pus is always intramuscular initially. Clinically it is characterized by localized muscle pain, swelling and tenderness. It generally occurs in the absence of a predisposing site of infection. Most cases occur in the tropics (tropical pyomyositis). In the U.S. it is very uncommon (only 100 cases reported over the past 20 years in North America), occurring both in persons who have recently emigrated from the tropics and in those who have always resided in a temperate climate. About 40% of cases in temperate climates lack any relevant underlying diseases, but the remainder may have possible predisposing conditions: diabetes mellitus, alcoholic liver disease, corticosteroid therapy, etc. Pyomyositis has been reported in patients with HIV infection due to *S. aureus*. The predisposition stems from the combination of defective bactericidal activity of neutrophils. The underlying cell mediated immuno-deficiency, and the potential muscle injury associated with this disease intravenous drug users are also at increased risk to develop polymyositis for the following factors: impaired cellular and humoral immunity, defective bactericidal activities of neutrophils, increased bacterial colonization of the skin, and injection of potentially contaminated materials. Pyomyositis can be divided into three clinical stages:

- Stage 1 is characterized by crampy local muscle pain, swelling and low-grade fever. Mild leukocytosis and induration of the affected muscles may be present. The muscle may have a "woody" texture on palpation. Fluctuation is absent, and muscle aspiration will not yield purulent material. Only 2% of patients present at this stage.
- Stage 2 occurs 10–21 days after the onset of symptoms and is characterized by fever, exquisite muscle tenderness, and edema. Marked leukocytosis is usually present, and eosinophilia is common in tropical pyomyositis. Aspiration of the affected muscle generally yields pus. Ninety percent of the patients are seen in this suppurative stage.
- Stage 3 is characterized by bacteremia and a toxic appearance. The affected muscle is fluctuant. Complications of S. aureus bacteremia may be present. The most frequent areas of involvement are the lower limb and trunk muscles.

The definitive diagnosis should be made by aspiration or surgical drainage of the abscess. Aspiration may be facilitated by localizing the site of muscle involvement by ultrasound or CT scan.

Stage 1 pyomyositis can be cured with antibiotics alone. Patients presenting with Stage 2 or 3 will require surgical drainage of all abscess plus antistaphylococcal antibiotics.

ANAEROBIC STREPTOCOCCAL MYOSITIS

Anaerobic streptococcal myositis is an indolent process involving muscle and fascial planes. It is usually associated with trauma or surgical procedures. The infection is characterized by severe local pain. The wound emits a brown foul smelling discharge. Bleb formation is common and gas may be present in surrounding tissues. However, inspection of the muscle reveals no myonecrosis or gangrene. This point differentiates benign streptococcal myositis from clostridial gas gangrene. A presumptive diagnosis of anaerobic streptococcal myositis is established by the appearance of the lesion and gram stain of exudate.

Treatment consists of incision and drainage of the wound and debridement and resection of subcutaneous tissue. The inflamed muscle should be spared whenever possible, since it can heal and become functional. Antibiotic therapy with intravenous Timentin, Augmentin, etc. is appropriate. Clindamycin is an alternative drug in penicillin allergic patients.

STREPTOCOCCAL MYOSITIS

Streptococcal myositis is an extremely uncommon Group A Streptococcal (GAS) infection. Adams et al. documented only 21 cases from 1900–1985, and Savane found only four cases in more than 20,000 autopsies. Severe pain may be the only early symptom, and swelling and erythema may be the only early physical findings, though muscle compartment syndromes may develop rapidly. Distinguishing streptococcal myositis from spontaneous gas gangrene caused by *C. perfringens* or *C. septicum* may be difficult, though crepitus or demonstration of gas in the tissue favors clostridial infection. Patients with *Streptococcal* TSS may have both necrotizing fasciitis and myositis. The case fatality rate for necrotizing fasciitis is 20–50%, whereas GAS myositis has a fatality rate of 80–100%.

Aggressive surgical debridement is extremely important for establishing a diagnosis and removing devitalized tissue.

SUMMARY

Skin and soft tissue infections account for a lot of visits to physicians and emergency rooms. Many of these infections are superficial and are treated with oral antibiotics and local care. However, others such as, group A beta hemolytic streptococcal gangrene, necrotizing cellulitis, and clostridial myonecrosis, are life threatening and require immediate medical and surgical care. Successful treatment of some of these infections depends on early recognition, appropriate intravenous antibiotics, and debridement of infected tissue in some cases. Adjunctive hyperbaric oxygen is needed in necrotizing fasciitis and clostridial myonecrosis.

DEDICATION AND ACKNOWLEDGMENTS

On October 25, 2002, Dr. Jon T. Mader, a pioneer and innovator in musculoskeletal infections passed away. He was a personal friend, colleague, and collaborator of mine for 29 years. He had many outstanding attributes, but what I will always remember about Jon is that "he cared." I dedicate this chapter to Jon's memory.

Dr. Le Frock would like to acknowledge Patti Reynolds and Gwen Wilson, Medical Librarians at Sarasota Memorial Hospital for their help in preparing this chapter.

REFERENCES

1. Adams EM, Gudmundsson S, Yocum DE, et al. Streptococcal myositis. *Arch Intern Med* 1985; 145: 1020-1025.
2. Baddour LM. Primary skin infections in primary care: An update. *Infect med* 1993; 10:42-46.
3. Baddour, LM. Extra intestinal Aeromonas infections, looking for Mr Sandbar. *Mayo Clin Proc.* 1992: 67:496-.
4. Bisno AL, Stevens DL. Streptococcal infections of skin and soft tissues. *N Engl J Med* 1996; 334:240- 245.
5. Casali RE, Tucker WE, Petrino RA, et al. Postoperative necrotizing fasciitis of the abdominal wall. *Am J Surg* 1980; 140:787-791.
6. Christin L, Sarosi, GA. Pyomyositis in North America: Case reports and review. *CID* 1992; 15:668-672.
7. Dellinger, PE. Severe necrotizing soft-tissue infections. Multiple disease entities requiring a common approach. *JAMA*, 1981; 246:1717-1721.
8. Eke N. Fournier's gangrene: A review of 1726 cases. *Brit J Surg* 2000; 87:718-728.
9. Elliot D, Kufera JA, Myers, RA. The microbiology of necrotizing soft tissue infections. *Am J Surg* 2000; 179:361-366.
10. Gary RD, Jon O, Banjamin O, et al. Pyomyositis. *Am Fam Physician* 1996; 54:565-568.
11. Gregory DW, Schaffner W. Pseudomonas infections associated with hot tubs and other environments. *Infect Dis Clin North Am* 1987; 1:635-640.
12. Holmstrom B, Grimsley EW. Necrotizing fasciitis and toxic shock-like syndrome caused by group B Streptococcus. *SMJ* 2000; 93:1096-1098.
13. Hejase MJ, Simonin JE, Bihrle R, et al. Genital Fournier's gangrene: Experience with 38 patients. *Urology* 1996; 47:734-9.
14. Kingston D, Seal DV. Current hypotheses on synergistic microbial gangrene. *Br J Surg* 1990; 77:260-264.
15. Kirsner RS, Pardes JB, Eaglstein WH, et al. The clinical spectrum of lipodermatosclerosis. *J Am Acad Dermatol* 1993; 28:623-627.
16. Lamothe F, D'Amico P, Ghosn P, et al. Clinical usefulness of intravenous human immunoglobulins in invasive group A streptococcal infections: case report and review. *CID* 1995; 21:1469-1472.
17. Le Frock JL, Joseph WS. Bone and soft-tissue infections of the lower extremity in diabetics. *Clin in Pod Med and Surg* 1995; 12:87-103.
18. Le Frock JL, Molavi A. Necrotizing skin and subcutaneous infections. *J Antimicrob Chemother* 1982; 9:suppl-A 183-192.
19. Lewis RT. Necrotizing soft-tissue infections. *Infect Dis Clin NA* 1992; 6:693-703.
20. Lipsky BA, Berendt AR, Deery HG, et al. Diagnosis and Treatment of Diabetic Foot Infections. *IDSA Guidelines CID* 2004; 39:885-910.
21. MacLennan J. The histotoxic Clostridial infections of man. *Bacteriol Rev* 1962; 26:177-274.
22. Majeski JA, Alexander JW. Early diagnosis, nutritional support and immediate extensive debridement improve survival in necrotizing fasciitis. *Am J Surg* 1983; 145:784-787.
23. Mathieu D, Neviere N, Lefebvre-Lebleu N, et al. Anaerobic infections in soft tissues. *Ann Chir* 1997; 51:272-287.
24. Miller LG, Perdreau-Remington F, Rieg G, et al. Necrotizing fasciitis caused by community-associated methicillin-resistant staphylococcus in Los Angeles. *N Engl J Med* 2005; 352: 1445-1453.
25. Mulla ZD, Leaverton FE, Wiersma ST. Invasive group A streptococcal infections in Florida. *South Med J* 2003; 96:968-973.

26. Oelschlager BK, Dellinger EP. Necrotizing soft-tissue infections. *Cont Surg* 2001; 57:526-531.

27. Rolston KVI. Infections involving the skin and soft-tissues of the lower extremities. *J Foot Surg* 1987; 265:525-529.

28. Sachs MD. The optimum use of needle aspirations in the bacteriologic diagnosis of cellulitis in adults. *Arch Intern Med* 1990; 150: 1907-1912.

29. Schmid M, Kossmann T, Duewell S. Differentiation of necrotizing fasciitis and cellulitis using MR imaging. *Am J Radiol* 1998; 170:615-620.

30. Stephens BJ, Lathrop JC, Rice WT, et al. Fournier's gangrene: Historic (1964-1978) versus contemporary (1979-1988) differences in etiology and clinical importance. *Am J Surg* 1993; 59:149-154.

31. Stevens DL, Bisno AL, Chambers HF, et al: Practice guidelines for the diagnosis and management of skin and soft-tissue infections in SA Guidelines. *CID* 2005; 41:1373-1406.

32. Stevens DL. Invasive group A streptococcus infections. *CID* 1992; 14:2-13.

33. Stevens DL, Musher DM, Watson DA, et al. Spontaneous, nontraumatic gangrene due to Clostridium septicum. *Rev Infect Dis* 1990; 12:286-296.

34. Stevens DL. Streptococcal toxic shock syndrome: spectrum of disease, pathogenesis, and new concepts in treatment. *Emerg Infect Dis* 1995; 1:69-78.

35. Stevens DL. Dilemmas in the treatment of invasive streptococcus pyogenes infections. *Clin Infect Dis* 2003; 37:341-343.

36. Swartz MN. Clinical practice. Cellulitis. *N Engl J Med*. 2004; 350:904-912.

37. The working group on severe streptococcal infections. Defining the Group A streptococcal toxic shock syndrome: Rationale and consensus definition. *JAMA* 1993; 269:390-391.

38. Voss LM, Rhodes KH, Johnson KA. Musculoskeletal and soft tissue Aeromonas infection: An environmental disease. *Mayo Clin Proc* 1992; 67:422- 427.

39. Waldor MK, Wilson B, Swartz M. Cellulitis caused by Legionella pneumophila. *CID* 1993; 16:51-53.

40. Wall DB, Klein SR, Black S, et al. A simple model to help distinguish necrotizing fasciitis from nonnecrotizing soft tissue infection. *J Am Coll Surg* 2000; 191:227-231.

41. Weinstein L, Barza M. Gas gangrene. *N Engl J Med* 1973; 289:1129-1131.

42. Weinstein L, Le Frock J. Does antimicrobial therapy of Streptococcal pharyngitis or pyoderma alter the risk of glomerulonephritis? *J Infect Dis* 1971; 124:229-231.

REVIEW QUESTIONS

1.) A disease that is sometimes confused with cellulitis:
   a. Acute dermatitis
   b. Gout
   c. Contact with an allergen
   d. Herpes Zoster
   e. All of the above

2.) Outcomes in necrotizing fasciitis are determined by the following EXCEPT:
   a. Early recognition of tissue necrosis
   b. Prompt surgical intervention
   c. Resuscitation and stabilization
   d. Appropriate antibiotics
   e. Adjunctive hyperbaric oxygen
   f. Sex
   g. All of the above

3.) The advantage of early HBO2 therapy for necrotizing wounds is:
   a. Life saving, stops the production of alpha-toxin
   b. Prevents major amputation or excision prematurely (except for opening of wounds)
   c. It clarifies the demarcation in 24–30 hours, so there is a clear distinction between dead and living tissue.
   d. All of the above

4.) Which of the following signs are NOT USED in the differential diagnosis of necrotizing infections of skin & subcutaneous tissues?
   a. Pain
   b. Tissue gas
   c. Skin changes
   d. Odor to exudates
   e. Systemic involvement
   f. Tissue hypoxia
   g. All of the above

5.) Polymicrobial necrotizing fasciitis is treated with the following antibiotics: Pipercillin / tazobactum or Imipenem
   a. True
   b. False

6.) Streptococcal necrotizing fasciitis is treated with penicillin and clindamycin.
   a. True
   b. False

7.) Clostridial anaerobic cellulitis is treated with penicillin
   a. True
   b. False

Answers: 1e, 2f, 3d, 4f, 5a, 6a, 7a.

NOTES

CHAPTER 31

Post-Operative Surgical Site Infections, Non-Necrotizing Skin, and Soft Tissue Infections

CHAPTER THIRTY-ONE OVERVIEW

Post-Operative Surgical Site Infections, Non-Necrotizing Skin, and Soft Tissue Infections

Jack L. Le Frock

INTRODUCTION

Skin and soft tissue infections are frequently the cause of visits to the doctor or emergency room. Most of these infections are superficial (impetigo, folliculitis, cellulitis) and are easily treated with antibiotics and local care. However, others such as group A B hemolytic streptococcal gangrene and clostridial myonecrosis are life threatening which require combined medical and surgical intervention.

Post-operative surgical site infections (SSIs) remain a major source of morbidity and mortality in surgical patients. They are the second most common nosocomial infection. Among surgical patients, SSIs are the most common nosocomial infection, accounting for 38% of nosocomial infections. It is estimated that SSIs develop in 2–5% of the 16 million patients undergoing surgical procedures each year. SSIs increase the post-operative length of hospital stay by 7–10 days, hospital charges increase by $2,000–$4,500. In these patients, death is directly related to SSI in over 75% of patients with SSI who die in the post-operative period.

This chapter will consider the different types of skin and soft tissue infections as well as SSI infections. Discussion will include the pathogenesis, predisposing factors, signs and symptoms, diagnosis, treatment, microbiology and prevention of them, where possible.

WOUND TYPES

Wounds can be classified as acute or chronic. Acute wounds are caused by external damage to intact skin. Some examples are: surgical wounds, bites, burns, abrasions, minor cuts, lacerations, crush, and gunshot injuries. Acute wounds generally heal rapidly within a predictable time period. However, treatment may vary according to type, site, depth and severity of the wound.

Wounds due to burns or gunshots will require surgical debridement, antibiotics, and wound care to enable healing.

On the other hand, chronic wounds are due to endogenous sources and pathophysiological abnormalities that compromise the integrity of dermal and epidermal tissue. Examples of chronic wounds are leg ulcers, foot ulcers and pressure sores.

The underlying factors which give rise to chronic infections are: peripheral vascular disease, venous hypertension and diabetes mellitus. Other factors that contribute to the development of chronic wounds are: obesity, smoking, poor nutrition, immunosuppression (steroids, chemotherapy, radiation therapy, AIDS). Chronic wounds lead to other complications, and heal slowly in an unpredictable manner.

WOUND CLASSIFICATION

A widely accepted wound classification system was developed over 35 years ago. This wound classification scheme, developed by the National Academy of Sciences and the National Research Council, was based upon the degree of expected microbial contamination during surgery. It stratified wounds as clean, clean-contaminated, contaminated, or dirty using the following definitions:

- Clean wounds were defined as uninfected operative wounds in which no inflammation was encountered and the wound was closed primarily. By definition, a viscus (respiratory, alimentary, genital, or urinary tract) was not entered during a clean procedure. SSI–1.3 to 2.9%.
- Clean-contaminated wounds were defined as operative wounds in which a viscus was entered under controlled conditions and without unusual contamination. SSI–2.4 to 7.7%.
- Contaminated wounds included open, fresh accidental wounds, operations with major breaks in sterile technique or gross spillage from a viscus. Wounds in which acute, purulent inflammation was encountered also were included in this category. SSI–6.4 to 15.2%.
- Dirty wounds were defined as old traumatic wounds with retained devitalized tissue, foreign bodies, fecal contamination, and wounds that involve existing clinical infection or perforated viscus. SSI–7.1 to 40.0%.

WOUND MICROBIOLOGY—SOURCE OF MICROBIAL COLONIZATION

Wound microorganisms originate from three sources: 1) The environment and other exogenous microorganisms in the air or those introduced by traumatic injury, direct contact with other humans, plants or animals harboring microorganisms, indirect contact with contaminated inanimate objects. 2) The surrounding skin (members of the normal skin flora, i.e., Staphylococcus epidermidis, micrococci, skin diphtheroids, propionbacteria, etc. 3) Endogenous sources (gastrointestinal, oropharyngeal and genitourinary mucosae). The normal flora of the endogenous sources are very diverse and abundant. Studies have shown a correlation between the normal flora of the oral cavity and gut and those found in the wound. Dental plaque, the gingival crevice, and the contents of the colon contain 10^{11} to 10^{12} microorganisms per gram of tissue, of which up to 90% of the oral microflora and 99% of the colonic microflora are anaerobes. Therefore, it would be reasonable to predict that wounds with a sufficiently hypoxic and reduced environment are susceptible to colonization by a wide variety of endogenous anaerobic bacteria.

However, based on clinical experience aerobic or facultative pathogens such as *Staphylococcus aureus, Pseudomonas aeruginosa,* and *beta-hemolytic streptococci* are the primary causes of delayed healing and infection in both acute and chronic wounds. This author's experience as well as other infectious disease clinicians is that endogenous anaerobic bacteria were the likely cause of post-operative infections when wound specimens failed to yield bacterial growth on routine culture.

Infectious agents are indirectly acquired by: 1) inhalation of contaminated aerosols, 2) ingestion of contaminated food or drink, 3) contact with contaminated inanimate objects (fomites) and 4), bites from insects that carry microorganisms. However, formites is the major potential source of infectious agents causing wound infections.

ORGANISMS COMMONLY FOUND IN WOUND INFECTIONS

When the disease-producing capabilities of microorganisms over power the defense systems of the host, wound sepsis occurs. Wound sepsis is defined by the U.S. Institute of Surgical Research as bacterial contamination exceeding 10^5 organisms per gram of tissue.

A recent study indicated that the most common pathogens involved in nosocomial infections in U.S. hospitals are *S. aureus, Escherichia coli* and *Pseudomonas aeruginosa*.

Bacteria from both endogenous and exogenous sources are commonly involved in post-operative wound infections (Table 1). *S. aureus* is the most common strain and *methicillin resistant S. aureus* (MRSA) is a growing concern for all healthcare facilities in the U.S. The source of MRSA infections is often the infected individual's own skin, anterior nares, or from healthcare workers.

Facultative gram-negative rods, commonly implicated in wound infections, include bacteria such as *E. coli, Proteus sp., Enterobacter sp.,* and *Klebsiella sp.* These organisms are usually endogenous bacteria causing infection when wounds become contaminated with intestinal contents. *Pseudomonas aeruginosa* may come from the intestine or from the hospital environment (sinks, hydrotherapy, inhalation equipment, hot tubs and whirlpools). Burn infections are commonly caused by either *P. aeruginosa* or *S. aureus*. Anaerobes are generally found in deep traumatic wounds or wounds contaminated with feces or soil.

Factors predisposing to microbial proliferation:

- Pathogenic properties of microbes
- Host defense mechanisms

TABLE 1. AEROBIC AND ANAEROBIC ISOLATES FROM ISOLATED ACUTE AND CHRONIC WOUNDS OF DIFFERENT ETIOLOGIES

Aerobic Gram-Positive Cocci	
S. aureus (MSSA, MRSA) *Coagulase negative Staphylococcus sp.* (MSSE, MRSE) *S.pyogenes*	*S. agalactiae* *Enterococcus faecolis* *Enterococcus faecium* (VRE)
Aerobic Gram-Negative Bacilli	
Enterbacteriaceae *E. coli* *Klebsiella sp.* *Enterobacter sp.* *Serratia sp.*	*Citrabacter sp.* *Providencia sp.* *Pseudomonas sp.* *Acinetobacter sp.* *Stenotrophomonas maltophilia*
Anaerobes	
Gram Negative Bacilli	
Bacteroides sp. *B. fragilis* *Prevotella sp.* *Pr. Melaninogenicus*	*Fusobacterium sp.* *F. necrophorum* *F. nucleatum*
Gram Positive Bacilli	
Clostridium sp. *C. septicum* *C. perfringens*	*C. Novyi* *C. histolyticum*
Gram Positive Cocci	
Peptostreptococcus sp. *Ps. magnus*	*Ps. anaerobius* *Actinomyces sp.*

Surgical wounds will heal rapidly if blood perfusion is maximized, thus delivering nutrients, oxygen, and cells of the immune system to the site of injury and thus reducing the opportunity for the microorganisms to colonize and proliferate.

Anal wounds are a perfect example of the above. The chances of wound healing increases if the tissue oxygen tension (pO_2) is >40 mm Hg, but healing is less likely to occur at levels of <20 mm Hg.

In contrast, chronic non-healing wounds are frequently hypoxic due to poor blood perfusion, and host and microbial cell metabolism contributes further to the lowering of the local pO_2. With low pO_2 tension in a wound, one sees cell death and tissue necrosis that are ideal growth conditions in which bacteria proliferate. This also leads to a low oxidation-reduction potential (Eh) which favors the proliferation of anaerobic bacteria.

Microbes possess a variety of mechanisms by which they can produce virulent factors that cause disease. *Streptococcus pneumoniae* and *Haemophilus influenzae* produce capsules that reduce their ability to be phagocytized. *S. aureus* and *Clostridium perfringens* produce leukocidins that are toxic to white blood cells including those that are phagocytic. Clostridium also produces other exotoxins. *P. aeruginosa* and *S. aureus* survive in phagocytic cells by interfering with lysosomal function which leads to the death of phagocytic cells. The encapsulated strain of *S. aureus* "M" is capable of evading phagocytosis by preventing opsonization. The slime of *P. aeruginosa* is composed of a glycoprotein which obviates phagocytosis, giving rise to a leukopenia. Group A B *hemolytic streptococci* is an extremely virulent organism. S. pyogenes not only produces hyaluronidase, but *streptolysin* S in a leukotoxic component that destroys polymorphoneutrophils by causing the disruption of the neutrophil granule. Group A *streptococci* also generates *streptolysin* O, a hemolysis that attacks red blood cells and induces them to lyse.

Not all microorganisms have the capability to produce virulent products, however, all microbes have the capability to inaugurate an infection.

A compromised host is one who cannot mount an adequate defense against infection or even contain the infection once it occurs. There are systemic as well as local factors that affect the immune system in warding off infection. Some of the systemic factors known to predispose an individual to infection are: congenital immunodeficiency diseases, HIV/AIDS, asplenic patients, malignancy, metabolic diseases (i.e., Diabetes mellitus), renal and hepatic failure, malnutrition, extremes of age, alcohol and tobacco abuse, and immunosuppressive drugs. Some local factors are: preoperative nasal carriage of *S. aureus*, venous stasis, arterial insufficiency, arteritis, radiation fibrosis, neuropathy, chronic lymphedema, obesity, presence of a remote focus of infection and duration of preoperative hospitalization.

SIGNIFICANCE OF MICROBIAL NUMBERS IN WOUNDS

The number of bacteria in a wound will determine the time it will take for a wound to heal. In 1964, Bendly and associates showed that a decubitus ulcer wound only heals if the bacterial load was $\leq 10^6$ CFU/ml of wound fluid. Other researchers doing counts on tissue biopsy cultures had similar findings. Later, a rapid gram stain technique was shown to reliably predict a microbial load of $\geq 10^5$ CFU/g of tissue if a single microorganism was seen on the slide preparation. Many investigators believe that acute or chronic infection exists when the microbial load is $\geq 10^5$ CFU/g of tissue. Pruitt and associates reported that quantitative cultures are incapable of differentiating between colonization and infection in a burn wound, and considered histological analysis to be the most effective way of determining burn wound infection. There are two schools of thought described in the literature. One group favors using surface sampling techniques and the other group uses deep tissue biopsy techniques. The scope of this chapter will not deal with these different schools, but some of the references are provided.

SIGNIFICANCE OF SPECIFIC MICROORGANISMS

The majority of wounds are polymicrobial, involving both aerobes and anaerobes. *S. aureus, P. aeruginosa* and *beta hemolytic streptococci* have been most frequently noted as the cause of delayed wound healing and infection. S. *aureus* is considered to be the most problematic microorganism in traumatic, surgical, and burn wound infections. In 1998, at a consensus meeting of the European Tissue Repair Society, a consensus was reached that the presence of *beta-hemolytic* (Group A) *streptococci* or *P. aeruginosa* in a chronic wound was an indicator for antimicrobial therapy. Contrary to widespread published data on the responsibility of specific microorganisms for a delay in wound healing, other investigators have shown that the resident micro flora has little effect on the outcome of wound healing. In reviewing all the papers, one can say that the role of specific microorganisms in many types of infected wounds is still uncertain. It is not possible to differentiate between pathogenic and non-pathogenic species in a polymicrobial infected wound. Therefore, diagnosis of infection in polymicrobial-infected wounds should be based primarily on clinical signs.

WOUND INFECTIONS

The intact skin and the mucous membranes are the most important defenses for humans. Any damage or injury to the integument disturbs this bastion and its equilibrium with the bacterial flora. Infection occurs when the bacteria accomplishes penetration of the subcutaneous tissue and achieves an acute number. Not only is quantity crucial, but conjoined virulence factors provide the microbes with an adjunctive armamentarium that magnifies their ability to alter the balance in their favor, thus inflicting grave damage to the host.

Another way to look at it is that infection occurs when the pathogenic properties of the microbes (virulence factors) in a wound out competes the hosts natural immune system (host defense mechanisms) and subsequent invasion and dissemination of microorganisms in viable tissue provokes a series of local and systemic host responses.

The first step in the establishment of an infection involves contact between a microbe and a susceptible host. Factors that determine the fate of the initial contact include the ability of the host to mount an adequate defense, the pathogenic potential of the microbe(s), and the number of organisms introduced into the site. Other factors to consider are the type, size and depth of the wound, level of blood perfusion to the wound, and the general health and immune status of the host. Based on multiple studies, it seems that the frequency of anaerobic bacteria in a non-infected wound is 38% and in an infected wound is 48%.

Types of wound infections include: 1) surgical wound infections (SSI's), 2) bite wound infections, 3) acute soft tissue infections, 4) burn wound infections, 5) diabetic foot ulcer infections and 6) pressure ulcer infections (leg and decubitus). In this chapter we will only discuss the first three types, the other three will be discussed in other chapters in this book.

SURGICAL WOUND INFECTIONS

All post-operative surgical infections occurring in an operative site are now termed surgical site infections (SSI's), which occur within 30 days of an operative procedure (or within 1 year if an implant is left in place). SSI's are further divided into superficial incisional (involving only the skin and subcutaneous tissues, deep incisional (involving fascial and muscle layers of the incision), and organ space (involving any part of the anatomy, i.e., organs or spaces.) Organ space SSI's include post-operative intra-abdominal abscesses, empyema, or mediastinitis.

The clinical criteria used to define a SSI include any of the following:

1. A purulent exudate draining from a surgical site
2. A positive fluid culture obtained from a surgical site that was primarily closed

3. The surgeon's diagnosis of infection
4. A surgical site that requires reopening

The risk of infection is generally based on the susceptibility of a surgical wound to microbial contamination. Rates of SSIs for individual procedures vary widely depending upon the patient population, size of hospital, experience of the surgeon and methods used for surveillance. Nonteaching hospitals generally have the lowest rates of SSI compared to small (<500 beds) or large (>500 beds) teaching hospitals (4.6 vs. 6.4 and 8.2%, respectively).

The type of procedure is also associated with different rates of SSIs. The highest SSI rates occur after abdominal surgery: small bowel surgery (5.3–10.6%), colon surgery (4.3–10.5%), gastric surgery (2.8–12.3%, liver/pancreas surgery (2.8–10.2%), exploratory laparotomy (1.9–6.9%), and appendectomy (1.3–3.1%). High volume surgeries are associated with higher rates of SSI and therefore more common infections include: coronary bypass surgery (3.3–3.7%), cesarean section (3.4–4.4%), vascular surgery (1.3–5.2%), joint prosthesis (0.7–1.7%), and spinal fusion (1.3–3.1%). Eye surgery is associated with an extremely low rate of SSI (0.14%).

Except for clean operative procedures, surgical wound infections are polymicrobial in nature, involving both aerobic and anaerobic bacteria. Reported wound infection rates following orthopedic surgery are relatively low (2–6.8%), generalized post-operative wound types reported 3.4% in 5,129 operations and 4.7% in 62,939 operations. Infection rates following clean surgery ranged from 1.5–5.9% and 40–52.9% following contaminated surgery. The CDC surgical site infection study has found *S. aureus, coagulase-negative staphylococci, Enterococcus sp., E coli, P. aeruginosa*, and *Enterobacter sp.* as the most frequently isolated pathogens.

The endogenous and exogenous microbial contamination must be minimized by ensuring good aseptic skilled surgical techniques, minimizing length of surgery, prophylactic antibiotics prior to surgery, and optimizing the local wound conditions (removing devitalized tissues, maintaining adequate perfusion to deliver oxygen, antibiotics, nutrients, immune cells, etc.).

BITE WOUND INFECTIONS

Human and animal bites and other orally contaminated wounds are relatively common. More than one million animal bites require medical attention each year and account for one percent of emergency room visits. The microbiology of bite wounds generally is polymicrobial reflecting the aerobic and anaerobic microbiology of the oral flora of the biter. Bite wounds include scratches, punctures, lacerations, and evulsions. These wounds can be clinically quite deceptive, because what initially appears to be a minor wound may involve the subjacent joint space or bone, resulting in serious complications (damage to a limb, or amputation and permanent disability). The reported infection rate for human bite wounds range from 10–50% depending on the severity and location of the bite, and up to 20% of dog bites and 30–50% of cat bites become infected.

Dog and cat bites occur mostly on the upper extremity. A dog's teeth are not sharp, but can exert a pressure of 200–450 psi. This pressure is strong enough to perforate sheet metal and result in a crush injury with much devitalized tissue, rather than a laceration. The average dog's mouth harbors more than 64 species of bacteria, including *S. aureus, Pasteurella multocida, anaerobic bacteria, alpha-, beta-*, and *gamma-hemolytic streptococci*, and several genera of gram-negative organisms.

P. multocida is isolated between 20 and 50% in dog bites and up to 75% in cat bites. Although *Pasteurella* species are the most common isolates, cat and dog bites contain an average of five different aerobic and anaerobic bacteria per wound.

Cats have slender and extremely sharp teeth that typically cause a puncture type injury with potential involvement of bone or joint. The overall rate of wound infection after cat bite is $\geq$50%, with a proportionate increase in the incidence of associated septic arthritis and osteomyelitis.

A good history and physical exam is important in a patient with a bite wound. It is important to document the presence or absence of more than one wound. Check for signs of wound infection (i.e., fever, localized cellulitis, pain, purulent discharge), or joint penetration (i.e., penetrating bite near a joint or pain, edema, or decreased range of motion).

Important issues to be considered in patients with uninfected wounds include rabies prophylaxis, tetanus immunization, and antibiotic prophylaxis. Wound cultures of uninfected wounds are unnecessary with the one exception for puncture wounds. Both puncture wounds and dog bites of the hand should not be closed primarily. Wounds with extensive crush injuries and wounds that require extensive debridement should not be closed primarily.

Rabies prophylaxis is administered if the dog or cat is rabid or suspected rabid. A healthy dog and cat should be observed for ten days. Because of the devastating effects of rabies virus infection in humans, many physicians recommend vaccination when the animal is not available for observation. The rabies vaccine is administered in five doses, one ml intramuscularly on days 0, 3, 7, 14, and 28. In addition one dose of human rabies immune globulin is given intramuscularly (20 IU/kg) on the first day. If anatomically possible, up to one-half of the dose should be infiltrated around the wounds.

Dog and cat bites should be treated with tetanus immunization. Tetanus-diphtheria toxoid (CTD) should be given to those who have completed their primary immunization and who have not received a booster immunization in the past five years. For anyone whose immune status is uncertain, a dose of tetanus toxoid (0.5 ml intramuscularly) and tetanus immune globulin (250 U intramuscularly) should be given.

Antimicrobial prophylaxis for dog bite wounds is controversial. The author feels it should be given in the following situations: 1) hand bite wounds, 2) deep puncture wounds, 3) wounds requiring surgical debridement, 4) older patients, 5) immuno-compromised patients, 6) bite wounds near a prosthetic joint. Table 2 gives empiric antibiotic therapy for bite wounds.

For someone who presents with an infected bite wound, one must consider rabies prophylaxis, immunize for tetanus, irrigate the wound with normal saline, take photographs to document the infection, obtain x-rays to evaluate the underlying bone status and presence of foreign material, and consult with a hand surgeon. Antimicrobial therapy should be directed against

TABLE 2. MICROBIOLOGY AND EMPIRIC THERAPY OF BITE ASSOCIATED INFECTIONS

Type of Bite	Usual Microbiology	Treatment	Penicillin Allergic
Dog	*Streptococci* *S. aureus* *Eikenella corrodens* *P. multocida* anaerobes	Oral: Amoxicillin/clavulante 500 mg three times daily Parenteral: Ampicillin/sulbactam 3 g every 6 hrs	Oral: Levofloxacin 500 mg once daily or Gatifloxacin 400 mg once daily
Cat	*P. multocida* *Streptococci* anaerobes	Oral: Amoxicillin/clavulanate 500 mg three times daily Parenteral: Ampicillin/sulbactam 3 g every 6 hrs	Either of above medicines PLUS Clindamycin 300 mg every 6 hrs or Metronidazole 500 mg every 6 hrs
Human	*S. aureus* *E. corrodens* *H. influenzae* anaerobes	Oral: Amoxicillin/clavulanate 500 mg three times daily Parenteral: Ampicillin/sulbactam 3 g every 6 hrs or Cefoxitin 2 g every 8 hrs	Parenteral: Levofloxacin 500 mg IV once daily or Gatifloxacin 400 mg IV once daily or Metronidazole 500 mg IV every 6hrs

the polymicrobial infection that frequently occurs following animal bite wounds.

Human bites tend to be more serious and more prone to infection than animal bites, in part because of the typical mechanisms of injury (i.e., clenched fist and occlusional injuries). Clenched fist injuries typically involve trauma to the metacarpophalangeal joints, and thus are at high risk for complications such as deep soft tissue infections, septic arthritis, and osteomyelitis. Soft tissue infections caused by "love nips" are typically seen in teenagers and young adults and can occur on any area of the body. Occlusional bites usually involve the upper extremities in males and breasts and genitalia in females.

Potential pathogens include *S. aureus, H. influenzae, Eikenella corrodens*, and *anaerobic bacteria* including strains that produce B-lactamase. Tetanus immunization status should be determined, saline irrigation should be performed in all wounds, debridement of all devitalized tissues, x-rays taken and antibiotics administered. *E. corrodens* is resistant to first generation cephalosporins, macrolides, clindamycin, and aminoglycosides. Thus, given a choice, remember intravenous treatment with ampicillin-sulbactam or cefoxitin is the best choice.

Remember the complications of bite wounds may include septic arthritis, osteomyelitis tendonitis, and subcutaneous abscess formation.

Complications of human bites are frequent and include tendon and nerve damage, fractures, septic arthritis, and osteomyelitis.

ACUTE SOFT TISSUE INFECTIONS

Acute soft tissue infections can be divided into non-necrotizing and necrotizing soft tissue infections. They range in severity from self-limiting localized inflammation to rapidly progressive, life and limb threatening necrosis with severe systemic toxicity. The non-necrotizing infections include: impetigo, erysipelas, folliculitis, ecthyma, furunculosis, carbunculosis, and cellulitis. Necrotizing soft tissue infections include the skin (clostridial and non-clostridial anaerobic cellulitis), subcutaneous tissue to the muscle fascia (necrotizing fascitis Type I & II) and muscle tissue (clostridial myonecrosis) (gas gangrene). Tables 3 and 4 summarize the microbiology, important facts (Table 3), and empiric treatment (Table 4) of the different types of non-necrotizing soft tissue infections or primary infections.

Primary infections of the skin, or pyodermas, are generally produced by the invasion of normal epidermis by a single species of bacteria. These infections include impetigo, ecthyma, skin abscess, folliculitis furuncles and carbuncles. Impetigo, folliculitis, furuncles and carbuncles have the following four things in common: 1) usually caused by *S. aureus*, 2) rarely require hospitalization, 3) may respond to local measures, 4) recurrence may be prevented by decreasing *S. aureus* skin carriage.

TABLE 3. ANATOMICAL OVERVIEW OF SOFT TISSUE INFECTIONS

Anatomy	Syndrome	More Frequent	Less Frequent	
Epidermis	Erysipelas	*S. pyogenes*	*S. aureus*	Edematous, red, indurated, spreading lesions; sharply demarcated, elevated margin. Most commonly on face. Pain, fever, systemic toxicity common.
	Impetigo	*S. pyogenes* *S. aureus*		Vesicopustular or crusted superficial skin infection. No pain or constitutional symptoms
	Ecthyma	*S. aureus* *S. pyogenes*	*Ps. aeruginosa*	Typically occur on lower extremities. Punched out ulcers appearing beneath adherent crusts
	Folliculitis	*S. aureus*	*Ps. aeruginosa*	Ostium of hair follicle typically on face, buttocks, extensor surface of extremity. Small tender erythematous papules or pustules, drains, becomes crusted, spontaneously heal
	Furunculosis Carbuncle	*S. aureus*		Tender, firm, erythematous nodules that become fluctuant. Moist area skin with hair follicles. More extensive multiloculated subcutaneous lesion
Dermis Superficial fascia	Cellulitis	*S. pyogenes* *S. aureus*	*H. influenzae* *P. multocida* *Aeromonas sp*	Diffuse infection of skin & subcutaneous tissue. Systemic toxicity is variable. Lesions hot red, diffuse or vague margins. S/S celsus
Subcutaneous fat, nerves, arteries, veins Deep fascia	Necrotizing fasciitis Type I Type II	Mixed aerobes & anaerobes *S. pyogenes*		Rapidly progressive infections with soft tissue necrosis. Systemic toxicity. Multi system organ failure may occur. Pain
Muscle	Myonecrosis (Clostridial and non-clostridial)	*C. perfringens* Mixed aerobes & anaerobes	*C. septicum*	Serious, rapidly progressive infection that poses eminent risk to limb & life. Presence of contaminated devitalized tissue

TABLE 4. EMPIRIC THERAPY OF NON-NECROTIZING SOFT TISSUE INFECTIONS

Syndrome	Treatment	Penicillin Allergy
Impetigo	Dicloxacillin, 250–500 mg QID or Cephalexin 250–500 mg QID or Topical mupirocin	Clindamycin 150–300 mg QID or Erythromycin 250–500 mg QID or Topical mupirocin
Erysipelas	Parenteral: Nafcillin, 2 g Q4–6 hrs or Cefazolin 1 g Q8 hrs Oral: Dialoxacillin 500 mg QID Cephalexin 500 mg QID	Parenteral: Clindamycin, 600–900 mg Q8 hrs or Vancomycin, 15 mg/kg Q12 hrs Oral: Clindamycin, 300 mg QID
Ecthyma S. aureus	Dicloxacillin 500 mg Q6 hrs or Cephalexin 500 mg Q6 hrs	Clindamycin, 150–300 mg QID
Ps. aeruginosa	Piperacillin 304 g IV Q6 hrs + Gentamicin or tobramycin 1.5 mg/kg Q8 hrs or Ceftazidime 1–2 gm Q8 hrs + 1- gentamicin or tobramycin	Ciprofloxacin 400 mg IV QD or 750 mg orally Q12 hrs
Cellulitis	Parenteral: Nafcillin 1-2 g Q4–6 hrs or Cefazolin 1 g Q8 hrs Oral: Dicloxacillin 500 mg QID or Cephlexin 500 mg QID	Parenteral: Clindamycin 600–900 mg Q8 hrs Vancomycin 15 mg/kg Q12 hrs Oral: Clindamycin 150–300 mg QID
Cutaneous Abscess	Parenteral: Nafcillin 102 g Q6 hrs or Cefazolin 1g Q8 hrs Oral: Dicloxacillin 250–500 mg QID or Cephalexin 250–500 mg QID	Parenteral: Clindamycin 600–900 mg Q8 hrs or Vancomycin 15 mg/kg Q12 hrs Oral: Clindamycin 150–300 mg QID
Furuncle	If associated cellulitis Dicloxacillin 250–500 mg or Cephalexin 250–500 mg QID	Clindamycin 150–300 mg QID
Carbuncle	Parenteral: Nafcillin 102 g Q6 hrs or Cefazolin 1 g Q8 hrs Oral: Dicloxacillin 500 mg QID or Cephalexin 500 mg QID	Parenteral: Clindamycin 600–900 mg Q8 hrs or Vancomycin 15 mg/kg Q12 hrs Oral: Clindamycin 300 mg QID
Folliculitis	Antimicrobial therapy	Generally not indicated

Dosage: For normal renal function, QID — Four times per day, Q — every

IMPETIGO

Impetigo is a superficial vesiculopustular skin infection occurring on exposed areas of the face and extremities usually caused by *S. aureus* and/or *S. pyogenes*. The infection remains superficial and generally doesn't result in ulceration or scarring. Fever or other constitutional symptoms are absent or minimal. Pruritis is very common and scratching of lesions can result in spread of infection to uninvolved areas. If the infection is caused by the nephritogenic strains of group A streptococci, it can result in post-streptococcal glomerulonephritis.

In spite of the fact that it may resolve spontaneously without antibiotic therapy, the author recommends treating it. Treatment leads to more rapid resolution, prevents the formation of new lesions, and prevents the evolution to cellulitis. Treatment choices are a ten-day course of oral dicloxacillin, cephalexin, clindamycin, or topical mupirocin.

Clinical entities that may be confused with impetigo are herpes simplex, insect bites, and contact dermatitis.

ECTHYMA

Ecthyma is a deeper form of impetigo that begins as a vesicle and progresses to a punched out ulcer that is surrounded by a violaceous border and covered by an adherent crust. It is most often caused by *S. aureus* or *S. pyogenes*. *P. aeruginosa* can produce similar lesions and bacteremia giving rise to ecthyma gangrenosum. The treatment is the same as for impetigo.

SKIN (CUTANEOUS) ABSCESS

Cutaneous abscess is a localized accumulation of polymorphonuclear leukocytes with tissue necrosis involving the dermis and subcutaneous tissue. They can be due to a variety of microorganisms and may be polymicrobial. The most common organism is *S. aureus*. These abscesses are seen in patients with nasal or skin carriage of *S. aureus*, and patients with diabetes mellitus, hidradenitis suppurativa, or immunologic abnormalities.

The most common findings are local pain, swelling, erythema and regional adenopathy. Fever, chills and systemic toxicity with skin abscess is unusual except with concomitant cellulitis.

Initial antibiotic therapy should always include coverage for *S. aureus*. Intravenous staphylococcus coverage is used in patients with associated cellulitis and systemic toxicity. Otherwise, oral antistaphylococcal agents can be given. Surgical incision and drainage should be done if the abscess feels fluctuant or has "pointed."

Complications of cutaneous abscesses include bacteremia and spread of infection into adjacent structures, including bone or joints. Cutaneous abscess can also arise as a complication of bacteremia, endocarditis, or osteomyelitis, sometimes creating difficulties in determining which entity occurred first.

FOLLICULITIS

Folliculitis is a pyoderma localized to hair follicles. This disease is due to bacteria or fungus (S. aureus, P. aeruginosa, candida in immunocompetent subjects). It is seen in people who have nasal carriage of *S. aureus*, exposure to whirlpools, swimming pools and hot tubs with inadequate chlorination, receiving antibiotics and corticosteroids. The lesions consist of small, tender erythematous papules or pustules that eventually drain, become crusted, and heal. Lesions in different stages of evolution are often present simultaneously.

Associated conjunctivitis and external otitis are seen in some cases caused by *P. aeruginosa*. HIV infected patients develop aeosinophilic pustular folliculitis. Anti-infective therapy is not indicated for folliculitis.

FURUNCLES/CARBUNCLES

Furunculosis is an inflammatory nodule involving the hair follicle that usually follows an episode of folliculitis and spreads to the subcutaneous layers of the skin. It presents as a tender, firm erythematous nodule that becomes fluctuant. Furuncles and carbuncles are found in moist areas of skin that contain hair follicles and are subject to friction (i.e., neck, axillae buttocks, face). Factors predisposing to the development of them are obesity, corticosteroid therapy, and defective neutrophil function. They are both almost always caused by *S. aureus*.

A carbuncle is a more extensive, multiloculated subcutaneous lesion that occurs most commonly at the nape of the neck, back, or thighs. It is generally quite painful, and cause fever and other systemic symptoms. With furunculosis, systemic symptoms do not occur.

Most patients with furuncles can be treated with warm compresses to promote spontaneous drainage. Large furuncles and carbuncles require incision and drainage as well as oral anti-staphylococcal therapy. Furuncles involving the nose and perioral area can be complicated by cavernous sinus infection. Staphylococcal bacteremia may occur with large carbuncles resulting in metastatic abscesses.

Infections Associated With Animal Contact

Infections associated with animal contact, although uncommon, are frequently severe, sometimes lethal, and diagnostically challenging. The potential use of *Bacillus anthracis, Francisella tularensis* and *versinia pestis* for bioterrorism has generated great interest in rapid diagnostic techniques because early recognition and treatment are essential. Doxycycline or Ciprofloxacin therapy is recommended for initial treatment in children older than eight years and non-pregnant females.

SOFT TISSUE INFECTIONS FOLLOWING ANIMAL CONTACT

Erysipeloid

Erysipelothrix rhusiopathiae, a thin pleomorphic gram-positive bacillus causes both a self-limited soft tissue illness (Erysipeloid) and a serious systemic infection. It is a zoonosis seen in persons who handle fish, marine animals, swine or poultry. It is also found in sheep, horses, dogs and cats.

The clinical spectrum of human infection includes: localized cutaneous infection; diffuse cutaneous disease, and systemic blood stream infection. The localized cutaneous form, known as Erysipeloid of Rosenbach usually involves fingers and/or hands. Initially, mild pain may occur at the site of inoculation, followed by throbbing pain, itching, burning, and tingling. One to seven days after exposure, a red maculopapular lesion usually develops on the fingers or hands. Erythema spreads centrifugally with central clearing. A blue ring with a peripheral red halo may appear giving the lesion a target appearance. In one third of the cases regional lymphangitis and/or lymphadenopathy occurs. Untreated erysipeloid resolved over 3–4 weeks, but treatment will probably hasten healing and reduce systemic complications.

Erysipeloid occasionally progresses to the diffuse cutaneous form in untreated patients. Eating contaminated meat has also been associated with this clinical picture. Bullous lesions at the primary or distant sites may be seen. These patients often have high fever, arthralgias and negative blood cultures.

Culture of a lesion aspirate and/or biopsy specimen establishes diagnosis. For cutaneous infection, penicillin (500 mg orally four times per day) or amoxicillin (500 mg three times per day) for 7–10 days seems to work. For patients allergic to penicillin cephalosporins, clindamycin or fluoroginolones also work.

Glanders

Glanders, caused by the aerobic gram-negative rod *Burkholderia mallei*, is a disease of horses, mules and donkeys. Infection is via inhalation or skin contact. Although different organs may be involved, pustular skin lesions, and lymphadenopathy with suppurative nodes may be the prominent presentation. Invitro testing suggests this organism is sensitive to ceftazidime, gentamicin, imipenem, doxycycline and ciprofloxacin.

Bubonic Plague

The plague appears primarily in three forms: bubonic, septicemic, and pneumonic. Bubonic plague (*Pestis bubonica*) is the most common form which occurs when *Yersinia pestis* causes an inflammation of the lymph nodes, making them tender and swollen. Pneumonic plague or pulmonic plague (*Pestis pneumonica*) is the second most common form of plague which occurs when the lungs are infected by *Yersinia pestis*. It may be a secondary infection, caused by bacteria spreading from the lymph nodes and reaching the lungs, but can also exist on its own, caused by inhalation of airborne bacteria. Septicemic plague (*Pestis septic(h)aemica*) is the third most common form which occurs when *Yersinia pestis* multiply in the blood. It is usually associated with hunting and skinning of animals, but can also occur secondary to bubonic and pneumonic plague. Plague most commonly presents in its bubonic form, representing 75% or more of modem clinical cases.

Yersinia pestis is principally a zoonotic infection affecting rodents (rats, mice, ground squirrels, prairie dogs, bobcats, cats, rabbits, and chipmunks). The organism is a pleomorphic gram-negative coccobacillus that is a facultative anaerobe. Humans are infected when they come in close contact with wild animal (sylvatic) sources of disease and are bitten by the particular (infected) rodent or animal flea, or they handle tissue, or they ingest contaminated animal meats. In modem times, airborne human infection from a pneumonic plague, transmission from man to man, and animal to man, occurs infrequently. Ninety percent of human cases in the USA have occurred in the following four states: Arizona, California, Colorado and New Mexico.

The disease is acquired from inoculation of the organism after the bite of an infected flea or exposure of cut or abraded skin to contaminated animal tissues or body fluids. The incubation period ranges from a few hours to tendays (average 3–6 days). Patients develop an abrupt onset of high fever (38.5– 40° C) with rigors, malaise, weakness and headache. Simultaneously with fever, the patients note the focal lymphadenopathy. A palpable bulbo in a single anatomic region will appear, sometimes initially painless, before rapidly becoming extremely tender, that patient with any movement that will simulate pain. Buboes are l cm to 10 cm, are oval and elevate the skin. Lymph nodes are commonly found in the groin (52–86%), femoral nodes more than inguinal nodes; axilla (9–16%), cervical nodes (5–33%). Axillary adenopathy results in abducting the shoulder and splinting the arm. When intra-abdominal nodes are involved, plague may mimic a surgical abdomen.

In the recovery period, some nodes may continue to enlarge, soften and if not incised will burst, discharging sometimes foul smelling pus. Peripheral edema, especially of the leg, is sometimes a sequela because of scarring of the lymphatics.

A small proportion of patients, either in early or late stages of the disease, have what looks like carbuncles. They actually are small patches of moist gangrenous skin that will become larger and may slough. A generalized popular rash of the hands, feet and pectoral regions may be seen in untreated patients.

Diagnosis can be made by blood cultures and by aspirating lymph nodes for staining and culture. No controlled comparative studies exist for the treatment of plague. Streptomycin has been the drug of choice, although tetracycline and chloramphenicol is considered appropriate therapy. Fluroquinolones are another option.

Tularemia

Tularemia ulceroglandular, glandular, or *glandular Francisella tularensis* is a fastidious, aerobic, gram-negative *coceobacillus*. Infection of humans follows a) contact with infected rabbits, b) bites by deer flies, dog or wood ticks, cats, coyotes, dogs, or skunks, c) skinning or dressing infected animals and d) ingesting contaminated meat (uncommon). Biting flies occasionally transmit the illness in the United States, whereas mosquitoes are common vectors in Europe. Five clinical forms of the disease have been described: 1) ulceroglandular, 2) glandular, 3) typhoidal, 4) pneumonic and 5) oculoglandular, or oropharyngeal. The glandular varieties are generally acquired by handling infected animals, by tick bites, and sometimes by animal bites, especially from cats.

Ulceroglandular tularemia is the most common form of the disease. Incubation period averages two to five days but may be as short as one or as long as ten days. The first manifestations are headache, chills, generalized aching, weakness and fever as high as 104°F (40°C). Most patients are severely ill. Within 36 to 48 hours, the site of inoculation of the organism becomes inflamed and tender. A papule then appears and is soon capped by a vesicle which postulates and becomes necrotic. The fully developed lesion is an ulcer covered by a black eschar; a scanty serous discharge is present. The draining lymphatics may become painful, and subcutaneous nodules may develop along the course of the lymphatic vessels connecting the lesion in the skin and the regional lymph nodes; the appearance is similar to that of sporotrichosis. The draining lymph nodes become enlarged and painful;

they remain hard, or suppurate and drain (thus the term "ulceroglandular"). Pustular petechial and vesicular rashes are observed on any area of the body in some cases. In some patients, the skin lesion is inconspicuous or healed by the time that they seek medical care, resulting in "glandular" tularemia. Confirmation of the diagnosis is usually accomplished by means of serologic testing. Results of routine cultures are often negative, unless cysteine-supplemented media are used.

No prospective controlled or randomized trials of therapy for tularemia have been performed, nor has the optimal duration of treatment been established, but many patients will require initiation of treatment before confirmation of the diagnosis. To date streptomycin is the drug of choice. Failures have been reported with ceftriaxone. With static drugs such as tetracyclines and chloroamphenicol, relapses may be more common. Not enough patients to date have been treated with fluorquinolones to give an opinion.

Cat-Scratch Disease and Bacillary Angiomatosis

Cat-scratch disease (CSD) is an infectious disease characterized by self-limited regional lymph-adenopathy. The manifestations of CSD, however, can include visceral organ, neurological, and ocular involvement. *Bartonella henselae* causes most cases of cat-scratch disease in immunocompetent hosts. *Bacillary angiomatosis*, seen in immunocompromised patients can occur from either *B. henselae* or *Bartonella quintana*. They are gram-negative, pleomorphic bacteria that stain very poorly in tissues using Gram's stain but will stain black with silver-impregnated stains, such as the Warthin-Starry stain. Most *Bartonella sp.* that cause human disease are associated with well-defined reservoirs, usually domestic (cats and dogs), and wild animals (rats, mice, dogs).

Cat-scratch disease most often (in 85 to 90% of children) presents as a localized cutaneous and lymph node disorder near the site of organism inoculation. In some individuals, the organisms disseminate and infect the liver, spleen, eye, and central nervous system. Patients with localized disease generally have a self limited illness, whereas those with disseminated disease can have life threatening complications.

Treatment of cat-scratch disease with antimicrobial agents has had variable, but rarely dramatic results. A single, double blind, placebo controlled study consisted of 29 patients, 14 of whom received azithromycin. The lymph node size had regressed 30 days after treatment more often in the azithromycin treated patients.

Cutaneous bacillary angiomatosis therapy has not been systemically examined. Based on case reports either erythromycin or doxycycline seems to work. Initial therapy should be at least four weeks.

Anthrax

Anthrax is an uncommon illness in the United States, although there is concern with its use as a bioterrorism weapon. Animals become infected with *Bacillus anthracis*, a sporulating gram-positive rod, by ingesting spores while grazing on contaminated grass or feed. Transmission to humans is accomplished through direct exposure to infected animals or animal products through skin exposure, ingestion, or inhalation.

The most common form of the disease is cutaneous anthrax, accounting for between 95 and 99% of human cases. Lesions are usually single and are associated with regional lymphadenitis. The initial lesion may consist of a small ring of vesicles that coalesce into a single large vesicle or as a pruritic papule. Papules will progress rapidly to vesicles containing serous or serosanguinous fluid. A central black eschar forms and is often surrounded by a ring of secondary vesicles called the "pearly wreath." Non pitting edema, sometimes described as "malignant edema," when there is extensive edema of the head and neck, develops in 36 hours.

Five percent of patients are bacteremic. In adults, there is mild fever and malaise. Lymphangitis and regional lymphadenitis are less frequent in the adult. Gram staining the vesicular fluid is essential, as bacilli are easily seen in cases of anthrax.

Untreated cutaneous anthrax has 20% mortality. The mortality rate in appropriately treated cases is less than 1% with treatment, edema resolves in 2–3 days, but progression of the eschar is unaffected. The eschar grows to 1–3 cm diameter in ten days and heals with scarring.

Cultures of untreated lesions, depending on the stage of evolution, have positive results >80% of the time. Methods of specimen collection for culture depend on the type of lesion. With vesicles, the blister should be unroofed and two dry swabs soaked in the fluid. At a later stage, two moist swabs should be rotated in the ulcer base or beneath the eschar's edge. Patients who have previously received antimicrobials or who have negative results of tests but still have suspected cutaneous anthrax should have a punch biopsy specimen obtained that can be submitted for special studies, such as immunohistochemical staining and/or PCR (polymerase chain reaction).

The recommended treatment for cutaneous anthrax is 2 million units of penicillin G intravenously every six hours until the edema subsides (usually for 2–4 days) followed by oral penicillin therapy for a total of ten days. Sixty days of treatment is recommended when infection is associated with bioterrorism because concomitant inhalation may have occurred. Doxycycline or erythromycin (4 grams daily) are considered alternative agents.

EVALUATION OF A PATIENT WITH A SOFT TISSUE INFECTION

When evaluating a patient with soft tissue infection the following sixteen things should always be considered:

1. Define the host (i.e., immune status, integrity of the integument)
2. Detailed patient history. Impaired cell mediated immunity (i.e., steroid therapy, HIV, or hematological malignancy may be susceptible for infection with an opportunistic pathogen).
3. Systemic toxicity (i.e., fever, chills, prostration).
4. Rate of progression of inflammatory process.
5. Presence or absence of significant pain in involved area.
6. Environmental exposure (i.e., sun, fresh or salt water, plants, insects, animal or human bite.
7. Precipitating event (puncture injury, bite).

8. Presence of an associated underlying disease. (i.e., necrotizing infections associated with advanced age or underlying co-morbidity, diabetes mellitus, malignancy, alcoholism, peripheral vascular disease, immunosuppressive therapy.)
9. Allergy to any antibiotics.
10. Amount of alcohol usually consumed per week.
11. Use of illicit drugs.
12. Currently taking steroids or any other immunosuppressive medications?
13. Any treatment received for this problem?
14. Any recent hospital or chronic care facility stay prior to or during the time that the symptoms began?
15. Is the infection related to any new or old injury?
16. Is it possible that there may be a foreign object in the wound?

PHYSICAL EXAM OF A PATIENT WITH A SOFT TISSUE INFECTION

Every patient with a soft tissue infection should be checked for the following:

1. Presence or absence of fever and other signs of systemic toxicity (i.e., hypotension, confusion, oliguria).
2. Assess for erythema, induration, fluctuans, crepitus, lymphangitis, tenderness, duskiness (evidence of ischemia) bullae, hemorrhagic lesions, presence and characteristics of any drainage.
3. Gas in tissue or not.
4. Try to figure which anatomic structures are involved which frequently gives a clue to the microbiology of the specific syndrome.
5. Measure the depth, length, width of wound, note type of drainage, and any odor.

LABORATORY STUDIES AND OTHER TESTS

The following laboratory studies should be done in patients with soft tissue infections:

1. Complete blood count.
2. BUN and creatinine. If elevated it may suggest hypoperfusion and incipient renal failure.
3. Creatinine kinase — if elevated may indicate myonecrosis secondary to necrotizing fasciitis.
4. X-rays to rule out foreign bodies or gas in the tissues.
5. Ultrasound or computed tomography to look for drainable collections.
6. Doppler vascular exam to rule out deep venous thrombosis.
7. Blood cultures.
8. Culture and sensitivity of the wound via tissue biopsy, curettage, needle aspiration, etc. depending on the type of wound.

Not all of the above tests are required for every patient with a wound. Based on the clinician's findings one, two, or all of the above tests should be ordered.

TREATMENT OF WOUND AND SOFT TISSUE INFECTIONS

The treatment of wound and soft tissue infections is multifocal including the following:

Surgical Debridement

Infected and non-infected, non-healing wounds can also benefit from surgical debridement, since devitalized tissue both obstructs the healing process and often forms the focus for microbial proliferation. Surgical debridement will significantly reduce the microbial load as well as exposing healthy tissue required for wound healing. Besides surgical debridement there is autolytic and enzymatic debridement, as well as biosurgical debridement. Debridement details will be discussed in the chapter by TM Emhoff and SA Ferro entitled, "Wound Debridement."

Pressure Reduction in Wounds

With the exception of burn wounds, pressure and duration of pressure application are key factors in the pathogenesis of the majority of wounds. Therefore, it makes sense to eliminate these factors for the healing of these wounds. Two major ways to accomplish this is off-loading and negative pressure wound therapy both of which will be discussed in another chapter.

Altering Abnormal Host Factors

Infections in the compromised host may involve the treatment of the underlying disease, such as control of blood sugar levels in the diabetic, get patients to stop smoking, stop drinking, improve nutrition, use vitamins, etc.

Hyperbaric Oxygen (HBO2) Therapy

HBO2 should be considered in the wound care in the compromised host. HBO2 at 2 ATA increases blood plasma and tissue fluid oxygen tensions ten fold, blood oxygen content by 125% and oxygen diffusion through tissues three fold. The hyper-oxygenation effects lead to secondary effects important in wound healing and infection control such as leucocyte oxidative killing, fibroblastic function (migration, proliferation, and secretion), neovascularization, toxin inactivation, and bacteriostasis. HBO2 is an adjunct form of therapy which will be discussed in details in another chapter by CE Fife entitled, "Hyperbaric Oxygen Applications in Wound Care."

Antimicrobial Agents

Antibiotics are used prophylactically to prevent post operative wound infections and are often used to treat soft tissue and wound infections that develop for multiple reasons. Antibiotics should not be administered for therapy unless signs of local or systemic spread of the infectious process are evident or the patient is severely immunocompromised. Characteristics of the infecting organism(s) and the host factors must be considered when selecting the appropriate antimicrobial agent to be used. Many factors have to be considered when choosing the most appropriate antibacterial agent.

Antibiotic therapy must be tailored to the individual infection. Things one has to consider: broad or narrow spectrum antibiotic, bactericidal or bacteriostatic agent, single agent or combination therapy, antimicrobial resistance, tissue penetration, drug interactions, host factors (renal or hepatic toxicity), spectrum of drug, route of administration, adverse reactions, etc. To make a logical systematic selection of the appropriate antibiotic in a given clinical situation, it is important to define the "drug of choice." In terms of antibiotic therapy, the agent that is selected should demonstrate three properties:

1. It is the narrowest spectrum agent available for the suspected or confirmed pathogen.
2. It is the least expensive.
3. It is the safest.

Tables 5, 6, and 7 show the initial choice of antibiotics for gram-positive (Table 5), gram-negative (Table 6), and anaerobic organisms (Table 7). Table 8 lists antibiotic choices for necrotizing soft tissue infections.

TABLE 5. GRAM-POSITIVE ORGANISMS: INITIAL CHOICE OF ANTIBIOTICS FOR THERAPY (ADULT DOSAGES)

Organism	Antibiotics of 1st choice	Alternative antibiotics
Methicillin-sensitive ***Staphylococcus aureus***	Nafcillin 2 g Q4 hrs or Clindamycin 900 mg Q8 hrs	Cefazolin Vancomycin
Coagulase-negative ***Staphylococcus sp.***	Nafcillin 2 g Q6 hrs or Clindamycin 900 mg Q8 hrs	Cefazolin Vancomycin
Methicillin-resistant ***Staphylococcus aureus***	Vancomycin 1 g Q12 hrs or Linezoid 600 mg Q12 hrs	SMZ-TMP or Minocycline + Rifampin
Coagulase-negative ***Staphylococcus sp.***	Vancomycin 1 g Q12 hrs or Linezoid 600 mg Q12 hrs	SMZ-TMP or Minocycline + Rifampin, Clindamycin
Group A streptococcus ***Strep. Pyogenes***	Penicillin G 2 x 10 U Q4 hrs or ampicillin 2 g Q6 hrs	Clindamycin, Cephalosporin Vancomycin
Group B streptococcus ***Strep. Agalactiae***	Penicillin G 2 x 10 U Q4 hrs or ampicillin 2 g Q6 hrs	Clindamycin Cephalosporin Vancomycin
Sensitive ***Strep. Pneumoniae***	Penicillin G 2 x 10 U Q4 hrs	Clindamycin, Erythromycin
Intermediate ***Strep. Pneumoniae***	Cefotaxime 1 g Q8 hrs Erythromycin	Clindamycin
Resistant ***Strep. Pneumoniae***	Vancomycin 1 g Q12 hrs or Levofloxacin 500 mg/day	Quinupristin & Dalfopristin, Linezolid
Sensitive ***Enterococcus sp.***	Ampicillin 1 g Q6 hrs Vancomycin 1 g Q12 hrs	Ampicillin-sulbactam Linezolid
Resistant ***Enterococcus faecium***	Quinupristin/dalfopristin 7.5 mg/kg Q8 hrs Linezolid 600 mg Q 12 hrs	Chloramphenicol and Rifampin

TABLE 6. GRAM-NEGATIVE ORGANISMS: INITIAL CHOICE OF ANTIBIOTICS FOR THERAPY (ADULT DOSAGES)

Organism	Antibiotics of 1st choice	Alternative Antibiotics
Acinetobacter sp.	Ceftazidime 1 g Q8 hrs + Levofloxacin 500 mg/day or Imipenem 500 mg Q6 hrs	Ampicillin-sulbactam
Enterobacter sp.	Cefotaxime 1 g Q6 hrs or Imipenem 500 mg Q6 hrs	Levofloxacin, mezlocillin, ticarcillin-clavulanate
Escherichia coli	Ampicillin-sulbactam 3 g Q6 hrs	Cefazolin, levofloxacin, gentamicin, SXT
Haemophilus influenzae	Cefotaxime 1 g Q8 hrs or Ampicillin-sulbactam 3 g Q6 hrs	Levofloxacin, SMZ-TMP ampicillin, azithromycin
Klebsiella sp.	Cefotaxime 1 g Q6 hrs or Levofloxacin 500 mg/day	Ampicillin-sulbactam Gentamicin
Proteus mirabilis	Ampicillin 1 g Q6 hrs or Levofloxacin 500 mg/day	Cefazolin, SMZ-TMP Gentamicin
Proteus vulgaris	Cefotaxime 2 g Q8 hrs or Imipenem 500 mg Q6 hrs	Mezlocillin, gentamicin
Proteus rettgeri	Cefotaxime 2 g Q8 hrs or Imipenem 500 mg Q6 hrs	Ticarcillin-clavulanate
Morganella morganii	Levofloxacin 500 mg/day	
Neisseria gonorrhoeae	Cefriaxone 125 mg, IM once + azithromycin 1 g, PO once	Levofloxacin and Azithromycin
Providencia sp	Cefotaxime 2 g IV Q hrs or Levofloxacin 500 mg/day	SMZ-TMP, amikacin, Imipenem
Pseudomonas aeruginosa	Cefepime 2 g Q12 hrs or Piperacillin 3 g Q6 hrs or Imipenem 500 mg Q6 hrs	Ticarcillin-clavulanate, Tobramycin, amikacin, Ciprofloxacin
Serratia marcescens	Cefotaxime 2 g Q6 hrs	Levofloxacin, gentamicin, Imipenem

Dosage: Q—every, PO—preferred orally

TABLE 7. ANAEROBIC ORGANISMS: INITIAL CHOICE OF ANTIBIOTICS FOR THERAPY (ADULT DOSAGES)

Organism	Antibiotic of 1st choice	Alternative antibiotics
Bacteroides fragilis group	Clindamycin 900 mg Q8 hrs or Metronidazole 500 mg Q8 hrs	Ampicillin-sulbactam, Ticarcillin-clavulanic acid
Prevotella sp.	Clindamycin 900 mg Q8 hrs or Metronidazole 500 mg Q8 hrs	Ampicillin-sulbactam, Cefotetan
Peptostreptococcus sp.	Clindamycin 900 mg Q8 hrs or Penicillin G 2 x 10 U Q4 hrs	Clindamycin, Metronidazole
Clostridium sp.	Clindamycin 900 mg Q8 hrs or Penicillin G 2 x 10 U Q4 hrs	Ampicillin-sulbactam, metronidazole

TABLE 8. ANTIBIOTIC CHOICES FOR NECROTIZING SOFT-TISSUE INFECTIONS

Single Agents	
Ampicillin/sulbactam Ticarcillin/clavulanate Piperacillin/Tazobactam Cefoxitin	Cefotetan Imipenem Meropenem
Combination Regimens	
Aerobic/Facultative	**Anaerobic Coverage**
Aminoglycoside Fluoroqinolone 3rd –generation cephalosporin Aztreonam	Clindamycin Metronidazole Pcn/B-lactemase inhibitor

Emerging antibiotic resistance among *Staphylococcus aureus* (methicillin resistance) and *Streptococcus pyogenes* (erythromycin resistance) are problematic, because both of these organisms are common cause of a variety of skin and soft-tissue infections and because empirical choices of antimicrobials must include agents with activity against resistant strains. Minor skin and soft-tissue infections may be empirically treated with semi-synthetic penicillin, first generation or second generation oral cephalosporins, macrolides or clindamycin. However, 50% of methicillin resistant S. aureus (MRSA) strains have inducible or constitutive clindamycin resistance. Most community acquired MRSA strains remain susceptible to trimethoprim-sulfamethoxazole and tetracycline, though treatment failure rates of 21% have been reported with doxycline or minocycline. Therefore, it is prudent to reevaluate patients taking these drugs in 24–48 hours to verify clinical response.

Perioperative antimicrobial surgical prophylaxis is recommended for operative procedures that have a high rate of post operative wound infection, when foreign materials must be implanted, or when the wound infection rate is low, but the development of a wound infection could result in a disastrous event. Prophylactic antimicrobial agents should be bactericidal, non-toxic, have invitro activity against the common organisms that cause post operative wound infection after a specific surgical procedure, have a long half life, and be inexpensive. Most physicians use cefazolin or another cephalosporin because they meet the above criteria.

The prophylactic antimicrobial agent should be administered at 30–60 minutes prior to surgery. Exceptions to this rule are cesarean procedures and oral antimicrobials for colonic and urologic procedures. The length of prophylaxis should not exceed 24 hours post operatively. Fifty-six hospitals from 50 states participated in the National Surgical Infection Prevention Collaborative study using the above rules, and collectively reduced the overall surgical infection rate from 2.28 to 1.65%. Prolonged prophylaxis leads to the selection of resistant organisms, increased chance of developing *C. difficile* colitis, unnecessary expense, added antimicrobial toxicity, and an increase in MRSA surgical site infections.

Use of vancomycin for prophylaxis is appropriate only when there is a true type I hypersensitivity to penicillin or when there is a high incidence of surgical site infections due to *methicillin resistant staphylococci*. Adherence to this practice will help to avoid the emergence of vancomycin resistant organisms and vancomycin related toxicity.

INFECTION CONTROL

The potential for wound infections to occur increases as the number of organisms introduced into the site increases. The goal of infection control is to reduce the number of organisms in the environment. There are three terms often used in wound care and infection control: sterilization, disinfection and antisepsis. Sterilization is defined as the total destruction of all forms of microbial life. Disinfection is the reduction of the number of organisms present on inanimate objects. Antisepsis should be used for procedures that inhibit or destroy microorganisms on skin or living tissue.

Antiseptics are chemical agents that are potentially toxic to both microbial and host cells. Therefore, their use is limited to topical application to wounds and intact skin. Topical antiseptics are often used in traumatic or chronic wounds that are heavily contaminated with a variety of microorganisms. Some commonly used antiseptics are: providone iodine, Dakin's solution, hydrogen peroxide, chlorhexidine and acetic acid. These will be addressed by Coe and Clark in the chapter entitled, "Infection Control in the Wound Care Setting."

CONTROL OF ENDOGENOUS ORGANISMS

Surgical wounds following abdominal surgery of the intestines and rectum are generally due to the endogenous bacteria. The best way to reduce the incidence of these post surgical infections (SSI's) are to reduce the intestinal flora prior to surgery by mechanical cleansing and antimicrobial agents pre-operatively. Antibiotics with activity against aerobes and anaerobes are given, such as, neomycin sulfate 1g plus erythromycin base 1g orally (after mechanical bowel preparation is completed) at 19, 18, and 9 hrs before surgery, and IV cephalosporin at surgery. Suppression of the intestinal flora with antibiotics is also useful in preventing wound colonization in patients with burns greater than 25%. Perioperative antimicrobial surgical prophylaxis is a key factor in prevention (discussed in a previous part of this chapter).

Preventing bacterial access to the wound may include preparation of the skin before surgery, using antiseptic solutions such as chlorhexidine or iodine, which reduces the number of bacteria on the skin. Post operatively the wound must be prevented from becoming contaminated. Mechanical cleansing of the wound using irrigation is of questionable value.

CONTROL OF EXOGENOUS ORGANISMS

To reduce environmental sources of infection, physical or chemical agents are used to inhibit or destroy microorganisms. Disinfectants and sterilization is used based on specific protocols to reduce infection. The increasing incidence of infections caused by MRSA in healthcare facilities has led to the development of protocols to prevent its spread. Hand washing is a method of infection control that is often overlooked and definitely under-used. Remember to "wash your hands and drown a bug." Care must be taken to prevent the transmission of microorganisms from an infected individual to the healthcare worker. Guidelines for healthcare workers are available in publications of the Centers for Disease Control (CDC) and the Occupational Safety and Health Administration (OSHA). Universal precautions are now used in taking care of wound care patients.

PREVENTION OF SURGICAL SITE INFECTIONS (SSI'S)

Application of knowledge concerning the pathogenesis of wound infection and strict adherence to the principles of wound care can prevent many infectious complications. Preventing infectious complications is far more practical than treating them.

The most important factors in the prevention of SSI's are: the general health of the patient (host factors—previously discussed), meticulous operative techniques, timely administration of pre-operative antibiotics (previously discussed), hand washing, hair removal, hyperglycemia and diabetes control, perioperative normothermia and supplemental perioperative oxygen.

Good surgical technique is fundamental to lowering SSI rates. These techniques include: gentle traction, effective hemostasis, removal of devitalized tissues, obliteration of dead space, irrigation of tissues by saline during long procedures to avoid excessive drying, use of fine non-absorbed monofilament suture material, judicious use of closed suction drains, and wound closure without tension.

The goal of antimicrobial prophylaxis is to eradicate the growth of endogenous micro-organisms (previously discussed). Clipping of the hair or use of depilatory creams should be used to remove hair just prior to the surgical incision. The use of razors and shaving should not be done the night before surgery.

Hypothermia causes numerous adverse outcomes, including morbid myocardial events, increased blood loss and transfusion requirement, post-surgical wound infections and prolonged hospitalization. (Perioperative normothermia should thus be maintained unless therapeutic hypothermia is specifically indicated). Mild perioperative hypothermia may promote SSI by triggering thermo-regulatory vasoconstriction that, in turn may decrease subcutaneous oxygen tension. One study randomized 200 patients undergoing colorectal surgery to routine intraoperative thermal (the hypothermia group) and found a lower rate of SSI in the normothermia group (19 vs. 6%). In a study of clean surgical procedures, wound infection was significantly more common in the hypothermia vs the normothermia group (14 vs. 5%).

TABLE 9. IMPORTANT FACTORS TO CONSIDER IN PREVENTING WOUND INFECTION IN PATIENTS

1. Pre-operative antimicrobial shaver
2. Remove hair (if at all) by clipping
3. No shaving immediately before surgery
4. Administer preventive antibiotics 30–60 minutes prior to surgery when indicated, keeping therapeutic levels during the entire operative procedure
5. Exercise vigilance for breaks in aseptic technique by operating room team
6. Prevent hypothermia and maintain normothermia during operation
7. Administer high intraoperative and postoperative inspired oxygen
8. Maintain normal glucose levels during surgery
9. Limit sutures and ligatures
10. Use monofilament sutures
11. Employ closed suction rather than open drainage; use no drainage if possible
12. Exercise meticulous skin closure
13. Surveillance of wound infection rate with review of preventive measures

Supplemental perioperative oxygen (inspired fraction of 80% instead of 30%) significantly reduces post-operative nausea and vomiting, diminishes the decrease in phagocytosis, and bacterial killing usually associated with anesthesia and surgery, and reduces the rate of post-operative wound infection among patients who undergo colon resection.

Maintaining the careful regulation of the blood glucose level reduces the rate of infection. The primary defense against surgical pathogens is oxidative killing by neutrophils. Oxygen is a substrate for this process, and the reaction critically depends on tissue oxygen tension as well as the glucose level. High blood sugar inhibits neutrophil killing.

Hand hygiene is the single most important measure to reduce transmission of microorganisms from one person to another or one site to another on the same patient. The problem with hand hygiene is not a paucity of good products, but rather the laxity of practice. More than 150 years ago, Ignax Semmelweis showed that the infectious organisms causing puerperal fever were spread from patient to patient via the hands of healthcare workers. Compliance with handwashing rarely exceeds 40% even under study conditions, and even in intensive care units. In 90% of cases the mean observed washing time is < 10 seconds, compared with the recommended 15–30 seconds.

The Hospital Infection Control Practices Advisory Committee (HICPAC) and CDC guidelines advise use of a plain (non-antimicrobial) soap with water for routine handwashing and with the use of an antimicrobial agent for specific circumstances. Alcohol containing hand disinfection is an excellent effective and practical alternative to standard soap and water. Alcohol based products have rapid antimicrobial effect and are equally effective against Gram positive and Gram negative organisms. Alcohol based preparations also require less time to effect a maximum reduction in bacterial counts and are at least as tolerable on skin as are antiseptic detergents. Table 9 summarizes the important factors to consider in preventing wound infection in patients.

SUMMARY

Post-operative surgical site infections (SSIs) remain a major source of morbidity and mortality in surgical patients. Among surgical patients, SSI's are the most common nosocomial infection. They increase hospital stay by 7–10 days and increase hospital charges by $2,000–4,500. *S. aureus* is the most common pathogen involved in SSI's and *methicillin resistant S. aureus* (MRSA) is a growing concern for all healthcare facilities in the United States. Surgical wounds will heal rapidly if blood perfusion is maximized. However the best treatment is through prevention. Some important preventive measures are: good infection control, administer prophylactic antibiotics 30–60 minutes prior to surgery and stop prophylactic antibiotics after 24 hours, maintain normal glucose levels during surgery, administer high intraoperative and post-operative inspired oxygen, prevent hypothermia and maintain normothermia during surgery. Last but not least, wash your hands and drown a bug.

ACKNOWLEDGMENTS

The author would like to acknowledge Patti Reynolds and Gwen Wilson, Medical Librarians at Sarasota Memorial Hospital for their help in preparing this chapter.

REFERENCES

1. Agger WA, Mardan Ali. Pseudomonas aeruginosa infections of intact skin. *CID* 1995; 20:302-308.
2. Anonymous – DHHS and CDC draft guideline for the prevention of surgical site infection. *Fed Regist* 1998; 33167.
3. Baddour LM. Cellulitis syndromes: An update. *Int J Antimicrob Agents* 2000;14:113-116.
4. Bass JW, Vincent 1M, Person DA. The expanding spectrum of Bartonella infections: A. Cat-scratch disease. *Pediatr Infect Dis J* 1997; 16:163-169.
5. Bisno AL, Steven SDL. Streptococcal infections of skin and soft tissues. *N Eng J Med* 1996; 334:240.
6. Bowler PG, Davies BJ. The microbiology of acute and chronic wounds. *Wounds* 1999; 11:72-79.
7. Bowler PG. The anaerobic and aerobic microbiology of wounds: a review. *Wounds* 1998; 10:170-178.
8. Bratzler DW, Houck PM, Richards C, et al. Use of antimicrobial prophylaxis for major surgery; baseline results from the National Surgical Infection Prevention Project. *Arch Surg* 2005; 140:174-182.
9. Bratzler DW, Houck PM, Antimicrobial prophylaxis for surgery: an advisory statement from the National Surgical Infection Prevention Project. *Clin Infect Dis* 2004; 38: 1706-1715.
10. Brook I, Frazier EH. Aerobic and anaerobic bacteriology of wounds and cutaneous abscesses. *Arch Surg* 1990; 125:1445-1447.
11. CDC NNIS System National Nosocomial Infections Surveillance (NNIS) report, data summary from October 1986-April 1998, Issued June 1998.
12. Classen DC, Evans RS, Pestotnik SL, et al. The timing of prophylactic administration of antibiotics and the risk of surgical-wound infection. *N Eng J Med* 1992; 326:281-286.
13. Cox SK, Everett ED. Tularemia, an analysis of 25 cases. *Mo Med* 1981; 78(2):70-4.
14. Dellinger EP, Gross FA, Barrett TL, et al. Quality standard for antimicrobial prophylaxis in surgical procedures. Infectious Diseases Society of America. *Clin Infect Dis* 1994; 18:422-427.
15. Dellinger EP, Hausmann SM, Bratzler DW, et al. Hospitals collaborate to decrease surgical site infections. *Am J Surg* 2005; 190:9-15.
16. Dixon TC, Meselson M, Guillemin J, et al. Anthrax. *N Eng J Med* 1999; 341:815-820.
17. Enron LJ. Targeting lurking pathogens in acute traumatic and chronic wounds. *J Emerg Med* 1999; 17:189-195.
18. Evans ME, Gregory DW, Schaffner W, etal. Tularemia: a 30-year experience with 88 cases. *Medicine* (Baltimore) 1985; 64(4):251-69
19. Fowler E. Wound infection: a nurse's perspective. *Ostomy Wound Manage* 1998;44(8):44-53.
20. Gaynes RP, Culver DH, Horan T, et al. Surgical site infection (SSI) rates in the United States, 1992-1998: the National Nosocomial Infections Surveillance System basic SSI risk index. *CID* 2001; 33 suppl. 2: S69-S77.
21. Goldstein EJ. New horizons in the bacteriology, antimicrobial susceptibility and therapy of animal bite wounds. *J Med Microbial* 1998; 47:95-97.
22. Greener M. The fifty year war against infection. *Pharm Times* 1998; June:34-37.
23. Griego RD, Rosen T, Orengo IF, et al. Dog cat and human bites: a review. *J Am Acad Dermatol* 1995; 33:1019-1029.
24. Harbarth S. Handwashing – the Semmelweis lesson misunderstood? *Clin Infect Dis* 2000; 30:990-991.
25. Heggers JP. Defining infection in chronic wounds: methodology. An historical review of the quantitative assessment of microbial flora in wounds. *J Wound Care* 1998; 7:452-456.

26. Heggers JP. Defining infection in chronic wounds: does it matter? *J Wound Care* 1998; 7:389-392

27. Heggers JP. Assessing and controlling wound infection. *Clin Plastic Surg* 2003; 30:25-35.

28. Hohn DC, Mackay RD, Halliday B, et al. Effect of O_2 tension on microbial function of leukocytes in wounds and in vitro. *Surg. Forum* 1976; 27: 18-20.

29. Hunt TK, Hopf HW. Wound healing and wound infection-What surgeons and anesthesiologists can do. *Surg Clin North Am* 1997; 77:587-606.

30. Jacobs RF, Schutze GE. Bartonella henselae as a cause of prolonged fever and fever of unknown origin in children. *Clin Infect Dis* 1998; 26:80-84.

31. Larson E. Skin hygiene and infection prevention; more of the same or different approaches? *Clin Infect Dis* 1999; 29: 1287-1294.

32. Lavery LA, Harkless LB, Felder-Johnson K, et al. Bacterial pathogens in infected puncture wounds in adults with diabetes. *J Foot Ankle Surg* 1994; 33:91-97.

33. LeFrock JL, Molavi A. Necrotizing skin and subcutaneous infections. *J Antimicrob Chemother* 1982; 9: suppl. A. 183-192.

34. LeFrock JL, Joseph WS. Bone and soft-tissue infections of the lower extremity in diabetics. *Clin. In Pod Med and Surg* 1995; 12:87-103.

35. Manian FA, Meyer PL, Setzer J, et al. Surgical site infections associated with Methicillin-resistant Staphylococcus aureus: Do post-operative factors play a role? *CID* 2003; 36:863-868.

36. McDonald M, Grabsch E, Marshall C, et al. Single-versus multiple dose antimicrobial prophylaxis for major surgery: A systematic review. *Aust NZJ Surg* 1998; 68:388-396.

37. Mayhall CG. Surgical infections including burns. In RP Wenzel (ed.), *Prevention and Control of Nosocomial Infections* 2nd ed. Baltimore, MD: Williams and Wilkins, 1993; 614-664.

38. Nichols RL. Surgical antibiotic prophylaxis. *Med Clin North Am* 1995; 79:509-522.

39. Nichols RL. Post-operative infections in the age of drug-resistant Gram-positive bacteria. *Am J Med* 1998; 104(5A): 115-165.

40. Nichols RL, Florman S. Clinical presentations of soft-tissue infections and surgical site infections. *CID* 2001: 33 (suppl 2) 584-593.

41. Pankey GA, Katner HP, Valainis GT, et al. Overview of bacterial infections of the skin and soft tissue and clinical experience with ticarcillin plus clavulanate potassium in their treatment. *Am J Med* 1985; 79 (suppl 5B): 106-115.

42. Park MK, Myers RAM, Marzella L. Oxygen tensions and infections: modulation of microbial growth activity of antimicrobial agents, and immunologic responses. *CID* 1992; 14: 720-740.

43. Periti P, Tonelli F, Mini E. Selecting antibacterial agents for the control of surgical infection. *J Chemother* 1998,10: 83-90.

44. Perry RD, Fetherstone JD. Yersinia pestis-etiologic agent of plague. *Clin Microbial Rev* 1997; 10:35-66.

45. Phillips D, Davey C. Wound cleansing versus wound disinfection: a challenging dilemma. *Perspectives* 1997; 21: 15-16.

46. Raahave D, Friis-Moller A, Bjerre-Jepsen K, et al. The infective dose of aerobic and anaerobic bacteria in post-operative wound sepsis. *Arch Surg* 1986; 121: 924-929.

47. Raahave D. Wound contamination and post-operative infection. A review. *Dan Med Bull* 1991; 38:481-485.

48. Reboli AC, Farrar WE. Erysipelothrix-rhusiopathiae: an occupational pathogen. *Clin Microbiol Rev* 1989; 2(4):354-359.

49. Robson MC. Wound infection. A failure of wound healing caused by an imbalance of bacteria. *Surg Clin North Am* 1997; 77:637-650.

50. Rotstein OD, Pruett TL, Simmons RL. Mechanisms of microbial synergy in polymicrobial surgical infections. R*ev Infect Dis* 1985; 7:151-170.

51. Sessler DI, Akca O. Non pharmacological prevention of surgical wound infections. *CID* 2002; 35: 1397-1404.

52. Sorensen TS, Sorensen AI, Bremmelgaard JJ. Orthopedic wound infections 182 cases after 8913 operations during an 8 year survey. *Acta Orthop Scand* 1997; 68:466-469.

53. Spach DH, Koehler JE. Bartonella-associated infections. *Infect Dis Clin North Am* 1998; 12(1):137-155.

54. Srinivasan A, Kraus CN, DeShazer D, et al. Glanders in a military research microbiologist. *N Engl J Med* 2001; 345:256-258.

55. Stevens DL. Invasive group A streptococcal infections: the past, present and future. *Pediatr Infect Dis J* 1994; 13:561-566.

56. Summanen PH, Talon DA, Strong C, et al. Bacteriology of skin and soft tissue infections: comparison of infections in intravenous drug users and individuals with no history of intravenous drug use. *CID* 1995; 20:S279-S282.

57. Talan DA, Abrahamian FM, Moran GJ, et al. Clinical presentation and bacteriologic analysis of infected human bites in patients presenting to emergency departments. *Clin Infect Dis* 2003; 37:1481-1489.

58. Zoutman D, McDonald S, Vethanayagan D. Total and attributable costs of surgical wound infections at a Canadian tertiary care center. *Infect Control Hosp Epidermiol* 1998; 19:254-259.

REVIEW QUESTIONS

1.) Human bites tend to be more serious and more prone to infection than dog or cat bites.
   a. True
   b. False

2.) Pyodermas have the following four things in common:
- Etiology S. aureus
- Rarely require hospitalization
- May respond to local measures
- Recurrence may be prevented by decreasing S. aureus skin carriage

   a. True
   b. False

3.) Every patient with a soft tissue infection should be checked for the following:
- Presence or absence of fever and other signs of systemic toxicity
- Assess for erythema, induration, crepitus, fluctuans, tenderness, duskiness, etc.
- Gas in tissue or not
- Measure depth, length, width of wound, note type of drainage, and any odor
- Try to figure which anatomic structures are involved which frequently gives a clue to the microbiology of the specific syndrome

   a. True
   b. False

4.) Most important factors in the prevention of SSI' s are:
General health of patient, meticulous operative techniques, timely administration of pre-operative antibiotics, hand washing, hyperglycemia and diabetes control, perioperative normothermia, and supplemental perioperative oxygen.
   a. True
   b. False

5.) Hypothermia causes numerous adverse outcomes including:
Morbid myocardial events, increased blood loss, post surgical wound infections, and prolonged hospitalization.
   a. True
   b. False

Answers: 1a, 2a, 3a, 4a, 5a

CHAPTER 32

ACUTE AND CHRONIC PAIN MANAGEMENT

CHAPTER THIRTY-TWO OVERVIEW

Acute and Chronic Pain Management

Lynda T. Wells

INTRODUCTION

Pain is the symptom that most commonly causes patients to seek medical advice. It is also described by both adult and pediatric patients as being one of the most distressing aspects of medical care. Defined by the International Association for the Study of Pain (IASP) as "an unpleasant sensory or emotional experience associated with actual or potential tissue damage or perceived in terms of such damage," pain is a complex experience incorporating physical (nociceptive), emotional, social, psychological and behavioral elements. Recent advances in the understanding of the pathophysiology of pain and in the application of pharmacologic and non-pharmacologic analgesic therapies have enhanced the physician's ability to treat acute, chronic and procedural pain.

PAIN CLASSIFICATIONS

None of the classifications of pain provide a comprehensive and unambiguous guide to clinical management.

The IASP has devised a universal pain classification system to facilitate scientific communication (1). The IASP classification codes pain by 5 axes: body region, body system, the pain's temporal characteristics (pattern of occurrence), the patient's statements of intensity (since time of onset of pain), and etiology. The etiological classification subsets are outlined in Table 1 and cover all types of pathology including congenital, organic, and psychological.

TABLE 1. IASP RECOGNIZED PAIN ETIOLOGIES

- Genetic/congenital disorders
- Trauma, surgery, burns
- Infective, parasitic
- Inflammatory (no known infective agent), immune reactions
- Neoplastic
- Toxic, metabolic (i.e., alcoholic neuropathy, anoxia, vascular, nutritional, endocrine), radiation
- Degenerative, mechanical (i.e., biliary colic, PDPH)
- Dysfunctional (including psychophysiological) i.e., migraine, irritable bowel syndrome, tension headaches
- Unknown/other
- Psychological origin (i.e., conversion hysteria, depressive hallucination)

Pain is also characterized by its duration of action, phenomenology, and etiology. When classified by its duration, pain is designated as either "acute" or "chronic." Acute pain (2) is defined as pain that lasts less than three months. It usually has an identifiable cause and the mainstay of treatment encompasses pharmacological, physical, and anxiolytic measures as well as interventions that improve the patient's comfort. Chronic pain is defined as pain that persists for longer than six months. Unlike acute pain, its onset and source is often less easy to determine. Thus, therapeutic interventions are geared towards the improvement of lifestyle, optimization of function, relief of depression, physical therapies, and both pharmacological and non-pharmacological measures. Whilst these measures may improve physical and psychological function, pain scores might remain unchanged. Nevertheless, both definitions of pain are inadequate because they do not always describe the underlying pathophysiology. For instance, the alleviation of acute pain should mirror the healing process. It is present while there is tissue damage and resolves when healing is complete. In contradiction to that definition, pain from a superficial skin cut that persists after two weeks is a chronic pain because it persists after tissue healing has occurred. Similarly, recovery from neurological injuries takes approximately 12 months. Pain lasting over six months is to be expected and does not constitute chronic pain per se. The classification of pain as acute or chronic is not directly meaningful to the provision of clinical care.

Pain can be classified etiologically based upon its pathophysiology or its site of anatomic origin. Pathophysiologically, pain is either inflammatory or neuropathic, and both types of pain can co-exist. Anatomically, the characteristics of the pain can be described by the structures that are affected irrespective of pathophysiology. For instance, pain arising from skin and mucous membranes in response to chemical, thermal, and mechanical stimuli is termed *somatic*. That arising from muscle, tendons, ligaments, periosteum, and joint capsule in response to chemical, thermal, mechanical, or ischemic stimuli is termed *deep somatic*. Pain arising from the viscera and peritoneum is termed *visceral*, and that arising from nervous tissue is termed *neuropathic*. Acute somatic, deep somatic and visceral pains are usually inflammatory in origin. Chronic and neuropathic pains are usually neuropathic in origin. Each of these pains has distinct qualities and characteristics that reflect their afferent neural pathways. Individual interpretation of pain and its consequent emotional, social, psychological and behavioral manifestations will shape how and when a patient seeks treatment and their therapeutic response (3). The drugs and interventions used in treatment are guided by the physiologic processes underlying the painful condition and the patient's response to their symptoms. Effective analgesia improves patient well-being and function. The opposite occurs when therapy is ineffective or inappropriate.

APPRECIATION OF PAIN

Pain is appreciated as true pain, epicritic pain, and cognitive/cerebral pain. True pain is localized poorly and transmitted by slow conducting, unmyelinated C-fibers. It has a dull, aching, dragging quality and persists after the stimulus is removed. Referred pain is true pain. It elicits motor and autonomic reflex activity (i.e., muscle rigidity/contraction, immobilization of the injury part) and is not suppressed by transection of the spinal cord. Neonates appreciate pain as true pain almost exclusively.

Epicritic pain is discriminatory and conducted by fast conducting, myelinated A-delta fibers. This type of pain allows accurate localization of impulses arising in the skin and identification of the nature and duration of the noxious stimulus. It is the mechanism by which one knows a thumb tack just went into the tip of ones left ring finger. Epicritic pain evokes protective reflexes (i.e., withdrawal of limb, fleeing) and is abolished by disruption of the spinothalamic and spinoreticular tracts. It increases with increasing myelination and is fully mature by the end of the second year of life.

Cognitive/cerebral pain is multi-factorial. It develops constantly throughout life leading to highly structured responses (pain behaviors). It is heavily influenced by societal, cultural, familial, educational and individual factors, i.e., previous experience. From approximately six months of age the cognitive/cerebral aspects of pain, which are the psychological, emotional and social implications of the painful event, cannot be separated from the physical aspects of the pain.

All three types of pain appreciation are intertwined and inseparable. In formulating a pain management plan the relative contributions of each type of pain appreciation should be evaluated and addressed.

IMPORTANCE OF PAIN CONTROL

Pain control is important for societal, psychological/behavioral, physiological and anatomical reasons. North American culture promotes the relief of suffering whenever it is practicable as a desirable behavior. Thus, the act of relieving painful conditions is valued by society. It is encouraged as the "humane" response.

Pain behaviors are learned. The memory of painful events is very strong especially in children. Many studies have shown that newborns who experience pain, with no recalled memory of painful events, show distinct behaviors in response to future painful events. Examples include Taddio et al's study (4) that showed that boys who were circumcised at birth without the use of analgesia demonstrated a much more profound pain response when receiving childhood immunizations than boys who had received analgesia prior to circumcision. The latter group's pain behaviors were comparable to those exhibited by girls. Schechter et al. (5) demonstrated learned pain behavior in children undergoing repeated painful procedures for oncologic therapy. Prior to the first painful intervention, children were assigned to an analgesic (fentanyl) or a placebo group. The painful procedure was performed and the severity of the pain was rated. The children in the analgesic group rated their pain as "mild" (visual analog scale (VAS) 2-4/10). The children in the placebo group rated their pain as "severe" (VAS 8-10/10). For all subsequent procedures all the children were aggressively medicated with fentanyl. Pain scores in the original analgesic group continued to be low. However, pain scores in the original placebo group continued to be extremely high despite analgesic interventions. The children in the placebo group knew what the procedure felt like and their perception was not changed by receipt of analgesia. This illustrates the importance of ensuring adequate analgesia prior to initiating painful procedures.

Unmodified, afferent, nociceptive stimuli that persist over time lead to physiological changes in the peripheral and central nervous systems known as "wind up." "Wind up" is characterized by enhanced afferent transmission, expansion of receptor fields and progressive facilitation of neuronal firing leading to hyperalgesia and allodynia. Hyperalgesia is an increased response to a stimulus that is normally painful. Allodynia describes pain experienced in response to a stimulus that does not normally induce pain, e.g. light touch. These sensations reflect changes in central transmission of afferent nociceptive impulses and are associated with increased transmission at N-methyl D-aspartate (NMDA) receptors. Persistent pain impulses from the periphery cause changes in the axons and dorsal horn of the spinal cord that allow "cross talk" between neurons. This means that stimuli that would usually be transmitted via spinothalamic and spinoreticular "pain tracts" are also transmitted via A-beta fibers. A-beta fibers usually transmit touch, pressure and proprioception, i.e. non-noxious sensations, hence the perception of non-noxious stimulation as painful.

NMDA receptor antagonists include ketamine, amantadine, methadone, propoxyphene and dextrometorphan. Opioids other than methadone and propoxyphene are not effective at reversing "wind up" because their site of action is more distal in the spinal cord. Methadone is unique in being a racemate of two analgesic drugs. S-methadone is an opioid receptor agonist comparable to morphine. R-methadone is an NMDA receptor antagonist comparable to S-ketamine. Propoxyphene has neurotoxic adverse effects and is not recommended. Local anesthetics stop "wind up" by blocking afferent neural transmission. This allows the central hypersensitization to reverse. "Wind up" can be prevented by pre-emptive, preventive analgesia. However, if left unchecked it can lead to gene induction.

Gene induction occurs in response to persistent or repeated noxious events and manifests as anatomical changes in the central nervous system (CNS). It results in increased synthesis of cellular mediators of pain that in turn leads to altered post-synaptic morphology. Anatomical changes can persist for up to six months after noxious stimulation ceases. An example of "wind up" and gene induction is commonly encountered in post-surgical patients. If post-surgical analgesia is inadequate, the area of skin surrounding the incision will become more and more sensitive until non-noxious stimuli such as light abdominal palpation cause pain. Patients who have experienced "wind up" and gene induction continue to experience functionally limiting pain for several months after tissue healing has occurred (6, 7).

The final reason for treating pain is related to the neuroendocrine stress response. Pain is a physiological stressor and causes neuroendocrine changes in the body. These changes are characterized by catabolism leading to a reduction in body mass and tissue reserve, immunosuppression, increased myocardial oxygen demand, diminished ventilatory function and increased thromboembolic risk. Overwhelming catabolism is fatal and is the mechanism by which pain kills. Neuroendocrine stress exacerbates the deleterious effects of systemic inflammation and vice versa. Systemic inflammation can lead to functional changes in the nervous system resulting in neurological dysfunction and further pain. Overall the neuroendocrine stress response is associated with increased morbidity and mortality. This in turn increases the cost of health care and is the basis for regulatory agencies mandating pain management activities in all accredited healthcare facilities.

SOURCES OF PAIN IN WOUND CARE PATIENTS RELATED TO PRE-EXISTING DISEASES AND TO ACUTE INJURY AND DISEASE

The majority of pain experienced by patients during wound care is of somatic origin, arising from skin edges, deep tissues and muscle. However, many patients who present for wound care have pre-existing pain either as a symptom of their underlying disease or as a consequence of trauma. This poses a therapeutic challenge as in order to treat procedural pain successfully it is necessary to optimize pre-existing painful conditions. Understanding the pathophysiology of pain states associated with diabetes mellitus, ischemia, burns and amputation allows rational analgesic therapies to be applied to optimize "background" pain. Neuropathic pain features in all these conditions. Somatic pain of inflammatory origin may also be present.

Neuropathic Pain

Peripheral and central neuropathic pain is characterized by neuronal excitability in damaged areas of the nervous system. Peripheral nerve pain arises from abnormal spontaneous and increased evoked discharges in damaged nerve endings due in part to an increase in, and novel expression of, sodium channels. This hyperexcitability spreads from the peripheral nociceptor to the dorsal root ganglion (DRG), dorsal horn of the spinal cord and brain (8). In addition to abnormal expression of sodium channels, there is increased activity at glutamate receptor sites, reduced GABA-ergic inhibition and altered calcium influx into cells (9). Activity at these sites forms the basis of the pharmacologic efficacy of anti-depressent, anti-convulsant and local anesthetic drugs in the treatment of neuropathic pain. For example, anti-convulsants modulate post-injury neural changes, and hence pain transmission, by suppressing sodium and calcium channel activity and antagonizing glutamate receptors at peripheral, spinal and supraspinal sites. Additionally, drugs such as gabapentin and pregabalin (10) are agonists at GABA-ergic receptors. Further discussion of analgesic therapies for neuropathic pain is presented later in this chapter.

Somatic Pain

Somatic wound pain arises from an inflammatory response to injury and repeated minor trauma, i.e., debridement and abrading during dressing changes. Local anesthetic, opioid and non-opioid anti-inflammatory drugs are effective analgesics for pain of this nature.

Diabetes Mellitus Induced Pain

Diabetes mellitus sufferers have pain syndromes unique to their disease. Hyperglycemia induces a painful neuropathy, usually of the feet, that can exist even in the presence of numbness. The primary, and most important, remedy is to ensure that the blood glucose is maintained within the normal range and at least below 200 mg/dl. Many patients with painful diabetic neuropathies experience resolution of their pain once adequate glycemic control is achieved. Optimal glycemic control is necessary in all diabetic patients regardless of whether they obtain analgesia with disease optimization alone because pharmacological interventions are less likely to succeed in hyperglycemic patients. Hyperglycemia is pro-algesic via its immunosuppressant effects. Changes in immune function are associated with the genesis and maintenance of neuropathic pain states.

Pain from Ischemia

Wounds of ischemic origin (i.e., arteriosclerosis, sickle cell disease) are frequently associated with pain of a mixed somatic and neuropathic character. This is in keeping with tissue loss and neuronal ischemia associated with these lesions. Analgesics aimed at alleviating both types of pain are frequently used in combination. It should be noted that the somatic pain associated with ischemia is often refractory to standard analgesic doses and that two to three times the opiate dose needed in post-surgical patients may be required to achieve pain relief.

Pain from Burns

As with pain of ischemic origin, high opioid doses may be needed in burned patients because they suffer profound systemic inflammation and CNS sensitization as a consequence of their injuries. Pain generating mechanisms include nociception, primary and secondary hyperalgesia and neuropathy. As direct neural injury occurs, many of the neuropathic pain regimens utilized in diabetic patients have a role in burned patients. The most important point in treating burn pain is to rapidly achieve analgesia (baseline and procedural) by whatever means available and to address the inflammatory response to prevent CNS changes and the onset of chronic pain. Local anesthetic techniques are particularly useful in this regard and nerve blocks and central axis blocks should be used when appropriate. Burn pain is particularly associated with psychological and functional difficulties. A multi-modal analgesic approach combining pharmacologic and non-pharmacologic analgesia works best to provide comfort and to optimize psychological and functional outcomes (11).

Background infusions of opioids or the equivalent from sustained release oral preparations are indicated in these patients. It has been shown that in equianalgesic doses all opioids provide equivalent analgesia. However, methadone has been shown to improve quality of life and sleep measures. Remifentanil infusions are associated with acute opioid tolerance and should be avoided. No route of administration has been found to be superior to another although for rapidity of onset intravenous administration is best. Recently topical morphine gel was found to be effective in the relief of painful inflammatory conditions (e.g. burns) in children (12). Opioid effectiveness can be improved by the use of various adjuvants including α2-adrenergic agonists, NMDA receptor antagonists, NSAIDs, CCK-antagonists, gabapetinoids and NK-1 receptor antagonists (13). The utility of the α2-adrenergic agonist, dexmedetomidine, which has sedative, anxiolytic and analgesic properties but less risk of respiratory depression than other sedatives has been confirmed in pediatric burns patients (14). In contrast to diabetic neuropathic pain, ketamine has been shown to be beneficial as an analgesic and for opioid sparing in burned patients. Its sedative and dissociative effects can also be beneficial especially in pediatric patients.

Pain and Amputations

Analgesic interventions in amputees focus on control of somatic and neuropathic pains. Stump pain is somatic; phantom pain is neuropathic. There is no definitive intervention to prevent or treat phantom pain. However, it is known that pain in the body part prior to amputation and pain in the amputation wound are etiological in the development of phantom pain (15, 16). Phantom sensation and pain can arise in any body region following amputation. Phantom sensation post-amputation is normal. Phantom pain is pathologic and is indicative of neurologic dysfunction. Although phantom pain is often referred to as "phantom limb pain," patients can experience phantom pain in any amputated body part, e.g. the breast after mastectomy or the rectum after abdominoperineal resection.

AN APPROACH TO PAIN MANAGEMENT

Analgesic therapy can provide relief of both anticipatory and actual painful experiences. Our understanding of the effects and utility of analgesics comes from knowledge of cellular inflammatory processes, animal models, and clinical practice. Hence, these advances in understanding the pathophysiology of pain have led to the development of multimodal therapies for its treatment.

Pathophysiology: Cellular and Inflammatory Processes

Our understanding of the role of inflammation and the immune system in the etiology and maintenance of neuropathy and neuropathic pain has evolved over the last 20 years. It is estimated that more than half the cases of neuropathic pain are due to inflammation or infection of the peripheral nerves and not nerve trauma. Postulated non-traumatic mechanisms of injury include antibody attack of peripheral nerves and immune attack upon peripheral nerve blood vessels (17). Targeting analgesic interventions to address these different etiologies forms the basis of development of specific classes of drug for the treatment of painful neuropathy (18). These include vasodilators, protein kinase C beta inhibition, antioxidants and novel aldose reductase inhibitors. However, in current practice analgesic therapies remain the same regardless of the pain's cellular evolution.

Macrophages and neutrophils are the key immune cells at the site of peripheral nerve injury, infection or inflammation (8). An excessive inflammatory response in defense of the host results in proinflammatory cytokines, nitric oxide and reactive oxygen species going beyond killing pathogens and causing increased nerve excitability, myelin damage and an impaired blood-nerve barrier. Tissue necrosis factor alpha (TNFα) is the prototypical proinflammatory cytokine and shows increased expression in both damaged and spared sensory neurons (8). This adds weight to the conclusion that neuropathic pain is a neurological disorder of the peripheral and central nervous systems. Local anesthetics are known to prevent this excessive inflammatory response while allowing protective inflammation to continue, i.e. local anesthetics do not cause immunosuppression. Etanercept is a TNFα-sequestering drug and can inhibit mechanical allodynia when given pre-emptively in animals. It has no analgesic effect once neuropathic pain is established. Its use as an analgesic for neuropathic pain of various etiologies in humans has not been evaluated. Analgesic therapies designed to target these immune mechanisms are being developed.

Animal Models

Animal models reveal that immune activation in and around nerve trunks, dorsal root ganglia (DRG), and the dorsal roots is hyperalgesic and that the immune system actively participates in creating and maintaining neuropathic pain of diverse etiologies. This is pathological and contrasts with physiological pain in which the immune system remains silent (8). Although it is well known that physical nerve damage activates the immune system and leads to changes in nociceptive function and pain perception, a similar chain of events can occur in the absence of direct nerve trauma. Within a nerve injured and uninjured axons have highly abnormal properties as a consequence of nerve damage and exhibit dysregulated gene expression and the generation of ectopic (spontaneous) discharges. These abnormal activities later impinge on the CNS and are crucial in generating neuropathic pain. It is clear that abnormal peripheral inputs feed into a spinal processing system that is disrupted in these neuropathic states.

Clinical Experience

Clinical experience has shown that patients undergoing wound care can experience various modalities of pain depending upon their stage of treatment. For instance, most wounds evince a combination of both neuropathic and somatic pain. Treatment of established wounds typically requires debridement and cleaning of the wound. This can necessitate extension of the wound edge leading to the emergence of an acute somatic pain over and above the existing mixed modalities of existing pain. Thus, appropriate treatment needs to be geared not only towards treatment of the established mixed pain states but also towards relief of the anticipated painful stimuli. In that sense, the lessons learned from both cellular-inflammatory processes and animal models can be translated into determining effective multi-modal analgesic strategies for the treatment of pain in humans. These lessons have been encapsulated within the World Health Organization recommendations, and extended into the clinical practice of delivering pharmacotherapy, psycho-social interventions, and adjunctive therapy either alone or in combination.

World Health Organization Recommendations

The World Health Organization (WHO) advocates an analgesic approach based upon the philosophy that "an essential principle in using medications to manage pain is to individualize the regimen to the patient." Their recommendation is to use oral medications whenever possible, to dose "by the clock" with additional medications available "as needed" for breakthrough pain, to titrate the dose, to use appropriate dosing intervals, to be aware of relative potencies and to treat side effects. Oral medications are recommended because they are generally cheaper, have a slower onset time that allows serious side effects to be identified and treated before they compromise the patient, e.g. oversedation preceding respiratory depression with opioids cannot be recognized with the rapid onset following intravenous administration, and are equally effective as drugs given by other routes. Individual responses to a given analgesic vary widely between individuals so dose titration is necessary to identify the optimal amount for each patient. Dosing intervals should be such that the patient does not experience a resurgence of their pain before the next dose is given. Knowledge of the duration of drug action allows the drug to be prescribed as a scheduled medication. All medications have side effects and these should be managed as indicated. If the incidence or severity of side effects limits the utility of a particular drug, it should be changed to another, or the analgesic modality altered. Knowledge of relative potencies facilitates changing from one drug to another while preserving analgesic efficacy.

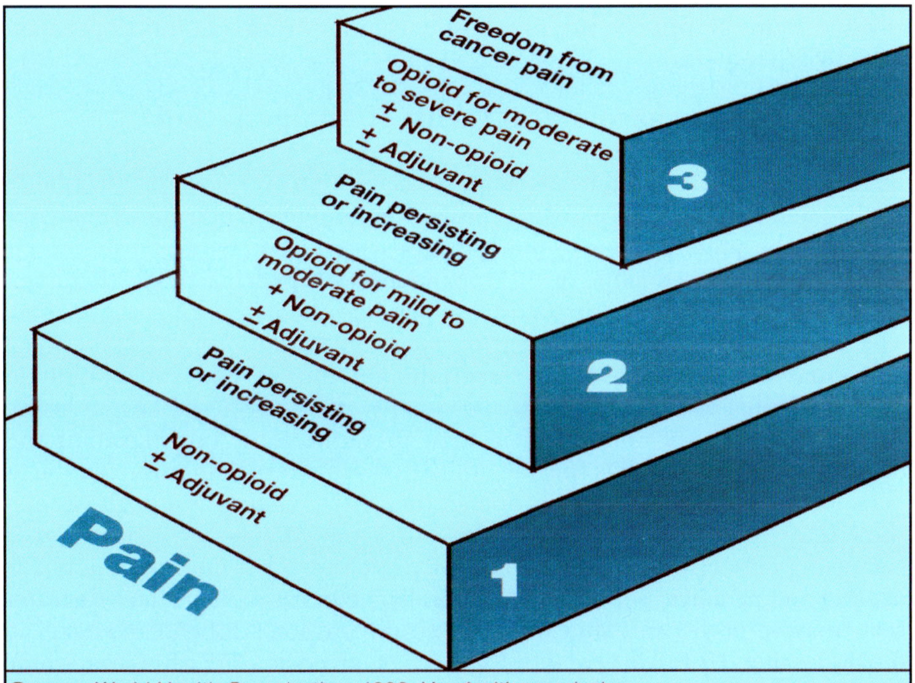

Source: World Health Organization, 1990. Used with permission.

Figure 1. WHO three-step analgesic ladder.

The WHO analgesic ladder provides a framework for drug choices (Figure 1). The 3 steps correspond to mild, moderate, and severe pain. The ladder was initially devised to facilitate treatment of cancer pain. Patients advance up the ladder as their disease progresses. Patients with acute pain have the opposite profile and start at the top of the ladder with severe pain initially and then move down the ladder as healing occurs.

Rapport (Psychosocial Relief of Pain)

A patient's mood and perceptions influence their pain appreciation. This is especially true of patient's who have poorly controlled background pain or who have had unpleasant experiences associated with therapeutic procedures in the past. Anxiety, depression, fear and anger are emotions associated with pain and are known to aggravate the symptom. Lack of information, fatigue, insomnia and discomfort are also recognized factors in decreasing the pain threshold. Factors known to increase the pain threshold and improve the patient's pain perception include restful sleep, effective coping skills, symptom relief, being informed, distraction, understanding and sympathy.

Acute pain is most commonly associated with anxiety. Establishing a good rapport with the patient is essential to diminish anxiety and allow the patient to become informed about and involved in their care. At least half of the analgesic efficacy in acute pain patients is achieved by establishing a therapeutic alliance based on honesty, trust, and information sharing. In patients who are extremely anxious, pharmacological anxiolysis may be helpful. Pharmacological anxiolysis should not be used as a substitute for provider/patient rapport. Depression is commonly present in patients with chronic pain. Rapport and professional supervision of anti-depressant therapy are required.

Other Non-Pharmacological Forms of Analgesia and Adjunctive Therapies

The goals of non-pharmacologic analgesic interventions are to relieve anxiety and increase the patient's sense of autonomy. When these goals are achieved the patient's perception of pain is reduced. Non-pharmacologic therapies can be used alone or in combination with pharmacologic therapies. When a physically painful procedure is planned the latter approach is used. The utility of different non-pharmacologic interventions varies between individual patients and needs a certain amount of experimentation to determine what works best.

The majority of non-pharmacologic therapies focus on relaxation and distraction. Distraction has specific utility because interpreting nociception as pain is a particularly attention-demanding task. Neurophysiologic studies show that when a patient engages in distraction the act of focusing on a competing sensory input causes pain to be perceived as less intense. This is true in adult and pediatric populations. Generally, pediatric patients derive greater relief than adults because they will more readily suspend disbelief to engage in the distraction. Hoffman et al. (19-23), at the University of Washington School of Medicine, have investigated this area of analgesia and pioneered a highly sophisticated immersive, interactive virtual reality (VR) that uses high sensory stimulation and attention-demanding distractive techniques. Patients wear a helmet that prevents them seeing the treatment room. The image inside the helmet completely surrounds the patient and changes in response to their eye movements, e.g. looking up reveals the sky, looking down the ground. The program used in burned patients is a snow world using cold to contrast with the heat of their injury. Patients use a joystick and keypad to navigate the snow world throwing snowballs at snow men and penguins. Their research demonstrated a 25-40 % reduction in procedural pain with VR and VR and pharmacologic analgesia combined compared to pharmacologic analgesia alone. This effect was maintained over repeated treatments. Less sophisticated hardware, such as video games on hand held devices, is also effective although the ability to distract is less complete.

Other non-pharmacologic analgesic therapies include guided imagery, biofeedback, mindfulness meditation, cognitive behavioral therapies, massage, therapeutic touch, acupuncture, aromatherapy and music. Patients who benefit from music should be encouraged to bring their own CDs and player to their wound care sessions. Aromatic essences can be provided by the patient or a selection can be available at the Wound Care Center. Massage of an area outside of the treatment area may be therapeutic. A mind/body therapy as simple as controlled breathing can be very useful. More sophisticated techniques, such as auto-hypnosis, will need to be learned and practiced by the patient. The presence of an empathetic individual to help coach the patient through their preferred analgesic technique is invaluable. This can be a member of the healthcare team or a friend or relative of the patient. Examples of non-pharmacologic analgesic interventions are provided in Table 2.

TABLE 2. NON-PHARMACOLOGIC ANALGESIC INTERVENTIONS

- Aromatherapy
- Acupuncture
- Books (children)
- Cold
- Control of breathing
- Empathetic distraction (i.e., avoids focusing the patient's attention on the painful procedure)
- Guided imagery
- Heat
- Hypnotherapy
- Massage
- Meditation
- Mobiles (children)
- Music
- Radio
- Television
- Toys (children)
- Video tapes
- Well informed about procedures

Sleep hygiene is particularly important. Poor sleep is associated with higher reported pain intensity and greater analgesic needs. The higher the pain and greater the need for analgesics the poorer the quality of sleep. Antidepressants can play a dual role in providing an improved sleep pattern and neuropathic analgesia.

Adjunctive analgesic therapies used to augment pharmacological treatments include psychosocial modalities (i.e., relaxation therapy, support groups), physical modalities (i.e., physical therapy, posture, exercise), chemotherapy, radiotherapy, biofeedback, implantable infusion pumps, and surgical interventions. They generally form part of a multi-modal, multi-disciplinary approach to pain management and disease treatment.

PHARMACOTHERAPY

Pre-emptive Analgesia

Pre-emptive analgesia (24) is defined as "the administration of analgesic agents prior to an injury in order to prevent the development of CNS hyper-excitability or sensitization" (wind up). CNS sensitization begins approximately 20 minutes after injury-induced inflammatory mediators are released. If analgesia is commenced prior to the release of inflammatory mediators and continued until their tissue concentration falls, CNS hypersensitivity does not occur. When analgesic interventions are initiated after CNS hypersensitivity has occurred, they must be continued for longer than pre-emptive interventions if hypersensitivity is to be reversed (Figure 2). Use of analgesic therapies to prevent CNS hypersensitivity is known as "preventive analgesia" when the therapy is initiated pre-emptively and deliberately continued for as long as inflammatory and neuroendocrine stress responses are present.

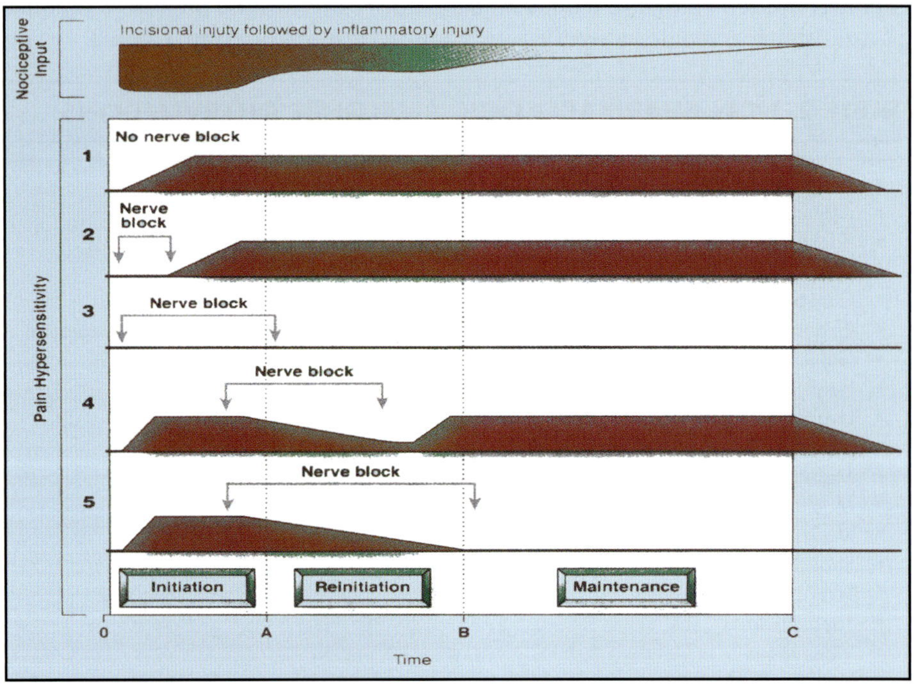

Figure 2. An illustration of the relationship between the intensity of inflammatory mediated nocieptive input, central hypersensitivity to pain ('wind up") and the effects of different premptive and non-preemptive analgesic interventions (in this example, a nerve block). Pre-emptive interventions should be of sufficient duration to prevent initiation and re-initiation of central hypersensitvity (line 2). Non-preemptive interventions must be of longer duration to prevent central hypersensitivity as re-initiation is more likely to occur in the context of prior sensitization (lines 4 and 5)(5).

Pharmacologic Interventions

In the acute setting, pharmacologic interventions rely mainly upon opioids, non-steroidal anti-inflammatory drugs and local anesthetics. The type of medication and dose required to provide analgesia is influenced by the character and intensity of the pain experienced by the patient, the efficacy of non-pharmacologic interventions and the quality of the existing analgesic regimen. If the patient has continuous pain from their wound or medical condition, the better the quality of their daily analgesic regimen the easier it will be to control their pain during wound care. Medications can be used alone or in combination.

The choice of analgesic intervention is based upon the following considerations: the type of pain, its severity, its anticipated duration, available routes of administration, side effects, metabolites, the physical status of the patient, whether the patient is an in-patient or out-patient and the availability of institutional resources. Mild to moderate pain will respond to simple analgesics, i.e., acetaminophen and NSAIDs, and weak opiates. Moderate to severe pain requires strong opiates, i.e., morphine. Local anesthetics are effective for all levels of pain. Ideally the duration of action of the analgesic intervention should equal the duration of discomfort experienced by the patient. Longer acting drugs are usually more convenient than shorter acting drugs as re-dosing during the procedure is less likely to be needed. However, short acting drugs are generally more rapidly titrated to effect and this may be advantageous in certain settings and individuals.

The safest, cheapest route of drug administration is oral. Oral medications take approximately 30–45 minutes to achieve a clinical effect. Parenteral administration is also frequently used as it has the advantage of a quicker onset of action. Clinical effect after intravenous administration generally occurs within 10 minutes; after subcutaneous administration (maximum 3 ml volume) within 15 minutes; and after intramuscular injection within 25 minutes. Other routes of administration include transmucosal, transdermal, rectal, epidural and intrathecal.

Knowledge of the adverse effects of various drug classes is pertinent to the choice of therapy.

Non-steroidal anti-inflammatory drugs and simple analgesics

Non-steroidal anti-inflammatory drugs (NSAIDs) inhibit production of cyclo-oxygenase type 1 (COX-1) and type 2 (COX-2) and are useful analgesics in relieving inflammatory pain. NSAIDs all have the following side effects. They can cause gastric erosions, platelet inactivation, high output renal failure and bronchospasm in "brittle" asthmatics. The use of cyclo-oxygenase type 2 inhibitors (COX-2s) reduces the risk for gastric erosions and does not cause platelet inactivation. However, this class of anti-inflammatory drug is more likely to cause sodium and water retention leading to an exacerbation of hypertension and congestive cardiac failure in susceptible individuals. NSAIDs and COX-2s should be used with caution in patients with renal insufficiency and any medical condition which would be aggravated by their mechanism of action.

Acetaminophen is an excellent analgesic with peripheral and central sites of action. It is not an anti-inflammatory drug but does have utility in the treatment of inflammatory pain. The maximum recommended daily dose in healthy adults is 4g/24h. The maximum recommended daily dose in patients with renal or hepatic dysfunction is 2g/24h. Treatment of side effects consists of stopping the drug and supportive management.

Opioid analgesia

Opioid analgesics are efficacious in the management of inflammatory pain and have recently been shown to have utility in treating neuropathic pain. As mentioned previously, some drugs in this class have particular indications and contra-indications in the management of certain pain states. They have various durations of action and can be administered by a variety of routes. The adverse effects of opioids include constipation, nausea, vomiting, dysphoria, pruritis, urinary retention, sedation and respiratory depression. Constipation is the only effect that occurs in 100% of patients using opioid analgesics. Respiratory depression, characterized by slow, deep ventilations, is always preceded by oversedation. It is unlikely to occur unless sedative drugs of different classes are used together, e.g. benzodiazepines, antihistamines. In a monitored setting this should not pose a significant risk. Opioid effects can be reversed by naloxone, an opioid antagonist, and adverse effects can be controlled by laxatives, antiemetics, etc. It is recommended that all patients maintained on opioid analgesia should use a bowel hygiene regimen concurrently to control constipation.

Agonist/antagonist and partial agonist opioids are not recommended for management of more than mild to moderate pain. All drugs in this class have an analgesic ceiling. Doses above those recommended merely lead to an increase in adverse effects. Pure agonists do not have an analgesic ceiling and increasing doses continue to provide increasing analgesia. However, pure agonist side effects are more likely at higher doses. Another disadvantage of this class of drug is that if the analgesic ceiling is reached and the patient still has pain it is extremely difficult to use pure agonist opioids effectively because of changes in receptor affinity. Agonist/antagonist opioids, e.g., nalbuphine, are kappa-receptor agonists and mu-receptor antagonists. Partial agonist opioids, e.g., buprenorphine, have partial agonism at mu-receptors.

Local anesthetics

Local anesthetics can be used as sole analgesic drugs or in combination with other drugs and analgesic modalities. They are extremely versatile and can be used topically (e.g., EMLA® cream, viscous lidocaine, patches), by infiltration, parenterally (lidocaine), in nerve blocks, plexus blocks and central axis blocks.

Local anesthetics act by inhibiting sodium channel activity and are effective in the treatment of neuropathic and somatic pain. Intravenous lidocaine has been shown to be equally as efficacious as tocainide, mexiletine and flecainide which have in turn been shown to have equal efficacy to opioids, gabapentin, amantadine and carbamazepine. Intravenous infusion of lidocaine 5 mg/kg given over 30 minutes was well tolerated and shown to be as effective as 225-750 mg of mexiletine (25). Topical local anesthetics such as viscous lidocaine, 5% lidocaine patches and EMLA® cream (a eutectic mixture of lidocaine 2.5% and prilocaine 2.5%) have also been used successfully to treat diabetic neuropathy. Systemic, and systemically absorbed, lidocaine may be analgesic via its anti-inflammatory effects on neutrophils and cytokines.

TABLE 3. DOSES OR LOCAL ANESTHETIC AGENTS

Agent	Plain Solution (mg/kg)	Solution with Epinephrine (mg/kg)
Chloropracaine	15	15
Procaine	10–15	10–15
Lidocaine	5	10
Mepivacaine	5	7
Etidocaine	3	3–4
Bupivacaine	3	3
Tetracaine	2	2
Prilocaine	5–7*	7–9

Local anesthestic adverse effects reflect the plasma concentration. As the plasma concentration increases the patient may experience circumoral numbness, a metallic taste, tinnitus, a feeling of impending doom, seizures, dysrhythmias, coma and cardiorespiratory arrest. The recommended maximum doses for local anesthetic drugs are shown in Table 3. The rate of absorption from the application site also influences the rate of increase of the plasma concentration. For example, local anesthestic injected to block an intercostal nerve is absorbed faster than when given by subcutaneous infiltration.

Adjunctive drugs

Adjunctive drugs are used to treat analgesic medication side effects or to augment analgesic therapy. They include laxatives, antiemetics, psychostimulants, antispasmodics, muscle relaxants, antidepressants, anticonvulsants, and corticosteroids. Laxatives, as part of bowel hygiene regimens, are prescribed routinely to patients maintained on opioid therapy. Antiemetics are useful in the small proportion of patients who experience opioid induced nausea. Tolerance to this side effect develops rapidly and patients rarely require antiemetics after 1–2 weeks. Psychostimulants are useful in patients in whom oversedation limits dose escalation. Antispasmodics and muscle relaxants are extremely useful in relieving painful muscle contraction, e.g., diazepam in patients with spastic neurological disorders such as cerebral palsy. Antidepressants are useful in improving sleep patterns and elevating mood. Both of these effects diminish the patient's perception of pain. Additionally, antidepressants such as amitryptiline are analgesic for neuropathic pain. Certain anticonvulsants are also efficacious in the relief of neuropathic pain. Corticosteroids are analgesic via their anti-inflammatory actions.

Anti-depressant and anti-convulsant analgesia

In the past, anti-depressants and anti-convulsants were considered to be pharmacological adjuncts in the treatment of pain. As our knowledge of the pathophysiology of pain has evolved and clinical experience using these drugs

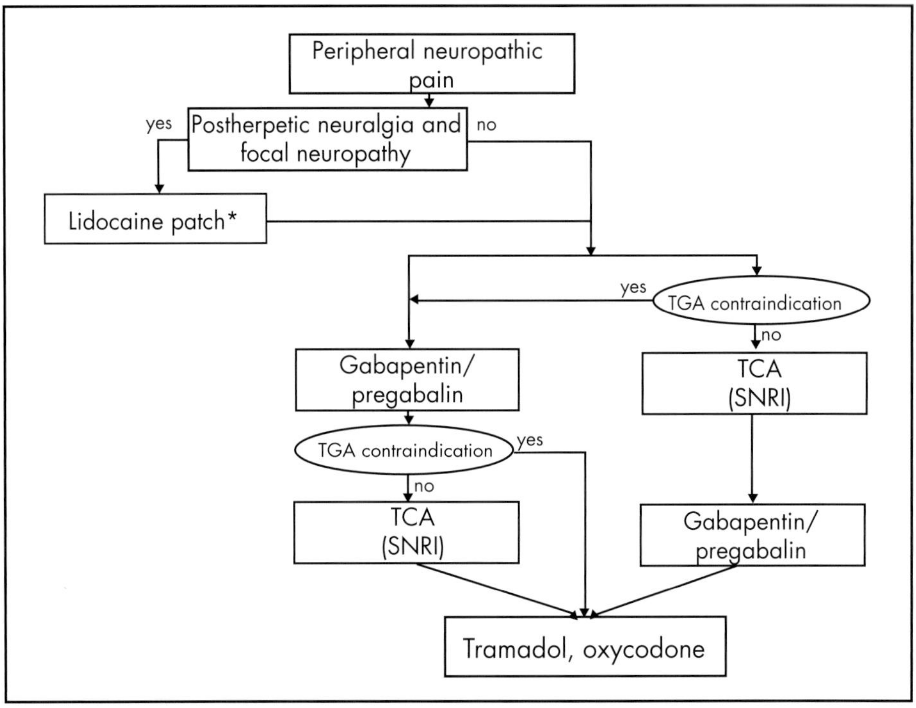

*Figure 3. Treatment algorithm. Proposed algorithm for the treatment of peripheral neuropathic pain. TCA, tricyclic antidepressants, SNRI, serotonin noradrenalin reuptake inhibitors. *Pain relieving effect of topical lidocaine has been shown in patients with allodynia.*

has increased, it is now apparent that these classes of drug are first line analgesics in certain neuropathic pain states.

Recent evidence based reviews have confirmed the utility of anti-depressant and anti-convulsant drugs in the treatment of neuropathic pain associated with diabetes and other pains of neural origin. Tricyclic anti-depressants (TCAs) in optimal doses are most efficacious in relieving neuropathic pain. The best evidence is for amitryptyline (26). In a review by McQuay et al. (27), of 100 patients taking anti-depressants as their primary analgesic for neuropathic pain 30 had a greater than 50% reduction in pain, 30 experienced minor side effects and 4 patients experienced major side effects and stopped therapy. TCAs with a more favorable side effect profile than amitriptyline include nortriptyline (its primary metabolite), imipramine and desipramine. Evaluation of the newer serotonin/norepinephrine reuptake inhibiting antidepressants, e.g. duloxetine, show promise with the number needed to treat (efficacy) being 4 compared to 2–3 for the TCAs (28). Tramadol, which has a similar mechanism of action and also has weak mu-opioid receptor agonist effects, has also been shown to be effective in neuropathic pain. It is particularly effective in the relief of paraesthesias, allodynia and touch evoked pain (29).

Although the data indicate that anti-convulsants and anti-depressant drugs are equally efficacious, anti-convulsants have a more favorable side effect profile. The most common side effects of anti-convulsants are sedation and cerebellar symptoms (nystagmus, tremor and inco-ordination). Tricyclic antidepressants can cause dry mouth, blurred vision, constipation, urinary retention, orthostatic hypotension, and cardiac dysrhythmias in overdose. Anti-convulsants and anti-depressants can be given together and combinations have been shown to provide greater analgesia than when used singly.

Gabapentin is considered to be preferable to carbemazepine and lamotrigine because it lacks drug-drug interactions. The dose should be reduced in the presence of renal insufficiency and renal failure.

Newer anticonvulsants have been evaluated for their analgesic utility. Oxcarbazepine, topiramate, zonisamide and levetiracetam are all effective in the relief of neuropathic pain. Unfortunately their side effects, including hyponatremia, nephrolithiasis, closed-angle glaucoma and cognitive dysfunction, limit their usefulness especially in the elderly. Thus they are recommended only when other therapies have failed. More randomized controlled trials are needed to determine their therapeutic role in the treatment of neuropathic pain.

An evidence-based algorithm for the treatment of neuropathic pain has been proposed (28) (Figure 3).

Miscellaneous adjunctive drugs

Analgesic therapies that have been evaluated in neuropathic pain and found to be of limited efficacy in a general population are topical capsaicin and ketamine. These are recommended as third line drugs in patients who have a poor analgesic response or significant side effects from other therapies. An exception is the use of ketamine in the treatment of burn pain.

Current data does not indicate the use of cannabinoids at this time. Randomized controlled trials are underway to determine their efficacy and safety.

Inhalational analgesia

Inhaled nitrous oxide in oxygen is a popular and effective analgesic outside of the United States. It is used frequently for analgesia during dressing changes, superficial wound debridement and other painful procedures.

Drug metabolism and excretion

The majority of drugs used for analgesia are metabolized by the liver and the metabolites are excreted by the kidneys. In patients with renal impairment, repeated doses of drugs may lead to accumulation of metabolites or unchanged parent drug. The metabolites of NSAIDs, COX-2s and local anesthetics do not have clinical effects. Acetaminophen has hepatotoxic metabolites in overdose. Opioid metabolites range from inactive, as with hydromorphone and fentanyl, to neurotoxic, as with meperidine and propoxyphene. This is one of the reasons why the latter drugs are not favored in pain management. Short duration of action and comparatively weak analgesic efficacy are others. Opioids such as methadone have potentially beneficial metabolites, i.e., normethadone has NMDA receptor antagonist activity. Morphine has potentially harmful metabolites. Morphine-6-glucuronide, a major metabolite, is ten times more potent than the parent drug as an analgesic, sedative and respiratory depressant. Morphine-3-glucuronide has been shown to be anti-analgesic in rodents and possibly in large doses in humans.

In patients in whom drug metabolism or excretion is impaired doses of the parent drug should be decreased. In patients in whom drug metabolism or excretion have been induced, larger doses or more frequent doses of the parent drug will be required to obtain the same clinical effect.

Physical status and drug selection

The physical status of the patient alters the pharmacokinetics and pharmacodynamics of analgesic drugs. Neonates and young infants have immature organ function associated with prolonged clearance. Toddlers have enhanced organ function associated with a shortened duration of action and the need for relatively more drug per kilogram body weight. Elderly patients have degenerative function associated with prolonged clearance. Concurrent illness in children has a more profound adverse effect on drug metabolism than in adults. Elderly patients are more sensitive to the central depressant effects of opioids and are more likely to suffer mental status changes in the adult therapeutic dose range.

Pharmacogenetics

Pharmacogenetics also plays a role in how individuals dispose of analgesic drugs. The mild opioids codeine, hydrocodone, and oxycodone are non-analgesic prodrugs. They have their clinical analgesic effects by being activated by the 2D6 subset of the cytochrome P450 system into morphine, hydromorphone and oxymorphone respectively (30, 31). This enzyme subset is non-inducible and has a bimodal distribution in Caucasian populations. Ninety percent of Caucasians are extensive metabolizers, and can activate the drugs, while 10% are poor metabolizers and cannot. Poor metabolizers do not obtain analgesia from these drugs but instead experience side effects from the parent compounds. These include headache, dizziness, irritability, and insomnia. The prevalence of poor versus extensive metabolizers varies within different racial groups and appears to be higher in Africans, Hispanics, and Native American peoples. As there is no ready way to identify who is an extensive metabolizer and who is not, it has been suggested that these prodrugs should be abandoned and replaced with analgesic regimens utilizing strong opioids (the active forms of these drugs) and simple analgesics.

Institutional resources

Availability of institutional resources dictates which pharmacological therapies are available and prudent to use. The pharmacy formulary should have a range of drugs sufficient to meet the needs of the patient population. Nursing and medical staff should have sufficient knowledge and understanding of the pharmacology of the drugs they use to ensure adequate monitoring of therapeutic and adverse effects. Additionally the expertise and ability to treat adverse effects must be available. All facilities where opioids, anxiolytics, and other central depressant drugs are used should have staff trained in basic or advanced cardiac life support. Patients should be monitored by a dedicated caregiver in addition to electronic monitoring as recommended in the American Society of Anesthesiologists guidelines on conscious sedation (32, 33). A hospital with ICU facilities should be immediately accessible if the need arises.

Patient disposition and analgesia

The choice of non-pharmacological and pharmacological drug

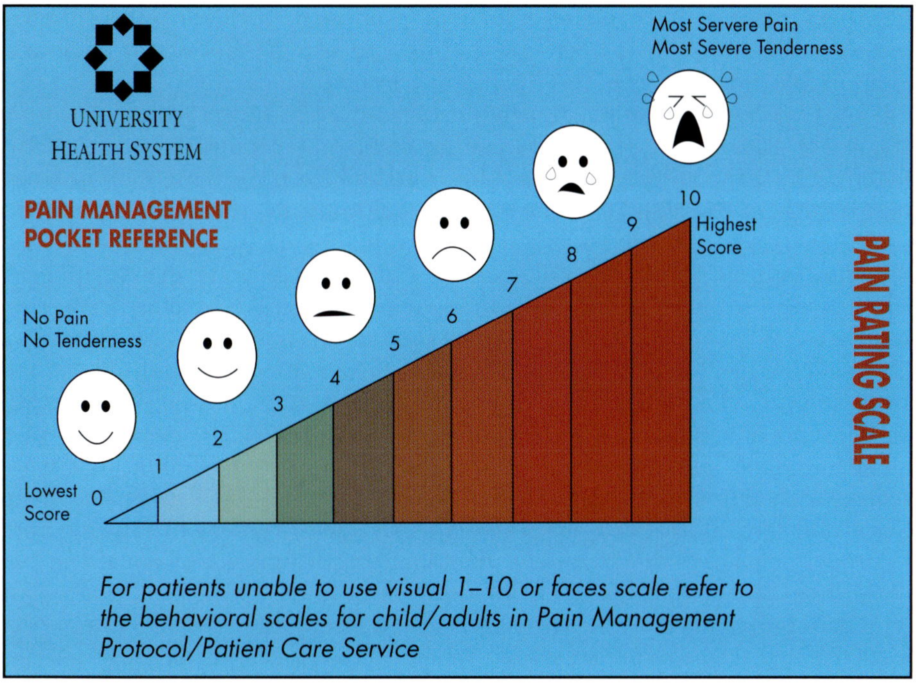

Figure 4. UHS pain scoring scale.

treatments can vary according to whether the patient is an in-patient or out-patient. Out-patients are most conveniently managed with oral drugs when needed and topical local anesthetics or local infiltration or nerve blocks. Patients should be advised to take their medications approximately one hour before their scheduled procedure. Patients should not drive themselves or travel unaccompanied to or from the Wound Care facility if the analgesic drugs impair cognition and motor performance. In-patients can be managed in the same way. In addition there is the opportunity to use invasive analgesic techniques such as parenteral opiates, nerve blocks, plexus blocks, and central axis blocks that utilize indwelling catheters. These allow for "top up" medications to be given prior to procedures.

Assessment of analgesic efficacy

Pain Scoring

The gold standard for pain scoring is self report. In adult populations, for the assessment of acute and procedural pain, visual analog scale (VAS) tools are popular and easily administered. Most scales are 10 cm long and are scored between 0 and 10/10. A VAS of 0 indicates no pain; 1–3 indicates mild pain; 4–7 indicates moderate pain; 8–10 indicates severe pain. It is important to enquire about pre-existing pain, discomfort and tenderness before the start of any procedures to identify their number, nature and severity. The efficacy of interventions can then be assessed. A typical aim of therapy is to maintain a VAS pain score of 3/10 or less.

Some patients are unable to comprehend the VAS concept. These patients will not be able to provide a pain score other than to indicate that the pain is small, medium or large. As pain and discomfort diminish, function improves. If the pain score does not fall in response to analgesic interventions, but function improves to set end points and the patient states they are comfortable, no changes to the treatment regimen are needed.

At University Hospital, San Antonio, Texas, a 4-in-1 VAS pain tool is used (Figure 4). Patients can score their pain by faces, numerically 0 through 10, by height of the bars or by intensity of color. This tool has proven useful in patients over a range of educational, socioeconomic, cultural and ethnic backgrounds.

VAS pain scores are less useful in the evaluation of therapeutic efficacy in patients with chronic pain. For example, a patient with severe peripheral vascular disease suffered from painful ischemic ulcers. His baseline VAS pain score was 10/10. Analgesic interventions relieved his pain to a 7/10. However, his quality of life, sleep pattern and functional state improved and the patient pronounced he had not felt so comfortable in years. In this case a pain score of 3/10 was not attained but the goal of therapy was achieved. In order to capture elements of analgesic efficacy other than pain intensity multi-dimensional pain scoring tools are used. The Brief Pain Inventory (34) and the Neuropathic Pain Scale (35) have both been advocated for the measurement of chronic and neuropathic pain. It would appear that as long as a multi-dimensional scoring tool is used, the actual scale is not so important.

Pain is dynamic and should be reassessed frequently.

Clinical Examples of Multi-Modal Analgesic Regimens

Case 1. Patient A self-administered oral vicodin (acetaminophen/hydrocodone) and ibuprofen at home approximately one hour prior to attending her wound care appointments. She had learned the art of auto-hypnosis and would entrance herself during the procedure. Topical lidocaine was applied to augment analgesia.

Case 2. Attending the hospital and undergoing procedures made patient B very anxious. The actual wound care treatment was not particularly painful but the patient found it difficult to tolerate because of his anxiety. Patient B self-administered oral lorazepam 1 to 2 hours prior to his arrival at the hospital.

Case 3. Patient C sustained a traumatic amputation of his left leg. He required hyperbaric oxygen therapy and negative pressure wound therapy (wound VAC) applications to his stump wound. Immediately after amputation he experienced stump pain and phantom limb pain. Epidural analgesia was contra-indicated. Therefore, the stump pain was controlled with oral methadone and the phantom limb pain with amitryptiline and gabapentin. However, he found the wound care therapy painful and would become very anxious anticipating the pain. He was managed with supplemental morphine IV and lorazepam IV administered in the wound care center. Initially moderately high doses of morphine were needed (0.3 mg/kg). As healing progressed and his wound VAC changes became more comfortable, patient C required less supplemental morphine but continued to need pharmacological anxiolysis in the form of lorazepam. Once dosing requirements were constant both medications were converted to oral administration and given one hour prior to Patient C's treatment. Additionally the Acute Pain Service nurse practitioner accompanied the patient to his wound care sessions to provide empathetic distraction in the form of guided imagery, assist with dose titration when IV drugs were used and to monitor his vital signs.

Case 4. Patient D sustained a crush injury to his hand involving all 5 digits. He described somatic pain associated with all his injuries and neuropathic pain in the ulna nerve distribution. A continuous axillary brachial plexus catheter was placed and analgesia of his somatic pain was achieved with a bupivacaine infusion. Patient D complained of neuropathic type breakthrough pain for which he received amitryptiline. He experienced somatic type breakthrough pain associated with his wound care. Patient D received a bupivacaine bolus to the axillary catheter 20 minutes prior to each wound care treatment. This successfully controlled his pain.

Case 5. Patient E complained of painful diabetic neuropathy in both feet which was poorly controlled with parenteral opioids. She experienced significant exacerbation of her pain during wound care treatment of an infected ulcer on the sole of her foot. Her blood sugar estimation was 350 mg/dl. Patient E's glycemic control was improved and her blood sugar estimation was 150 mg/dl. Her painful neuropathy resolved as a consequence, opioid analgesics were discontinued and she no longer experienced significant pain during wound care therapy.

SPECIAL POPULATIONS

Pediatric

All humans, from approximately 24 weeks post-conceptual age, can feel pain. All the neurotransmitters and receptors associated with pain modulation are present at birth and will respond to exogenous drugs. Pain serves as an innate protection. Children born with congenital analgesia die at an early age from infective and inflammatory processes. Premature infants and term infants less than 6 months old may experience greater discomfort for a given stimulus because descending, inhibitory pathways which modify afferent, excitatory, nociceptive input do not mature until 4–6 months of age. They are unable to "gate" painful sensory input. The degree of physiological maturity at different ages dictates the pharmacokinetic and pharmacodynamic effects of analgesic medications. The pediatric population can be subdivided based on physiological maturity into:

preterm
neonate (first month of life)
young infant (1–3 months)
older infant (4–12 months)
toddler (1–3 years)
child (3–12 years)

Children over 12 years old metabolize drugs in the same way as adults. However, they remain psychologically and emotionally immature. Illness in children will alter drug effects to a greater extent than in adults. Acetaminophen and pure agonist opioids can be used for all ages, as can local anesthetics. NSAIDs are not recommended for analgesia until after 3 months of age. Ketorolac in repeated doses is not recommended in children under 16 years. Preterm babies, neonates, and young infants have lower opioid requirements than older children and adolescents. Toddlers often require a higher mg/kg/day dose of opioids than children at other ages.

The gold standard for pain scoring is self report. Babies and very young children do not have sufficient vocabulary or understanding of the concept of pain scoring to provide a report. Pain scoring in these children is based upon physiological measures and behaviors. Scoring systems exist for each developmental age group (36). None of the systems available is considered the model. The choice of pain scoring tool used is based upon what seems to work best for the patient population and those care providers administering the scale. Self report usually starts at about 3–4 years old. Younger children have difficulty choosing between too many options. The optimal number of choices for 3–6 year olds appears to be 4. Older children and adolescents use distraction as a means to distance themselves from their pain. Outwardly these patients appear to be comfortable when they are not. Therefore, it is extremely important that patients who can communicate are asked specifically about their pain and discomfort.

Geriatric

Elderly patients have degenerating organ function. They metabolize and clear drugs less readily than younger adults. Consequently, these patients require smaller doses or less frequent doses than younger adults in order to achieve a given clinical effect. Additionally oversedation and confusion are more likely in the elderly in response to recommended drug doses. Paradoxically, uncontrolled pain causes confusion and increasing analgesia will restore the patient to normal function. Long acting drugs with active metabolites should be used with caution in elderly patients. Elderly patients who cannot communicate meaningfully should be assessed using a standardized non-verbal behavioral pain scoring tool.

Non-verbal/Cognitively Impaired

Patients who are non-verbal, severely dysarthric, or cognitively impaired may be unable to provide a pain self-report. In these situations care givers should be asked to describe which behaviors are manifested during painful experiences. If the care giver can be present during the wound care treatment this may help to provide non-pharmacological anxiolysis through distraction and empathy in addition to identifying pain behaviors. Cognitively impaired individuals may become disinhibited when given sedative/anxiolytic drugs. A careful drug history should be taken to avoid use of drugs that can make the patient's behavior unmanageable during treatment. The response to analgesic medications is usually the same as that of an individual in the same physical condition without cognitive impairment. Recently, pain scoring tools designed especially for the evaluation of cognitively impaired individuals have been introduced. They are more sensitive to the nuances of the cognitively impair patient's behavior than standard non-verbal pain assessment tools.

Drug-Addicted and Substance-Abusing Patients

Care of drug-addicted or substance-abusing patients can be very challenging (37). Thirty three percent of the population of the United States has used illicit drugs and 6–15% of the population has a substance use disorder at any given time. Consequently, substance-abusing individuals form a significant proportion of the patient population. Substance abusers commonly experience injuries and infections associated with poor wound healing. This is often compounded by the immunosuppressive effects associated with chronic illicit opioid use and HIV infection.

The American Medical Association defines addiction as a chronic disorder characterized by "the compulsive use of a substance resulting in physical, psychological or social harm to the user and continued use despite harm." Drug seeking, drug tolerance and physical dependence alone are not indicators of addiction. The latter two reflect pharmacological properties of drugs. The former is appropriate behavior in one who has pain that can be relieved by medications. This behavior has been termed pseudo-addiction and is defined as "drug seeking behavior that is observed in the setting of uncontrolled pain and disappears when analgesic interventions, often including increasing doses of an opioid, became effective."

Data confirm that the therapeutic use of opioid drugs does not lead to drug addiction. Thus, opioid analgesics should not be withheld or limited because of fears of causing addiction in non-addicts. Equally, there is no evidence to support the belief that patients with a remote history of drug addiction are more likely to become addicted to therapeutic opioids than individuals without such a history. Fears that opioid analgesics will aggravate the disease in those individuals currently addicted are unsubstantiated. The need for opioid analgesics can be minimized by optimizing the use of local anesthetics, NSAIDs and non-pharmacological therapies whenever possible.

Drug-abusing individuals frequently have significant psychopathy and often exhibit antisocial and dysfunctional behaviors. This can impede therapeutic advances as compliance is often poor. The psychological component to pain may be greater in drug addicts and they often manifest higher levels of anxiety than non-addicted patients. Anxiolytic measures, both pharmacological and non-pharmacological, may prove especially beneficial in the comfort of these patients. Establishing a therapeutic contract with the patient based upon frank discussion of the expectations of therapy and what constitutes acceptable behavior is often helpful. Referral to a psychiatrist for addiction treatment and for advice on how best to manage individual patients in the wound care center may be helpful. When opioid medication is used it may be preferable to supervise dose administration at the wound care facility rather than allow the patient to keep drugs at home for self-medication prior to their scheduled procedure. Opioids with slow onset and offset times tend not to cause a "buzz." Methadone is especially bland in this regard even after intravenous administration. Regardless of the strategies adopted, drug addicted patients require analgesia for painful procedures in the same way as non-addicts. Drug-addicted patients may or may not require higher doses than their non-addicted counterparts and medications should be titrated to effect. Extreme care must be exercised in giving analgesic and sedative drugs to patients who present in an intoxicated state and therapy should be postponed until the patient is sober.

SUMMARY

Identifying and understanding the sources of pain in patients allows a customized therapeutic analgesic regimen to be implemented. A multi-modal, multi-disciplinary approach utilizing pharmacological and non-pharmacological interventions, and optimizing pain-provoking disease states usually provides the best results.

REFERENCES

1. Mersky H, Bogduk N. Classification of Chronic Pain: descriptions of chronic pain syndromes and definitions of pain terms prepared by the International Association for the Study of Pain, Task Force on Taxonomy. Seattle, WA:IASP Press, 1994.
2. Carr DB, Goudas LC. Acute Pain. *Lancet* 1999; 353:2051-2058.
3. Eccleston C. Role of psychology in pain management. *Br J Anaesth* 2001; 87:144-52.
4. Taddio A, Katz J, Ilerisch A, et al. Effect of neonatal circumcision on pain response during subsequent routine vaccination. *Lancet* 1997; 349:599-603.
5. Schechter NL, Weisman SJ, Rosenblum M, et al. The use of oral transmucosal fentanyl citrate for painful procedures in children. *Pediatrics* 1995; 95:335-339.
6. Kehlet H, Holte K. Effect of postoperative analgesia on surgical outcome. *Br J Anaesth* 2001; 87:62-72.
7. Macrae WA. Chronic pain after surgery. *Br J Anaesth* 2001; 87:88-98.
8. Marchand F, Perretti M, McMahon SB. Role of the Immune System in Chronic Pain. *Nature Reviews* 2005;6:521-532
9. Jensen TS. Anticonvulsants in neuropathic pain: rationale and clinical evidence. *Eur J Pain* 2002; 6 suppl A:61-68
10. Jaaskelainen SK. Pregabalin for painful neuropathy. *Lancet Neurol* 2005; 4(4):207-8
11. Gallagher G, Rae CP, Kinsella J. Treatment of pain in severe burns. *Am J Clin Dermatology* 2000; 1(6):329-35
12. Watterson G, Howard R, Goldman A. Peripheral opioids in inflammatory pain. *Archives of Disease in Childhood* 2004; 89(7):679-81
13. Kalso E. Improving opioid effectiveness: from ideas to evidence. *Eur J Pain* 2005; 9(2):131-5
14. Walker J, Maccallum M, Fischer C, et al. Sedation using dexmedetomidine in pediatric burns patients. *Journal of Burn Care and Research* 2006; 27(2):206-10
15. Nikolajsen L, Jensen TS. Phantom limb pain. *Br J Anesth* 2001; 87:107-16.
16. Ramachandran VS, Hirstein W. The perception of phantom limbs. The D. O. Hebb lecture. *Brain* 1998; 121:1603-1630.
17. Watkins LR, Maier SF. Neuropathic Pain: The Immune Connection. *Pain clinical updates* 2004;XII (1):1-4
18. Krishnan ST, Ravman G. New treatments for diabetic neuropathy:symptomatic treatments. *Curr Diab Rep* 2003; 3(6):459-67
19. Hoffman HG, Doctor JN, Patterson DR, et al. Virtual reality as an adjunctive pain control during burn wound carae in adolescent patients. *Pain* 2000; 85:305-9
20. Hoffman HG, Patterson DR, Carrouogher GJ, et al. The effectiveness of virtual reality beased pain control with multiple treatments. *Clin J Pain* 2001; 17:229-235
21. Hoffman HG, Patterson DR, Magula J, et al. Water-friendly virtual reality pain control during wound care. *J Clin Psychol* 2004; 60:189-195
22. Hoffman HG, Richards TL, Coda BA, et al. Modulation of thermal pain-related brain activity with virtual reality: evidence from fMRI. *Neuro Report* 2004; 15:1245-1248
23. Hoffman HG, Sharar SR, Everett J, et al. Manipulating presence influences the magnitude of virtual reality analgesia. *Pain* 2004; 111:162-168
24. Kissin I. Preemptive Analgesia. *Anesthesiology* 2000; 93:1138-43.
25. Kalso E, Tramer MR, McQuay HJ, et al. Systemic local-anesthetic-type drugs in chronic pain: a systemic review. *Eur J Pain* 1998; 2(1):3-14
26. *Cochrane Database System Rev* 2005; 20(3):CD005454

27. McQuay HJ, Tramer M, Nye BA, et al. A systemiatic review of antidepressants in neuropathic pain. *Pain* 1996; 68(2-3):217-27

28. Finnerup NB, Otto M, McQuay HJ, et al. Algorithm for neuropathic pain treatment; an evidence based proposal. *Pain* 2005; 118(3):289-305

29. Hollingshead J. *Cochrane Database Systematic Review* 2006; 3:CD003726

30. Wilcox RA, Owen H. Variable Cytochrome P450 2D6 Expression and metabolism of codeine and other opioid prodrugs: implications for the Australian Anaesthetist. *Anaesth Intensive Care* 2000; 28:611-619.

31. Otton SV, Schadel M, Cheung SW, et al. CYP2D6 phenotype determines the metabolic conversion of hydrocodone to hydromorphone. *Clin Pharamacol Ther* 1993; 54:463-472.

32. Practice Guidelines for Sedation and Analgesia by Non-Anesthesiologists. *Anesthesiology* 1996; 84:459-71.

33. Guidelines for Monitoring and Management of Pediatric Patients During and After Sedation For Diagnostic and Therapeutic Procedures. *Pediatrics* 1992; 89:1110-1115.

34. Cleeland CS, Ryan KM. Pain assessment: Global use of the brief pain inventory. *Ann Acad Med Singapore* 1994; 23(2):129-38

35. Galer BS, Jensen MP. Development and preliminary validation of a pain measure specific to neuropathic pain: the neuropathic pain scale. *Neurology* 1997; 48(2):332-338

36. Finlay GA, McGrath PJ, eds. Progress in Pain Research and Management Volume 10: Measurement of Pain in Infants and Children. Seattle, WA:IASP Press, 1998.

37. Portnoy RK, Payne R. Acute and Chronic Pain. In: Lowenstein JH, Ruiz P, Millman RB, eds. Substance Abuse: a comprehensive textbook. Baltimore, MD: Williams and Wilkins, 1992; 691-72.

Additional resources:

Anderson CTM, Zeltzer LK, Fanurik D. Procedural Pain. In: Schechter NL, Berde CB, Yaster M,eds. *Pain in Infants, Children and Adolescents*. Baltimore, MD: Williams and Wilkins, 1993; 435-458.

Walco GA, Cassidy RC, Schechter NL. Pain, Hurt, and Harm – The Ethics of Pain Control in Infants and Children. *N Engl J Med* 1994; 331(8):541-544.

Ferrante FM, VadeBoncouer TR, eds. *Postoperative Pain Management* Churchill Livingstone, 1993.

US Department of Health and Human Services. Acute Pain Management: Operative or Medical Procedures and Trauma, 1992; AHCPR Publication No. 92-0032.

REVIEW QUESTIONS

1.) Non-pharmacological analgesia in the form of distraction techniques can reduce pain perception by:
   a. 10%
   b. 30%
   c. 60%
   d. 90%
   e. distraction does not change pain perception

2.) The following class(es) of analgesic drug(s) is(are) effective in the treatment of neuropathic pain:
   a. opioids
   b. anti-depressants
   c. anti-convulsants
   d. local anesthetics
   e. all of the above

3.) The single most important intervention in the management of painful diabetic neuropathy is:
   a. Supportive psychotherapy
   b. Non-steroidal anti-inflammatory drugs (NSAIDs)
   c. Relaxation techniques to reduce stress
   d. Glycemic control with optimal blood sugar concentration 80 – 150 mg/dl
   e. Cannabinoids

4.) The following statement is CORRECT regarding analgesic management in special populations:
   a. Confusion in elderly patients can be a sign of inadequate pain control and may be resolved by giving more analgesia
   b. Patients with a history of substance abuse should not be given parenteral analgesics
   c. Multi-modal analgesic therapies are not appropriate for use in children
   d. Tricyclic antidepressants are contraindicated in patients over 65 years of age
   e. Non-pharmacologic analgesic therapies are not effective in drug addicted patients

5.) The following opioid analgesic is considered to have greatest utility in the treatment of persistant somatic and neuropathic pain because of its agonist activity at mu-receptors and antagonist activity at NMDA receptors:
   a. Morphine
   b. Methadone
   c. fentanyl
   d. remifentanil
   e. hydromorphone

Answers: 1b, 2e, 3d, 4a, 5b

CHAPTER 33

WOUND PAIN MANAGEMENT: A WOUND CARE SPECIALIST'S PERSPECTIVE

CHAPTER THIRTY-THREE OVERVIEW

NOTES

Wound Pain Management: A Wound Care Specialist's Perspective

Diane L. Krasner

INTRODUCTION

Whether a wound is acute or chronic, simple or complex, the pain that the person experiences is typically a complex, multidimensional phenomenon (1, 2). It usually involves procedural pain (such as pain from debridement, dressings, or therapies) as well as non-procedural pain (such as body image changes, loss of function, suffering or ache and anguish) (3, 4). Only in the past decade and a half has the importance of the wound pain experience been truly appreciated by wound care providers (5–8). If the person is also receiving hyperbaric oxygen therapy, additional factors may contribute to the pain experienced, including the pain associated with transfer, transport, and immobility. The wound care specialist must anticipate, assess and address the wound pain as well as other wound healing issues (9).

To date, only a handful of wound centers have algologists or anesthesiologists on the interdisciplinary team. The evidence suggests that wound pain management in hospitals still leaves much to be desired (10). Wound centers that have hyperbaric oxygen therapy capability may be more fortunate in that they may have more ready access to anesthesiologists who can consult on patients' wound pain problems. In an ideal world, pain specialist doctors and nurses would be part of every wound care team. When that is not feasible, having a pain specialist who can be regularly consulted may be the next best thing. Another option may be to designate the member of the wound care team who has the most interest in pain management to be the watchdog, to coordinate pain management efforts, and to advocate for the appropriate pain plans of care for patients. Whichever approach you choose, attending to wound pain is no longer an option—pain management is essential for advanced wound caring (11).

While research has not yet conclusively demonstrated that decreasing wound pain will improve the time to healing of wounds, it seems intuitively likely to be the case. Decreasing a person's pain response is an important and quantifiable outcome measure of care that wound care specialists will find useful in this age of outcome imperatives. Painful wounds often frustrate both patient and caregiver. They may represent failed expectations from the point of view of the patient, the providers—or both. They may be palliative wounds that will never heal. Painful wounds are much more, therefore, than mere physical damage to skin and tissue. The psychological aspects of managing wound pain—addressing the suffering, the ache and anguish—are as essential as relieving the physical pain. Changes in body image, activities of daily living, productivity and functional status are usually significant contributors to the overall wound pain experience.

During interviews for this author's dissertation, a phenomenological study that explored the lived experience of chronic wound pain (12), Mr. Beech (a pseudonym), a tough truck driver with a seven year history of a non-healing venous ulcer, said to me one day, "Do you know how much courage it takes to come back to this clinic every week, knowing I'm going to be tortured?" Would you go to the dentist for a root canal without an anesthetic? Of course, not! But this is the expectation for far too many wound patients. Even our language reflects our bias in common phrases such as "Bite the bullet," "No pain, no gain," and "Grin and bear it."

We can do better. We must do better. By opening our eyes and our ears to the issue of wound pain (13) and employing the strategies that will be discussed in this chapter, we can reduce the pain and suffering that far too many patients with painful wounds still experience.

> The real voyage of discovery
> consists not in seeking new landscapes,
> but in having new eyes.
>
> – Marcel Proust

> When wounds are painful,
> They are trying to communicate that something is wrong.
> All we have to do is listen.
>
> – Lia van Rijswijk

ACUTE AND CHRONIC WOUND PAIN

Interest in chronic wound pain has evolved slowly in contrast to interest in acute and burn pain or to the science of wound healing both of which have grown by leaps and bounds. Pain experienced by chronic wound suffers was occasionally mentioned in the chronic wound literature prior to the 1990's (14, 15). The 1990's saw an emerging interest in the phenomenon with the publication of various descriptive studies addressing the experiences of leg ulcer patients in pain (16–18), as well as the impact of the wound pain experience on health-related quality of life (19, 20). Interventional research on the subject is just reaching the chronic wound research agenda. So, at the beginning of the 21st century, it is fair to say that our research-base for practice related to chronic wound pain is spotty and superficial. There is certainly much more room for research into this important area of practice.

CLASSIFICATION OF WOUND PAIN

Pain has classically been categorized in several different ways:

- Nociceptive (tissue injury) versus neuropathic (nerve injury)
- Procedural versus non-procedural
- Acute versus chronic
- Acute versus Chronic Malignant versus Chronic Non-Malignant

In every case, it is recognized that the pain experience is multidimensional and that people commonly experience more than one type of pain, either sequentially or concurrently (21). The implication of this for the wound care specialist is that frequently multiple approaches and/or poly pharmacy are required for a person to achieve an acceptable level of pain relief.

In 1995 this researcher, after experiencing three surgeries, each of which involved wound complications (22–25), developed a model entitled The Chronic Wound Pain Experience Model. This model is based on empirical experience and makes a distinction between acute non-cyclic wound pain, acute cyclic wound pain and chronic wound pain (26) (Figure 1). This author suggests that in the real world, distinguishing between one-time or very limited painful stimuli (such as one time debridement or drain tube removal) versus cyclic painful stimuli (such as daily dressing changes) versus chronic painful stimuli (such as the continuous burning or throbbing of a wound) can help clinicians to distinguish the type of pain-reducing interventions that may be needed for a particular individual. So, for example, the patient with a painful diabetic foot ulcer with osteomyelitis who is receiving daily hyperbaric treatments with dressing changes and PRN debridements, may need all of the following strategies to address all three dimensions of his chronic wound pain experience:

For Acute Non-Cyclic Wound Pain secondary to debridement:

- EMLA® topically under a transparent film dressing 1 hour prior to the debridement
- Oral analgesia following the procedure

For Acute Cyclic Wound Pain secondary to hyperbaric treatments, exudate build-up, and dressing changes:

- Oral analgesia before and after transfer and transport to the wound center
- Wound cleansing
- Pain-reducing dressings
- Reduced dressing change schedule by employing advanced wound dressings
- Periwound skin barriers

For Chronic Wound Pain secondary to neuropathic pain:

- Antidepressant medication for neuropathic pain

RESOURCES

Several excellent sources for information on pain (generally) and wound pain (specifically) are worthy of mention. In 1992, the Agency for Health Care

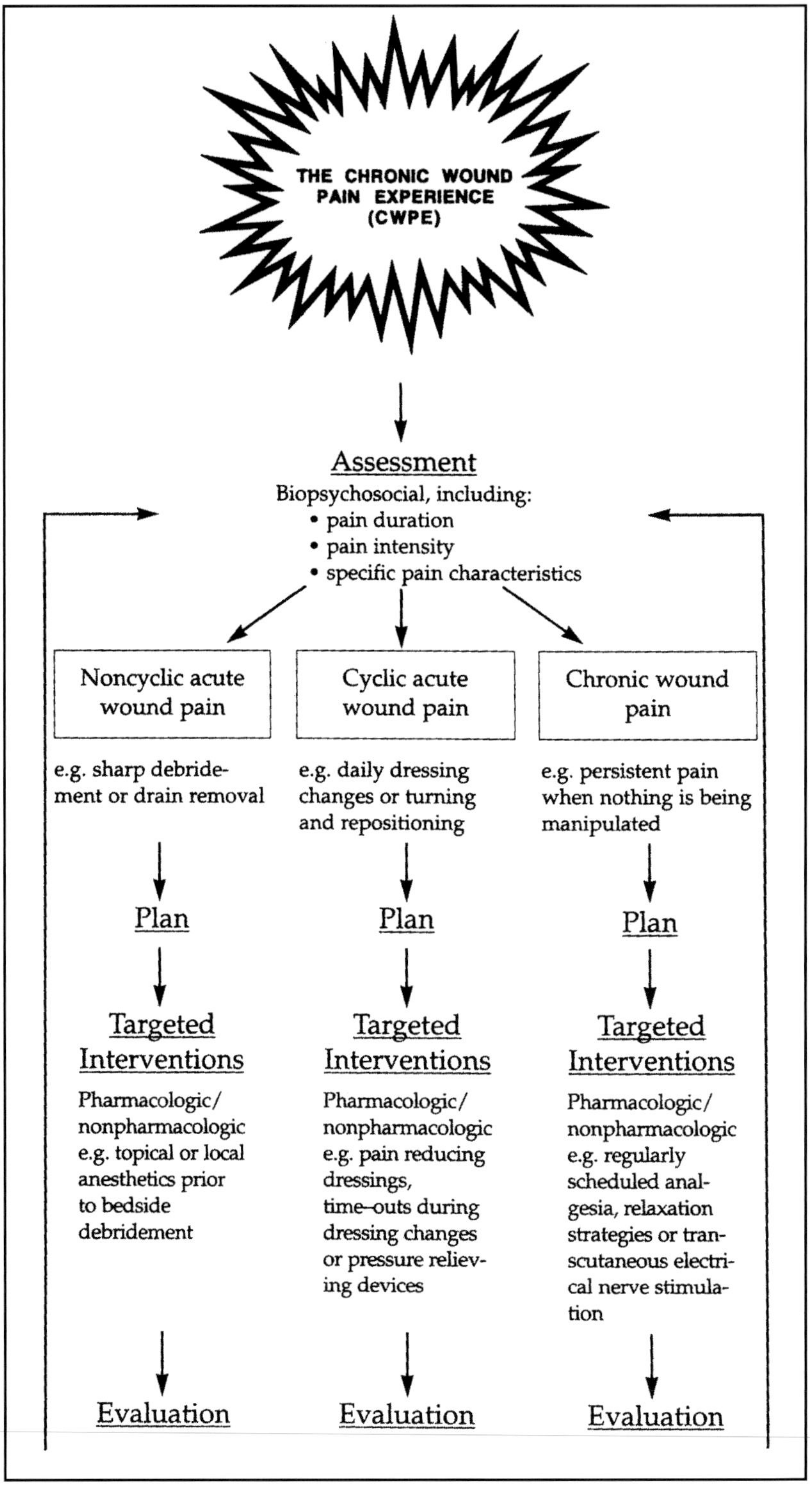

Figure 1. Proposed model of the chronic wound pain experience (CWPE). ©1995 Diane L. Krasner. Used with permission.

Policy & Research (AHCPR) published the first in a series of Clinical Practice Guidelines entitled Acute Pain Management: Operative or Medical Procedures and Trauma (27). In 1994, Guideline #9 was published entitled Chronic Malignant Pain (28). Both of these guidelines provide excellent starting points for clinicians interested in standards of care for pain management in general.

In 1994, the AHCPR also published a guideline addressing The Treatment of Pressure Ulcers (29). This guideline briefly mentions pressure ulcer pain, recommending:

- Assess all patients with pain related to the pressure ulcer or its treatment.
- Manage pain by eliminating or controlling the source of pain (i.e., covering wounds, adjusting support surfaces, repositioning).
- Provide analgesia as needed and appropriate.
- Prevent or manage pain associated with debridement as needed.

In 2002, the European Wound Management Association (EWMA) published a position document on wound pain at wound dressing changes (30). This excellent resource consists of a series of review articles on the following topics:

- Pain at wound dressing changes. CJ Moffatt
- Understanding wound pain and trauma: an international perspective. CJ Moffatt, PJ Franks, H Hollingworth
- The theory of pain. H Wulf, R Baron
- Pain at wound dressing changes: a guide to management. M Briggs, JE Torra, I Bou
- The EWMA position document on wound pain can be downloaded from the Internet at *www.tendra.com*

In 2004, the World Union of Wound Healing Societies released a Principles of Best Practice document entitled "Minimizing pain at wound dressing-related procedures: A consensus document" (31). This document can be downloaded in five languages from the World Union website (*www.wuwhs.org*).

WOUND PAIN ASSESSMENT

Wound pain comes from a variety of sources, most commonly secondary to tissue trauma, treatments, devices, swelling, infection, and nerve damage. The presence of new or increased pain, often signals complications, such as infection, a Charcot arthropathy, or vascular compromise. As with all types of pain, it is a subjective phenomenon defined and experienced by the individual. McCaffery captured this important recognition in her 1972 definition of pain: "Pain is whatever the experiencing person says it is and exists whenever he /she says it does" (32). Many other definitions of pain exist and the reader is referred to the extensive literature on pain for further definitions.

It has been suggested that pain be viewed as the Fifth Vital Sign. Routine assessment of pain, along with temperature, pulse, respirations and blood pressure is advocated by many. Following the pain initiative in 2001 by the Joint Commission on the Accreditation of Healthcare Organizations in the USA, many facilities added pain scores to their vital signs flow sheets.

Pain Tools and Scales

The pain assessment tools in general use today range from simple visual analogue scales to complex multidimensional instruments. All have their purpose and place. Because of the subjective nature of the pain experience, it is only appropriate for the person experiencing pain to determine his/her own score. It is never considered appropriate for a healthcare professional to rate a person's pain level for him, unless he is nonresponsive and then a specialized tool can be used. The AHCPR Panel on Acute Pain Management emphasized this in the strongest terms in the 1992 AHCPR Clinical Practice Guideline #1: The single most reliable indicator of the existence and intensity of acute pain—and any resultant affective discomfort or distress—is the patient's self report (33).

This mandate presents challenges for those wound patients who, due to stroke or other illnesses, are unable to express themselves. In such cases, this author recommends relying on expert knowing (34) and experience and intuiting the person's level of pain from your prior experience with similar patients with the given type of wound/etiology and pain. The reader is referred to articles by Herr & Mobily (35, 36) for further discussion of this topic and information about the assessment of pain in the elderly.

The gold standard for measuring pain for research and clinical purposes is the 10 mm horizontal visual analogue scale (VAS). On this scale the left anchor marks "No pain" and the right anchor marks "Pain as bad as it can be." The person is asked to point to the place on the line representing the intensity of his pain at the current moment, known as Present Pain Intensity (PPI). This scale can also be used to measure pain distress. Visual analogue scales may not be intuitive or easily comprehended by all people. In such situations, an alternative scale, such as a numeric scale, a descriptor scale or the Faces Pain Scale (37) may be used. Dallam et al. showed a good correlation between the VAS and the Faces scales in their study of hospitalized elderly patients with pressure ulcer pain (38).

Pain assessment should be done on a regular basis. Enlightened clinicians often routinely measure pain prior to and following procedures that are known to cause pain, such as debridements or dressing changes, to assure that adequate pain control has been achieved. Some clinicians advocate asking the person a second question, "Where do you want your pain level to be" and using that level as the target for treatment and level for measuring effectiveness of the interventions. For people experiencing on-going pain, it is often helpful to have them keep a pain diary in order to understand the full extent and daily variation in the pain experience. In-depth pain assessment can be obtained using the McGill Pain Questionnaire or the Short Form-McGill Pain Questionnaire (39). Other pain descriptors that are often assessed include pain duration (i.e., periodic, intermittent, persistent) and pain characteristics (i.e., descriptors such as sharp, burning, etc.).

Management Tactics at the Time of Dressing Change

Dressing change pain, which is classified as procedural or acute cyclic pain, is often cited by wound patients as the worst pain they experience.

This may illustrate the problems caused by using antiquated dressings, such as gauze wet-to-dry dressings, that are ripped out of the wound and reinjure it with each dressing change—starting the wounding process all over again. Many strategies can be employed to minimize wound dressing change pain (40) including:

1. Using pain reducing dressings that cover the wound bed and exposed nerve endings, adhere as little as possible and leave minimal residue behind. Examples include hydrogels, foams, non-adherent dressings, or specialty absorptive dressings like hydrofibers or alginates. Dressings that cause pain should be avoided, such as wet-to-dry gauze and adhesive dressings on certain areas of the body.
2. Managing wound exudate properly, so that it does not pool in the wound bed causing local pressure and pain or leak out of the wound bed macerating or denuding the surrounding skin. If wound margins become macerated or denuded, cover them to prevent pain and further damage with a moisture barrier ointment (i.e., petrolatum, zinc oxide) a hydrocolloid or thin hydrocolloid dressing (that will stick to denuded skin) or a special wound barrier dressing.
3. Avoiding the use of cytotoxic agents, such as full strength povidone-iodine, which in and of themselves often cause pain when applied to wounds.
4. Minimizing the frequency of dressing changes by selecting advanced wound dressings that require daily or every other day changes (as opposed to twice a day or three times a day dressing changes)
5. Selecting a time of day for the dressing changes when that individual can best tolerate the dressing change (i.e., mornings for morning people, evenings for night owls)
6. Giving the person permission to call time-out if the pain gets to be too great. Burn research has demonstrated that giving people this control reduces pain scores related to dressing changes (41).
7. Allowing people who are able to change their own dressings, which often cause less pain than when someone else does it.
8. Using diversionary tactics at dressing changes to help reduce the pain experienced, such as conversation, music, or imagery.

Device Application and Removal

The application and removal of specialty devices, such as tubes, drains and the Negative Pressure Wound Therapy (NPWT, such as the V.A.C.®, KCI, San Antonio, TX) can cause pain or exacerbate preexisting pain. The planned used of anesthetics and analgesia can offer considerable relief. Preventive dosing is always more effective than addressing the pain when it is already peaking.

The application and removal of the NPWT on a painful wound poses special challenges for healthcare providers. Specific strategies can be implemented to reduce NPWT-related wound pain. These are reviewed in detail in an article published in "Ostomy/Wound Management," 2002, by this author (42). Some of the strategies include:

1. Instilling normal saline or lidocaine solution into the NPWT tubing for one-half to one hour prior to sponge removal
2. Lining the wound bed with a non-adherent impregnated gauze (i.e., Adaptic®), white NPWT foam, an amorphous hydrogel or for heavily draining wounds an alginate dressing prior to applying the gray NPWT sponge
3. Preventing periwound maceration by applying a skin sealant, a hydrocolloid or thin hydrocolloid dressing to the wound margin before applying the NPWT drape;
4. Premedicating the patient in sufficient time for the analgesic to have its peak effect at the time of dressing change
5. Covering exposed tissue with normal saline moistened gauze during the procedure to minimize dehydration of the tissues
6. Using sufficient personnel to minimize the time it takes to perform the NPWT dressing change
7. Taking the person for the NPWT dressing change to a special procedures room or the OR for more intense pain management if the above measures do not control the person's pain.

Other Strategies for Reducing Procedural Pain

Other procedures that often elicit wound pain, especially for the person undergoing hyperbaric treatments, include turning and repositioning, transferring and transporting. These procedures are essential, of course, for accessing hyperbaric chambers and for overall well-being, maintenance of function and prevention of pneumonia and other immobility-related disorders, and should not be eliminated due to pain unless the person is terminal and a decision for palliative care has been made. Rather, every effort should be made to reduce the pain experienced by the use of timely premedication, pressure-relieving or reducing devices, splints, immobilizers, abdominal binders and so on, all of which can help reduce the pain experienced. Using lift sheets to lift and move patients, instead of draw sheets (that drag) helps to prevent painful friction and shear injuries. For many patients, splinting or immobilizing the wounded area (i.e., the use of an abdominal binder for a mid-line incision or wound) can offer significant comfort.

Strategies for Managing Non-Procedural Pain

Common sources of non-procedural pain in people with wounds include swelling, inflammation and infection. Edema can be controlled by thoughtful positioning (i.e., elevation of swollen extremities as much as possible) as well as the appropriate selection of dressings, compression therapy, offloading and devices to reduce edema. The etiology of wound inflammation or infection should be identified and treatment initiated to address the cause(s).

Changes in body image, activities of daily living, sleep patterns, and productivity are commonly seen with wound patients and contribute to the psychological suffering that many patients experience. Depression is not uncommon and warrants referral to a trained healthcare professional.

SPECIAL CONSIDERATIONS

Non-healing chronic wounds or palliative wounds occur due to malignancy, host immunocompromise, or the inability of the host to muster the energy needed for wound healing (43,44). For these types of wounds, where healing is not the goal of care, pain management and prevention of infection or wound deterioration often become the key objectives. Frequently these patients will require extraordinarily high levels of analgesia to control their pain, especially as tumors in wounds grow and increase in size and depth. Creative dressing strategies can go a long way towards alleviating the pain and suffering associated with these types of wounds. Odor control and exudate management are usually key factors to be addressed.

In 2004 the International Palliative Wound Care Initiative developed a consensus statement entitled "Palliative Wound Care: Managing Chronic Wounds across Life's Continuum (45)." This document defines the problem, concepts and related terms and discusses opportunities and challenges for implementing palliative wound care. The document is reprinted in its entirety in Figure 2 and may be reproduced and distributed for non-commercial educational purposes when the copyright statement is displayed.

CONCLUSION

In today's healthcare environment, where measuring outcomes has become the gold standard, a reduction in wound patients' pain scores can be used as a quantitative measure of the effectiveness of the wound care in addition to "time to healing" measures. For those patients with palliative, non-healing wounds for whom healing is not a realistic outcome, reduction in pain may be the most realistic outcome measure.

No one can argue the importance of reducing pain and suffering for improving a person's health-related quality of life. From the suffering person's perspective, wound pain and its sequelae are often their most significant problems. So, we must remember these words of wisdom from an ancient Greek epigrapher, as we strive to provide the best in modern wound care for our patients:

To cure — occasionally.
To relieve — often.
To comfort — always.

Palliative Wound Care
Managing Chronic Wounds Across Life's Continuum

A Consensus Statement from the International Palliative Wound Care Initiative

Frank D. Ferris, MD (Chair)[1]; Ahmad Abdullah Al Khateib, MHA MSN[2]; Isabelle Fromantin[3]; Linda Hoplamazian, RN BSN MHA WCC[4]; Theresa Hurd, RN BScN CCRN MScN APN[5]; Diane L. Krasner, PhD RN CWOCN CWS FAAN[6]; Vincent Maida, BSc MD CCFP[7]; Patricia Price, BA PhD AFBPsS CHPsychol[8]; Louanne Rich-vanderBij, MSc BScN RN CWCN COCN[9].

From [1]San Diego Hospice & Palliative Care, San Diego, California; [2]King Hussein Cancer Center, Amman, Jordan; [3]L'Institut Curie, Paris, France; [4]excelleRx Inc., Philadelphia, Pennsylvania; [5]Niagara Regional Community Senior Services, Fort Erie, Ontario; [6]York Hospital Wound Healing Center, York, Pennsylvania; [7]William Osler Health Centre, Toronto, Ontario; [8]University of Cardiff, Wales; [9]Sunnybrook & Women's College Health Sciences Centre, Toronto, Ontario

The Problem

Worldwide, individuals of all ages (from neonates to elders) and all socioeconomic groups develop chronic wounds.* This is particularly true for people living with advanced/end-stage chronic illnesses associated with arterial or venous insufficiency/edema (eg, diabetes mellitus, peripheral vascular disease), central and peripheral neurological disorders causing motor dysfunction and/or sensory deficits (eg, dementia, stroke, Parkinson's disease, neurodegenerative disorders), cancers and other diseases leading to cachexia, immunocompromise, chronic infections or an impaired ability to heal. Even with the best of nursing care, these patients may develop chronic wounds.

While wound care has historically focused on curing the underlying disease and healing the wound(s), healthcare professionals now recognize that chronic wounds are frequently associated with multiple concurrent issues that cause suffering for the patient and her/his family.† If these are not managed, they may delay wound healing.

While most chronic wounds will eventually heal if managed appropriately, some will not. In patients with non-healable wounds, therapies that aim to heal the wound may not be in anyone's best interest.

Palliative Wound Care

Palliative wound care is the evolving body of knowledge and skills that takes a holistic approach to relieving suffering and improving quality of life for patients and families living with chronic wounds, whether the wound is healable, or not. While palliative care‡ was initially reserved for terminally ill patients at the end of their lives (often called hospice care), the potential for palliative care to improve wound healing and the quality of life for patients and families living with chronic wounds is now being recognized.

Palliative wound care is an extension of both palliative care[1-5] and wound care.[6] It encompasses all of the therapeutic interventions that aim to:

- guide effective communication, decision-making and care delivery
- stabilize the wound
- minimize the risk of infection and further progression of the wound
- manage the multiple issues that cause patients and families suffering
- optimize the patient's function and quality of life for as long as possible.

From the onset of an illness, patients and their families are encouraged to actively participate in all aspects of their care. Information is shared respectfully. Goals of care and treatment priorities are negotiated with each patient based on the stage of the underlying disease process and the potential for available therapeutic options to be beneficial and meet personal preferences.

Initially, most patients choose therapies intended to cure the underlying disease and heal their wound(s). Concurrently most patients also want to integrate therapies to 'palliate' the multiple concurrent issues that cause suffering and impact the quality of their lives, including symptom management, nutritional support, physical and occupational therapy, counselling and spiritual support.

Over time, if the patient's health status deteriorates and/or therapies to heal the wound prove to be ineffective, the focus of care usually shifts to focus on therapies that aim to stabilize the wound, minimize the risk of infection and further progression, maintain function and relieve suffering for as long as possible. Many patients also want to prepare for the end of their lives and ensure that family members will be safe and well cared for after they die.

The Opportunity

For wound care: Palliative wound care can be integrated into day-to-day wound care if an interdisciplinary team of wound care professionals§ is skilled in the basics of palliative care. When the issues become complex, additional expertise can be provided by palliative care consult services and hospices.

For palliative care: Similarly, the core skills of palliative wound care can be integrated into the day-to-day activities of palliative care practitioners with consultative support from wound care experts.

LEGEND

***Chronic wound** = a break or ulceration of the skin and underlying tissues that does not respond to medical or surgical interventions.

†**Family** = those closest to the patient in knowledge, care and affection.

‡**Palliative care** = therapies to relieve suffering and improve quality of life (has evolved from the Latin word *palliare* = to cloak; cover up).

§**Interdisciplinary care** = typically includes input from physicians, nurses, pharmacists, social workers, chaplains, physiotherapists, occupational therapists, dietitians, psychologists and volunteers appropriate for the issues that the patient and family are experiencing.

Figure 2. Palliative Wound Care: Managing Chronic Wounds Across Life's Continuum

The Challenges

To this end, strategies are needed to:

1. increase awareness of the problem, the magnitude of the need and the potential for palliative wound care to enhance healing and quality of life
2. advocate for changes in policy, regulations and reimbursement guidelines that may be limiting palliative wound care practice
3. increase the knowledge and skills
   a. of core palliative care skills in wound care practitioners[7,8]
   b. of core wound care skills in palliative care practitioners
4. integrate collaborative palliative wound care practice and consultative expertise into acute, home and long-term healthcare services.

The International Palliative Wound Care Initiative

The International Palliative Wound Care Initiative is a global group of palliative care, wound care and continuing education professionals.

Mission
To promote the advancement of effective palliative wound care by developing information and strategies to care for patients and families living with chronic wounds, and disseminating these resources internationally.

Vision
The complex issues faced by patients and families living with chronic wounds will be appropriately addressed and managed through the integration of palliative care throughout their wound care experience.

Goals
The Initiative recognizes that the expertise and skills in palliative wound care can improve the quality of life of all individuals living with or affected by healing and non-healing chronic wounds. It is guided by the philosophy that the opportunity exists to negotiate personalized goals of care to optimize quality of life through an interdisciplinary approach to care.

The Initiative is exploring ways to increase awareness and change attitudes through advocacy; enhance knowledge and skills through education; influence day-to-day behaviour through norms of practice and preferred practice guidelines; and evaluate outcomes for individuals, organizations, and society.

For more information on the International Palliative Wound Care Initiative please visit www.palliativewoundcare.info.

Disclosure: The work of the International Palliative Wound Care Initiative is supported by The Medicine Group through an unrestricted educational grant from Smith & Nephew Inc.

Printed in Canada.

References

1. Ferris F, Balfour H, Bowen K, et al. A model to guide patient and family care. Based on nationally accepted principles and norms of practice. *J Pain Symptom Manage* 2002;**24**:106-123.
2. Ferris FD, Balfour HM, Bowen K, et al. A model to guide hospice palliative care. [online]. Ottawa, ON: Canadian Hospice Palliative Care Association, March 2002 [cited November 18, 2004]:
   English version <http://www.chpca.net/publications/norms_of_practice.htm>,
   French version <http://www.acsp.net/publications_et_ressouces/normes.htm>.
3. WHO definition of palliative care. [online]. Geneva, Switzerland: World Health Organization, 2003 [cited November 18, 2004]: <http://www.who.int/cancer/palliative/definition/en/>.
4. Doyle D, Hanks G, Cherny NI, Calman K (eds). *Oxford Textbook of Palliative Medicine*. New York, NY: Oxford University Press, 2003.
5. Ferrell BR, Coyle N (eds). *Textbook of Palliative Nursing*. New York, NY: Oxford University Press, 2001.
6. Krasner DL, Rodeheaver GT, Sibbald RG, eds. *Chronic Wound Care: A Clinical Source Book for Healthcare Professionals*. 3rd ed. Wayne, PA: HMP Communications, 2001.
7. Emanuel LL, von Gunten CF, Ferris FD. The education on palliative and end-of-life care (EPEC) curriculum [online]. Chicago, IL: The EPEC Project, Northwestern University, 2003 [cited November 26, 2004]: <http://www.epec.net>.
8. The End of Life Nursing Education Consortium (ELNEC) Project, 2000 [online]: <http://www.aacn.nche.edu/elnec/>.

REFERENCES

1. Wall P, Melzack R (eds). Textbook of Pain. 2d ed. Edinburgh, Scotland: Churchill Livingstone, 1994.
2. Rice A. Pain, inflammation and wound healing. *J Wound Care* 1994; 3(5):246-249.
3. Morris DB. The Culture of Pain. Berkeley: University of California Press, 1991.
4. Price P. Quality of life. In: Krasner DL, Rodeheaver GT, Sibbald RG, eds. Chronic Wound Care: A Clinical Source Book for Healthcare Professionals. Wayne, PA: HMP Communications, 2001:91-97.
5. Walsche C. Living with a venous ulcer: A descriptive study of patients' experiences. *J Adv Nursing* 1995; 22:1092-1100.
6. Hofman D, Ryan TJ, Arnold F, et al. Pain in venous leg ulcers. *J Wound Care* 1997; 6(5):222-224.
7. Krasner D. Painful venous ulcers: themes and stories about living with the pain and suffering. *J WOCN* 1998; 25(3): 158-168.
8. Krasner D. Painful venous ulcers: themes and stories about their impact on quality of life. *Ostomy/Wound Management* 1998 44(9): 38-49.
9. Broussard CL. Hyperbaric oxygenation and wound healing. *JWOCN* 2003 30(4):210-216.
10. Dallam L, Smyth D, Jackson B, et al. Pressure ulcer pain: assessment and quantification. *J WOCN* 1995; 22(5): 211-218.
11. Krasner DL, Rodeheaver GT, Sibbald RG. Interprofessional Wound Caring. In: Krasner DL, Rodeheaver GT, Sibbald RG. Chronic Wound Care: A Clinical Source Book for Healthcare Professionals. Wayne, PA: HMP Communications. 4th edition. 2007:3-9.
12. Krasner DL. Carrying on despite the pain: living with painful venous ulcers: a Heideggerian hermeneutic analysis. Doctoral dissertation. Ann Arbor, MI: UMI, 1997.
13. van Rijswijk. Wound pain. In: McCaffery M, Pasero C. Pain Clinical Manual. St. Louis, MO: Mosby, 1999.
14. Thomas S. Pain and wound management. *Community Outlook* 1989; July:11-15.
15. Callam MJ, Harper DR, Dale JJ, et al. Chronic leg ulceration: socio-economic aspects. *Scottish Medical J* 1988; 33:358-360.
16. Phillips T, Stanton B, Provan A, et al. A study of the impact of leg ulcers on quality of life: financial, social and psychologic implications. *J Am Adac Dermatol* 1994; 31(1): 49-53.
17. Pieper B. A retrospective analysis of venous ulcer healing in current and former drug users of injected drugs. *J WOCN* 1996; 23(6):291-296.
18. Pieper B, Rossi R, Templin T. Pain associated with venous ulcers in injecting drug users. *Ostomy/Wound Management* 1998; 44(11): 54-66.
19. Franks P, Moffatt C, Connolly M, et al. Community leg ulcer clinics: effect on quality of life. *Phlebology* 1994; 9:83-86.
20. Hamer C, Cullum N, Roe B. Patients' perceptions of chronic leg ulceration. In: Proceedings of the 2nd European Conference in Advances in Wound Management. London, England: Macmillan Magazines, Ltd, 1992.
21. Wall P, Melzack R (eds). Textbook of Pain. 2d Ed. Edinburgh, Scotland: Churchill Livingstone, 1994.
22. Krasner D. Using a hydrogel, foam and dressing retention sheet. *Ostomy/Wound Management* 1992; 38(3):28-33.
23. Ponder R, Krasner D. Gauzes and related dressings. *Ostomy/Wound Management* 1993; 39(5):48-60.
24. Krasner D. Treating postoperative wounds with an amorphous hydrogel. *Journal of Wound Care* 1993; 2(3).

25. Krasner DL, Papen J, Sibbald RG. Helping patients out of the SWAMP©: Skin and Wound Assessment and Management of Pain. In: Krasner DL, Rodeheaver GT, Sibbald RG. Chronic Wound Care: A Clinical Source Book for Healthcare Professionals. Wayne, PA: HMP Communications. 4th edition. 2007:85-97.

26. Krasner D. The chronic wound pain experience: a conceptual model. *Ostomy/Wound Management* 1995; 41(3): 20-27.

27. Acute Pain Management Guideline Panel: Acute pain management: Operative or medical procedures and trauma. Clinical Practice Guideline #1. AHCPR Pub. No. 92-0032. Rockville, MD: Agency for Health Care Policy and Research, Public Health Service, U.S. Department of Health and Human Services, February 1991.

28. Jacox A, Carr C, Payne R, et al.: Management of cancer pain. Clinical Practice Guideline No. 9. AHCPR Publication No. 94-0592. Rockville, MD: Agency for Health Care Policy and Research, U.S. Department of Health and Human Services, Public Health Service, March 1994.

29. Bergstrom N, Bennett M, Carlson C, et al: Treatment of pressure ulcers. Clinical Practice Guideline, No. 15. AHCPR Pub. No. 95-0622,Rockville, MD: U.S. Department of Health and Human Services, Public Health Service, Agency for Health Care Policy and Research,1994.

30. Pain at wound dressing changes. Position Document. European Wound Management Association. London: Medical Education Partnership, 2002. Downloadable from the Internet at *www.tendra.com*

31. Minimizing pain at wound dressing-related procedures: A consensus document. World Union of Wound Healing Societies, 2004. *www.wuwhs.org*

32. McCaffery M. Nursing management of the patient with pain. Philadelphia, PA: Lippincott, 1972.

33. Acute Pain Management Guideline Panel: Acute pain management: Operative or medical procedures and trauma. Clinical Practice Guideline #1. AHCPR Pub. No. 92-0032. Rockville, MD: Agency for Health Care Policy and Research, Public Health Service, U.S. Department of Health and Human Services, February 1991.

34. Benner P. From Novice to Expert: Excellence and Power in Clinical Nursing Practice. Menlo Park, CA: Addison Wesley, 1984.

35. Herr K, Mobily P. Pain assessment in the elderly: clinical considerations. *J Gerontological Nurs* 1991; 17(4):12-19.

36. Herr K, Mobily P. Comparison of selected pain assessment tools for use with the elderly. *Appl Nurs Res* 1993; 6(1):39-46.

37. Wong DL. Whaley & Wong's Essentials of Pediatric Nursing (5th edition). St. Louis, MO: Mosby 1997.

38. Dallam L, Smyth D, Jackson B, et al. Pressure ulcer pain: assessment and quantification. *J WOCN* 1995; 22(5): 211-218.

39. Melzack R. The McGill Pain Questionnaire: major properties and scoring methods. *Pain* 1975; 1:277-299.

40. Krasner DL, Sibbald RG. Wound Management: Best Chronic Wound Care Practices for the Hyperbaric Practitioner. In: Kindwall EP, Whelan HT, eds. Hyperbaric Medicine Practice (second edition). Flagstaff, AZ: Best Publishing Company, 1999: 395-429.

41. Acute Pain Management Guideline Panel: Acute pain management: Operative or medical procedures and trauma. Clinical Practice Guideline #1. AHCPR Pub. No. 92-0032. Rockville, MD: Agency for Health Care Policy and Research, Public Health Service, U.S. Department of Health and Human Services, February 1991.

42. Krasner D. Managing wound pain for patients with vacuum-assisted closure devices. *Ostomy/Wound Management* May 2002; 48(5), 38-43.

43. Barton P, Parslow N. Malignant wounds: Holistic assessment and management. . In: Krasner DL, Rodeheaver GT, Sibbald RG, eds. Chronic Wound Care: A Clinical Source Book for Healthcare Professionals. Wayne, PA: HMP Communications, 2001: 699-710.

44. Rolstad BS, Nix D. Management of wound recalcitrance and deterioration. . In: Krasner DL, Rodeheaver GT, Sibbald RG, Eds. Chronic Wound Care: A Clinical Source Book for Healthcare Professionals. Wayne, PA: HMP Communications, 2001:731-742.

45. Ferris FD, et al. Palliative Wound Care: Managing Chronic Wounds Across Life's Continuum© A consensus statement jointly held by The Medicine Group and the International Palliative Wound Care Initiative, 2005.

REVIEW QUESTIONS:

1.) Which of the following types of pain is MOST OFTEN associated with procedures?
   a. Nociceptive
   b. Neuropathic
   c. Persistent
   d. Chronic

2.) A person with diabetes with a neuropathic foot ulcer, undergoing a debridement and dressing change following a hyperbaric treatment, complains of burning and stabbing pain. Analgesia should address which of the following pain problems:
   a. Procedural pain of debridement
   b. Diabetic neuropathic pain
   c. Cyclic acute dressing change pain
   d. All of the above

3.) Implementing a palliative wound care plan would be MOST appropriate for which of the following patients?
   a. An osteoradionecrosis patient undergoing HBO2 therapy
   b. A venous ulcer patient with a ten year history of recurrent ulcerations
   c. A nursing home resident with a Stage 4 sacral pressure ulcer who is cachetic and on tube feedings
   d. A terminal cancer patient with a granulating pressure ulcer of the trochanter

4.) Common sources of non-procedural pain in people with wounds include;
   a. Swelling
   b. Inflammation
   c. Infection
   d. All of the above

5.) For palliative wounds, which of the following is NOT a key objective?
   a. Heal it
   b. Manage the pain
   c. Prevent infection
   d. Prevent wound deterioration.

Answers: 1a, 2d, 3c, 4d, 5a

NOTES

CHAPTER 34

ROLE OF THERAPY IN WOUND MANAGEMENT

CHAPTER THIRTY-FOUR OVERVIEW

NOTES

Role of Therapy in Wound Management

Philomena C. Broussard, Elizabeth Ann Pickett

Wound care for military personnel in World War I was a primary impetus for the development of therapy as a profession. Historically the armed services assembled a group known as Reconstructive Aides to treat the amputees and burned victims returning from war zones. Between World War I and World War II, the non-military professions of Physical and Occupational Therapy were created, using the model of the Reconstruction Aide (1). Wound care is part of the history and the heart of therapy.

Rehabilitation therapists in a comprehensive wound center can provide primary wound care and can manage the functional limitations imposed by wound healing. Involvement varies because of the overlap of function between the therapist and the nurse, and the overlap among the therapists themselves. The therapist is well qualified to play a primary role in wound care through the application of treatment modalities, including debridement, pulsed lavage, or electrical stimulation. In some facilities, however, their role is to protect and restore function as the nurse manages wound healing. The distinction between Physical and Occupational Therapy has also become less demonstrable. Occupational Therapists now use physical agents. Certified Hand Therapists can be either Physical or Occupational Therapists. Often the extent of the therapist's role is a function of the facility's organization. Sometimes it is a matter of who got there first, or who is more assertive in marketing their product.

Concerning the issue of primary wound care; therapists are trained in wound care, including debridement, as part of their master's curriculum or advanced education in their chosen specialty area. Therapists practicing wound care management are educated in the normal cellular activity of wound repair and the physiologic effects of therapy intervention on cellular response (2). All therapists have the goal of protection and/or restoration of function as the ultimate dictum of their training.

Hopefully, this chapter will provide the reader with an overview of the contribution that Physical and Occupational Therapy provide to comprehensive wound management. There is an obvious need for Physical and Occupational Therapy, whether primarily in wound healing or secondarily in functional restoration. As patients often consider maintenance of bipedal ambulation and hand function to be equally important to wound healing, the therapist's role should not be understated. Success in a comprehensive wound management center often comes first, in developing a true interdisciplinary approach and then capitalizing on the individual talents of each member.

THE ROLE OF THERAPY IN WOUND MANAGEMENT

Primary Wound Care

The therapist is trained to provide the full range of wound care services, which include the following:

- Sharp and Mechanical Debridement
- Pulsed Lavage
- Whirlpool
- Electrical Stimulation
- Ultrasound
- Noncontact, Normothermic Wound Therapy
- Negative Pressure Wound Therapy
- Heterographs
- Wound Dressing
- Edema Management
- Scar Management

Functional restoration

The ultimate goal of therapy is to protect and restore function. This is accomplished by maintaining range, strength and endurance, while adapting the activities of daily living to accommodate physical limitations. Functional modalities include:

- Exercise, passive and active
- Splinting
- Activities of daily living
- Training, including adaptive equipment
- Gait training, including assistive devices, pressure relief

Physical modalities

Therapists traditionally apply physical agents, i.e., heat, sound, pressure and electricity, to facilitate healing. The resulting histamine reaction, increased circulation, muscle relaxation, or pain modulation has been used more typically in rehabilitation of musculoskeletal injuries. This discussion of physical modalities will delineate their use in wound management.

Whirlpool hydrotherapy

Whirlpool is perhaps the first physical modality used in wound care. (Figure 1) This modality provides both mechanical debridement and thermal effects. Its usage became standard therapy long before clinical trials had proven its efficacy. Presently, the use of whirlpool is declining. Issues of public water quality and cross contamination may require additives that would be cytotoxic in excessive concentrations. Outside the issue of cytotoxicity, issues of high turbulence and excessive water temperature must be regulated to prevent delicate tissue injury. When wounds are clean with signs of granulation and epithelialization, continued whirlpool application may be contraindicated. Furthermore, allowing an extremity to hang dependent in warm water for 20 minutes can increase venous stasis.

When appropriately used, however, whirlpool can effectively debride necrotic tissue, soak off adherent dressings, and cleanse the wound of dirt, foreign contaminants and toxic residues. Providone-iodine diluted to a 0.001% concentration is bactericidal to Staphyloccoccus aureus, yet non-cytotoxic to cultured human fibroblasts. Chloramide-T as a whirlpool additive, 200 parts per million, is less irritating and cytotoxic than sodium hypochlorite (3). A tepid whirlpool (80–92°F) for only five minutes is effective in cleansing when venous stasis is a problem. Whirlpool has a definitive place, particularly early on in the care of the necrotic wound. It, like any other modality, must be prescribed according to a critical decision process that considers the desired effect and the patient's needs.

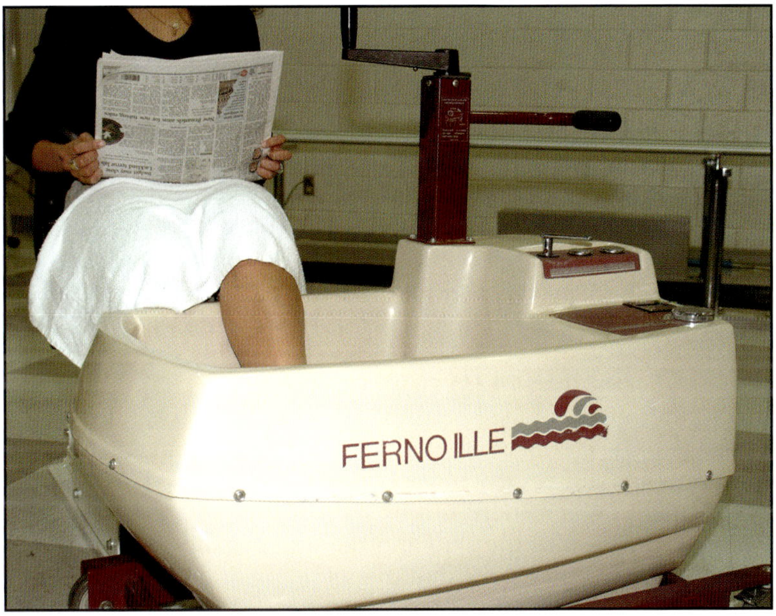

Figure 1. Whirlpool.

Pulsed lavage hydrotherapy

Pulsed lavage is the newest form of hydrotherapy that uses pulsating, pressurized jets of water to irrigate and debride wounds (4). It is often used in conjunction with suction to remove debris, bacteria and necrotic tissue from a wide variety of wounds (5). Unlike whirlpool the treatment area is specific and the water pressure can be specifically controlled. Recommended pressures are 8–15 psi. This pressure is sufficient to cleanse the wound but does not cause tissue injury. Special tips allow access to tunneling or undermining wounds. Pulsed lavage systems use IV fluids as a water source, eliminating the dependency on questionable public water sources. Any medication that can be mixed in an IV solution and is suitable for wound care can be used during the pulsed lavage treatment, i.e., using a weak Dakins solution (0.25) early on in the treatment of a malodorous, infected wound. Contraindications are few.

Because of the small size of the treatment tip, pulsed lavage of large burns is not practical. As with whirlpool, continuation of hydrotherapy should be reassessed when the wound is red, free of necrotic tissue and granulating. Pulsed lavage is indicated for cleaning and/or debriding burns, venous leg ulcers, diabetic ulcers, wounds with significant debris or bacteria, infected surgical sites, amputation sites, and pressure ulcers, as well as other type of wounds (5).

For more details about whirlpool and pulsed lavage hydrotherapy see the Vaughn chapter entitled "Physical Therapeutic Modalities in Wound Healing."

Noncontact normothermic wound therapy

Thermal issues in hydrotherapy have already been addressed. Dropping the temperature of the wound environment can slow leukocytic and mitotic activity. Sussman indicates that it takes three hours for a chilled wound to rewarm and resume normal cellular activity (6). While the use of infrared heat has been the mainstay of dermatology, the issue of heat for wound care has recently been popularized through noncontact normothermic wound therapy (NNWT). An elevation in nitric oxide has been suggested as a mechanism of action (7). Polarized light is very popular in Eastern European countries. An article on polarized light therapy, suggests alignment of fat and protein molecules on the cell membranes as the mechanism that promotes cell regeneration and healing (8). The Centers for Medicare & Medicaid Services (CMS) has determined that there is insufficient clinical or scientific evidence to consider Noncontact Normothermic Wound Therapy as reasonable or necessary. Please refer to CMS bulletin HOSP 2002-42 and HOSP 2002-43.

Electrical stimulation therapy

One of the oldest modalities in the therapist's repertoire is electrical stimulation (9). It is relatively new to wound management. Electrical stimulation therapy mimics the bioelectric mechanism the body employs as a response to injury. When there is a break in the skin, the body's bioelectric system communicates with the skin and the other tissues of the body. Repair cells are called to the injured site and the secretion of fluids, so vital to wound healing is enhanced, as cell membrane permeability changes (10). Cell structures orient along electrical fields. This has been called the current of injury between the skin and inner tissues and is necessary for healing. A rationale for applying electrical stimulation is that it mimics the natural current of injury and will jump-start or accelerate the wound healing process (6). In 1994, the Agency for Health Care Policy and Research panel issued Treatment of Pressure Ulcers, Clinical Practice Guideline, Number 15. The panel indicated, Consider a course of treatment with electrotherapy for Stage III and IV pressure ulcers that have proved unresponsive to conventional therapy (11). On April 1, 2003 the Centers for Medicare and Medicaid Services (CMS) recognized electrical stimulation for chronic Stage III or Stage IV pressure ulcers, arterial ulcers, diabetic ulcers and venous stasis ulcers. Chronic ulcers are defined as ulcers that have not healed within 30 days of occurrence. HCPCS Code G0281 may be used as long as both the stage and chronicity requirements have been met. The electrical stimulation must be performed by a physician, or therapist, or be incident to a physician service.

The best source for application techniques is Carrie Sussman, PT, who wrote the Wound Care Collaborative Practice Manual for Physical Therapists and Nurses. Her chapter, Electrical Stimulation for Wound Healing has become the definitive guide for the application of electrical stimulation to wounds (6). Sussman advocates high voltage pulsed current (HVPC) as the most tested and safest type of stimulation. Application of HVPC directly to the wound has better outcomes than using the whirlpool to conduct current. Amorphous Hydrogel is used for conduction and can be used as the moist wound dressing following stimulation. Treatment duration is approximately 60 minutes; frequency is daily and continues as the wound progresses through inflammation, proliferation and remodeling phases. Treatment settings are as follows:

Inflammation:	Negative Polarity	30pps	100–150 volts
Epithelialization:	Alternate Polarity (3days)	100–128pps	100–150 volts
Remodeling:	Alternate Polarity daily	60–64pps	100–150 volts

Contraindications for electrical stimulation are the same as with any electrical modality: electrodes tangential to the heart, presence of demand pacemaker, phrenic nerve or carotid sinus stimulation, malignancy, electrodes placed over the laryngeal musculature. Wound care adds two specific contraindications, osteomyelitis and heavy metal residue, including Mercurochrome and Providone Iodine.

Electrical stimulation's effect does not appear to be specific to certain pathologies. On all wounds the stimulation controls infection, initiates wound repair, stimulates fibroblasts, and stimulates wound contraction and epidermal reproduction. The beneficial effects therefore occur at all stages of wound repair and electrical stimulation has been effective in moving the chronic wound through the healing process. (Figure 2)

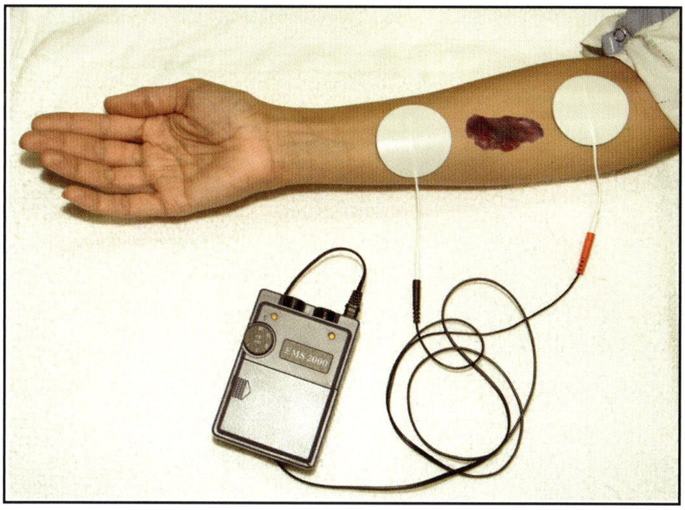

Figure 2. Electrical Stimulation Therapy.

Ultrasound therapy

Ultrasound is a mechanical vibration delivered at a frequency above the range of human hearing. Clinical ultrasound units deliver ultrasound at frequencies of 1 and 3 MHz with duty cycles ranging form 20–100%. (Figure 3) Duty cycles less than 100% are usually termed pulsed ultrasound while a 1005 duty cycle is referred to as continuous ultrasound (12). The evidence to support ultrasound as an adjunct to wound management is mixed. Efficacy studies have been both positive and negative (13). In 1995, Dyson reported the following physiological effects of ultrasound: increased fibroblastic activity, increased capillary permeability, accelerated mast cell and macrophage release, increased oxygen uptake with thermal effects and increased angiogenesis (14). Recommended treatment procedure according to Kloth is pulsed ultrasound directly to the wound or indirectly to the peri-wound area, 20% duty cycle, 0.5–1.0 W/cm^2, 1–3 MHz, 5–10 minutes (15). Overall, the application of ultrasound is easier than electrical stimulation. The shorter treatment time is certainly more attractive. However, there is insufficient documentation to support ultrasound's efficacy. Ultrasound's definitive response is a localized histamine reaction. As with electrical stimulation, membrane permeability and local circulatory changes result. Ultrasound does not have the polarity issue of electrical stimulation and therefore, may not be as applicable throughout the phases of healing. Hopefully, future research will delineate its appropriate use in wound management. This modality, while gaining in popularity, is not a Medicare covered service according to TriSpan, the Southern Regional Carrier for CMS.

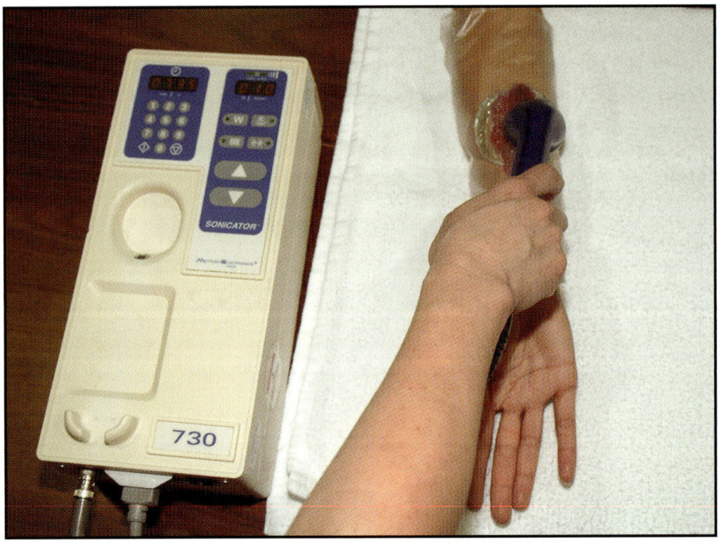

Figure 3. Ultrasound Therapy.

DEBRIDEMENT

Debridement is the removal of necrotic and devitalized tissue from a wound. The two types of debridement are selective and nonselective. Selective debridement can be performed by surgical excision, by facilitating autolysis in a moist environment, and through the topical application of enzymes.

Biologic agents such as maggots are reportedly selective in their debridement process. Nonselective debridement techniques include whirlpool, pulsed lavage, mechanical scrubbing and the effervescent action of topical hydrogen peroxide.

The earliest debridement of the acute wound takes place during the inflammatory phase. Migrating leukocytes and polymorphonuclear leukocytes and later macrophages debride as part of the natural healing process. In chronic wounds, necrotic tissue often impedes the formation of granulation tissue and prevents epithelial cell migration (3). Sharp debridement will remove both necrotic tissue and many of the microorganisms that feed on the tissue. Sharp debridement is effective in converting a chronic wound into an acute wound to accelerate the healing process. Sharp debridement is indicated to remove any buildup of circumferential tissue, which prevents the migration of epithelial cells. A sloped edge around the circumference of the wound will facilitate epithelialization and closure. Care must be taken to prevent sepsis and bleeding, particularly in patients with low platelet counts or those on anticoagulants. Chemical debridement is considered selective as the enzymes can be selected to work on denatured proteins (fibrinolysin and deoxyribonuclease) or undenatured collagen (collagenase). Application of enzymatic ointments is often three time per day. A thin layer is applied and covered with moistened gauze packing. For very thick eschar, cross-hatching may be needed to allow the enzyme to permeate. Autolytic debridement must be facilitated by occlusive dressings to allow normal phagocytic activity of white blood cells. It is the most selective form of debridement (3).

For more on debridement techniques see the chapter by Emhoff and Ferro entitled "Wound Debridement."

NEGATIVE PRESSURE WOUND THERAPY

Negative pressure wound therapy (NPWT) is the controlled application of subatmospheric pressure to a wound using an electrical pump to intermittently or continuously convey subatmospheric pressure to the wound. A specialized wound dressing includes a resilient, open-cell foam surface dressing, sealed with an occlusive dressing that is meant to contain the subatmospheric pressure at the wound site and thereby promote wound healing. Drainage from the wound is collected in a canister (16). The application of controlled subatmospheric pressure causes mechanical stress to tissues, mitosis is stimulated, new vessels are formed and the wound is drawn closed (17). Stagnant fluid is removed and laser Doppler flow studies have shown an increase in blood flow adjacent to a wound receiving negative pressure as a result of decreased peripheral edema (18). According to Kinetic Concepts, Inc., the Vacuum Assisted Closure (VAC®) equipment manufacturer, contraindications include wounds with necrotic tissue, untreated osteomyelitis, fistulas to organs or body cavities, placement directly over exposed veins or arteries, and malignancies. While frank necrosis is a contraindication, clinicians are reporting success in using selective enzymatic debriding agents prior to sponge application, to control thin layers of slough or fibrin buildup. Complaints of pain are usually low, but may be a limiting factor to NPWT use. Guidelines for use are delineated in the VAC® manual and in the previously referenced article by Susan Mendez-Eastman (17). Preparation of the wound and the periwound skin is critical to seal the occlusive drape. Foam dressing comes in two types, black polyurethane and white polyvinylalcohol (PVA). The black polyurethane has larger pores and is more effective in stimulating granulation and wound contraction. PVA soft foam is denser with smaller pores and is generally recommended when granulation needs to be restricted or for patient comfort.

For more details on NPWT see the chapter by Smith and Bozzuto entitled "Advanced Therapeutics: The Biochemistry and Biophysical Basis of Wound Products."

EDEMA MANAGEMENT

Edema is a normal and, when localized, it is a desirable occurrence in the inflammatory stage of wound healing. When chronic or uncontrolled, however, edema can be the mechanism of tissue destruction. Vascularization, oxygen supply, nutrient supply and lymphatic flow can be compromised by edema. Risk of infection and decreased motion is greater when edema persists. Varicose vein insufficiency can lead to ulceration (19). The risk of wounding by prolonged edema is described by Kimbrell and Larson-Lohr in their chapter entitled "Venous Disease."

Those patients who are not candidates for surgical ligation or sclerotherapy have options for conservative management. The gold standard of conservative management consists of cleansing, elevation, and compression. As previously mentioned in this chapter, McCulloch and Hovde reiterate that exercise is not contraindicated for venous stasis. They advocate compression during exercise and post-exercise elevation until the heart rate returns to normal (12).

McCulloch has suggested the following lower extremity treatment regime for venous stasis:

- Gentle cleansing lavage. Whirlpool is not the treatment of choice due to issues of heating in a dependent position. A tepid whirlpool for five minutes may be substituted.
- Intermittent compression pump on the extremity; pressure is less than diastolic and tolerance may be a deciding factor; cycling 90 seconds on/ 30 seconds off; variable treatment duration approximating one hour.
- Application of a non-elastic dressing immediately following intermittent external compression.
- Girth measurements should be taken at periodic intervals until a plateau has been reached. At this point, measurements for custom-fitted, gradient compression stockings can be taken.

Compression therapy can reduce superficial vein distention, capillary filtration, edema and reflux. It can improve the calf muscle pump function and ultimately improve healing rates. Compression therapy can take the form of intermittent pressure pumps, compression wraps and gradient support garments for the upper and lower extremities.

Pneumatic pumps are effective in temporarily reducing distal extremity edema that is typical in venous stasis. Distal fluid is easily moved into the non-congested, proximal circulation. These same pumps will not be effective in the quadrant edema that is so characteristic of chronic lymphedema.

Pneumatic pumps have evolved since the first full extremity lymphedema pumps. Pressure can be single compartment, sequential with pressure equal in each compartment, or sequential with gradient compartmental pressure. Sleeves can be full length or designed for the distal extremity only. Choosing a pump can be confusing. The difference in temporary distal edema reduction is often insignificant. Backflow of lymphatic fluid into the distal extremity has been reported with use of the single compartment pump in the post-mastectomy lymphedema patient (20). Equipment vendors have research that proves the efficacy of their product, but these studies are not truly independent. It is always important to note that the biological model is not sequential. The gastroc-soleus complex does not contract in a distal to proximal direction. Directionality is dependent upon one-way valves in the venous system. In pathology, incompetent valves and calf pump failure will lead to distal venous stasis. This pathology will not prevent the non-sequential pump from temporarily removing distal edema, in preparation for compression wraps. Sequential gradient pumps are apparently the current choice in clinical practice.

The two most common types of compression wraps are single, calamine and zinc oxide impregnated wraps, with an elastic bandage or the four-layered dressing system. They are both applied for single use by the clinician. While the four-layered system is more than three times the cost of the single layer impregnated bandage, the four-layered design is usually recommended and reduces application time. The four-layer bandage system provides 40 mm Hg of compression at the ankle, graduating to 17 mm Hg below the knee. It is able to control heavy drainage and requires less frequent changing.

The CircAid® system of non-elastic bands is a multi-use system of Velcro bands (21). The neoprene anchor distributes pressure and provides comfort. Patients are instructed to apply and adjust the system independently. In the educated and compliant patient, the adaptability of the CircAid® system allows gradient compression adjustments as the extremity size changes. Non-compliant patients, however, can easily loosen bands, disrupting gradient counter pressure.

Compression garments are classed according to ankle pressure. Class I garments provide 20–30 mm Hg of compression and is used for mild edema or varicosities and thromboembolism prophylaxis. Class II, 30–40 mm Hg of compression, is used in chronic venous insufficiency and post-surgically following sclerotherapy, stripping or SEPS. Severe, chronic venous insufficiency and mild lymphedema are treated with the 40–50 mm Hg provided by class III support stockings. Class IV garments provides greater than 50 mm Hg and are used in lymphedema (22). Patients should be measured for compression garments after girth measurements have stabilized through the use of compression pumps and wraps. Custom garments are preferable, although significantly more expensive. The unusual leg shapes of patients with edema can make the issue of custom fabrication a necessity. Donning of higher compression garments can be a challenge to the elderly and functionally challenged patient. Donning devices or family assistance is often required.

Zippers can often be added to custom garments, although they can sometimes be sources of pressure areas. As of October 1, 2003, the Center for Medicare and Medicaid Services (CMS) classified compression garments, those that provide greater than 30–50 mm Hg, to be a covered service. This eliminates Class I and Class IV garments from reimbursement. Appropriate Healthcare Common Procedure Coding System (HCPCS) codes are L8110 and L8120 for lower extremity stockings. Medicare bulletin HOSP 2003-168 covers the use of compression garments for venous stasis ulcers.

Therapeutic management of edema in the upper extremity includes evaluation techniques, controlled motion when possible, bulky dressings applied during the inflammatory stage, and compressive garments to maintain edema control. Coban wraps will control edema in digital wounds.

The previous discussion of edema has mainly addressed venous stasis. Those patients with secondary lymphedema have significantly greater issues of severity and complications. The buildup of large protein molecules in the interstitial space creates sufficient osmotic pressure to congest, not only the distal extremity, but also the entire quadrant. Pneumatic pumps and distal extremity compression garments become ineffective if the proximal circulation is also congested. Persistent swelling and stagnant protein eventually lead to fibrosis and provide an excellent culture medium for infection. Description of the disease and management of lymphedema patients are contained in the Fife chapter entitled "Lymphedema: An Epidemic Hidden In Plain View."

The current method of treatment for chronic lymphedema is a combination of massage, compression wrapping, and exercise. The Foeldi Technique, known as Complete Decongestive Physiotherapy (CDP), involves:

1. Meticulous skin and nail care;
2. Manual lymph drainage, following the Vodder technique of lymphatic massage (23);
3. Multilayer low-stretch bandaging immediately following manual lymph drainage;
4. Active range of motion exercises while bandaged.

Treatment is usually daily in the initial phase, over 1–4 weeks. The 90-minute treatment is performed only by specially trained therapists. The treatment phase is followed by a maintenance phase, which significantly depends upon patient compliance. Patients wrap at night and use compression garments during the day. Exercises are performed independently. Although CDP has obvious limitations of access to therapists, time constraints and patient compliance in the maintenance period, it appears to be more successful than other modalities in the treatment of lymphedema (20).

SCAR MANAGEMENT

Early on in wound healing, scar management consists of controlling variables that could lead to infection, an exaggerated inflammatory state, or dehydration. Control of these variables will help to minimize fibrosis and hypertrophic scarring (2). Therapeutic intervention consists of application of stress to realign collagen fibers. Scar management techniques include pressure garments, serial casting, motion, elastomer molds, silicone gel sheeting, splinting (low-load, long duration application of stress), deep friction massage, and mechanical vibration (24).

Hand Therapists are most familiar with silicone gel sheeting and elastomers as pressure techniques. Silicone gel sheets are purchased in various sizes and are applied with tape or can be placed under splints. They are occlusive in nature with a water vapor rate lower than that of the skin. Researchers postulate that the reduction in water vapor loss may decrease capillary activity thereby reducing collagen deposition and scar hypertrophy. Silicone gel sheeting was found to significantly inhibit the formation of hypertrophic scaring of surgical incisions when used at least 12 hours daily for two months (2). An alternate scar management technique is application of a silicone elastomer mold. The silicone foam is mixed with a catalyst, formed to the involved part, and secured by an elastic wrap (25).

Massage is defined as the method of manipulation of the body by rubbing, pinching, kneading, tapping, etc. Therapists use massage as effective means of freeing soft tissue restrictions that limit motion (26).

It is important that only gentle massage be performed on newly healing wounds to avoid skin breakdown and blister formation. As healing progresses and skin is thicker, greater pressure can be applied by massaging along the scar in a rotary motion. Non-water based creams such as lanolin are recommended for massage. Massaging over small open areas should be avoided. Massage is recommended at least twice daily to be effective (25).

Studies on tissue gases in normal dermis in hypertrophic scars have found that pressure of approximately 25 mm Hg is believed to decrease the blood flow to rapidly metabolizing collagenous tissue. According to the study, hypoxia does not appear to result in cell death but does indirectly affect the metabolic pathway of scar growth or maturation.

Pressure should be applied only after skin grafts are adherent to the wound closure. The purpose is to inhibit vascular and lymphatic pooling as well as inhibit scar contracture and hypertrophy. If interim pressure garments are used over small open wounds, light dressings will protect the fragile skin against the shearing forces of pressure bandages and gloves.

There are a variety of elastic bandaging materials commercially available that can be used until a commercially made custom garment is fitted to the patient. Interdigital web spaces and thumb web spaces should be guarded using soft lambs wool. Commercially made custom-fitted pressure garments are available from several companies. Each company varies in material used and measuring instructions. The requirements of the patient will dictate the selection of material and design. Specification may include open fingertips, zippers, Velcro closures, all of which depend on how fragile skin is and how the patient will tolerate the pressure of the material. These specifications, including pressure, should be discussed with the manufacturer. Commercially made custom-fitting garments are to be worn 24 hours daily until scar maturation and removed only for bathing, skin care, and range of motion exercises. The child's need of sensory and motor experiences requires more time out of the glove. It is important to have two garments so one can be washed and air dried while the other is being worn. The elastic properties of these garments meet the needs for scar pressure for about two months, and then need to be replaced.

Other reasons for replacement of garments, are decreased edema, weight changes, and growth in children. Manufacturers of garments and gloves that provide specific dynamics of pressure include: Barton Carey, Bio-Concepts, Gottfried, Jobst®, and Medical Z. Silicone molds that can be worn under the garment or in an insert are used on concave palmer surface wounds. With use of any compression garment, the skin must be checked routinely for breakdown (25).

EXERCISE

Movement affects both wound contraction and function contractures. Contraction occurs as the pre-existing tissue moves centripetally during wound healing. Collagen formation begins in random patterns. It is stress and strain on the tissue that cause functional alignment of the collagen fibers. Movement and prescribed exercise can provide the appropriate strain to strengthen and secure wound healing at an earlier date (15).

A contracture is loss of range of motion in a joint. The contracture may be the result of contraction itself or the concomitant adaptive shortening and adhesion that follows disuse. Active and gentle passive exercises are crucial to maintaining flexibility, while healing occurs. Minimal repetitive use is necessary to maintain normal viscoelasticity of connective tissue (27).

Resistance exercise of the peri-wound joints is not indicated. Extreme exercise can cause exacerbation of the inflammatory phase of wound healing (28). Application of high-force, short duration load creates more of an elastic response rather than tensile strengthening. It can result in less remodeling with greater risk (27). Exercises that cause gapping of wound surfaces in acute phase should also be avoided. Exercises that are timely and appropriately prescribed, however, can assist with remodeling and prevent functional loss, without hindering the healing process.

Exercise, such as walking, is not absolutely contraindicated in patients who have venous insufficiency. Muscle contraction is the pump for venous return. Control of edema is the prescription determinant. Therefore, frequency and duration should be within the limits of edema control if the exercise is performed in a dependent position. For edema management, compression garments should be worn during exercise, and the lower extremities should be elevated after exercise until the heart rate returns to normal (15).

Discussion of exercise would not be complete without mentioning the uninvolved extremities. Offloading of involved extremities places a significant burden on the remaining extremities. The loaded lower extremity may not be strong enough to handle full body weight. We often ask our patients to use assistive devices if they are without sufficient upper extremity strength. Strengthening the uninvolved extremities is a commitment to care of the total patient. Unfortunately, it may not be reimbursable unless the therapist can document functional deficits.

Patients want complete wound healing, but not at the sacrifice of function. Successful outcome measurement should be based on both wound healing and the maintenance of a functional state. Wound healing and function are not contradictory goals. A comprehensive exercise program to

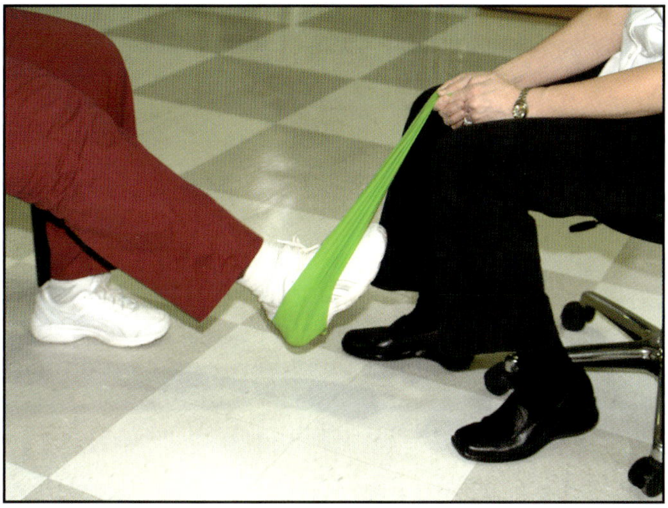

Figure 4 A-C. Hamstring strengthening exercise therapy.

(A) Start of hamstring strengthening exercise cycle with resistive exercise band.

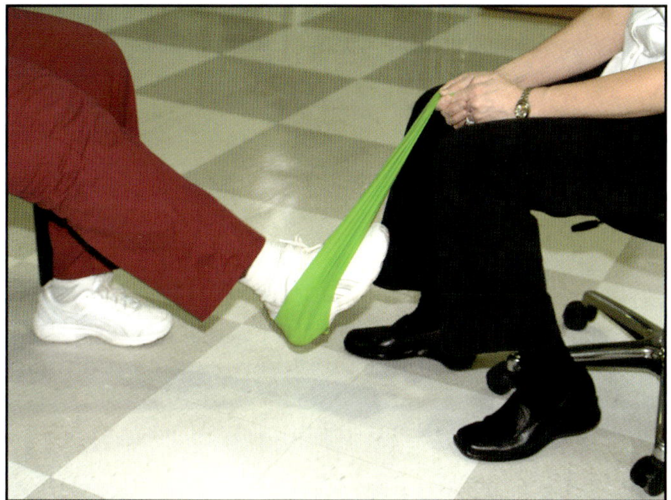

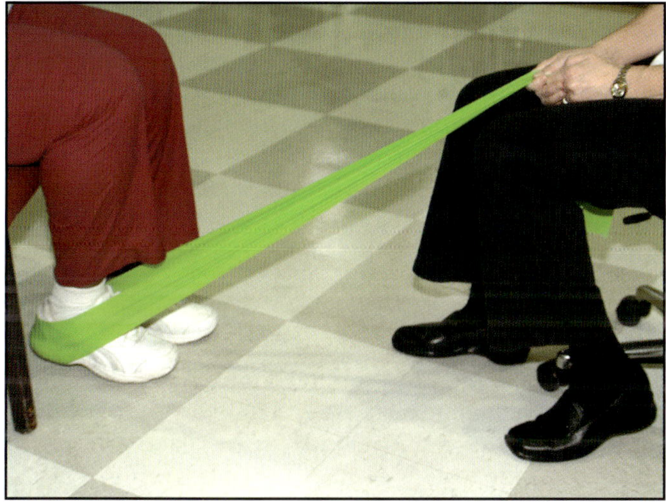

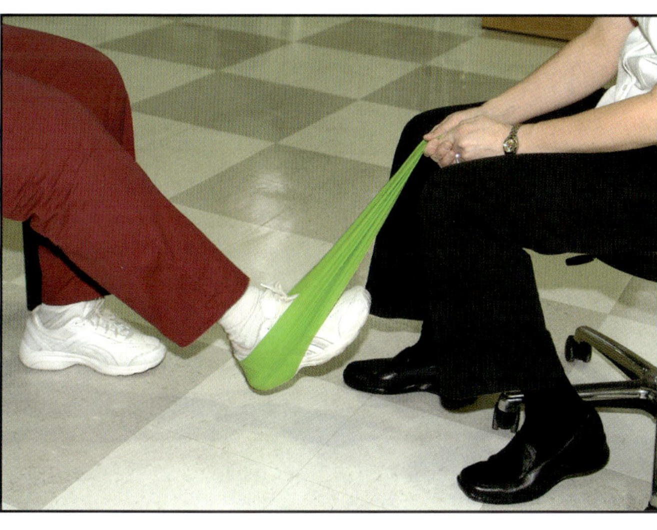

(B) End of flexion.

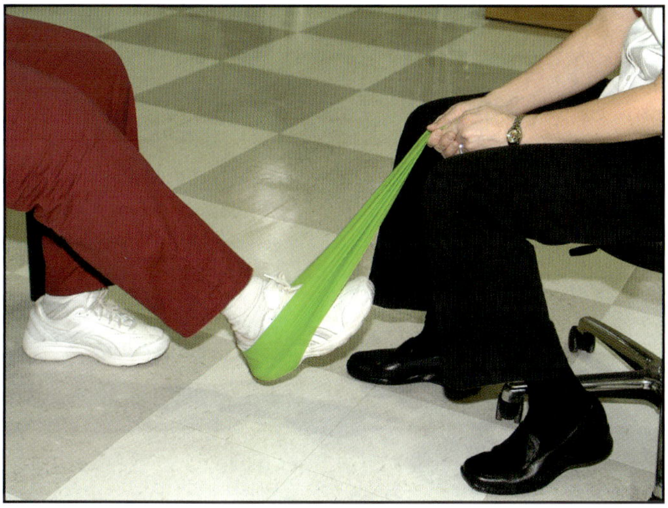

(C) Completion of repetition. It is important that the full cycle be performed slowly.

assist wound healing may have some of the following components:

- Active and passive; concentric or eccentric exercises to the peri-wound joints
- Passive mobilization to the peri-wound joints
- Conservative aerobic exercise
- Strengthening of the uninvolved extremities (Figure 4 A–C)

SPLINTING

Upper Extremity Splinting

Splints have been used since the time of Hippocrates. Among the factors that have influenced splint development and evolution are disease, political conflict, advancements in medicine and technology, and development of a splint classification system. Splinting to affect scar repair and remodeling requires close communication between surgeon, therapist, and patient.

Splints, braces, and orthosis vary slightly by definition, but are terms often used interchangeably. They are all a form of support. In the case of the mobilization splint, the support and mobilization component co-exist (29).

The purpose of splinting is to apply controlled gentle forces to soft tissue for sufficient lengths of time to induce tissue remodeling (30). When appropriately applied, detrimental microscopic disruption of cellular structures can be avoided. The six most cited reasons for splint application include: 1) increase function, 2) prevent deformity, 3) correct deformity, 4) protect healing structures, 5) restrict unwanted motion and 6) allow tissue growth or remodeling. Splinting is geared to specific type of tissue involved and physiologic stage of wound healing (29).

In the late 1960's low-temperature thermoplastic materials were introduced. Major advancements in materials and technology, as by-products of the rapid developments in combat and aerospace technology, have evolved (29). Most contemporary splinting materials are specialized blends of polycaprolactones with the exception of Orthoplast, which is an isoprene, or rubber based material. Enhanced accessory products and tools add to the endless potential for splinting.

Immobilization splints are used in the inflammatory and early fibroplastic phases of healing. In post-operative tendon repairs of the hand, specific motion parameters for controlled early passive or early active motion programs can be applied (26).

Mobilization splints apply very low-load controlled forces that influence scar remodeling by encouraging the development of tendon adhesions that are sufficient length to allow normal tendon glide, especially in the upper extremity. Splinting programs must be closely monitored and adapted as wound healing progresses.

Dynamic splinting may be used to correct joint contractures. An understanding of the mechanical forces involved in splinting and an understanding of soft tissue remodeling is emphasized when applying any splints on healing tissue. Soft tissue adapts to the presence or absence of prolonged gentle force by, respectively, increasing or decreasing in size (29).

Foot Orthotics

Orthotics are typically prescribed to apply low-load prolonged stress to increase viscoelasticity during healing. (Figure 5) This stress, or load per unit area, can remodel connective tissue so that both strength and elongation are possible for functional movement. This is especially true in the hand, and applies to the foot and ankle region. However, the concomitant goal of pressure off-loading is a significant issue in the foot that is not a component of upper extremity splinting.

Orthotics is discussed in the chapter entitled "Orthotics and Prosthetics in Wound Care" by GW Bosker and J LaFontaine. Thus, this section will focus on stress and function.

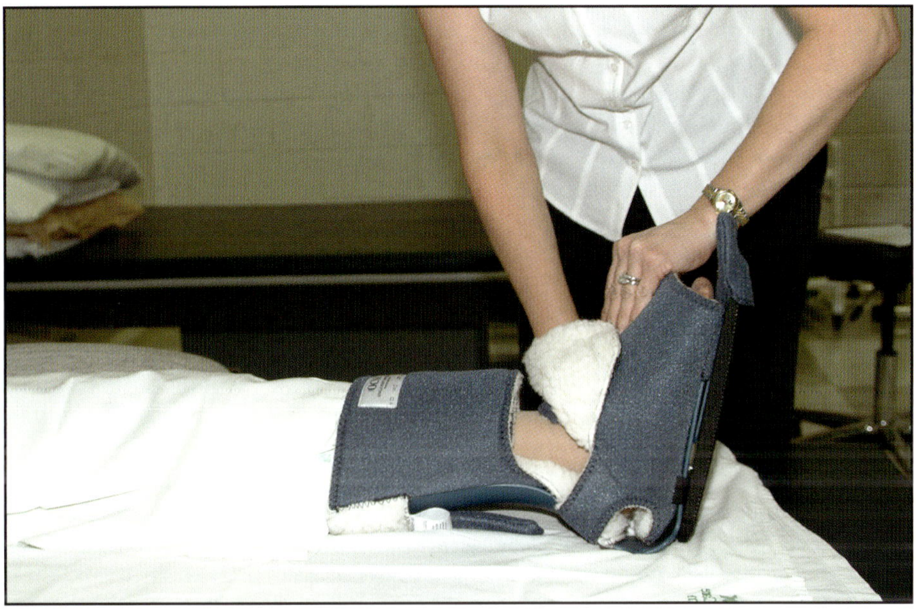

Figure 5. Foot orthotics device.

Stress and function

The anatomy and physiology of the foot and ankle complex forces the therapist to diligently guard function during the healing process. The size and strength of the Achilles tendon makes it a formidable structure to stretch after contracture has developed. The rear foot must be rehabilitated to absorb forces greater that body weight at heel strike. The power produced during propulsion phase of gait must be transmitted appropriately through the complex, and sometimes delicate, forefoot region.

The ankle foot region best demonstrates the need for combined low-load prolonged stress and exercise. During periods of bed rest or non-weight bearing, the ankle must be supported to prevent Achilles tendon contracture. This can be done quite easily without contact on a healing ulcer, by using prefabricated foam blocks or posterior splints. Significant care must be taken to prevent pressure areas from edges, straps, etc. Active ankle pumps will assists with the appropriate orientation of collagen fibers, and special attention to forefoot range of motion can be given through joint mobilization and exercise.

Offloading

The concomitant issue of off-loading presents a significant challenge for the wound care team. Issues of diabetic shoes, casts, and walkers are addressed elsewhere in this book and are often the responsibility of other team members. Therapists that are trained to mold low temperature thermoplastic shoe inserts most often play a role in preventing reulceration of the insensitive foot. In the months after a neuropathic ulcer is healed, to avoid re-injury the patient should be evaluated for both protective footwear and the slow reintroduction of activity. Custom molded orthotics can accommodate for mild or early mechanical and structural problems.

Gait deviations

Most of problems occur because of gait deviations. During gait, weight-bearing forces must be absorbed at the posterior lateral aspect of the calcaneus during heel strike or contact. The center of weight bearing forces then progresses distally to reach the first metatarsal head during toe-off of the propulsion phase. The change from soft shock absorber to rigid lever for power occurs because of significant rotational forces as the subtalar joint moves from pronation to supination and back (31). Any pathophysiology between rearfoot and forefoot function or any anatomical anomaly can change this cycle and result in increased pressure loading.

Plantar ulcerations

Most plantar ulcerations of the foot occur at the forefoot, particularly toes and metatarsal heads (32). This results from high stresses acting on the forefoot during the propulsive phase of gait. Reaching toe-off places significant rotational torque and shearing forces on the medial aspect of the normal forefoot. If the pathophysiology of a forefoot varus is added to this scenario, then excessive force is applied too medially. This facilitates hallux valgus deformities and breakdown at the first metatarsal head. Should pathological foot biomechanics prevent weight bearing forces from reaching the first metatarsal head, then callus formation and plantar ulcerations can occur under the more lateral metatarsal heads. An uncompensated plantar flexed first ray can significantly increase pressure and shearing forces on the first metatarsal head. Heel ulcers can result from sustained pressure in the non-ambulatory patient, trauma, or abnormal pressure from ankle calcaneus deformity (32).

Custom molded orthotics

Custom molded orthotics can reduce the abnormal rotational and sheering forces that occur during the gait cycle as a result of mild pathophysiology. Custom fabrication, using soft thermoplastics, can spread weight-bearing forces, control excessive rotation and still provide cushion support. Pressure relief can be added intrinsically, inside the orthotic, or extrinsically. Either option can reduce point pressure, while maintaining full contact through the top cover. See the chapter entitled "Orthotics and Prosthetics in Wound Care" by Bosker and LaFontaine.

Gait analysis in conjunction with applied biomechanical analysis of the foot and ankle complex can provide early detection of pressure sites in the insensitive foot. In mild cases or for those patients who are not candidates for surgical correction, custom molded orthotics can be an adjunct in preventing reulceration.

ACTIVITIES OF DAILY LIVING AND AIDES FOR DAILY LIVING

In an efficient rehab, the physical and occupational therapists are in constant contact during each phase of the patient's rehab. While both are capable of retraining in activities of daily living (ADL), and assessing function, it is standard practice for the occupational therapist to provide a range of alterations to tools and utensils that are used to perform daily tasks. Visits to the home and work site are made to study the actual work conditions, and advise on alterations of the living space or work conditions (33).

With the occupational therapist's skills in the use of tools and materials and knowledge and understanding of physical function, they are called upon to fabricate devices to assist with ADL. Even with increased availability of commercially supplied devices, the occupational therapist's key role is evaluating devices and training in use of the devices that meet the patient's functional need. Analyses of the patient's ADL needs will include weakness, loss of range of motion, loss of co-ordination, sensory deficiencies, and orthotic devices worn. Progression of skills is important, and gross activities are begun first (34).

A variety of aids and gadgets are available to assist the patient during weakness and limited range that resulted from the traumatic wound. Most household assistive aids are for adaptive use with one hand. For clothing, Velcro fasteners, dressing sticks, sock aids, and reachers are the most common types of aids used. For activities outside of the home, tools are adapted with secure grip and large grip handles (33).

ASSISTIVE DEVICES FOR AMBULATION AND PRESSURE RELIEF

Prescribing partial and non-weight bearing gait patterns can place increased physical demands on a patient who is not capable of compliance. A three-point, non-weight bearing gait can require energy expenditure between three and four times as much as a normal gait pattern (35). Patients must be evaluated for their ability to elevate the involved extremity, accept full body weight on the uninvolved extremity, achieve single-leg balance, and combine scapular depression with upper extremity extension to use an assistive device. Realistic goals for some may be assisted standing-pivot transfers and wheelchair pressure relief exercises. Others may need to use the assistive device over ramps, curbs, and stairs in the community. An individually designed exercise program that provides the strength and endurance for gait is a critical prerequisite to the prescription of altered gait patterns. Appropriately chosen assistive devices will meet the patient's need for both increased base of support (balance) and weight bearing relief. If the arms are too weak to assist, then passive upper extremity assistance through the forearm can replace active upper extremity push off, with the addition of forearm trough or platform attachments. There is a wide range of assistive devices on the market. The appropriate device will provide balance and weight-bearing support, be maneuverable enough for the patient's environment, and ultimately increase off-loading compliance.

Pressure relief cushions, mattress pads and beds must be used thoughtfully rather than habitually, even in the patient who is at minimal risk. No pressure relief device (PRD) on the market should instill the belief that a patient is no longer at risk or that healing will become automatic. The chance for product failure or misuse is too great. A wound complication in a debilitated individual is serious enough to be life threatening (3). Bed and wheelchair mobility training along with an appropriate pressure relief device are important adjuncts to complete wound management.

The variety of PRDs on the market can be confusing. Ultimately the goal is reduction in pressure to below 32 mm Hg in capillaries that permeates tissues covering bony prominences (3). Of particular interest is pressure relief over the sacrum, ischial tuberosities and greater trochanters. Product reports about pressure interface measurements can be misleading if testing was performed on healthy subjects. Maklebust and coworkers reported that a two-inch convoluted foam, Biogard foam pad, a Sof*Care bed cushion and a conventional hospital mattress all provided sufficient pressure relief at the sacrum in healthy subjects. However at the greater trochanters only the Sof*Care relieved pressure to less than 32 mm Hg and none of the products were able to reduce the mean pressure at the heels to less than 32 mm Hg. Their finding suggest that even though a support surface may provide adequate pressure relief for the sacrum and the trochanters, the heels may still be at risk (3, 36).

There are numerous types of PDR's:

1. Foam padding or convoluted foam should be used only when the patient is at minimal or no risk for developing a pressure sore. The patient should be ambulatory and transferring independently. Foam padding can increase skin temperature and it easily soils.
2. Water flotation devices can effectively disperse weight. These devices are heavy to handle and cold. It is critical to fill them appropriately. Overfilling or underfilling reduces the dispersive capacity of the device. Water flotation PRD can be used when the patient is at minimal risk, or has a manageable ulcer located in a site other than the heel or greater trochanter.
3. Gel PRDs are partially and temporarily displaced under pressure. They do not bottom out, and when not under a load, will return to their original shape. Manufacturers indicate that gel devices prevent shear and disperse heat. They can be used on patients with minimal to moderate risk, who are ambulating and transferring independently.
4. Static air PRDs are constructed so that as the patient shifts weight, air flows through channels present between two layers of air cushions and assists in redistributing the weight over the cushion. This product is especially popular with wheelchair cushions. They can puncture but can be patched with repair kits. Overinflation and underinflation are still issues, although some cushions come preinflated. Static air PRDs can be used on patients with minimal to moderate risk and on persons who have manageable ulcers. Independent mobility, particularly independent wheelchair pressure relief, is still a requirement.

5. Dynamic air PRDs are composed of compartments that are alternately inflated and deflated by an air pump that cycles repeatedly. This affords a shortened time span during which tissues are subjected to constant pressure. Proper maintenance to assure that all compartments inflate and deflate is critical. These PRDs can be used on patients with moderate risk and who are mobility dependent.
6. Specialty beds can be low air loss or air fluidized PRDs. They are prescribed for patients with moderate to maximum and maximum risk, respectively. Patients are mobility dependent and have hard to manage ulcers. Turning schedules, where possible, are still important adjuncts to pressure relief beds (3).

Compliance with off-loading is always an issue in wound care. Maintenance of function while providing off-loading for healing dictates that the patients have sufficient strength, balance and endurance to use assistive gait devices, and that they are properly trained. Wheelchair and bedridden patients, or their significant others, must be trained to perform bed mobility techniques, chair push-ups, and other pressure relief exercises. In instances of prescribed complete or partial immobility the appropriate PRD is essential to prevent further breakdown and to promote healing.

CONCLUSION

We have tried to provide an overview of the contribution that Physical and Occupational Therapy can provide to a comprehensive wound management center. Therapists bring a unique perspective to both primary wound care and functional restoration. This is not an all-inclusive chapter, as emphasis has been placed on those issues unique to therapy. New ideas and new uses for traditional modalities are forthcoming. Technology is constantly changing. It is important for clinicians to stay abreast of the new technology. Concerning references to third-party reimbursement, the information provided is current at the time this chapter was written. Reimbursement is the area that will probably see the most variability. All clinicians are urged to become familiar with the website of their local Medicare/Medicaid carriers. Websites that we consider helpful include:

- *www.medscape.com*
- *www.worldwidewounds.com*
- *www.medicaledu.com*
- *www.ahcpr.gov*
- *www.medicare.gov*
- *www.cms.gov*

REFERENCES

1. Bair, J. Occupational Therapy Defined. *American Journal of Occupational Therapy* May 1991: 45(5).
2. Evans RB, McAuliffe JA. Wound classification and management. In Hunter JM, Mackin EJ, Callahan AD. (Eds.). Rehabilitation of the hand: Surgery and therapy. (4th Ed.). St. Louis, MO: Mosby-Year Book. 1995; 217-235.
3. Feedar JA, Kloth LC. Conservative Management of Chronic Wounds. Kloth & McCulloch, Editors: Wound Healing: Alternatives in Management. Philadelphia, PA: F.A. Davis Company, 2002.
4. Loehne HB. Wound Debridement and Irrigation. Kloth & McCulloch, Editors: Wound Healing: Alternatives in Management. Philadelphia, PA: F.A. Davis Company, 2002.
5. Edwards SP. Pulsed lavage offers significant benefits over other wound treatments. Baystate Health System. 2002; 14:22:35.
6. Sussman C. Wound Care Collaborative Practice Manual for Physical Therapists and Nurses. Chapter 16, Electrical stimulation for wound healing, Gaithesburg, MD: Aspen Publishers: 1998.
7. Website: Horwitz LR. Augmentation of wound healing using monochromatic infrared energy, *http://www.bioscanlight.com*
8. Website: Light Therapy for Wound Healing, *http://www.ligtmask.com/Polar.htm*
9. Website: Electrical Stimulation for the Treatment of Wounds. *http://www.medicarenhic.com/articles/elecstim_0303.htm*
10. Blakeley EK. Wounds May Benefit From Electrical Stimulation, Wounds 1.com. March 14, 2001. *http://www.wounds1.com/news/tech_pf.cfm?newsarticle=2*
11. ACHPR Treatment Guidelines For Pressure Ulcers, U.S. Government Printing Office 1994. *www.ahcpr.gov*
12. Website: McCulloch J. Ultrasound in Wound Healing, Wound Care Information Network. *http://www.medicaledu.com/ultrasound.htm*
13. Website: Lepak V. Modalities and Wound Care, *http://moon.ouhsc.edu/llepak/wounds/modalities/modalities.ppt*
14. Dyson, M. Ultrasound management for wound management. P.P. Gogia Editor: Clinical Wound Management. Thorofare, NJ: Slack.1995; 197-204.
15. Kloth, LC. Adjunctive interventions for wound healing. Kloth & McCulloch, Editors: Wound Healing: Alternatives in Management. Philadelphia, PA: F.A. Davis Company, 2002.
16. DMERC Supplier Manual, Region B. Chapter 17-Medical Policy, Negative Pressure Wound Therapy Pumps. Revision 30 – June, 2002.
17. Mendez-Eastman S. Guidelines for using negative pressure wound therapy. advances in skin & wound care: The Journal for Prevention and Healing. November/December 2001,14 (6): 314-322.
18. Morykwas M. Vacuum assisted closure: a new method for wound control and treatment. *Ann Plastic Surgery* 1997; 38: 553-62.
19. Goulet C. Ulceration related to varicose vein insufficiency. Wound Care Institute Newsletter, Fall, 1996. *http://woundcare.org/newsvol1n3/ar7.htm*
20. Petrek JA. Diseases of the Breast. Chapter 69, Lymphedema. Philadelphia, PA: Lippincott Williams & Wilkins. 2000; 1033-1040.
21. Website: CircAid Innovative CircAid technology helps people get better faster. And stay that way. *http://www.circaid.com/about us.htm*
22. Smith APS. Venous stasis ulcers, evaluation and treatment. Hyperbaric Medicine Team Training. Education Department, International ATMO, Inc. San Antonio, Texas. July 13-19, 2003. (Seminar material)

23. Ko SC. Effective treatment of lymphedema of the extremities. *Archives of Surgery* April 1998; 133: 452-458.

24. Anthony MS. Wounds In Clark, Gaylord L. Editor, Hand Rehabilitation. New York, NY: Churchill Livingstone. 1993; 9-11.

25. deLinde LG, Miles WK . Remodeling of scar tissue in the burned hand. In J.M. Hunter, Editor. Rehabilitation of the Hand: Surgery and Therapy. (4th Ed.) St.Louis, MO: Mosby-Year Book. 1995; 1267-1294.

26. Colditz C. Therapist's management of the stiff hand. In J.M. Hunter, Editor. Rehabilitation of the Hand: Surgery and Therapy. (4th Ed.) 1995; pp 1267-1294. St.Louis, MO: Mosby-Year Book.

27. Cyr LM, Ross RG. How controlled stress affects healing tissues. *Journal of Hand Therapy* 1998; 11: 125-130.

28. Hunter JH, Makin E, Callahan AD. Rehabilitation of the Hand: Surgery and Therapy, St. Louis, MO: Mosby—Year Book, Inc. 1995: Chapter 74, page 1274. (Seminar material)

29. Fess EE, McCollum M. A history of splinting: To understand the present, view the past. *Journal of Hand Therapy* April-June, 2002; 97-131.

30. Fess EE, McCollum M. The influence of splinting on healing tissues. *Journal of Hand Therapy* 11, 1998; 157-161.

31. Hoke B, Stan S. When the feet hit the ground ... Everything changes. American Physical Rehabilitation Network. Sylvania, OH. 2000. (Seminar material)

32. Hampton G, Birke J. Treatment of wounds caused by pressure and insensitivity. Kloth & McCulloch, Editors: Wound Healing: Alternatives in Management. Philadelphia, PA:F.A. Davis Company, 2002.

33. Parry CBW. Rehabilitation of the Hand, London/Boston. *Butterworths* 1978; 252-260

34. Willard HS. Occupational Therapy, Chapter 17 Occupational Therapy in the A.D.L. Program, Zimmerman, Muriel. Philadelphia and Toronto: J.B. Lippencott Co. 1963.

35. Kottke F, Stillwell K, Lehmann J. Gait analysis: diagnosis and management. Krusen's Handbook of Physical Medicine and Rehabilitation. Philadelphia/London/Toronto. W.B. Saunders Company, 1982.

36. Maklebust J, Mondoux L, Sieggreen M. Pressure relief characteristics of various support surfaces used in prevention and treatment of pressure ulcers. *J Enterostom Ther* 1986; 13:85.

REVIEW QUESTIONS

1.) The ultimate goal of therapy is to
   a. Apply wound dressings
   b. Debride the wound
   c. Construct orthotics
   d. Protect and restore function

2.) Whirlpool hydrotherapy:
   a. Mechanically debrides the wound
   b. Is increasingly used in wound care
   c. Does not damage delicate tissue
   d. Should be continued until the wound is healed
   e. Is usually prescribed for venous stasis ulcers

3.) Any medication that can be mixed in an IV solution and is suitable for wound care can be used during the pulsed lavage treatment.
   a. True
   b. False

4.) Scar management consists of controlling:
   a. Variables that could lead to infection
   b. An exaggerated inflammatory state
   c. Dehydration
   d. All of the above
   e. A and b but not c

5.) Which of the following statements about wound healing is FALSE?
   a. Collagen formation begins in random patterns.
   b. Functional alignment of the collagen fibers is caused by stress and strain on the tissue.
   c. Movement and exercise retards wound healing.
   d. Exercise can strengthen and secure wound healing at an earlier date.

Answers: 1d, 2a, 3a, 4d, 5c

CHAPTER 35

Physical Therapeutic Modalities in Wound Healing

CHAPTER THIRTY-FIVE OVERVIEW

NOTES

Physical Therapeutic Modalities in Wound Healing

Misty M. Vaughn

INTRODUCTION

For more than 75 years, physical therapists have worked to address loss of function, pain, disease, and disability. Today's therapists can choose from over nineteen specialty sections in which to practice. Those interested in wound management are a largely specialized group. The therapist's role in wound management is to assess the physical condition of the skin, and the functional limitations that have occurred as a result of integumentary impairment. Following an evaluation, the therapist will determine appropriate treatment interventions, based on the anticipated goals for the patient. Choices for treatment interventions can include a variety of therapeutic modalities for wound management. Effectiveness of the treatment is determined by the selection of the appropriate modality, based on wound characteristics and underlying etiology. In this chapter, we will discuss traditional therapeutic modalities such as hydrotherapy, electrical stimulation, ultrasound, and ultraviolet light. We will also focus on newer and emerging therapies such as negative pressure wound therapy and normothermic wound therapy.

HYDROTHERAPY

Historically, the use of hydrotherapy has been reported in literature dating back to ancient times. In recent times, the whirlpool has become the most commonly recognized and utilized method of hydrotherapy.

Whirlpool

For years, a whirlpool has been a fixture in every physical therapy department. Often, "whirlpool" has become synonymous with "wound management" in physical therapy. Physician orders written as "PT for Whirlpool" usually mean more than just placing a patient in a tank of water. The implication is that the patient will be evaluated by a physical therapist, the wound cleansed, the appropriate dressing regimen will be determined, and the patient's pain and emotional distress will also be addressed—all of this falls under the veneer of "whirlpool."

There are two basic types of whirlpools: portable and fixed units. An example of a fixed unit would be a typical Hubbard Tank, attached to the floor. Whirlpool tanks come in a variety of shapes and sizes. Tank selection is based on patient mobility, the location and extent of the skin impairment. For example, a patient with multiple wounds to the trunk and legs may require full body immersion and a larger tank needed. Whereas, a patient with a neuropathic foot ulcer may only require immersion in a small portable extremity tank. All tanks require a hot and cold water source and a method to mix the water, usually a turbine attached to the tank, or incorporated into the wall of the unit (similar to a commercial hot tub). The turbine can be regulated to adjust the water and air intake, which in turn, controls the turbulence during treatment: the more aeration, the greater the turbulence and pressure.

Reputed effects of whirlpool include mechanical debridement (i.e., the reduction of wound contaminants, softening and/or removal of loosely adherent necrotic debris and exudates) and thermal effects (i.e., increasing local tissue perfusion; stimulating cellular activity; facilitating pain relief). Reduction of wound contaminants (i.e., foreign matter, cellular debris, bacteria) will indirectly support wound healing by decreasing bacterial counts and lowering the overall wound bioburden. It should be noted that the physical effects of immersion in water have little or no effect on adherent fibrous tissue and other methods of debridement should be considered. Whirlpool treatments are often the precursor to other debridement methods (sharp, enzymatic, autolytic) because soaking the tissues can result in saturation and loosening of necrotic tissues.

Use of the whirlpool for mechanical debridement can facilitate removal of necrotic tissue and decrease the overall levels of bacterial contamination in the wound base. Current research informs us that high levels of bacterial contamination and devitalized tissue in the wound base can contribute to a prolonged inflammatory process. In turn, this results in delayed wound healing. In theory, mechanical debridement should result in more rapid healing rates. However, the use of turbulent water to achieve this result may damage healthy tissue, as well as non-viable tissue. Positioning the wound too close to the high-pressure jet of the whirlpool may damage fragile granulation and epithelial tissue. Trauma from these mechanical forces may also cause prolonged inflammation and delay the normal healing cascade. Care should be taken to minimize trauma to healthy tissues through correct positioning in the whirlpool. Hydrotherapy should be discontinued when the goals of treatment have been achieved (i.e., a clean wound bed).

The thermal effects of whirlpool (Table 1) are directly related to the body's response to heating of the tissues. Studies have demonstrated that heat applied to an area for 20 minutes will cause vasodilation during treatment. Additionally, the highest levels of increased blood flow are actually achieved within an average of 46 minutes following the treatment period. This local vasodilation will cause an increase in local tissue perfusion. This is a simple and effective method of increasing blood flow and oxygen tension in the tissues. Increased oxygen tension facilitates collagen deposition and makes the tissue more resistant to bacterial invasion. It also improves the delivery of nutrients, growth factors, macrophages, and neutrophils while removing waste products from the tissues. For patients with poor tissue oxygenation, increased

TABLE 1. TERMINOLOGY DESCRIBING WATER TEMPERATURE, THE PHYSIOLOGICAL EFFECTS, AND RECOMMENDED UTILIZATION

Descriptive Terminology	Temperature	Physiological Effects	Appropriate Wound Patient
nonthermal/ tepid	80–92°F (27–33.5°C)	local vasoconstriction, decreased oxygen uptake, tissue cooling	venous disease for debridement
neutral warmth	92–96°F (33.5–35.5°C)	endothelial cell proliferation	peripheral vascular disease, sensory impairment, full body immersion
normothermal	98.6°F (37°C)	optimize cellular functions, increased enzymatic and biochemical functions, increased circulation, increased pulse rate, increased blood pressure	cardiovascular or pulmonary disease
hot	98–104°F (36.7–40°C)	increased circulation, increased pulse rate, increased blood pressure	higher temperatures are not recommended due to physiological stress

perfusion can be beneficial. However, in individuals with venous insufficiency, increased tissue perfusion and vasodilation can lead to additional tissue damage. Patients with venous insufficiency have difficulty managing fluid levels in the tissue. The increased vasodilation that occurs during and after the whirlpool treatment will lead to increased venous hypertension and vascular congestion. Local vasodilation with the limb in a dependent position should be considered a contraindication to the management of wounds with venous insufficiency. There are other methods for wound cleansing that are more appropriate for this particular etiology and will be discussed later in this chapter.

There are a number of cellular effects within the tissues that have been studied in recent years. Some of the specific findings will be discussed later in this chapter under Normothermic Wound Therapy. In general, an increase in temperature has the effect of stimulating cellular division, neutrophilic activity, clotting cascade activity, phagocytosis, and cellular repair. Heating the chronic wound fluid has been demonstrated to have a positive effect on the production and activity of fibroblasts. These cellular effects, attributed to tissue heating, can be achieved with temperatures ranging from 33–38°C.

Precautions

Because of the circulatory and cellular responses to temperature changes, precautions should be utilized during whirlpool treatment. 1) In patients with peripheral vascular disease, the water temperature should not exceed 34°C. 2) In patients with cardiovascular or pulmonary disease, water temperature should not exceed 38°C (the increased vasodilation can in turn cause increased cardiac output and additional work load on the heart). 3) Temperature extremes should be avoided in patients with loss of sensation.

In addition, the following situations should be considered when choosing a hydrotherapy modality: 1) presence of granulation tissue; 2) presence of new epithelial tissue; 3) fresh skin grafts; 4) recent tissue flaps; 5) clean neuropathic ulcers. Each of these situations presents with its own set of considerations and should be evaluated for the potentially detrimental effects of mechanical trauma related to whirlpool. Contraindications for the use of whirlpool have included the following: moderate and/or severe edema in the extremities; lethargy/unresponsiveness; maceration of tissues; compromised cardiovascular or pulmonary status; acute phlebitis; renal failure; dry gangrene; and fecal or urinary incontinence.

The use of whirlpool additives (antiseptic agents) with hydrotherapy is very controversial. Studies have demonstrated in vitro toxicity to cells related to tissue repair, specifically fibroblasts. Following the Agency for Health Care Policy and Research (AHCPR, now known as the AHRQ—Agency for Health Care Research and Quality) recommendation that antiseptic agents (i.e., povidone-iodine, iodophor, sodium hypochlorite solution, hydrogen peroxide, and acetic acid) not be used in clean ulcers, there has been increased attention to the utilization of these agents. However, it should also be noted that healing can be delayed when bacterial counts are greater than 10^5 colony forming units per gram of tissue. Appropriate utilization of whirlpool additives to decrease bacterial counts may be beneficial to wound healing. Bohannon (3) demonstrated further reduction of bacteria by vigorously rinsing the body/extremity with warm water after removal from the whirlpool. In clean wounds, continued use of antiseptic agents, even at appropriate dilutions, may result in impaired rates of healing due to their cytotoxic effects.

Historically, the frequency and duration of hydrotherapy was associated with dressing changes on burn units to facilitate the removal of topical creams and ointments. Wounds with copious exudate or infection have traditionally received whirlpool treatments twice daily. However, there have been no clinical trials that demonstrate the effectiveness of one treatment regimen over another. Daily treatments are now deemed sufficient. Consideration should be given to the cost of dressing supplies utilized during treatment, the associated labor costs, and the effects of frequent dressing changes on the wound environment. Treatment should be discontinued when a clean wound bed is present or when there is a lack of healing response.

Selecting the Parameters

In the past, hydrotherapy has been the therapeutic modality of choice for wound management. The theoretical and scientific basis behind the utilization of whirlpool is noteworthy (i.e., decrease bioburden and optimize cellular function). Conversely, treatment efficacy with whirlpool has not been demonstrated to date. There have been only two controlled clinical trials that directly studied the effects of whirlpool on wound healing. Yet, both of these studies contain considerable design flaws. The resulting data is of minimal significance and does not adequately demonstrate a beneficial effect on wound healing. While the science behind whirlpool as a therapeutic modality may be sound, further study is warranted to identify the best frequency, temperature, and treatment regimen to facilitate wound healing.

Pulsatile Lavage with Suction

More recently, alternative methods for irrigation and cleansing have been developed, such as syringe and needle irrigation, jet lavage, and other wound irrigation systems. Pulsatile lavage with suction (PLWS) is the only method to combine cleansing and debridement with suction to remove the irrigant and wound debris. This use of negative pressure may also enhance wound healing (negative pressure will be discussed in more detail later in this chapter).

In the early 1980's, physicians began utilizing high-pressure pulsatile irrigation units during surgery to remove necrotic material, debris, and bone residue. Studies indicated that high-pressure pulsatile irrigation could potentially damage bone and other tissue structures. These pressures were too high for wound management. In the late 1980's physical therapists began to use low-pressure systems for irrigating and debriding open wounds.

The typical low pressure PLWS unit is either battery powered, electrically or air driven. A suction source (suction canister and regulator at 60–100 mm Hg continuous suction) and irrigation fluid are attached to the hand unit. The hand unit controls the delivery of fluid and the removal of irrigant and debris through suction. Each company has devised a different method for controlling pressure levels usually recorded in pounds per square inch (psi). Some units allow variable psi levels through the hand control—with preset maximum and minimum impact psi levels. Other units will allow the user to control psi levels at the electronic console, but have digital readings to allow incremental psi adjustment for treatment of different tissue types.

While the science behind utilization of PLWS is sound, there have been limited studies to demonstrate the effectiveness of PLWS over whirlpool. Haynes (8) reported an increase in the production of granulation tissue 2.5 times more rapidly with PLWS over whirlpool. Though the study sample size was small (n=13), the study was relatively well designed. The author concluded that treatment with PLWS promoted wound closure at a faster rate than did sterile whirlpool.

Aside from increasing granulation tissue production, PLWS has proven to be an effective method to remove necrotic tissue from the wound. Necrotic tissue is a medium for bacterial growth. Bacterial infection and/or colonization are major factors in delayed wound healing. Products that facilitate removal of devitalized tissue can help to speed wound healing. Studies in the literature suggest that pulsating irrigation decreases the presence of wound contaminants, resulting in fewer wound infections.

The AHCPR (now AHRQ) Guideline #15 emphasizes use of "enough irrigation pressure to enhance wound cleansing without causing trauma to the wound bed." Several studies demonstrated that an irrigation pressure of at

TABLE 2. THERAPUTIC EFFECTS OF KNOWN IRRIGATION PRESSURES

PSI	Therapeutic Effects
< 4	Not effective to remove bacteria for wound cleansing
4–8	Safe, effective irrigation: removes bacteria, atraumatic to granulation tissue; lower pressures recommended for tunneling and undermining where tissue is not easily visualized
9–15	Safe, effective irrigation; removes bacteria, effective debridement of necrotic tissue or debris
> 15	Not recommended for routine use; may traumatize wound and drive bacteria into tissue

least four pounds per square inch (psi) was required to effectively remove bacteria from the wound surface (Table 2). Conversely, irrigation pressures greater than 15 psi were reported to cause trauma to the wound bed and drive bacteria into the tissues. An irrigation pressure of 8 psi was found to effectively remove bacteria, cleanse the wound, and reduce the risk of trauma and wound infection. There are a variety of devices on the market today that can be utilized for wound irrigation and it is important to know the impact pressures delivered by the unit. For example, Water Pik® (Teledyne, Fort Collins, CO) at the middle setting delivers an impact pressure of 42 psi—much too high for typical wound cleansing. Currently, there are three companies manufacturing PLWS units for use in acute/chronic wound management: Davol, Inc (Simpulse PLUS, Simpulse Varicare), Stryker Instruments (SurgiLav Plus, Interpulse), and Zimmer (Pulsavac, Pulsavac III, Var-a-Pulse). Each company's products come in a variety of power sources with different types of tips.

One aspect of the use of PLWS that has not received much attention from the general wound management community is the idea of using high pressure irrigation as an effective method of delivering specific solutions into the tissues. Surgeons and the military have utilized high pressure irrigation to deliver solutions of Vancomycin, Streptomycin, and Tetracycline to reduce bacterial counts within the tissues. Patients with infected neuropathic ulcers showed bacterial levels $<10^5$ colony forming units (CFU) per gram of tissue and surgeons were able to close the wounds with grafts or flaps. With a serious concern for the over-utilization of antibiotics, culture and sensitivity should be performed prior to using an antibiotic solution as an irrigant.

PLWS is considered to be an effective method of nonselective mechanical debridement. The pulsatile function of the irrigant works to loosen debris. The pulse-interpulse phase of the unit works to compress, then decompress, the tissues. Possibly, this is one mechanism by which the tissue is loosened from the wound base. Depending on the state licensing agency, certain health care practitioners would be prohibited from using this system. Be sure to check with your licensing board to ensure your ability to perform debridement. Currently, there are no states that prohibit debridement by a licensed physical therapist.

Aside from the benefits of debridement and reduction of bacterial counts, PLWS has a number of other advantages over whirlpool as the preferred method of hydrotherapy. Bedside treatments are possible with PLWS. This decreases transportation time to/from the hydrotherapy area. It also reduces safety risks associated with transferring a patient into/out of the whirlpool tank and patient comfort is improved. Because of the decreased bacterial levels and wound debridement, surgery can often be avoided, reducing associated hospital costs. Tunnels and undermining are easily treated with the appropriate pulsed lavage tip. One other significant benefit to the health care worker is the time savings associated with PLWS over whirlpool. A typical treatment using PLWS will take 15–30 minutes from set up to clean up. A whirlpool treatment can take longer than 60 minutes. Using PLWS there is no need to drain, clean, or fill the whirlpool. The transportation times are eliminated, and the clean up times are reduced because the products are disposable. This allows the therapist to schedule more patients in the same period of time, thereby increasing efficiency and productivity. If done in an outpatient setting, this can also increase revenue. Lastly, since there are no known contraindications for PLWS, it can be performed in instances where whirlpool would be contraindicated (i.e., lethargic or unresponsive patients, incontinence, venous insufficiency, cardiopulmonary compromise).

Precautions

Even though there are no known contraindications, therapists should be aware of certain precautions. A major concern is the fact that you are debriding tissue. You should be very familiar with the anatomy of the area in which you are debriding. Having a reference book available is beneficial. Also, know how to contact the physician in case of an emergency. Just as with any other method of debridement, precautions should be taken with patients on anticoagulants, insensate wounds, and the presence of tunneling and/or undermining. Treatment precautions should be taken if major vessels, pericardium or peritoneum are exposed, any exposed subcutaneous structure, or recent grafts or flaps.

One precaution in particular that has recently arisen is the issue of aerosolization of microorganisms during PLWS. There have been at least two reports of the spread of microorganisms that have been traced back to pulsed lavage treatments (12, 13). In one case, the outbreak was of a multiple-drug resistant bacteria (*Acinetobacter baumannii*) and some patients died. Based on these outbreaks, the US Centers for Disease Control and Prevention (CDC) has made the following recommendations for treatments using PLWS:

- Staff members should use appropriate personal protective equipment, including fluid-resistant gowns, gloves, surgical masks, eye protection, and shoe and hair covers
- Patients receiving pulsatile lavage treatment should wear surgical masks
- All intravenous lines and other wounds must be covered during the treatment.
- The procedure should be performed in a private room with the door closed, with easily washable surfaces, only essential equipment in the room, and no open supply shelves.
- All horizontal surfaces must be cleaned and disinfected following each procedure and at the end of the day.
- As with any medical procedure, all staff performing pulsatile lavage treatment should be thoroughly trained in proper technique for use of the device.
- Each single patient use item should be properly discarded immediately following treatment
- Suction canisters should be discarded or emptied following each procedure.

Selecting the Parameters

The recommended frequency and duration of treatment have not been scientifically established through research. However, as with whirlpool, patients with acute wounds are usually treated once a day. In an outpatient setting, treatment 2-3 times a week is recommended if the wound is clean, granulating and there are no signs or symptoms of infection present. PLWS can be used as an adjunct to other debridement options such as sharp, autolytic, or enzymatic debridement. The suggestion to discontinue treatment with a clean wound bed is somewhat controversial at this time. It is theorized that the negative pressure associated with the suctioning of the irrigant and wound debris can contribute to mechanical deformation of the wound and promote increased granulation. Therefore, treatment should be discontinued with wound closure, if there are no changes noted after one week, or if the wound appears to worsen.

Because of the decreased labor costs associated with PLWS over whirlpool, increased staff productivity and efficiency, avoidance of cross contamination, and enhanced debridement, PLWS is an optimal strategy for wound cleansing and debridement.

ELECTRICAL STIMULATION

Since the early 1960's, electrical stimulation (ES) has been utilized for the treatment of chronic wounds. Today, there are a variety of therapeutic devices on the market capable of delivering a medical current that is appropriate for wound healing.

Guidelines

In 1994, the AHCPR (now AHRQ) published guidelines for pressure ulcer treatment and prevention (14). Following an extensive review of literature, ES was the only therapeutic modality that received a recommendation by the panel of experts. The recommendation was given a "strength of evidence" rating of "B" in the Clinical Practice Guideline. This strength of evidence rating means that two or more controlled clinical trials on pressure ulcers in humans provide direct support for the recommendation, or two or more controlled animal trials provide indirect support. The guidelines recommend that one should, "consider a course of treatment with electrotherapy for Stage III and IV pressure ulcers that have proved unresponsive to conventional therapy. Electrical Stimulation may also be useful for recalcitrant Stage II Ulcers" (14).

In 1998, the Guidelines were reviewed and additional studies were evaluated. Based on the additional studies that had been conducted in the four years since the publication of the original guidelines, Ovington (11) changed the rating of "B" to a new strength of evidence rating of "A"—meaning the "results of two or more randomized controlled clinical trials on pressure ulcers in humans provide support" for the usage of ES in the treatment of pressure ulcers. In 2000, the Health Care Financing Administration (HCFA) (now CMS) Medical and Surgical Procedures Panel (15) unanimously voted that this form of therapeutic intervention was more effective than standard care alone. In accordance to that vote, national coverage guidelines have been established and in 2003, HCFA put two new HCPCS codes into effect related to electrical stimulation. Two of these codes are directly related to the treatment of chronic wounds. This overturns a previous ruling by HCFA that excluded reimbursement for all forms of electrical therapy for wound management.

Terminology

Before examining the evidence related to ES, a brief overview of the terminology and theories behind medical electricity should be beneficial. Charge, polarity, current, amperage, galvanotaxis, voltage, charge density, and waveforms are all terms that will be identified.

Charge

All forms of matter contain some type of electrical charge (Q). The charge can be positive, negative, or electrically neutral. Electrons are negatively charged particles. Neutrally charged matter losing electrons will become positively charged. Alternately, neutral matter gaining electrons will become negatively charged. Electrical charge is measured in units called coulombs (C), and represents a very specific number of electrons (1 C = 6.28 x 1018 electrons). To enhance wound healing, the amount of charge delivered to the tissues is in the range of microcoulombs (mC).

Polarity

Polarity refers to the property of having two oppositely charged poles (i.e., electrodes) in one device. The negative pole (cathode) is the source, or supply, of electrodes. The positive pole (anode) is the depository for the electron flow. The anode lacks electrons and will attract the electrons from the negative pole.

Current and amperage

This transfer of electrons between the oppositely charged poles creates an electrical current (I), which is measured in time (seconds). In the tissues, the flow of current is carried by charged ions (Na+, K+, Cl+). The rate of electron flow is measured in Amperes (A). The human body generates bioelectric tissue currents in the range of milliamperes (mA).

Galvanotaxis

Galvanotaxis is the attraction of positively or negatively charged cells toward an electric field of opposite polarity. There is a large body of evidence to support the influence that polarity has on certain cell types (Table 3). During the inflammatory phase of wound healing, neutrophils, lymphocytes, platelets, and macrophages are all present. In the presence of infection, neutrophils are attracted to the negative pole. Lymphocytes and platelets are also attracted to the negative pole. If infection is not present, the neutrophils are attracted to the positive pole, along with the macrophages. Autolytic debridement and phagocytosis are mediated by the neutrophils and macrophages. Treatment options for the infected wound should start with the negative pole over the wound. Once the infection is resolved, and necrotic tissue remains, the polarity should be switched to positive for autolytic debridement. In proliferation, the predominant cell type is the fibroblast. Negative polarity attracts the fibroblast and stimulates collagen synthesis and fibroblast proliferation. The remodeling phase has two components: scar contraction and epithelialization. During contraction, the myofibroblasts are present, and are attracted to the negative pole. Epithelial cells, however, are attracted to the positive pole. During remodeling, studies have demonstrated

TABLE 3. RECOMMENDED TREATMENT PARAMETERS DURING THE NORMAL PHASES OF WOUND HEALING

Phase of Healing	Cellular Attraction	Treatment Polarity	Pulse Rate (frequency)	Intensity	Frequency and Duration
Inflammatory Phase	Attracts Neutrophils, Macrophages, Platelets, Leukocytes	Positive (Negative for infection)	30–50 pps	100–150 V	60 min; QD
Proliferative Phase	Attracts Fibroblasts	Negative	100–128 pps	100–150 V	60 min; QD
Remodeling Phase	Attracts Epithelial Cells and Myofibroblasts	Alternate Positive and Negative every three days	60–64 pps	100–150 V	60 min; 3 times/week to daily

that alternating the polarity every three days enhanced wound contraction, tensile strength, and epidermal closure.

Voltage

Voltage (V) is a measure of the force of the flow of electrons (as opposed to amperage which is the rate of flow). The voltage between two electrodes is created when one electrode has an excess of electrons in comparison to the other. The electrodes become "polarized" with respect to one another. When the voltage is turned up, the current will also rise. Ohm's Law ($V = I R$, where V = voltage, I = current, and R = resistance) mathematically describes the relationship between voltage and current. In wound healing, the amplitude is increased until a slight tingling sensation is felt by the patient. If the individual is insensate, the voltage is increased until a muscle fasciculation, or contraction, is noted. The voltage is then turned down until the contraction is no longer visible. Usually an amplitude of 75–150V is sufficient to achieve this result with High Volt Pulsed Current, a type of waveform commonly used for wound management.

Waveforms

Waveforms are graphical representations of a current on a current/time plot. Different currents have characteristically different waveforms. Figures 1-5 are examples of waveforms. Current flow is uni- or bi-directional. Some of the more common waveforms are direct current (Figure 1), monophasic pulsed current (Figure 2), twin-peaked monophasic pulsed current (Figure 3), symmetrical biphasic current (Figure 4), and asymmetrical biphasic current (Figure 5). Sometimes, it is easier to understand the current by being able to view the associated waveform. Waveforms with symmetric or balanced phase characteristics have a net charge of zero, meaning there is not a build-up of electrical charge in either phase (the positive or negative phase).

Charge Density

As the electrical current enters the tissues, it interacts with a cross-sectional area of tissue that comes into contact with the electrode. Current density, also called charge density, is a measure of the electrical charge per unit

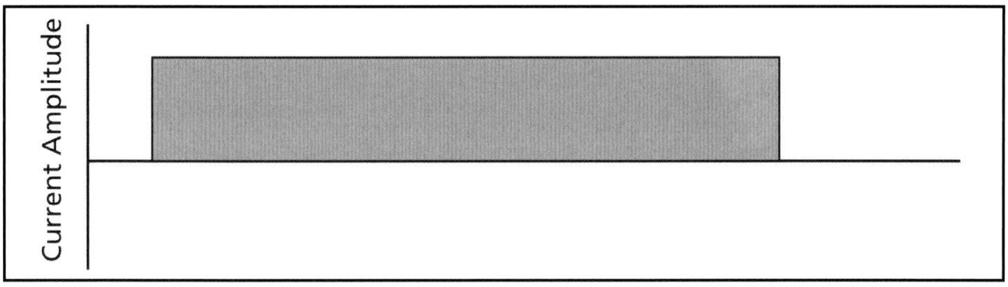

Figure 1. Direct Current Waveform.

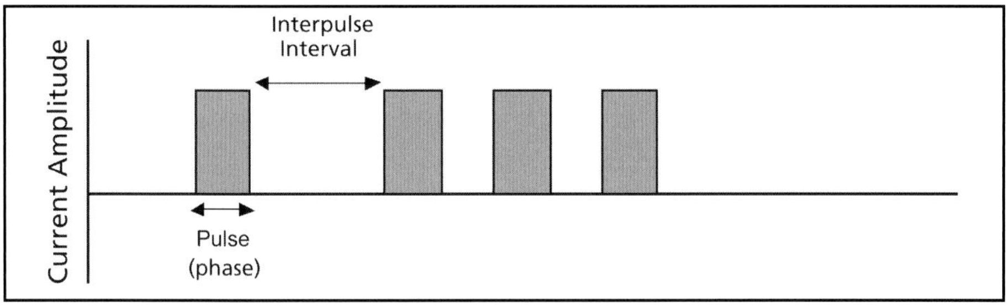

Figure 2. Monophasic Pulsed Current Waveform.

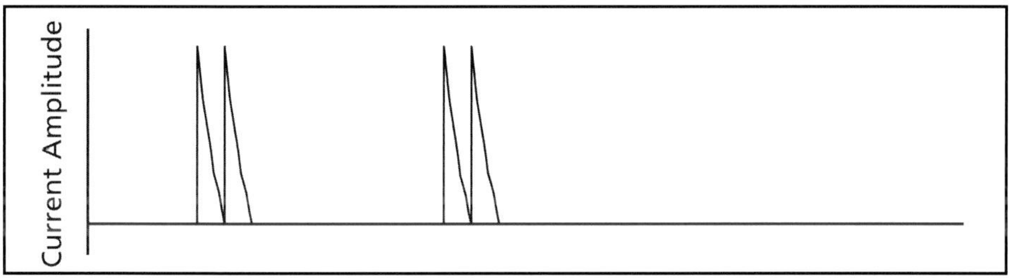

Figure 3. Twin-Peaked Monophasic Pulsed Current Waveform (Typical waveform of high-voltage pulsed current).

of

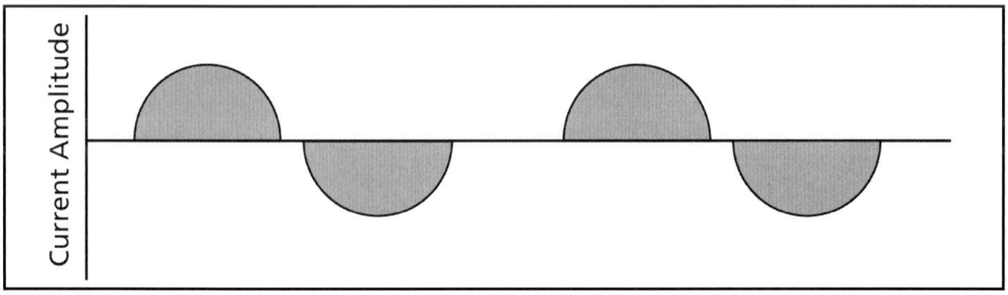

Figure 4. Symmetric Biphasic Current Waveform.

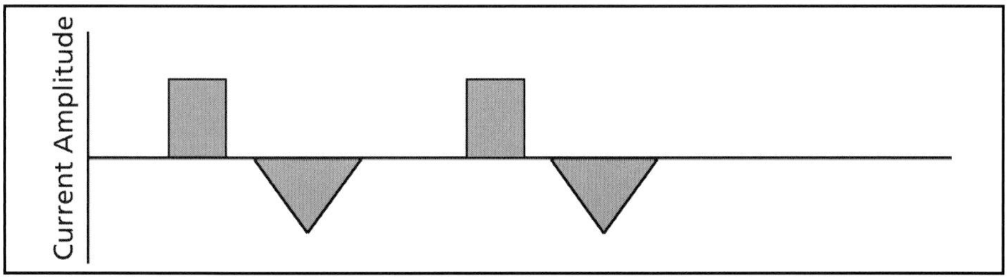

Figure 5. Asymmetric Biphasic Current Waveform.

cross-sectional area (cm^2). Current density is inversely related to the size of the electrodes (i.e., the larger the electrode, the smaller the current density, and vice versa). Current density has not been closely considered in past studies. However, Brighton et al. (16) studied new bone formation in relation to current density. Using a constant direct current (see Figure 1) at 20μC they achieved optimal bone formation. Increasing currents up to 80μC caused gradual cellular necrosis. Pulsed direct current (see Figure 2), reproduced the amount of bone formation, but only when the total charge delivered to the tissues approached that of the constant current. Therefore, the total charge delivered for optimal bone healing has been established and should be considered in future studies for soft tissue healing.

In order to generate an electrical current for soft tissue management, an electric circuit must be created. To do this, at least two electrodes must be in contact with the soft tissue. The electrodes must be connected to an electron source (negative jack) and an electron depository (positive jack). Electrodes are then applied to the surface of the tissues (skin/wound bed) with a wet conductive medium. When this contact occurs, it is described as capacitive coupling. The electrodes can either be placed in the wound bed using a monopolar technique, or straddling the wound using a bipolar technique. The bipolar technique is advantageous because it does not disrupt fragile tissues, wound hypothermia does not occur, and exogenous contaminants are avoided.

The human body produces its own measurable electrical current. This bioelectrical system has been measured since 1945 when electropositive voltages were discovered in the dermis and electronegative charges were discovered on the skin surface. Charges of 10–60mV are reported on human skin depending on the location. In addition, it was discovered that the skin contains an average negative (-) charge potential of -23.4mV with respect to the deeper tissue layers. When wounding occurs, the electrical current is "short-circuited" and the normal electrical potential surrounding the wound decreases significantly. In dry, desiccated wounds, the electrical potential is not measurable. However, Cheng and associates (17) were able to demonstrate that the use of moist wound healing maintained the normal electrical potential of the skin surrounding the wound.

There are two basic types of electrical currents described with ES: direct and alternating currents. Direct current (DC) is a continuous, uninterrupted flow of electricity (Figure 1). The direction of the current is determined by the polarity chosen for treatment. Direct current has also been delivered in the form of a "pulsed" current (Figure 2). This has been adopted in terminology as a "medical current" by the American Physical Therapy Association Clinical Electrophysiology Section. There are currently no wound related studies using alternating current (AC), so the discussion of AC will not be addressed in this chapter.

The pulsed current (PC) can either be uni- or bidirectional. This is described as mono- or biphasic. Each pulse (on phase) is separated by an interpulse interval (off phase). The monophasic PC waveforms used in soft tissue healing have been described as rectangular or twin-peaked. The twin-peaked form is traditionally used with the High-voltage PC (HVPC) (Figure 3).

Evidence Related to ES

Several studies have demonstrated either bacteriostatic or bactericidal properties related to ES in wound management. It is widely accepted that wound healing is delayed in the presence of infection. The results of the ES studies suggest these bactericidal and bacteriostatic properties are one mechanism by which ES can facilitate wound healing. A number of studies have been conducted using different amperages (milli- and microamperage), direct or pulsed current. One supposition is that pH related changes in the tissues kill bacteria. However, in one study, while no pH change was noted, bacterial growth was inhibited when exposed to anodal and cathodal HVPC for two hours at 250V. Szuminisky and colleagues (19) studied the in vitro effects of HVPC on four common species of bacteria and were unable to determine the direct mechanism by which the bacteria were killed. They were unable to ascertain if pH changes, local mechanical factors, increased heat generation, or mobilization of specific antimicrobial factors were responsible. Further studies on the antimicrobial effects of ES are warranted.

Animal studies have been helpful in determining the cellular effects of ES. Pig and rat models are commonly used for ES research. Studies have been conducted that demonstrate increased ATP production, increased angiogenesis, increased collagen synthesis, increased epithelialization, and increased fibroblast production. Along with increased collagen synthesis, an increase in tensile strength was noted by Nikolaew and colleagues (21).

Human studies have demonstrated many of the same effects. In addition, recent technological advances, such as Laser Doppler Imaging, have made it possible for researchers to quantify microcirculatory changes in humans. Hecker and colleagues (20) showed a trend toward increased blood flow with higher frequencies (32–128Hz) using negative polarity. Results from Cramp et al. showed a significant increase in blood perfusion during the treatment period in comparison to controls. Kaada (22) was able to demonstrate that a 15–30 minute treatment period would induce a vasodilation response not only during treatment, but also for several hours after.

An increase in blood flow will also increase oxygen transportation to the tissues. Tissue hypoxia can lead to cellular death and cessation in the metabolic processes related to wound healing. Gagnier and colleagues measured $TcpO_2$ levels 30 minutes before treatment, during a 30-minute treatment period and 30 minutes after the cessation of treatment, which used three different waveforms of ES. The $TcpO_2$ increased significantly from baseline during and after treatment, but no difference between waveforms was appreciated. A number of other investigators have been able to reproduce similar results using a variety of waveforms and parameters. These results have been repeated in animal models, healthy individuals, neuropathic foot ulcers, and spinal cord injuries. The greatest effects were seen with low-frequency stimulation.

Selecting the Parameters

While there have been over 100 studies that directly, or indirectly, evaluated the value of ES as it relates to wound healing, the most important treatment variables remain unclear. Many studies report similar results, but utilize different parameters to achieve those results. Returning to Brighton's original work, Kloth (25) reviewed additional studies and determined that the charge quantity, or total "dosage" is a common factor among all treatments. In his review, he found that the total dosage falls into a narrow window of 200–600 mC. This is one particular area that needs further study and review to help ameliorate the confusion associated with ES treatment parameters.

With all the confusion related to choosing the appropriate parameters, the clinician should take into consideration galvanotaxis, circulation, antimicrobial effects, and cellular processes when choosing protocols for ES. Characteristics of the wound responding favorably to ES have been autolysis, inflammation, contraction, and epithelialization. While both chronic and acute wounds have responded well, Medicare is currently only providing reimbursement for chronic wounds of greater than 30 days in duration, that have not demonstrated a measurable response to conservative treatment.

There are no significant treatment precautions related to ES for wound management. Skin irritation and mild discomfort have been reported in various trials. Also, children under the age of three should not be treated using ES if only because of questionable benefit to the patient.

Contraindications for treatment are:

1. Known malignancy in the treatment area (use of local ES away from the area of malignancy could be considered a precaution);
2. Active osteomyelitis (recent studies have demonstrated successful treatment of patients with osteomyelitis; however, manufacturer guidelines and text books include ES as a contraindication, so further research may be warranted);
3. Demand-type pacemakers (Reports of interference with pacemaker signals are inconsistent. Studies in 51 patients without interference were reported. Chen et al. (24) reported that while dysfunction did not show up on electrocardiogram, it did appear with extended observation using a Holter monitor. Therefore, contacting the cardiovascular physician and discussing the potential benefits of treatment should be considered);
4. Application of electrodes in a manner that the current flow would pass through the heart, carotid sinus, parasympathetic nerves, ganglia, laryngeal muscles, or phrenic nerve;
5. Directly over topical substances containing metal ions (Silver sulfadiazine, cadexamer iodine, povidone-iodine, zinc are all common topical agents in wound management. Direct current is used in iontophoresis to transfer ions into the tissues and could potentially cause tissue toxicity if used in conjunction with these topical agents);
6. Directly over pregnant uterus.

Electrode Selection and Placement

Once the treatment parameters have been decided, the clinician faces several more decisions. The size and shape of electrode will affect the current density. Larger electrodes will have a lower current density. Picture trying to force 100 gallons of water through a hose in a short period of time. If the hose has a one-foot diameter, the water pressure would be fairly low.

Conversely, 100 gallons passing through a one-inch hose in the same period of time would have a higher pressure. The same theory applies to current density. A smaller electrode will concentrate the current and have a stronger effect on the tissues.

Placement of the electrodes is also a consideration. Using a monophasic stimulator, there are two electrodes: the active and dispersive. The distance between the two electrodes should be 20–30cm. The farther apart the electrodes are placed, the deeper the current will flow. For more superficial wounds, electrodes can be placed in close proximity.

Using a monopolar technique, the active pad is placed in the wound bed over a wet, conductive medium. The dispersive pad is placed over intact skin at a distance from the wound bed, also using a wet, conductive medium. Current research indicates that it may be beneficial to alter the placement of the dispersive pad with each treatment to allow the current to flow into the wound from different areas.

With a bipolar technique, the two electrodes are situated to straddle the wound. The electrodes are placed on areas of intact skin using a wet, conductive medium. The current will flow between the two electrodes through the wound. Again, the proximity of the electrodes will determine the depth of the current flow. Current thinking indicates that the direction of the electrodes should be altered with each treatment just as with monopolar placement.

Electrical Stimulation for wound healing is supported by clear, strong evidence for its efficacy. ES can be utilized in every phase of wound healing, and can be utilized to initiate the healing process in chronic wounds. In conjunction with standard care, ES has been demonstrated to enhance wound healing through a variety of methods. Future studies should give consideration to the "dosage" or charge quantity in order to help establish more definitive parameters.

Electromagnetic Fields

There has been an increasing utilization of exogenous pulsed electromagnetic fields (PEMF) and pulsed radio frequency (PRF) in physical therapy in the past several years. Traditionally, these modalities have been utilized for musculoskeletal injuries such as sprains, strains, tendonitis, and even delayed and non-union fractures in orthopedic settings.

PEMF are usually low frequency fields with specific shape and amplitude. There are a fairly large number of commercially available devices and comparing the specific signals is the primary factor that impedes a direct clinical comparison of the physiological results from different units. PRF devices in the USA utilize the frequency of 27.12 MHz for soft tissue stimulation. If utilized in a continuous mode, a deep heating of the tissues occurs. If pulsed, (usually 65 microsecond pulse bursts) the tissue is only affected by the incident magnetic field.

Studies have demonstrated that small electrical currents can have significant physiological response in the tissues. One recent double-blind study by Kloth et al. (25) demonstrated a statistically significant decrease in wound size compared to placebo using PRF. The results achieved were similar to studies with HVPC, with the advantage of being a non-contact application with the PRF device.

With electrical stimulation and electromagnetic fields, as with many therapeutic treatment modalities, it has often been thought that if "a little is good, a lot is better." There is a significantly growing body of evidence that indicates that "less is more" in many instances. Low frequency electrotherapy and low frequency ultrasound have both demonstrated the ability to have profound effects on tissues and healing responses. Certainly, further clinical study in these areas is warranted to help determine the mechanism of action for the positive effects that are being noted in the clinical setting.

NEGATIVE PRESSURE WOUND THERAPY

Negative Pressure Wound Therapy (NPWT) is a relatively new treatment modality, having been approved by the FDA in 1995 for commercial marketing. NPWT is currently delivered by two devices in the USA: Vacuum-Assisted Closure (VAC), a product manufactured by Kinetic Concepts Inc (VAC®, KCI, San Antonio, TX) and the Versatile 1™ by Blue Sky Medical Group (V1™, La Costa, CA). NPWT involves the placement of a porous, collapsible material (such as a foam or gauze) into the wound base, covering with an occlusive dressing, and then applying a controlled subatmospheric (negative) pressure to the entire wound.

The application of negative pressure has been proven to remove excess edema fluid and cellular debris from interstices in/around the wound bed. The removal of excess wound fluid will restore local blood flow to vessels which may have been compressed by excess pressure. Chronic wound fluid also contains substances that can impede or halt wound healing (i.e., matrix metalloproteinases). Lastly, the mechanical deformation of the tissues has been demonstrated to increase cellular division, neovascularization and protein synthesis.

When negative pressure is placed on the wound through a closed system, it increases tension on the cells and alters the shape of the cells. This results in cellular division and a uniform contraction that pulls the edges of the wound toward the center of the defect. Mechanical stretching has been demonstrated to stimulate cellular proliferation in vivo and in vitro in a variety of cell types (endothelial cells, fibroblasts, vascular smooth muscle cells) and structures (nerve, blood vessels, and skin).

There have been a number of clinical studies that have demonstrated clinically and statistically significant results. NPWT was demonstrated superior to controls in all studies. One study in particular by Joseph and colleagues (31) randomized 36 patients (18 treatment and controls). The treatment group received NPWT therapy for six weeks (treatment parameters were not given). Blinded, independent evaluators took measurements at the beginning, and week three and six of the study. The most significant results were that of a decrease in total volume (78% with NPWT versus 30% with standard care) and change in depth (66% for NPWT and 20% for standard care). All wounds in the treatment group developed granulation tissue; whereas, granulation was not achieved in the entire control group.

NPWT is indicated to promote increased granulation and wound closure in chronic, full-thickness wounds (i.e., stage III and IV pressure ulcers).

NPWT has also been proven beneficial in acute and subacute wounds, dehisced surgical wounds, meshed skin grafts, and muscle flaps. Recently, the FDA has given approval for the treatment of enteric fistulas, which was previously considered a contraindication and off-label use.

One problem has been the issue of granulation tissue becoming "trapped" within the open cellular structures utilized within the wound cavity. Several clinicians, in an effort to decrease this problem have utilized a number of different contact layers within the wound base. A study by Jones, Banwell, and Shakespeare (34) demonstrated that different contact layers can decrease the negative pressures recorded by the device. Clinicians should note that by utilizing these contact layers, pressures may be lower than indicated on the device.

Precautions

Caution should be used with a patient on anticoagulants or with difficult wound hemostasis because of the potential for bleeding when the open-cell foam is removed from the wound bed. Contraindications would include presence of necrotic tissue; untreated osteomyelitis, malignancy in the wound or wound margins, and fistulas to organs or body cavities (other than the aforementioned enteric fistulas).

Selecting the Parameters

In the US, current research has been predominantly conducted utilizing the Kinetic Concepts Inc VAC®, until the past 2–3 years when the FDA cleared BlueSky's Versatile 1™ Wound Vacuum System for marketing. Recommended pressure settings for the VAC are 50–125 mm Hg below ambient pressure. For the first 48 hours, it is recommended that continuous negative pressure be applied. Subsequent treatments are an intermittent therapy with recommended five minutes on then two minutes off, for 24 hours a day. The target pressure is 125 mm Hg for all wounds other than chronic ulcers. There is a concern that negative pressure above 50–75 mm Hg will draw too much fluid from the chronic wound and desiccate the tissues. The dressings are changed every two days, unless infected, and then every 12 hours thereafter.

Papers published in 1987 by Usopov and Yepifanov (Russia) (32) indicated that a subatmospheric pressure of -75 to -80 mm Hg had the most distinct effect on drainage without damaging vessels. Negative pressures (vacuum) of -120 to -125 mm Hg were demonstrated to cause extensive tissue edema and greater vacuum caused fresh hemorrhage and coagulated vessels. Pressures of -35 to -40 mm Hg were shown upon histological evaluation to have increased cellular infiltration and insignificant tissue edema. Additional papers demonstrated that treatment times of 2.5–3 hours reduced bacterial load, reduced time to healing, and decreased septic complications for the patients.

There are a number of additional questions that should be addressed in regards to NPWT.

- What is the most efficacious time frame for treatment?
- Is continuous negative pressure as effective as intermittent negative pressure?

- If continuous negative pressure is efficacious, would two hours be sufficient—or would 20 achieve the best results?
- Can the same results be achieved with intermittent (i.e. periodic) negative pressure?

If only a few hours of therapy might be required, then costs of pump rentals might be decreased dramatically with several patients sharing the same pump, and it being rotated between patients for treatment. There is no clear consensus regarding frequency of dressing changes, intermittent or continuous therapy.

From an equipment cost standpoint, the NPWT is an expensive modality. Average daily costs can be up to $150 depending on which device is utilized. However, considering current research that demonstrates increased granulation and faster rates of healing, studies have demonstrated that, on average, NPWT may be a cost-effective treatment, especially for wounds with large, deep defects. Equipment costs and reimbursement will vary according to state and caregivers are advised to contact their local fiscal intermediary and insurance providers for coverage determination.

ULTRASOUND

Since the development of ultrasound (US) technology in the 1950s, several papers have been presented on its efficacy. These papers fall into two broad categories—pain control (musculoskeletal dysfunction) and tissue repair. The results of several meta-analyses by different groups are that US for pain management in musculoskeletal disorders lacks firm evidence and well controlled studies. The findings for the use of US for tissue repair were more positive, but contained mixed results. Studies were able to demonstrate a significant treatment effect over placebo, but the variables and parameters in the studies were not well documented. Therefore, it is difficult to come to a definitive conclusion on the efficacy of US in tissue repair. In 1993 a review of literature by the AHCPR determined that there was not sufficient evidence to support the inclusion of US in the Clinical Practice Guidelines for Pressure Ulcer Treatment, reporting a strength of evidence rating of "C" that was based on expert opinion and descriptive studies. Further investigation and additional clinical trials with known variables are warranted to determine the efficacy of this modality.

Although the current literature does not unequivocally conclude that US is effective, the theory and science behind the modality has good evidentiary support. US is defined as a mechanical vibration that is transmitted at a frequency above the limit of human hearing (>20 kHz). During application, sound waves pass into the tissues and the resulting mechanical energy that is transferred to the tissues causes the molecules to oscillate. This back-and-forth movement of the tissues can theoretically accelerate tissue healing.

The number of oscillations a molecule undergoes within 1 second defines the frequency of the sound wave and this is expressed in units of Hertz (Hz; 1 Hz=1 cycle per second [cps], 1 kHz=1000 cps; and 1 MHz=1 million cps). High frequency US (20–40 MHz) devices are utilized diagnostically to assess periwound skin, wound bed, and underlying soft tissue components.

Most of the historical research related to US in tissue healing focused on the non-thermal aspects of the treatment. There are two non-thermal ultrasound effects: cavitation and acoustic streaming. Cavitation is the production and vibration of micron-sized gas bubbles within the coupling medium and fluids within the tissues. These bubbles will collect and condense (decrease in size). As they decrease in size, stable cavities may occur. At sufficiently high intensities, the bubbles within the US field can collapse (implode), which may result in the destruction of tissue close to the bubbles of the US applicator. This temporary cavitation may be one mechanism that contributes to the increased lysis of fibrin on the wound surface.

The effect known as acoustic streaming causes an increase in circulation and fluid movement in the treated tissues. The fluid movement is very small, and has been termed microstreaming, which results in a fluid gradient in close proximity to cellular membranes. Theoretically, this may alter cellular structure and activity. For example, low frequency US treatments (kHz) have been demonstrated to temporarily increase collagen production by fibroblasts. Other notable possibilities are increased cell membrane permeability, increased nitric oxide production, improved perfusion, increased protein synthesis, and increased growth factor production. All of these effects have been demonstrated in current literature (Table 4).

TABLE 4. EFFECTS OF ULTRASOUND DURING WOUND HEALING PHASES

Inflammatory Phase	vasodilation, chemotaxis, & macrophage stimulation
Proliferative Phase	stimulates fibroblasts to produce collagen, increases contraction, increases endothelial cell activity, mast cells release angiogenic factors
Remodeling Phase	strengthens scar tissue, increases elasticity

A new theory, called frequency resonance theory, has been proposed. In general, it is believed that the energy from an ultrasound wave is absorbed by individual protein molecules which cause structural changes. Signal-transduction pathways are also stimulated by this energy, which can have sweeping cellular effects and can directly impact wound healing. Examples of these cellular effects are: growth factor production, collagen production, increased angiogenesis, increased fibrinolysis, and increased nitric oxide production.

In the inflammatory phase, a single US treatment can stimulate histamine release and other chemotactic agents that attract neutrophils and macrophages to the wound site. US performed within the first 24–48 hours of the inflammatory phase can stimulate platelets, mast cells, and macrophages to release growth factors that stimulate fibroblast and endothelial cell production. Treatment parameters during the acute inflammatory process are typically non-thermal. However, a single thermal treatment has been shown to produce an acute inflammatory response in a chronic wound. Early US intervention could theoretically be utilized to enhance the acute inflammatory process and accelerate the onset of the proliferative phase.

Approximately 72 hours after injury, the proliferative phase begins and overlaps with the inflammatory phase. The proliferative phase is characterized by fibroplasia and contraction. US treatment has been demonstrated to stimulate fibroblast migration and proliferation during this phase of healing. Endothelial cells are also affected by US during the proliferative phase. Chronically ischemic muscle tissue treated with US will develop signs of angiogenesis and accelerate wound healing. Late in the proliferative phase, wound contraction begins. The cell primarily responsible for wound contraction is the myofibroblast. US stimulation may cause the myofibroblasts to develop earlier, and accelerate wound contraction.

During remodeling, collagen fibers align to form more regular pattern. Structurally, the scar that is formed with wound healing is weaker and less elastic than the uninjured tissue. Several researchers have demonstrated that the application of thermal US increased collagen deposition, tensile strength, and elasticity. However, US treatment must be initiated during the inflammatory phase to achieve these effects. When US is started later in the healing process, it is less effective.

Precautions

A list of precautions for US is as follows: 1) acute infection; 2) epiphyseal plates; 3) cranium; 4) areas of anesthesia (use of a pulsed current, without a thermal effect will reduce the risk associated with possible equipment malfunction); 5) bony prominences; 6) subcutaneous major nerves (use of pulsed current will decrease associated risk).

The list of absolute contraindications with US has decreased in the recent past. Many of the contraindications have not been verified in research and should be considered for study. The following list of contraindications should be considered when choosing US treatment: 1) over pregnant uterus; 2) over the eye; 3) over reproductive organs; 4) over cancerous, or precancerous, lesions; 5) on spinal cord following laminectomy (or any other tissue of the central nervous system); 6) on patients with vascular abnormalities (i.e., DVT, Thrombophlebitis, emboli); 7) over cardiac area, particularly in the presence of a pacemaker.

Selection of the Parameters

When choosing ultrasound as a treatment modality for wound healing, one must first determine the goals of the therapeutic intervention (Table 5). This will drive the treatment parameters utilized in therapy. One of the first parameters that should be addressed is which frequency sound head to use. Frequency refers to the number of times per second that a displaced molecule completes a full cycle of movement and returns to its original position. Frequency of 1 Hz is equal to 1 cycle per second. Typical US machines will have 1 MHz and 3 MHz sound heads available. The US wave will penetrate into deeper tissues with a frequency of 1 MHz, therefore 3 MHz is recommended for treatment of superficial wounds.

The intensity of treatment is the amount of energy (W) delivered per unit of area, per unit of time (expressed in W/cm^2). This is the amount of energy delivered to the tissues. The amount of energy, if delivered in a continuous fashion, will cause a temperature increase in the attenuated tissues. This thermal effect can be unwelcome in soft tissue healing. To eliminate the

TABLE 5. RECOMMENDED TREATMENT PARAMETERS FOR SOFT TISSUE HEALING

	Chronic Inflammation	Proliferation	Bruising/ Hematoma	Tissue Ischemia	Undermining / Tunneling	Acute Inflammation
Frequency	1 MHz	0.75 MHz	1 MHz	1 MHz or 3 MHz	1 MHz	1 MHz or 3 MHz
Pulse Duty Cycle	20%	20%	pulsed 20%	continuous	20%	20–50%
Intensity	0.5 W/cm^2	0.1 W/cm^2	0.5 W/cm^2	1.0–1.4 W/cm^2	0.5 W/cm^2	0.1–0.2 W/cm^2
Treatment Frequency	Daily	Daily	Daily	Daily	Daily	3x/week
Time	5 minutes to periwound area	5 minutes to periwound area	5–10 minutes; depending on size resonated	*5–10 minutes; depending on size resonated	5 minutes to periwound area	1 min/cm^2; max 15 minutes total

* Expected changes following one treatment are; lysis of necrotic tissue, signs of acute inflammation, and temperature changes associated with increased circulation. If these signs are present after one treatment, change parameters to 0.5 W/cm^2, 20% duty cycle, 3–5x/week; otherwise, continue with single higher intensity treatments until signs of increased circulation are present, then follow with lower intensity treatments.

thermal effect, the sound wave can be interrupted with a pulsed current. This pulsed current can be further characterized by specifying the percentage of time the sound wave is present during one pulse cycle. Duty cycles of 20% and 50% are commonly used in soft tissue management.

The last parameter that should be considered is the BNR, or beam nonuniformity ratio. The ultrasonic beam is not homogenous, and this results in areas of higher peak intensities, or "hot spots" within the beam. In a perfect machine, the BNR would be a 1:1 ratio, meaning that the maximum intensity is the same at every point within the beam. A machine with a BNR of 6:1 would indicate that when the intensity was set at 1.0 W/cm^2, points within the beam would reach an intensity of 6.0 W/cm^2. This is an important consideration if using a continuous wave, because the thermal effects can cause tissue irritation, inflammation, and even necrosis if the temperature elevation is too high.

The human trials published for review using traditional MHz US have shown mixed results. Many of the studies have combined US with other modalities, making the results of the studies unreliable. Several of the controlled clinical trials did not publish all the treatment parameters, making it difficult to reproduce the outcomes of the five studies that looked at the use of US with venous healing, one of the controlled trials did not produce a therapeutic effect. There is sufficient evidence to support the continued use of US as a wound healing modality from the theoretical aspect. As with all therapeutic treatments, further research in this area is warranted.

Ultrasound for Debridement

Historically, Ultrasound has been utilized in the clinical treatment of the periwound tissues. Recently, there has been a shift toward the use of low-frequency ultrasound (kHz) to achieve bone healing, vascular vasodilation, and antimicrobial effects. There are two low-frequency ultrasound devices currently on the market being utilized for wound debridement (Sonoca 180, Soring, Inc, Fort Worth, TX and MIST Therapy Ultrasound, Celleration, Inc, Eden Prairie, MN). These devices operate at 25-45 kHz with a treatment intensity of 0.1–1.0 W/cm^2 depending on the device utilized.

Recent research has demonstrated that low-frequency US at 50-60 kHz effectively removed particulate debris and bacteria in rat models (McDonald and Nichter (42). Other investigators have reported antibacterial effects of low-frequency ultrasound as well, possibly attributing the effect to transient cavitation.

It has been theorized that the implosion of the gas bubbles caused by transient cavitation is one mechanism by which both debridement and bacterial destruction occurs. Another theory may be that the mechanical movement of water at the tips of the US device may promote fibrinolysis as it is moved across the wound surface. The slow movement also prevents the build-up of heat (thermal energy) and helps the US penetrate the tissues in a more efficient manner.

Because of the possibility of aerosolization of fluids, the clinician should don appropriate personal protective equipment (fluid-proof gowns, gloves, shoe covers, hair covers, masks, and face shield). The patient should also wear a mask during the procedure. It is possible that sensate patients may require a topical analgesic to help with any discomfort experienced with the treatment when higher output levels are utilized to lyse adherent necrotic tissue or fibrin.

NORMOTHERMIA

The theory that all biological, physiological, and chemical processes are optimized at normal body temperature (37 ± 1°C) is referred to as normothermia. Many wounds are hypothermic, an average of 5.6°C cooler than normal body temperature. Hypothermia can contribute to vasoconstriction, tissue hypoxia, decreased collagen production and deposition, increased risk of infection, and a delay in the normal wound healing process. Studies have demonstrated that warming of patients during surgery decreased the development of post-operative pressure ulcers by 50%. Warming the tissues to core body temperature increases vasodilation and increases oxygen delivery to the tissues.

Currently, the only FDA approved device is Warm-Up® Active Wound Therapy System (Augustine Medical, Inc, Eden Prairie, MN). This device is designed to deliver controlled, moist heat, by way of an infrared warming card placed in a noncontact, semiocclusive dressing. The system contains a temperature control unit; a sterile wound cover dressing; and a warming card that delivers the radiant heat to the wound bed. The dressing is designed to be noncontact, semi-occlusive, water resistant, and latex free. The wound cover will remain in place for up to three days and is disposable. The dressing also insulates the wound, protecting the tissues from heat loss when the warming card is not active. When activated, the warming card raises the temperature to 38°C.

The protocol for treatment is to apply the wound cover dressing, according to manufacturer guidelines, insert the warming card and turn the temperature control unit on for one hour. After the treatment is concluded, remove the warming card from the dressing. Repeat the treatment two additional times within a 24-hour period, with a minimum of two hours between each treatment. If necrotic tissue is present, it should be debrided prior to application of the wound cover dressing. Case studies have shown that with the use of Warm Up wound therapy, it is not necessary to pack tunneling/undermined wounds. However, when choosing a cover dressing, it is necessary to select a wound cover that encompasses the entire area of the tunneling/ undermining. Typically, the clinician can expect to see increased exudate during the first 7–10 days of treatment. This may indicate the transition of the wound into the inflammatory phase and would be a part of the normal healing process.

In 2000, Price and associates (48) published a randomized controlled trial in which 50 patients were divided into two groups. The study lasted six weeks and the experimental group received warming therapy for one hour daily. The dressings were changed daily. The control group received standard moist dressings (calcium alginate) changed as needed. At the end of the study period, the control and experimental group achieved a 22.8% and 54.6% reduction in mean area, respectively. Another aspect studied was the time it took for the wound to decrease to 25% of its original wound area. The results indicated that the experimental group achieved this reduction significantly faster than the control group ($p = 0.05$). Normothermia has been demonstrated to facilitate wound healing. However, as with all clinical modalities, our practices would be better served with additional studies in this area.

Precautions

As a precaution with any electrical device, always follow the manufacturer's guidelines for use. Do not apply the warming card directly to the periwound area, or wound bed. Use an appropriately sized dressing cover. As with many other modalities, precautions include: untreated osteomyelitis, or infection; fistulas, sinus tracts, or extensive undermining; dry, stable ischemic ulcers; and third degree burns (contraindication).

Since the first publication of this text, Centers for Medicare and Medicaid Services denied coverage for this device. There have only been a handful of additional studies that have been conducted and most of them have been outside the US with this device. While financial reimbursement is not readily available, the concept of normothermia has been carried into all aspects of wound management, from choosing the appropriate dressings, to warming saline before pulsed lavage.

ULTRAVIOLET LIGHT

The use of sunlight in the treatment of infection and skin disease has a history dating back to the times of cavemen. In the 1700s, it was discovered that a lack of exposure to the sun was correlated with the development of rickets. In the 1800s, the bactericidal properties of light were discovered. In the early 1900s, Ultraviolet (UV) light was discovered to be bactericidal to specific bacteria and was used to treat tuberculosis of the skin (Table 6).

TABLE 6. BACTERIAL EFFECTS OF UVC RADIATION

	Exposure time required for 99.9% kill	Exposure time required for 100% kill
MSRA	5 seconds	90 seconds
VRE	5 seconds	45 seconds
S.aureus	5 seconds	45 seconds
S. pyogenes **(group A strep)**	4 seconds	not achieved with 180 second exposure

UV light is a component of sunlight (radiant energy) that encompasses the wavelengths between 180 and 400 nanometers. It can be broken into three spectral bands: UVA (nonionizing and produces the most tanning effects), UVB (nonionizing, but produces more skin erythema, blistering, and is more carcinogenic), and UVC (ionizing, bactericidal, virucidal). In this chapter, while the focus is on the use of UVC light for its bactericidal effects, it should be mentioned that it is also believed that UV light can stimulate the healing process by causing an aseptic inflammatory response in the tissues.

Over 100 years ago, documentation was present to support the bactericidal effects of UV light. Regardless of a specific mechanism, UV light is lethal to bacteria and rapidly results in a clean wound bed. Questions arose concerning the effects of UVC on antibiotic resistant bacteria. Conner-Kerr and colleagues (49) delivered UVC for 30 seconds daily for eight days and monitored wound closure rates in control and experimental groups. At the end of the study, there was no bacterial growth in either the control group, or the treatment group. Tissue biopsy indicated that wound closure rates were not affected by the UVC treatments.

Another study by Conner-Kerr and associates (50) demonstrated UVC kill rates on MRSA were 99.9% at a five-second exposure and 100% at a 90-second exposure. Similar kill rates for Enterococcus faecalis and Stapholococcus aureus were found. Sullivan and associates (51) looked at the effects of UVC radiation on group A streptococcus (a cause of type II necrotizing fasciitis) and were able to produce a 99.9% kill rate at a four-second dosage to UVC light. However, they were not able to achieve 100% kill rates even at 180 seconds of UVC exposure.

Although significant experimental data exists to support the use of UV radiation in wound healing, very few clinical studies have been conducted. Based on current research, the protocol for the treatment of infected wounds for a bactericidal effect is fairly simple. The periwound area should be prepared (draped or apply a UV blocking lotion with an SPF of 30) and the patient and clinician should be provided with UV-protective eyewear. The UVC lamp should be placed one inch (2.54 cm) from the wound. Irradiate the wound for at least 30 seconds daily if the wound is either highly colonized or infected with antibiotic susceptible bacteria. If the wound is infected with MRSA, treat for 90 seconds, daily. If the wound is infected with antibiotic resistant E. faecalis, use a 45 second exposure time, once daily. Group A strep alone requires a treatment time of four seconds, but with concomitant S. aureus infection, increase daily treatment time to 120 seconds.

In several experimental studies, the bactericidal and wound healing effects have been noted. However, controlled clinical studies have not been able to adequately duplicate these findings. The opportunity to find an alternative method for bacterial control other than through the use of antibiotics is a powerful justification for conducting further research in this area. The increasing reports of MRSA, VRE and other antibiotic resistant bacteria make this an appealing treatment modality. Additional clinical research is also warranted with UVB light and its efficacy in promoting healing in chronic wounds.

Precautions

Contraindications for UV treatment commonly include: diabetes, pulmonary tuberculosis, hyperthyroidism, systemic lupus erythematous, cardiac, renal, hepatic disease, and carcinoma. Typical precautions for treatment are: photosensitizing medications and foods; recent x-ray therapy; photosensitivity (fair complexion); and eye exposure.

CONCLUSION

While there are certainly additional adjunctive modalities that can be discussed, the evidence and science behind those treatments are not well substantiated. Today's clinician has an assortment of therapeutic modalities that are available to stimulate every phase of wound healing, decrease necrotic tissue, decrease bacterial counts, promote angiogenesis and granulation tissue, enhance tissue oxygenation and vasodilation of tissues, promote collagen deposition and organization, and epithelialization. All of these things will help to bring a chronic wound back into balance and stimulate an acute wound for accelerated healing. The practitioner must first determine the goals of treatment, and understand what physiological effect he/she is trying to achieve. With that understanding, comes the enlightened choice for the most appropriate modality, or combination of modalities, that will enhance good local wound care. Lastly, it must be remembered that although we may use negative pressure wound care, we do not work in a vacuum. We must address the whole patient, and utilize all the members of the treatment team to achieve the goal of wound healing. Therapeutic modalities are but one integral part in the management of the wound care patient.

REFERENCES

Hydrotherapy

1. Bergstrom N, Bennett MA, Carlson C, et al. Treatment of Pressure Ulcers. Clinical Practice Guideline No. 15. Rockville, MD: Agency for Health Care Research and Quality (AHRQ), formerly known as the Agency for Health Care Policy and Research (AHCPR), US Public Health Service (PHS), US Department of Health and Human Services (DHHS); AHRQ Publication No. 95-0652. December 1994; 8,45-65.

2. Walsh M. Hydrotherapy: the use of water as a therapeutic agent. In: Michlovitz S, ed. Thermal Agents in Rehabilitation. Philadelphia, PA: FA Davis, 1990:109-132.

3. Bohannon R. Whirlpool versus whirlpool and rinse for removal of bacterial from a venous stasis ulcer. *Phys Ther* 1982; 62:304-308.

4. Cardany CR, Rodeheaver GT, Horowitz JH. Influence of hydrotherapy and antiseptic agents on burn wound bacterial contamination. *J Burn Care Rehabil* 1985; 6:230-232.

5. Loehne HB. Pulsatile Lavage with Suction. In: Sussman C, Bates-Jensen BM. Wound Care: A Collaborative Practice Manual for Physical Therapists and Nurses. Aspen, Gaithersburg, MD. 1998: 643-660.

6. Juve MB. Whirlpool therapy on postoperative pain and surgical wound healing: An exploration. *Patient Educ Couns* 1998; 33(1):39-48.

7. Burke DT, et al. Effects of hydrotherapy on pressure ulcer healing. *Am J Phys Med Rehabil* 1998; 77(5):394-398.

8. Haynes LJ, Handley C, Brown MH, et al. Comparison of pulsavac and sterile whirlpool regarding the promotion of tissue granulation. (abstr). *Phys Ther* 74(Suppl 5):S4, 1994.

9. Bhaskar SN, Cutright DE, Hunsuck EE, et al. Pulsating water jet devices in debridement of combat wounds. *Milit Med* 1971; 136:264-266.

10. Rodeheaver GT. Pressure ulcer debridement and cleansing: A review of current literature. *Ostomy/Wound Manage* 1999; 45(Suppl):80S-85S.

11. Ovington L. Dressings and adjunctive therapies: AHCPR Guidelines Revisited. *Ostomy/Wound Manage* 1999; (45A)99S-100S.

12. Maragakis L, et al. An Outbreak of multidrug-resistant Acinetobacter baumannii associated with pulsatile lavage wound treatment. *JAMA* 2004; 292(24):3006-3011.

13. Loehne, HB, Streed SA, Gaither B, et al. Aerosolization of microorganisms during pulsatile lavage with suction. Abstract presented at: Symposium on Advanced Wound Care and Medical Research Forum on Wound Repair; Baltimore, Md; April 29, 2002.

Electrical Stimulation

14. U.S. Department of Health and Human Services. Treatment of pressure ulcers (AHCPR Pub No 95-0652). Rockville, MD: US Government Printing, Office, 1994. *www.ahcpr.org*

15. Medical and Surgical Procedures Panel. Medicare Coverage Policy MCAC: Electrical Stimulation for the treatment of wounds. Baltimore, MD: Health Care Financing Administration; 2000:1-73.

16. Brighton CT, et al. Electrically induced osteogenesis: relationship between charge, current density, and the amount of bone formed: introduction of a new cathode concept. *Clin Orthop Relat Res* 1981; 161(124):131.

17. Cheng K, et al. Confirmation of the electrical potential induced by occlusive dressings. Abstract 28 presented at the Eighth Annual Symposium on Advanced Wound Care, April 1995, San Diego, CA. Health Management Publications, Wayne, PA, 1995.

18. Kincaid CB, Lavoie KH. Inhibition of bacterial growth in vitro following stimulation with high voltage, monophasic pulsed current. *Phys Ther* 69:651, 1989.

19. Szuminsky NJ, et al. Effect of narrow, pulsed high voltages on bacterial viability. *Phys Ther* 74:660, 1994.

20. Hecker B, et al. Pulsed galvanic stimulation: effects of current frequency and polarity on blood flow in healthy subjects. *Arch Phys Med Rehab* 1985; 66;35-37.

21. Nikolaew U, et al. Use of a sinusoidal current of optimal frequency to stimulate skin wound healing. New York, NY: Plenum, 1984; p812.

22. Kaada B. Vasodilation induced by transcutaneous nerve stimulation in peripheral ischemia (Reynaud's phenomena and diabetic polyneuropathy). *Eur Heart J.*1982; 3(4):303-314.

23. Rasmussen MJ, et al. Can transcutaneous electrical nerve stimulation be safely used in patients with permanent cardiac pacemakers? *Mayo Clin Proc* 1988; 63:443-445.

24. Chen D, et al. Cardiac pacemaker inhibition by transcutaneous electrical nerve stimulation. *Arch Phys Med Rehabil* 1990; 71(1):27-30.

25. Kloth LC, et al. 1999. Effect of pulsed radio-frequency stimulation on wound healing: a double-blind pilot clinical study. Electricity and Magnetism in Biology and Medicine. Bersani F, ed. Plenum, New York. 875-878.

26. Milgram, J, et al. The effect of short, high intensity magnetic field pulses on the healing of skin wounds in rats. *Bioelectrics* 2004; 25:271-277.

27. Kenkre JE, et al. A randomized controlled trial of electromagnetic therapy in the primary care management of venous leg ulceration. *Family Practice* 1996; 13: 236-241.

Negative Pressure Wound Therapy

28. Morykwas MJ, Argenta LC. Nonsurgical modalities to enhance healing and care of soft tissue wounds. *South Orthop Assoc* 6:279, 1997.

29. Morykwas MJ, et al. Vacuum-assisted closure: a new method for wound control and treatment: Animal studies and basic foundation. *Ann Plast Surg* 38:553, 1997.

30. Bates-Jensen BM, Sussman C. Wound care: a collaborative practice manual for physical therapists and nurses. Gaithersburg, MD: Aspen Publishers, 1998.

31. Joseph E, et al. New therapeutic approaches in wound care: a perspective randomized trial of vacuum assisted closure versus standard therapy of chronic non-healing wounds. *Wounds* 2000; 12(3):60-67.

32. Usupov YN, Yepifanov MV. Active Wound Drainage. *Vestkin Khirugii* 1987; 4:48-52.

33. Davydov YA, Malafeeva AP, Smirnov AP. Vacuum therapy in the treatment of purulent lactation mastitis. *Vestnik Khirurgii* 1986; 9:18-21.

34. Jones SM, Banwell PE, Shakespeare PG. Interface Dressings Influence the Delivery of Topical Negative Pressure Therapy. *Plast Reconstr Surg* 2005; 116:1023-1028.

Ultrasound

35. Young S. The effect of therapeutic ultrasound on the biological mechanisms involved in dermal repair. PhD Thesis, University of London, 1988.

36. Fyfe MC, Chahl LA. Mast cell degranulation: a possible mechanism of action of therapeutic ultrasound. *Ultrasound Med Biol* 8(Suppl 1):62, 1982.

37. Dyson M, Small D. Effects of ultrasound on wound contraction. In Millner R (ed) Ultrasound Interactions in Biology and Medicine. Plenum, New York, 1983, p 151.

38. Dyson M, et al. Stimulation of healing of varicose ulcers by ultrasound. *Ultrasonics* 14: 232, 1976

39. Lundeberg T, et al. Pulsed ultrasound does not improve healing of venous ulcers. *Scand J Rehab Med* 22:195, 1990.

40. Stansic MM, et al. Wound Debridement with 25 kHz Ultrasound. *Advances in Skin and Wound Care* 2005; 18(9):484-490.

41. Johns LD. Nonthermal effects of therapeutic ultrasound: the frequency resonance hypothesis. *J Athl Train* 2002; 37(3):293-299.

42. McDonald WS, Nichter LS. Debridement of bacterial and particulate-contaminated wounds. *Ann Plast Surg* 1994; 33:142-7.

Normothermia

43. Abramson D, et al. Changes in blood flow, oxygen uptake and tissue temperature produced by the topical application of wet heat. *Arch Phys Med Rehabil* 1961; 42:305-317.

44. Wessman HC, Kottke FJ. The effect of indirect heating on peripheral blood flow, pulse rate, blood pressure and temperature. *Arch Phys Med Rehabil* 1967; 48:567-576.

45. Rabkin JM, Hunt TK. Local heat increases blood flow and oxygen tension in wounds. *Arch Surg* 1987; 122: 221-225.

46. Michlovitz, S. Thermal Agents in Rehabilitation, 2nd Ed. Philadelphia, PA.: FA Davis Co,1990. 140-141.

47. Kloth L, et al. Effects of a normothermic dressing on pressure ulcer healing. *Adv Skin Wound Care* March/April 2000; 13(2):69-74.

Ultraviolet Light

48. Price P, et al. The effect of a radiant heat dressing on pressure ulcers. *J Wound Care* 9: 203, 2000.

49. Conner-Kerr T, et al. The effects of ultraviolet radiation on antibiotic resistant bacteria in living tissue. (abstract). *Ostomy/Wound Manag* 45:84, 1999.

50. Conner-Kerr T, et al. The effects of ultraviolet radiation on antibiotic resistant bacteria in vitro. *Ostomy/Wound Manag* 44:50, 1998.

51. Sullivan PK, et al. The effects of UVC irradiation on group A streptococcus in vitro. *Ostomy/Wound Manag* 45:50; 1999.

REVIEW QUESTIONS

1.) When utilizing low frequency ultrasound for wound healing, the effect known as microstreaming causes:
   a. Increased circulation and fluid movement in close proximity to the cellular membranes
   b. Implosion of stable gas bubbles and destruction of tissues
   c. Antibacterial and antiviral effects at the cellular level

2.) When using high frequency ultrasound for wound healing, what are the anticipated effects during the remodeling phase of wound healing?
   a. Vasodilation, chemotaxis, and macrophage stimulation
   b. Stimulating fibroblasts and increasing wound contraction
   c. Increasing endothelial cell activity and releasing angiogenic factors
   d. Strengthening of scar tissue and increasing tissue elasticity

3.) Using pulsatile lavage with suction, a psi setting of ______ will result in tissue trauma and bacteria being driven into the tissues, potentially leading to infection?
   a. <4 psi
   b. 8 psi
   c. 10 psi
   d. > 15 psi

4.) Which modality has been demonstrated to remove excess edema fluid and cellular debris from interstices in/around the wound bed?
   a. Electrotherapy
   b. Hydrotherapy
   c. Negative Pressure Wound Therapy
   d. Ultrasound

5.) Which spectral band of ultraviolet light has been demonstrated to be ionizing, bactericidal and virucidal?
   a. UVA
   b. UVB
   c. UVC
   d. UVD

Answers: 1a, 2d, 3d, 4c, 5c.

NOTES

CHAPTER 36

Orthotics and Prosthetics in Wound Care

CHAPTER THIRTY-SIX OVERVIEW

NOTES

ORTHOTICS AND PROSTHETICS IN WOUND CARE

Gordon W. Bosker, Javier LaFontaine

INTRODUCTION

In the United States alone, it is estimated that over 17 million people are affected with diabetes with more than 12 million remaining undiagnosed. Of the total diabetic population, approximately 15% will develop foot ulcerations with 6% continuing on to some manner of foot or lower limb amputation. Such outcomes are frequently the consequence of repetitive or traumatic foot tissue injury in the presence of peripheral neuropathy (PN) and/or peripheral vascular disease (PVD), both conditions being closely associated with diabetes.

PN/PVD of the lower extremities, with its inherent lack of sensory feedback, may lead to seemingly subtle yet less-adaptive gait patterns that cause foot tissue impact and injury. Such tissue injury, if undetected, ignored or mismanaged, promotes the formation of ulcers. Neuropathic ulceration is highly identifiable by its characteristic very red base (granulation tissue) surrounded by white hyperkeratotic tissue (Figure 1).

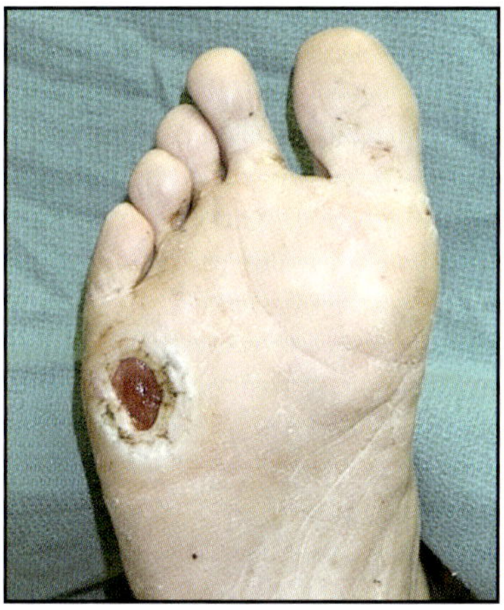

Figure 1. Showing formation of ulceration. Also note the dryness of the skin.

Foot ulcers can develop in any location of the foot. They are more common under the metatarsal heads, hallux, heel or other weight-bearing areas. Foot ulcers may also develop as a consequence of poor footwear fit creating undue pressures, frictions or irritants. The mechanism of injury is commonly described as moderate pressure with repetitive trauma. Offloading is the key for healing the neuropathic ulceration. Nonetheless, once ulceration occurs management usually falls into three stages: debridement of callus, eradication of infection, and reduction of weight bearing forces.

In terms of the PN/PVD ulcer and reduction of weight bearing forces, several acceptable modalities exist. These may include but not limited to extra-depth shoes with specific modifications, extra-depth shoes with inserts whether they are "off-the-shelf" or custom, total contact cast, or other types of off-loading orthoses.

However, when applying any type of orthosis or cast, one must be aware of the biomechanics of the gait cycle to accmplish the proper off-loading and protection of the ulcer site and foot while not generating other complications. One must remember that pathophysiologic alterations and adaptations of the foot will be progressively changing as PN/PVD continues to decrease the normal protection and gait function of the foot and ankle. So, understanding normal gait is a prerequisite to understanding the pathophysiologic alterations and adaptations that could occur with musculoskeletal and neurological disorders. While the next next section will focus on gait patterns associated with the foot and ankle, its concepts are also relevant to the knee and hip.

NORMAL GAIT PATTERNS

Requirements/Overview

Normal adult gait is a complex, efficient, biomechanical movement with feedback from visual, vestibular and proprioceptive systems. To better conceptualize normal gait and thereby comprehend the implications of deviations one must know:

a. the phase of a typical gait cycle that characterize the temporal features of normal and abnormal gait patterns;
b. the patterns and approximate magnitudes of the motion that occur at the major joints in order to relate a patient's available joint range of motion (ROM) to that needed for more efficient walking;
c. when muscle groups are active and how they function to control motion or propel the body forward. This allows one to predict and understand the deficits that occur from various forms of weakness and abnormal motor control;
d. how to systematically analyze a gait—this usually requires observation of both overall movement symmetry and pattern of trunk progression as well as detail observation of each joint throughout the gait cycle; and
e. how to report and describe one's finding in an effective and clear manner.

Phases of the Gait Cycle

Basic definitions

Initial contact: is an instantaneous point in time only and occurs the instant the foot of the leading lower limb touches the ground. Most of the motor function that occurs during initial contact is in preparation for the loading response phase that will follow. This phase represents the beginning of the stance phase.

Loading response: is the phase that occupies about 10% of the gait cycle and constitutes the period of initial double-limb support. During loading response, the foot comes in full contact with the floor, and body weight is fully transferred onto the stance limb.

Midstance: represents the first half of single support, which occurs from the 10% to 30% periods of the gait cycle. It begins when the contralateral foot leaves the ground and continues as the body weight travels along the length of the foot until it is aligned over the forefoot.

Terminal stance: constitutes the second half of single limb support. It begins with heel rise and ends when the contralateral foot contacts the ground. Terminal stance occurs from the 30% to 50% periods of the gait cycle. During this phase, body weight moves ahead of the forefoot. The term heel off (HO) is a descriptor useful in observational analysis and is the point during the stance phase when the heel leaves the ground.

Pre-swing: is the terminal double-limb support period and occupies the last 12% of stance phase, from 50% to 62%. It begins when the contralateral foot contacts the ground and ends with ipsilateral toe off. During this period, the stance limb is unloaded and body weight is transferred onto the contralateral limb.

Initial swing: begins the moment the foot leaves the ground and continues until maximum knee flexion occurs, when the swinging extremity is directly under the body and directly opposite the stance limb. It is a period of rapid acceleration of the swing leg coinciding with weight acceptance to mid-stance of the opposite limb. The initial one-third of the swing period, from the 62% to 75% periods of the gait cycle is spent in initial swing.

Mid-swing: occurs in the second third of the swing period, from the 75% to 85% periods of the gait cycle. Critical events include continued limb advancement and foot clearance. This phase begins following maximum knee flexion and ends when the tibia is in a vertical position.

Terminal swing: In the final phase of terminal swing from the 85% to 100% periods of the gait cycle, the tibia passes beyond perpendicular, and while the knee fully extends deceleration of the swing limb prepares for initial contact.

Stance Phase Events

As stated earlier the stance phase begins with initial contact of a limb, and progresses through pre-swing of that same foot. Within stance phase are several meaningful, temporal events: the point of application of the ground reaction force (GRF) is forced to move forward with each successive rocker, thus allowing the center of mass to move forward with it (Figure 2).

a. Initial response and loading response is otherwise known as the period of weight acceptance. It is the demand for immediate transfer

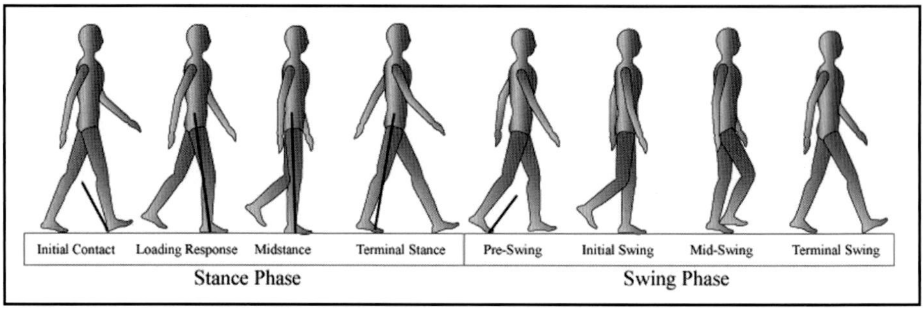

Figure 2. Showing the different phases of gait and the ground reaction forces that take place (GRF). The GRF represents the net effect of the mass and acceleration of the body as you push against the ground during walking. It can be conceptualized as a vertically directed force extending upward from the center of pressure (the point of force application) as shown for the different phases of the stance phase. At various times throughout the gait cycle it may pass either in front of or behind the joints of the lower extremity. This force creates moments (torques) about the joints that will want to force the joint to rotate. In this example, it shows the different GRF that may pass behind or in front of the ankle joint, which would create a moment wanting to plantarflex or dorsiflex the ankle. The lower extremity response is to activate the dorsiflexors or plantiflexors muscles that create forces and moments that oppose the effect of the GRF. The net effect depends on which moment is larger.

Different authors adopt different points of view about the force and moments though the emerging trend is to view gait events from the perspective of what the muscles are doing.

of body weight on to the limb as soon as it contacts the ground. This requires initial limb stability and shock absorption while simultaneously preserving the momentum of progression.

b. Midstance is a period of single support and balance as the opposite limb swings through. It is the time when the contralateral side is entering the swing period and the total body weight is exclusively supported on the stance limb. It accomplishes forward progression of body weight over the foot while maintaining stability. This is the single limb support and we must have stability to maintain proper gait.

c. Terminal stance and pre-swing: At pre-swing the knee flexes, ankle plantarflexes, first ray plantarflexes, first MPJ dorsiflexes. Inside the ankle subtalar inversion occurs which causes the axes of the talonavicular and calcaneocuboid to diverge. This locks the midtarsal joint in a relative plantar flexion (high arch). Then the foot has the intertarsal stability to support all of the body weight on the forefoot. Pre-swing usually coincides with termination of the opposite limb's swing and a period of double-support (both feet in contact with the ground) during which the stance leg prepares to swing forward.

Characteristics of Normal Gait

Temporal/spatial measures

a. Normal gait is symmetric—temporal, joint and force measures are not grossly different between limbs.

b. Stance phase lasts about 60%, swing about 40% and double support about 10% of the gait cycle.

c. Average adult self-selected walking speeds are about 80 meter/sec and remain fairly constant until age 60 when they gradually fall to around 60 meters/sec.
d. Average cadence is about 110 steps/min.
e. Stride length ranges from 1.28m for women and 1.46m for men.
f. Walking at the self selected speed requires peak muscle force generation of approximately 30–40% of maximal force. This corresponds to a score of 3+ on manual muscle testing (MMT).

Ground Reaction Forces (GRF), and Center of Pressure (COP) Patterns in Gait

When walking, you apply a force to the ground. Since force = mass x acceleration, the force you apply to the ground is the net result of your body mass being accelerated against both gravity and the work done by muscles as they speed up and slow down body segments. The ground reaction force (GRF) is the force the ground exerts against you and is simply equal in magnitude but opposite in direction to the force you apply to the ground. For example, consider the vertical GRF as it occurs during stance phase. In this case, the magnitude of the vertical GRF exceeds body weight at two points in the gait cycle. The first peak is reflective of weight acceptance as the body's downward motion and velocity is slowed (early stance). Next, the second peak (late stance) describes the acceleration of the body (especially the leg) upward in preparation for push-off (Figure 3).

It is very important that one know where the GRF is applied to the foot. This point of application is referred to as the center of pressure (COP) and its vector is directed toward the body's Center of Mass (COM), roughly several cm

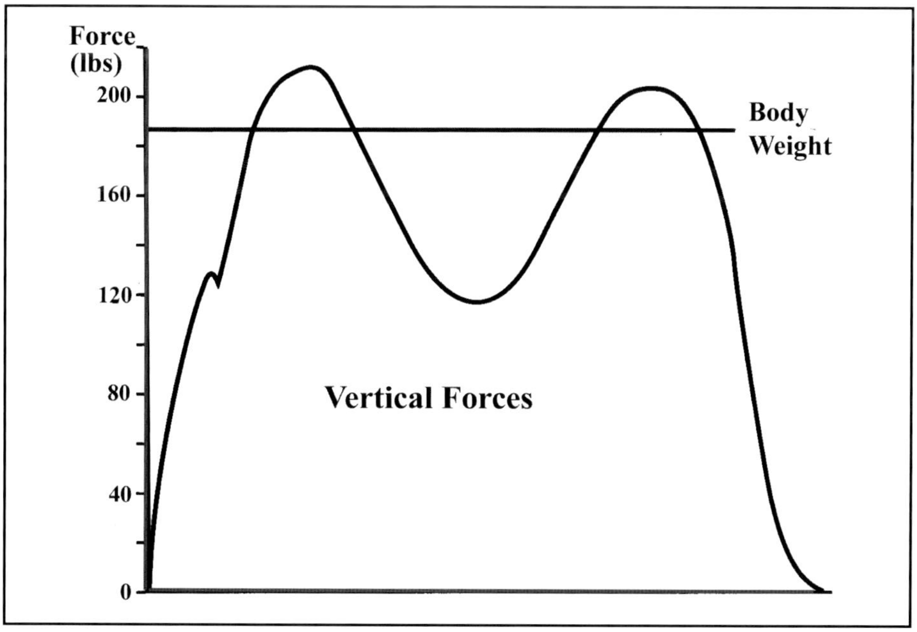

Figure 3. Showing the first and second peak of weight acceptance in a normal healthy adult.

anterior to the sacrum. As would be expected, there is a progressive displacement of the COP from the heel, along the lateral border of the foot to the medial forefoot as the gait cycle progresses from heel strike to push-off. As this force vector (COP) progresses, it may pass either in front of or behind the joints of the lower extremity. This force creates moments (torques) about the joints that will induce the joint to rotate. For example, as the GRF passes behind the ankle joint it creates a moment wanting to plantarflex the ankle. The lower extremity responds to this by activating the dorsiflexory muscles which will create forces and moments that oppose the effect of the GRF. The net effect depends on which moment is larger.

The Action of the Foot/Ankle During Normal Gait

The foot is in a neutral position at heel strike and then rapidly plantarflexes until foot flat occurs. The GRF vector passes from its COP location at the heel posterior to the ankle creating a tendency for the ankle to plantarflex (a dorsiflexion moment) To control and slow the rapid early stance plantarflexion, the dorsiflexory muscles are active but because the GRF induced moment is larger, they undergo an eccentric contraction. The ankle then progressively dorsiflexes during midstance as the tibia and trunk advance forward over the foot. The ankle plantarflexor muscles become active at this time, functioning to control the forward advancement of the tibia. The plantarflexors are eccentrically contracting.

It is during midstance that the ankle requires its greatest amount of dorsiflexion range (~10°). Limited ankle dorsiflexion ROM makes it difficult to advance the tibia and trunk forward during stance. As terminal stance phase is reached, the heel rises and the ankle enters a phase of rapid plantarflexion. Plantarflexion muscle activity peaks during late stance as they change their function from one of controlling midstance ankle rotation to one of rapid concentric contraction and energy generation to accelerate the limb forward into stance.

Weakness of the plantarflexor muscles manifest themselves as excessive ankle plantarflexion during midstance, a shortened step length on the contralateral side (because the trunk can not advance forward over the weak leg safely) and a reduced walking speed. The ankle plantarflexors are the single biggest generators of energy during the gait cycle. Contrary to popular belief, during push-off they actually have a negligible effect on trunk energy. Essentially all of the plantarflexor muscle push-off work is used to accelerate the limb forward so that swing phase can be completed.

Even in normal gait, the magnitude of the pressures and shears experienced at the heel and across the metatarsal heads are relatively high. Hence, one can comprehend the predisposition for breakdown over these areas given a neuropathic foot with its potentially altered foot biomechanics and sensory loss that are confounded by the occurrence of repetitive and concentrated pressures about boney prominences (Figure 4).

Many of the gait abnormalities that result from contracture and weakness reflect more the change in the location of the COP rather than significant changes in the magnitude of the GRFs. Likewise most of the interventions we use, especially upper extremity (UE) walking aids, ankle foot orthosis (AFOs), and custom inserts largely work by altering the position of or the manner in which the COP advances.

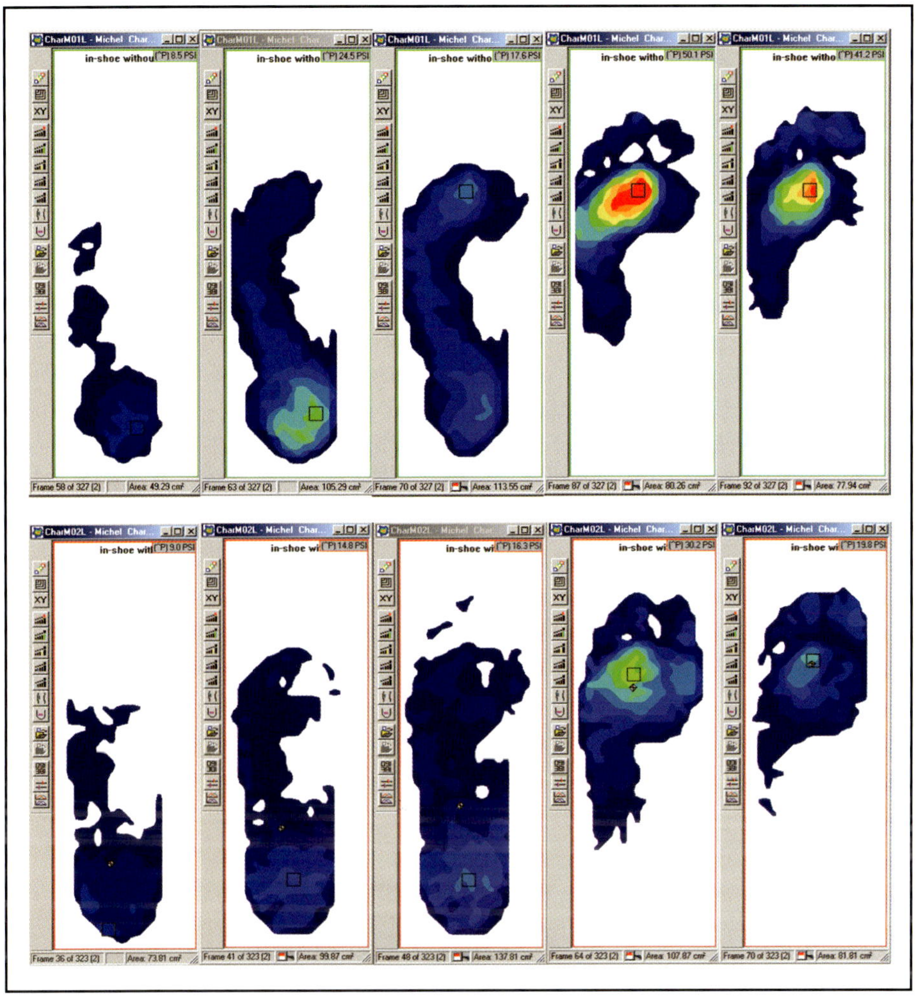

Figure 4. FSCAN images of foot in shoe during gait cycle—initial contact to pressing without a custom molded insert.

PREVENTIVE / PROTECTIVE MANAGEMENT

Shoes

Approximately half of diabetes-related amputations have been attributed to poorly fitting footwear. To protect the foot from the repetitive or undue GRF's, a proper shoe should be:

a. measured for foot width and length;
b. chosen after considering any foot deformities and their implications; and
c. fitted by a qualified specialist.

If the deformities are too extreme for off-the-shelf shoes then custom molded shoes should be considered—especially in the case of wound prevention, protection or healing. Because of an insensate foot a diabetic patient will wear a shoe that is actually too tight, inadvertently causing wounds on the medial, lateral or dorsal side of the foot. Given a neuropathic foot, many patients declare some sense of improved proprioception with a tightly fitted shoe and will not complain of expected pain or discomfort from the shoe. This presents a challenging clinical scenario in which the patient may determine that a shoe is too large when the proper shoe is fitted to the patient on the basis of foot shape and size, rather than a sense of snug "containment." Footwear should provide the following protective benefits:

a. high, wide toe box—sufficiently high and wide space in the toe area to accommodate bunions, claw toes, hammer toes, mallet toes, ulceration, etc;
b. extra depth with removable insoles for fitting flexibility and the option, if necessary, to insert orthotics and achieve total contact of the foot's plantar surface;
c. shock absorbing soles to reduce impact shock;
d. Lycra type material or heat moldable for toe box area to accommodate toe deformities such as bunions, claw toes, hammer toes, mallet toes, ulceration, etc (Figure 5);
e. rocker soles designed to reduce pressure on the plantar surface of the metatarsal area and toe area (Figure 6);
f. long medial heel counter to support the heel and medial arch; and
g. the more proximal the partial foot amputation the higher the shoe.

Shoe manufactures are progressively improving the style of extra depth shoes, which helps the patient to become more compliant in their wear.

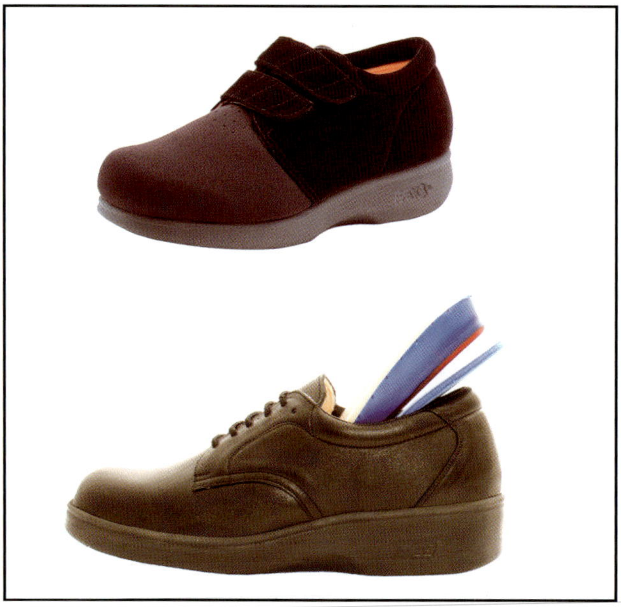

Figure 5. Top shoe shown could be used for hammer or claw toes (Lycra top). Bottom shoe shows inserts that come with shoe. In both extra depth shoes the inserts could be replaced with custom molded inserts.

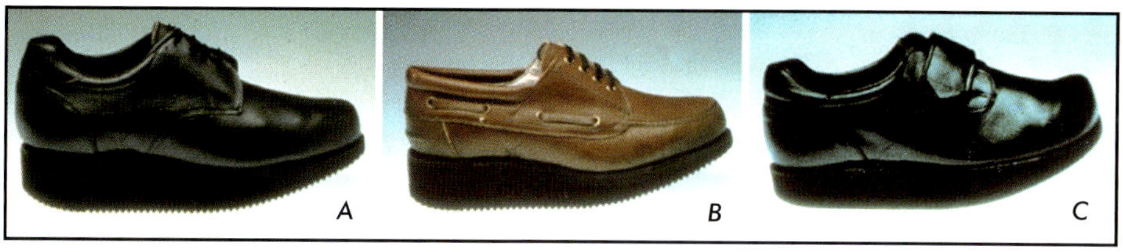

Figure 6 (A–C). Different Rockers added to the sole of the shoe will assist in healing of ulcers and other complications.
A. This type of rocker sole is shaped with a more severe angle at both the heel and toe. It is intended to aid propulsion at toe-off, decrease heel-strike forces on the calcaneus and decrease the need for ankle motion.
B. The toe rocker angle is only at the toe with the midstance extending to the back end of the sole. This rocker sole increases weight bearing proximal to the metatarsal heads, provides a stable midstance, and reduces the need for toes dorsiflexion on toe-off.
C. Shaped with a rocker angle at the toe and has a negative heel, this rocker sole positions the heel lower than or even with ball of the foot when the patient is standing. The negative heel rocker sole can accommodate a foot that is fixed in dorsiflexion and shift forefoot pressure to the hindfoot and midfoot.

Inserts

Inserts are made from several different types of material and can be either off-the-shelf, customized (heat molded to the foot) or custom molded to a cast of the foot. Their purpose is to relieve areas of excessive plantar pressure, reduce shock, reduce shear, accommodate deformities, stabilize and support deformities or control joint motion of the foot (Figure 7).

Custom molded inserts are made from a foot impression foam block, a computer aided design system, or a cast of the foot. First a "negative" mold of the foot is derived from impressions or casts of the foot, and then poured with plaster or, in the case of computer-aided systems, imported as computer files. The positive model is then modified for any correction or relief. These types of insert usually consist of soft and medium density plastizote with a third layer of shock absorbance material with a custom arch support.

Off the shelf inserts for the diabetic usually consist of a top layer of soft or medium density plastizote, a middle layer for shock absorbance, and an optional bottom or third layer to improve the longevity of the insert. As a consequence of compression and heat during wear, the plastizote will conform to the shape of the plantar surface of the foot. For this reason, it is suggested to have at least three sets of inserts so while one is being worn the other is rebounding from wear. The custom molded or off-the-shelf inserts can be pulled from the shoe, inspected briefly, evaluated, and modified as necessary to off-load any high pressure or wound areas.

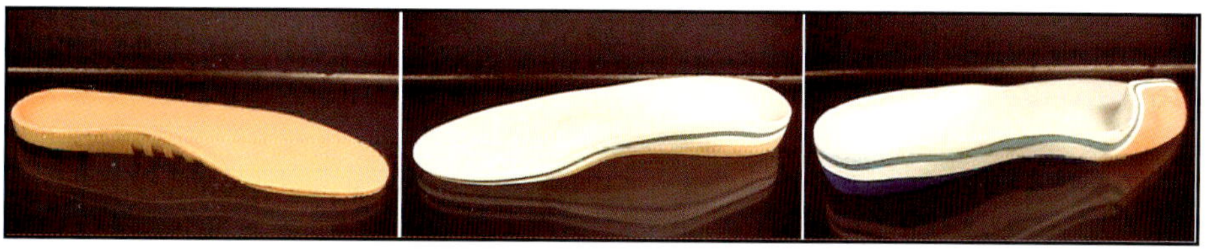

Figure 7. Inserts ranging from off-the-shelf (left) to custom (center) and custom with toe filler (right).

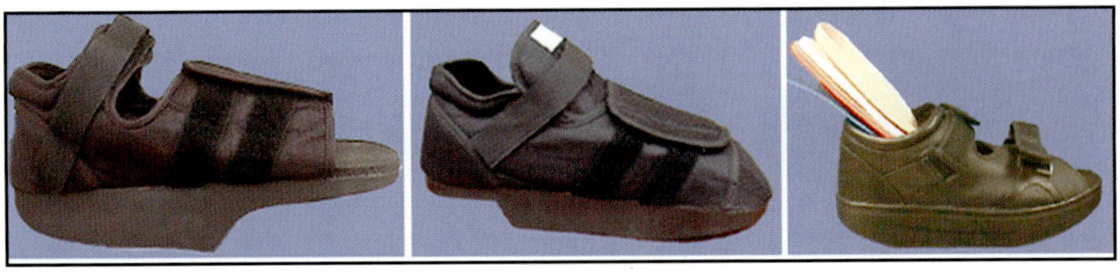

Figure 8. Showing half shoes (left) and Wound Care Shoe (center). Note the depth of inserts in Wound Care Shoe (right). This allows for a custom molded insert to be placed in the shoe.

Off Loading Shoes

The most common half shoes were specifically designed for the treatment of forefoot ulceration and only provide support under the rear and mid-foot—the IPOS and DARCO half shoes. Other half shoes have been designed for treatment of heel ulceration and provide support under the front and mid-foot (Figure 8).

The Integrated Prosthetic and Orthotic System (IPOS, Niagara Falls, New York) half shoe was formally referred to as the Barouk Post-Op shoe and has fairly recently been modified to increase durability. The shoe is designed with a 10° dorsiflexion incline decreasing pressures of the metatarsal heads and digits during weight-bearing phases of the gait cycle stance. This particular shoe also comes with an optional protective shield.

The DARCO half shoe (Darco International, Huntington, West Virginia), as the IPOS shoe, is specifically designed to protect the forefoot. The unique designs makes these shoes a natural for the treatment of diabetic forefoot ulcerations and serves as an outstanding post-op shoe, appropriate for use after surgeries to correct hallux valgus, hammer toes, Tailor's bunions and other osteotomies with or without pins.

The Wound Care Shoe System™ (Darco International, Huntington, West Virginia), is recommended for the treatment of open and closed ulcerations as well as other foot conditions requiring redistribution of weight and pressure about specific areas. The circumferential counter of the shoe forms a deep pocket in the sole to permit the use of a variety of insoles under the ulceration or area of pressure. The insole material is placed below the level of the top of

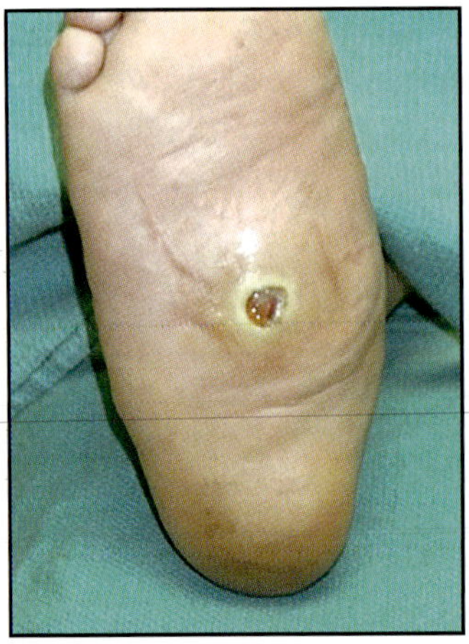

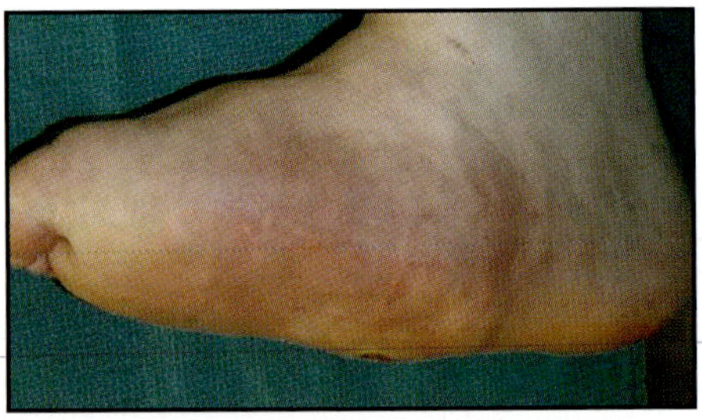

Figure 9. Charcot's foot showing ulceration and rocker type foot with midfoot being lowest point.

the circumferential counter, providing greater stability for the foot by preventing the layered insoles from shifting within the shoe.

Total Contact Cast and the Charcot Restraint Orthotic Walker (CROW)

Charcot neuroarthropathy is one of the most devastating complications of diabetes. In most cases, the collapse of the mid-foot leads to a rocker bottom deformity, thereby concentrating the entire body weight on a small area of the foot's plantar surface. (Figure 9) Charcot's foot is frequently misdiagnosed as a bone infection since there is no definitive diagnostic test that confirms its presence. Nonetheless, certain indicative warning signs exist that should be noted and followed:

a. localized swelling;
b. pain although patient is neuropathic;
c. temperature difference >4° F (2.2°C) between the feet; and
d. erythema in the absence of an open wound.

In the presence of such clinical signs, the foot should be immobilized and non-weight bearing until signs of healing becomes apparent. In protecting Charcot's foot there are two devices utilized successfully—the Total Contact Cast (TCC) and the Charcot's Restraint Orthotic Walker (CROW).

The TCC is considered to be the gold standard for several reasons (Figure 10):

a. it allows complete rest of the foot by forcing compliance;
b. it alters temporal gait patterns (decreases cadence, shortens stride length, reduces activity) thereby reducing the magnitude and duration of plantar pressures while the patient remains mobile;
c. it protects the foot from trauma and infection;
d. it controls edema which can often impede healing; and
e. it has a 70%–100% proven success history.

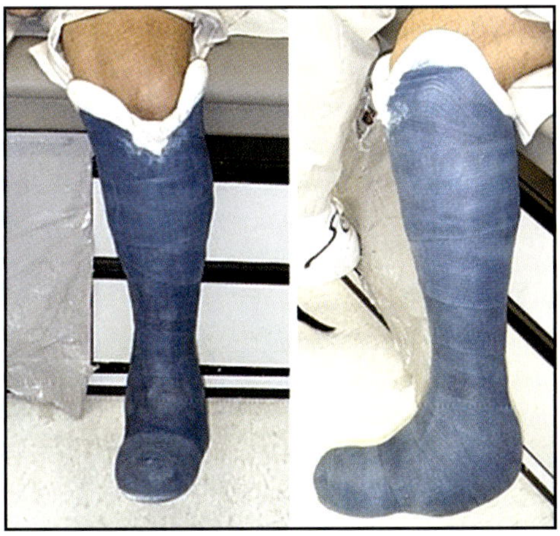

Figure 10. Total Contact Cast—the gold standard.

Nonetheless, there are distinct limitations and disadvantages of the TCC to include:

a. difficulty in proper fitting;
b. inability to inspect the wound on a daily basis;
c. certain wound healing modalities that require daily applications cannot be employed;
d. patient comfort—it is a cast, heavy & bulky; and
e. need for frequent cast changes (usually weekly).

Alternatively, the CROW orthosis or neuropathic walker is an ankle-foot-orthosis (Figure 11). Once swelling and erythema resolve and radiographic stability is achieved or if lower extremity edema is not controlled by the TCC, use of the CROW orthosis is highly applicable.

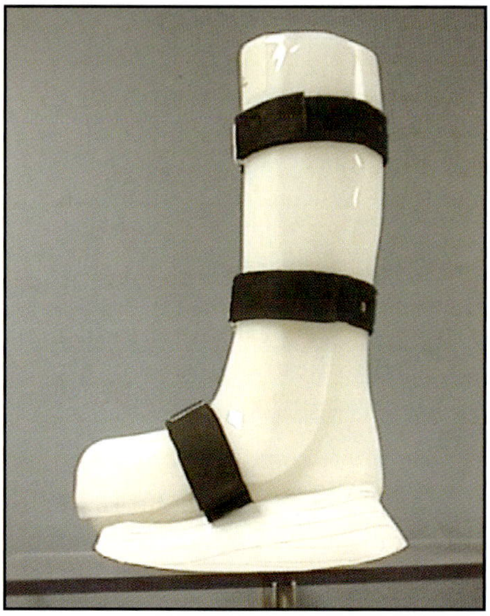

Figure 11. CROW orthosis.

The CROW orthosis is custom made and acts similarly to the TCC. It is not unusual for this orthosis to be used for six months to two years or until a stable foot is obtained. Conveniently, the CROW is easily removed for wound inspections, showers and sleeping, achieving high patient satisfaction relative to the TCC. However, the "ease of removal" is actually somewhat of a disadvantage by removing the "forced compliance" element associated with the TCC.

Removable Cast Walkers

Because of some of the inherent disadvantages/limitations associated with the TCC or CROW, some physicians prefer using off-the-shelf removable cast walker or cam walkers such as the DH Walker (Figure 12).

The DH Pressure Relief Walker (Royce Medical Corp, Camarillo, California), is a modified cast walker device that consists of an insole with small hexagonal foam columns that can be removed to provide pressure relief for an ulcer. Results from a gait study (Figure 13) completed at the University of

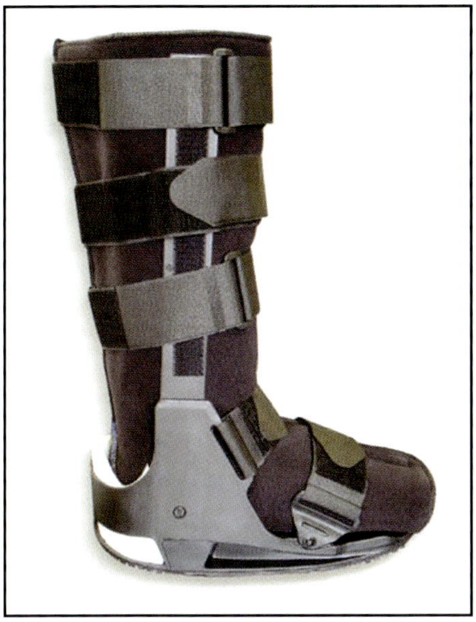

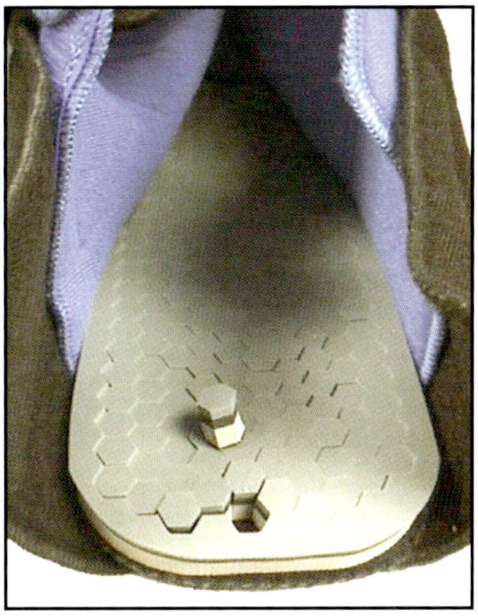

Figure 12. DH Walker and close-up of the hexagon padding that can be removed under ulcerated area.

Texas Health Science Center at San Antonio suggested that the cast walker was as effective as the total contact casts in reducing peak plantar pressure with great-toe ulcers and more effective for ulcers located under the ball of the foot. Again, as with the CROW, the main disadvantage of a removable cast walker is the loss of the "force compliance" element.

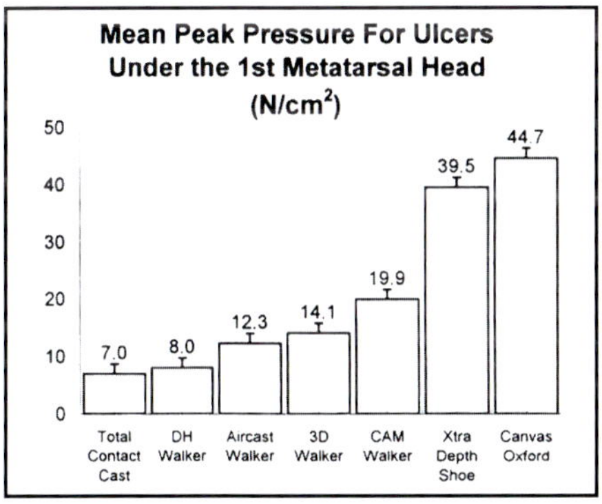

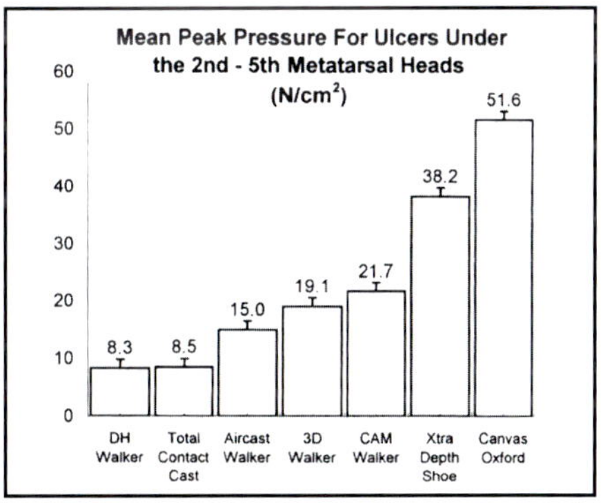

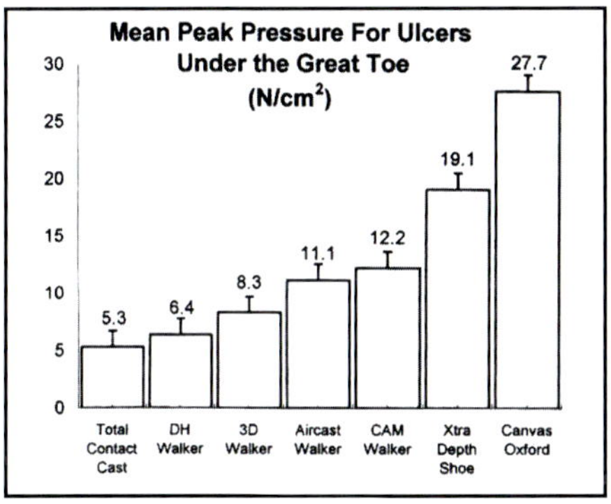

Figure 13. Research results of TCC vs. DH Walker and other devices showing that the DH Walker has less peak pressure on the 2nd to 5th metatarsal heads.

Armstrong and colleagues describe (8) an "instant total contact cast" by using a removable cast walker and plaster. Basically, the removable cast walker is applied and then covered with 2–3 layers of plaster. The physician then has an offloading device that has the same capability as the TCC but enjoys the ease of application of the cast walker and forces compliance in the patient.

It is suggested that a key element of the efficacy of the TCC, CROW, and Removable Cast Walker devices is the fact that they limit the function of the plantarflexory muscle groups at the ankle. Locking of the ankle allows a reduction of forefoot pressures and can minimize the pathologic influence of equinus. An additional noted mechanism of action for these devices is the transfer of weight bearing pressures from the device directly onto the leg. The shape of these devices maximizes the ability to offload pressures onto the leg by conforming to the calf and leg muscles.

Partial Foot Amputations

Ray resections, transmetatarsal and toe amputations

Toe amputations, ray resections, and transmetatarsal amputations are highly functional amputations that require minimal prosthetic/orthotic intervention. Accommodative shoes with custom insoles, arch supports and toe fillers are usually adequate to protect and/or help to relieve pressure of the foot. More active individuals with a transmetatarsal amputation may benefit from orthotic modifications that better substitute for the lost anterior foot lever arm. Options include the addition of carbon fiber or spring steel sole shanks, rocker soles, or short ankle foot orthosis.

Tarsal-metatarsal and transtarsal amputations

Partial foot amputations at the tarsal-metatarsal and transtarsal levels (e.g. Lisfranc, Chopart) are relatively uncommon and have historically been associated with equinovarus contracture of the hindfoot increasing the likelihood of skin breakdown over the plantar surface of the foot (Figure14). However, improved surgical techniques that include Achilles tendon lengthening/resection and anterior tibialis and peroneus tendon transfers have reduced equinovarus deformities to result in a functional and useful amputation level. Prosthetic/orthotic devices for the individual with a proximal

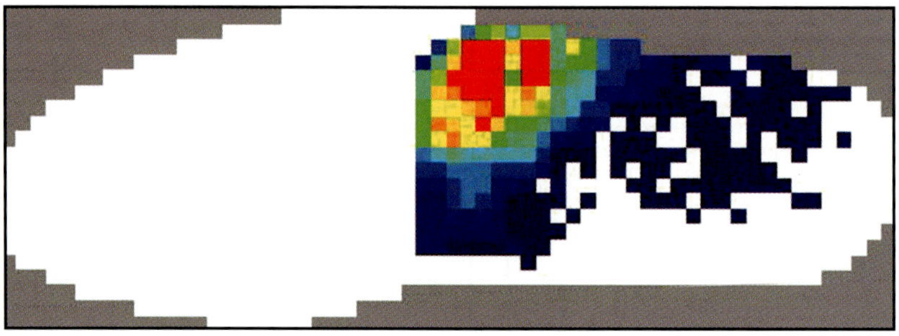

Figure 14. FSCAN showing peak pressure on partial foot amputation trans-metatarsal and possible breakdown.

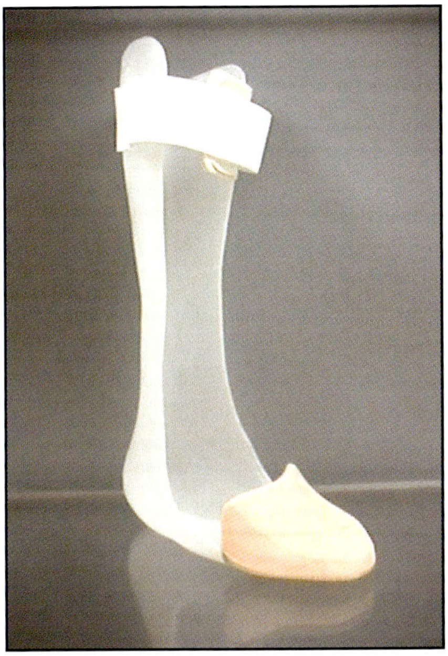

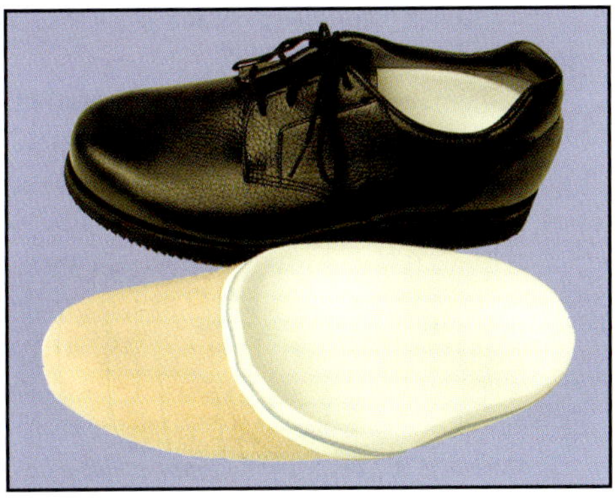

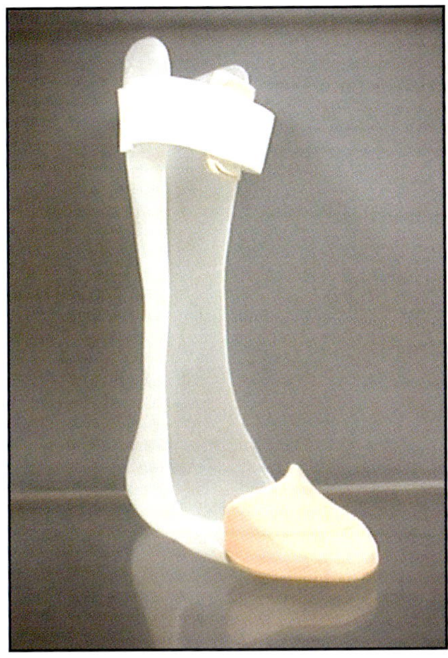

Figure 15. Ankle Foot Orthosis (AFO) with toe filler (left) and shoe with custom insert with toe filler (right).

partial foot amputation need to supply medial-lateral stabilization of the hindfoot and substitute for the lost forefoot lever. Options include

a. an extra depth shoe with toe filler, steel shank and rocker bottom modifications (Figure 15);

b. custom posterior leaf-spring ankle foot orthosis with toe filler; or

c. a custom prosthetic foot with a self-suspending rear opening split socket.

A major advantage of all partial foot amputations is the ability to be fully end bearing, allowing ambulation without any devices.

CONCLUSION

These and many more offloading techniques are available for management of diabetic neuropathic ulcerations, but other variables must be considered in any attempt to facilitate the healing of the neuropathic ulcer, such as patient acceptance, cost, compliance and accessibility. It has become very important to utilize a team approach in managing the diabetic patient. Certainly, the key factor to ensure proper healing and improvement is both patient and physician education. As specialists and clinicians, we have all become educators continually striving to improve health care and research.

In this capacity we understand the significance and necessity of patient monitoring and follow-up care both as part of treatment and preventive care. Armed with a cadre of applications, tools and devices, individualized care is feasible and beneficial. Sadly, the most disappointing factor and challenging barrier to a good outcome is the patient's noncompliance to prescribed care and footwear.

REFERENCES

1. Perry J. Gait Analysis—Normal and Pathological Function, Thorofare, NJ:Slack Inc, 1992.
2. Mundermann A, Stefanyshyn. Wakeling JM, Nigg BM, et al. Foot orthoses affect frequency components of muscle activity in the lower extremity, Apr Gait & Posture. 2006; 23(3):295-302
3. Reiber GE, Smith DG, Wallace C, et al, Effect of therapeutic footwear on foot reulceration in patients with diabetes – a randomized controlled trial. *JAMA* 2002; 287:2552-2558.
4. Burns J. Crosbie J. Ouvrier R. Effective orthotic therapy for the painful cavus foot: a randomized controlled trial. *J Am Podiatr Med Assoc* 2006 May-Jun; 96(3):205-11
5. Margan JM, Biehl WC 3rd, Wagner FW Jr., Management of neuropathic arthropathy with the Charcot Restraint Orthotic Walker. *Clin Orthoop* 1993 Nov; (296):58-63.
6. Mueller MJ, Lott DJ, Hastings MK, et al. Efficacy and mechanism of orthotic devices to unload metatarsal heads in people with diabetes and a history of plantar ulcers. *Physical Therapy* 2006 Jun; 86(6):833-42.
7. McGuire JB. Pressure redistribution strategies for the diabetic or at-risk foot: Part II. Review] [12 refs] - *Advances in Skin & Wound Care* 2006 Jun; 19(5):270-277.
8. Armstrong DG, Stacpoole-Shea S. Total contact casts and removable cast walkers–mitigation of plantar heel pressure. *J Am Podiatr Med Assoc* 1999 Jan; 89(1):50-53.
9. Boike AM, Hall JO, A practical guide for examining and treating the diabetic foot – Cleveland Clinic. *J Med* 2002 Apr; 69(4):342-348.
10. Leibner ED, Brodsky JW, Pollo FE. et al. Unloading mechanism in the total contact cast. *Foot & Ankle International.*, 2006 Apr; 27(4):281-5.
11. Armstrong DG, Nguyen HC, Lavery LA, et al. Off-loading the diabetic foot wound: A randomized clinical trial. *Diabetes Care* 2001 Jun; 24(6):1019-1022.

REVIEW QUESTIONS

1.) During the gait cycle, the body weight is fully transferred onto the leading limb during:
  a. Initial contact
  b. Loading response
  c. Midstance
  d. Terminal stance

2.) Functional tasks of gait include:
  a. Loading response, single limb support and foot clearance
  b. Weight acceptance, single limb support, and foot clearance
  c. Weight acceptance, single limb support, and swing limb advancement
  d. Loading response, midstance, swing limb advancement

3.) Foot ulcers only develop in the metatarsal heads, hallux, heel or other weight-bearing areas
  a. True
  b. False

4.) It is recommended to give a diabetic patient three pair of inserts during the initial fitting.
  a. True
  b. False

5.) Practitioners are using the removable cast walker as an "instant total contact cast."
  a. True
  b. False

Answers: 1b, 2c, 3b, 4a, 5a.

NOTES

CHAPTER 37

Modern Wound Dressings-Principles, Form and Function

CHAPTER THIRTY-SEVEN OVERVIEW

NOTES

Modern Wound Dressings-Principles, Form and Function

Valerie Larson-Lohr, Cynthia A. Fleck

HISTORICAL ROLE OF DRESSINGS

The use of dressings in wound management can be traced back to the Egyptians. In 1862, a papyrus, dating back to 3000–2500 BC, was discovered by American Egyptologist Edwin Smith. When the papyrus was finally translated in 1930, a variety of dressings were recorded. The dressings included grease, resin, honey, lint, and fresh meat. Wounds were closed by the use of linen strips to which sticky gum had been applied. Antiseptics were made from green copper pigment and chyrsoedla were used in open wounds.

From 25 BC to 37 AD, Roman writer Celsus wrote extensively on medicine. He was the first to describe rubor, tumor, calor, and dolor (redness, swelling, heat, and pain) as cardinal symptoms of infection. Celsus advocated the removal of foreign bodies before closure and expected the wound to become purulent.

Galen (129–200 AD) was a Greek surgeon who tended gladiators in Pergamun. He is famous for his "laudable pus" theory. Galen advocated that wounds needed to become infected and form pus before healing would ensue. As a result, clean uninfected wounds were inoculated with a variety of substances to induce infection. This theory persisted for more than a thousand years (1).

Renaissance French physician, Dr. Ambrose Paré followed the theory of his times and used boiling oils as cautery for amputation of limbs and wounds. During a great battle he ran out of boiling oils used to treat the soldiers. Dr. Paré began applying egg yolks, oil of roses, and turpentine. At the conclusion of the battle, he found the soldiers to whom the egg yolk mixture had been applied were making better progress than those soldiers that had boiling oil applied to their wounds. Dr. Paré began to question the theory of "laudable pus" and changed his practice (2).

During World War I, the use of topical antiseptics such as Dakins, iodine, carbolic acid, and mercury was used to prevent infection in battlefield wounds. British soldiers were advised to carry iodine and immediately apply it to gunshot wounds. Unfortunately, many developed dermatitis as a result of indiscriminate use. It was also in this era a dressing called *tulle gras* was developed by Lumiere. This was gauze that had been impregnated with paraffin (3).

Through World War I, the task of changing dressings was in the realm of physicians and medical students. In the 1930s, the changing of dressings was given over to experienced nurses and became recognized as a nursing task. For the next 40–50 years the mainstay of wound coverings were gauze, cotton wool pads, impregnated gauze, absorbent cotton, and adhesive pads. The 1960s were the start of a change in dressings and the philosophy of their use.

CHANGING PHILOSOPHY

Early work in the 1960s started to define the idea of moist wound care and the benefit in optimizing wound healing. The concept of moist wound care began to receive serious consideration in the late 1970s and 1980s. Prior to this time, drying of the wound was accomplished by several mechanisms. The use of betadine as a drying agent, heat lamps, wet-to-dry dressings, and leaving the open wound exposed to air (4). Transparent film dressings and hydrocolloids were the first widely used dressings that addressed moisture retention. Throughout the 1980s and early 1990s there was an explosion in the realm of dressing products. Alginates, hydrogels, and foams appeared on the market in a wide variety of products. The concept of passive dressings began to change. Dressings were becoming active in their role to change the wound milieu in the healing process. The advent of growth factors and other biosynthetics such as collagen began the movement to an interactive dressing.

Today, research and development is being focused at the cellular level. Interactions of the cellular components within the chronic wound environment and how interactive dressings can alter the wound milieu is putting dressing technology on the cutting edge. What is next may be limited only by our understanding of how the body changes from a normal healing environment to a chronic wound environment, our technological ability to create products, and our imagination on how to get there.

DRESSING CATEGORIES

For more than two decades we have taught practitioners to learn categories of dressings in order to understand how they work and when to use them (Table 1). The classic categories are gauze, films, alginates, foam, hydrogels, hydrocolloid, and composite dressings. Today, there is such an expanse of dressing products that the seven classic categories no longer are adequate. In order to embrace the new dressings, an eighth category was created called interactive dressings.

Hand-in-hand with dressing selection is the question of frequency of dressing change. The frequency of a dressing change will first and foremost be based on sound clinical judgment. If the dressing is soiled,

TABLE 1. DRESSING CATAGORIES

Category	Advantages/Disadvantage	Examples	
Gauze Mechanically debride Permeable to gases Fills dead space Economical Readily available Absorptive	Can damage granulation tissue on removal May dehydrate the wound Permeable to fluid and bacteria May require more frequent dressing changes	Kerlix Kling Nu-Gauze Sof-wick Tendersorb Mirasorb	
Impregnated Gauze Less adherent to wound bed May keep wound moist	Requires secondary dressing Less absorptive than plain gauze	Xeroform Vaseline gauze	Adaptic DermAssist
Films Semipermeable Retain moisture Waterproof Allow wound visualization	Do not use on infected wounds May tear fragile skin May dislodge in high friction areas	Bioclusive Flexfilm Tegaderm	Opsite Polyskin II Cutifilm
Hydrocolloids Impermeable to bacteria Facilitates autolytic debridement Conformable Water resistant Self adhesive Reduces pain Can be used under compression dressings	Can not be used in moderate to heavy exudate Do not use on infected wounds Softens and looses shape with heat and friction Caution if there is fragile skin surrounding wound	Duoderm Replicare Restore	Tegasorb Cutinova
Hydrogels Soothing and reduces pain Rehydrates wound Extends period time between dressing changes Can fill dead space Comes in amorphous gels, sheets, freeze dry forms	Requires secondary dressing Sheets may be difficult to secure Can cause periwound maceration minimal absorption	NU-GEL Curasol Safe-gel Carrasyn	Hypergel Gentell Vigilon Cearsite
Foams Highly absorption Non-adherent Conformable Protects wound and periwound against trauma Thermal insulation Can be used under compression dressing	May require secondary dressing May macerate wound edge if dressing becomes saturated Not effective for wounds with dry eschar	Allevyn Flexan	Lyofoam PolyMem
Alginates Form moist gel in wound Highly absorptive Fills dead space Controls heavy exudate	Can not be used in dry wounds or wounds with minimal exudate Can dehydrate wound bed Reports of burning sensation on application with certain products Requires secondary dressing	Sorbsan Kaltostat Curasorb Algisite	Tegagen HG AlgiDERM Seasorb Melgisorb
Composite Combines 2 or more physically distinct products for better outcomes	Can be expensive Provider must have good understanding of properties of dressing Generally requires intact skin border for anchoring dressing	Fibrocol (collagen & alginate) Versiva (foam & hydrofiber)	Tielle (foam & polyurethane covering) Safe-Gel (hydrogel & alginate)
Biologics & Biosynthetics Combats bioburden and superficial infection	Wide variety, need to look at effectiveness and appropriate use	Silverlon Silver Cel Aquacel AG SIlvaSorb	Argales Acticoat Cadexomer Iodine AMD
Collagen Available in sheets, gels, particles. Stimulate and recruit specific cells to enhance wound healing	Require secondary dressing	Medifil particles/pads BGC Matrix Celerate Gel & powder	Fibrocol Oasis Promogram

loose, slipping or curling at the edges it is obvious that a dressing change is needed. If there is accumulation of fluid and debris that saturates the dressing, it will need to be changed. If infection is present, there may be a need for increased frequency of dressing change. All dressing products come from the manufacturer with recommendations for frequency of change or how long a particular dressing is expected to maintain its action. These recommendations should be used as guidelines.

Gauze Dressings (Figure 1)

Gauze dressings are dry woven or non-woven sponges and wraps with varying degrees of absorbency, based on design. Fabric composition may include cotton, polyester or rayon. They are available as sterile or nonsterile, in bulk, and with or without adhesive border. The gauze may be impregnated with other products.

Transparent Films (Figure 2)

Thought to be the very first advanced wound care dressing (5), transparent films are polymer membranes of varying thickness with adhesive coatings on one side only to allow adherence to the skin. These dressings are impermeable to liquid and microbes but permeable to moisture vapor and atmospheric gases like oxygen. Visualization is easy since you can see the wound through the dressing. They are comfortable to wear because they can stay firmly on the skin for an extended period of time making them both an excellent secondary dressing for long wear time as well as a good primary dressing for lacerations, skin tears, and I.V. sites. Other varieties offer an island configuration with a soaker pad of non-adherent gauze, alginate pad or other component. Films have been shown to have a lower overall infection rates associated with their use than traditional gauze dressings (6). It is important to select the correct dressing size to allow for approximately 1-inch of dressing contacting the intact periwound skin. To remove, gently pull up just the edge of the dressing and pull/stretch the dressing at a parallel angle to the skin, breaking the seal. Do not pull straight up as this can cause damage to the epidermis.

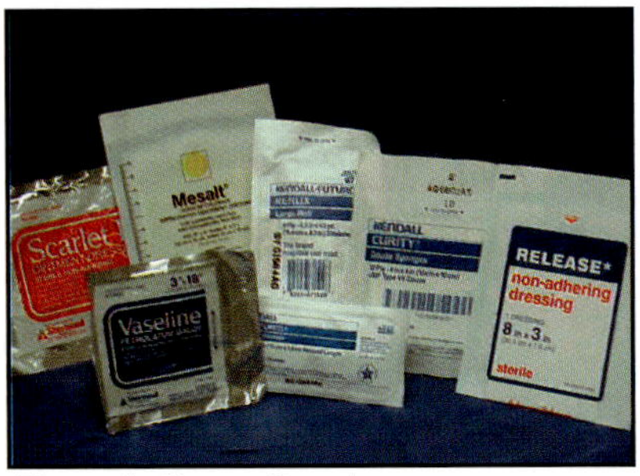

Figure 1. Gauze Dressings

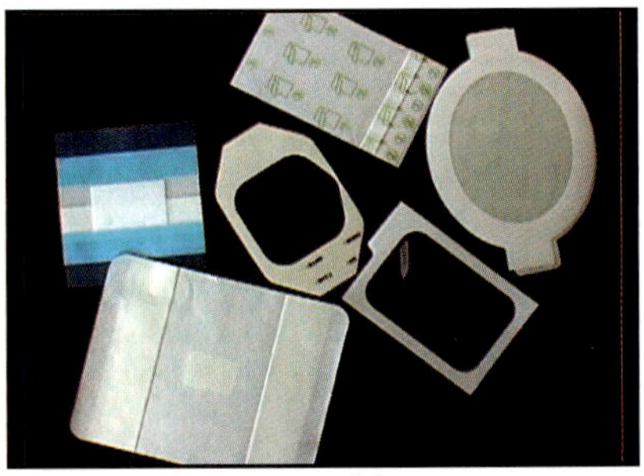

Figure 2. Transparent Films

Alginates (Figure 3)

Calcium-alginate, calcium-sodium-alginate, and collagen alginate dressings are natural fiber dressings derived from processed seaweed. These dressings are highly absorbent and conform readily to wounds of various shapes and sizes. The chemical reaction between the dressings and the wound

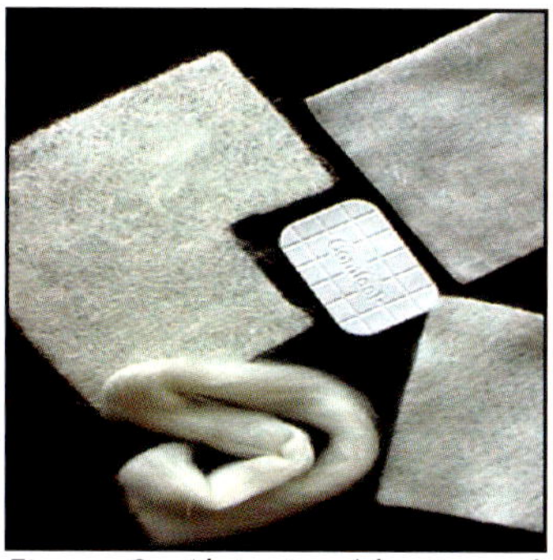

Figure 3. Alginates (sheets and ropes)

exudate creates a gel-like substance. The gel in turn assists in maintaining a moist wound-healing environment. An alginate can absorb up to 20 times its weight. Most alginates come in both sheet and rope form. Because alginate dressings are very porous and have no adhesive properties, secondary dressings must be used to secure them (7).

Hydrogels (Figures 4 and 5)

By far one of the most versatile dressings on the market, hydrogels are primarily water and/or glycerin in composition. They are three-dimensional networks of hydrophilic polymers prepared from materials such as gelatin, polysaccharides, cross-linked polyacrylamide polymers, polyelectrolyte complexes and polymers or copolymers derived from methacrylate esters (8). Their function depends on their form, for instance amorphous (literally meaning "without form") hydrogels donate moisture to the wound and offer gentle application and removal. This type also provides a good option for autolytic debridement and substitution for moist gauze. Additionally, some amorphous hydrogels additionally have the sophisticated capability to absorb and/or donate, depending on the wound's needs. Other forms include impregnated dressings such as gauze and sheet, strand or semi occlusive varieties. The latter offers soothing, cooling relief and gentle healing to wounds such as skin tears (8–10). These dressings can and should be cut to fit the wound.

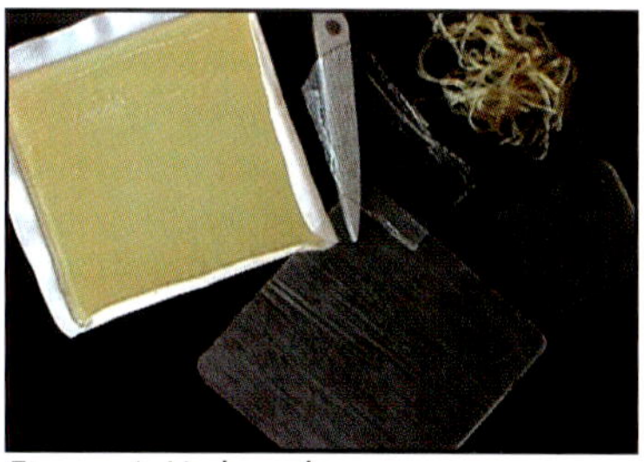

Figure 4. Hydrogels

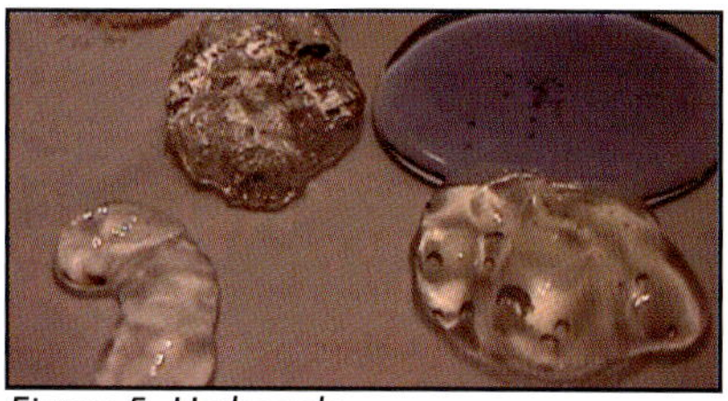

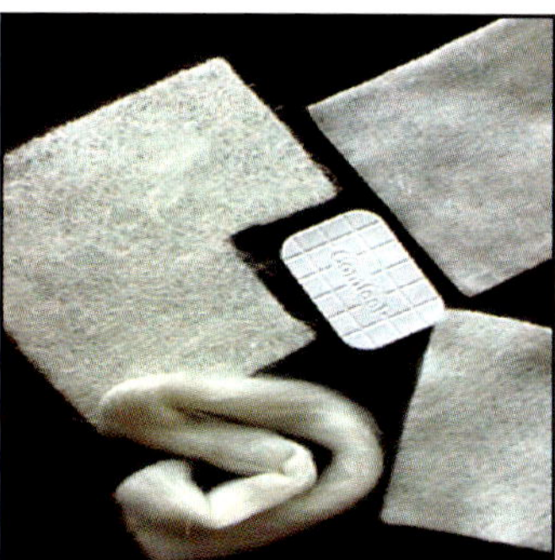

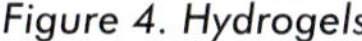

Figure 5. Hydrogels

Hydrocolloids (Figure 6)

One of the initial advanced wound care dressings to come to market (5), hydrocolloids are occlusive and semi occlusive dressings composed of carboxymethylcellulose, pectin, or gelatin, and have different absorption capabilities depending on their thickness and composition. The original hydrocolloids were developed from the adhesive flanges used for the long term protection of skin surrounding stomas (8). The barrier produced when the dressing comes in contact with the tissue, prevents excretions and exudate from eroding or denuding the skin surrounding the wound. As exudate is absorbed by the dressing, it develops a thick colloidal gel in the wound bed that increases the moist healing environment necessary for granulation, epithelialization, and autolysis.

These wafers come in a variety of sizes and shapes such as the "butterfly" design or sacrum shape that are "hinged" to fit the gluteal fold of the buttocks. Look for tapered, low profile edges that decrease the chances of rolling up and a smooth satin-like outer coating to decrease friction and shear.

Although considered a low-tech option for chronic wound care, in many settings hydrocolloids remain the most heavily utilized moist dressing option for wound management (11).

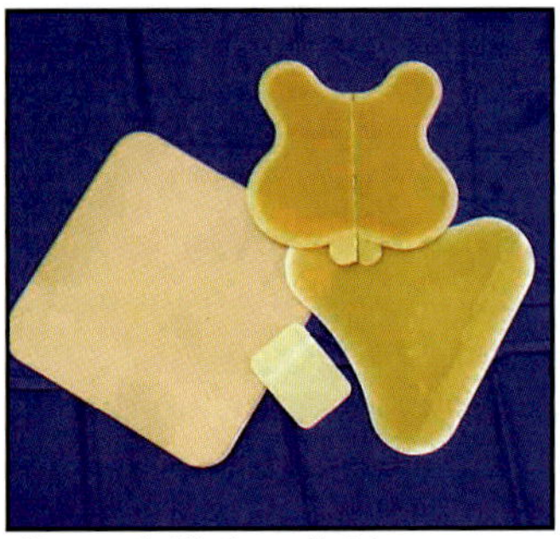

Figure 6. Hydrocolloids

Foams (Figure 7)

Foams are non-adherent, absorbent dressings that vary in thickness and are obtainable in adhesive vs. non-adhesive varieties. They are composed of polymers like polyurethane with small open cells that trap moisture. They are appropriate for partial- and full-thickness wounds, provide for moist wound healing, thermoregulation and protection. Look for varieties that offer superior moisture management, micropores for low adherence to the wound bed, decreasing pain and disruption of healing and a water-proof backing to prevent strike-through bacterial penetration. Absorbency and moisture vapor permeability are varied either by a physical alteration or by uniting the foam with an added sheet element.

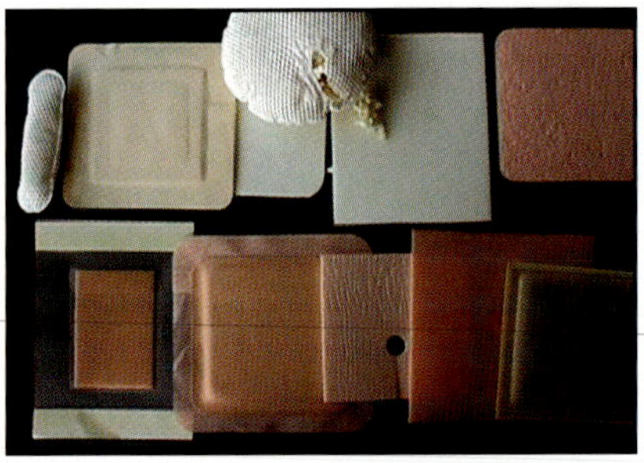

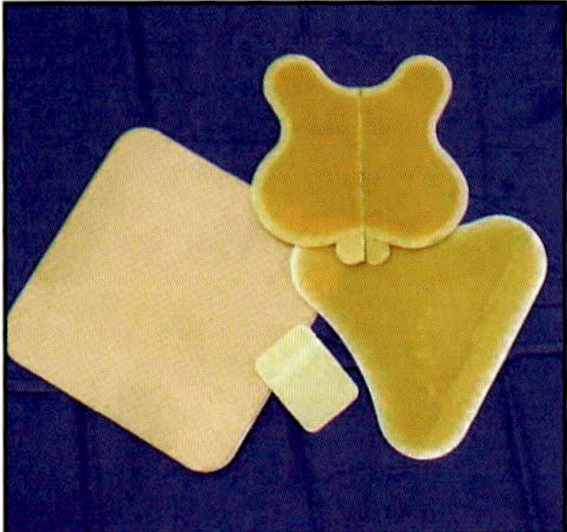

Figure 7. Foams

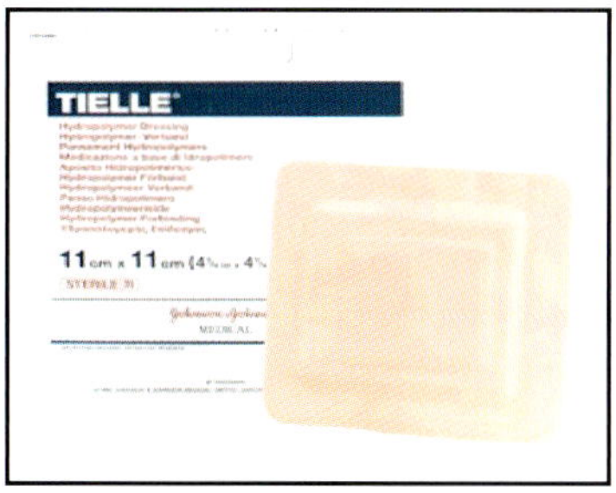

Figure 8. Composite

Composite (Figure 8)

Composites combine two different types of dressings with several functions in one single dressing that can address different needs. They can be used as a primary and/or secondary dressing and feature an absorptive layer, an adhesive border and a strike-through barrier. These dressings are versatile and convenient offering options for both partial and full thickness wounds. Their water-proof nature makes them a popular choice for areas prone to moisture assault from incontinence. These versatile dressings provide a barrier to bioburden while offering a simple "Band-Aid" type application and removal.

Interactive

Dressings that interact with the wound bed components to assist in producing an improved wound healing milieu. They can accomplished this via reducing colonization count, reducing the level of exudates, improving wound bed moisture retention, improving wound collagen matrix, removal of cellular products or providing protection for the epithelializing bed. Interactive dressings come in various forms.

Antimicrobials (Figure 9)

Antimicrobial dressings contain agents such as silver, iodine and polyhexethylene biguanide (PHMB) to help combat bioburden and superficial infection or keep such microbes at bay by eliminating pathogens that come into contact with the antimicrobials in the dressing. Both in vitro as well as clinical observations support the utilization of various biocide and antimicrobial products. Several of these products are outlined below.

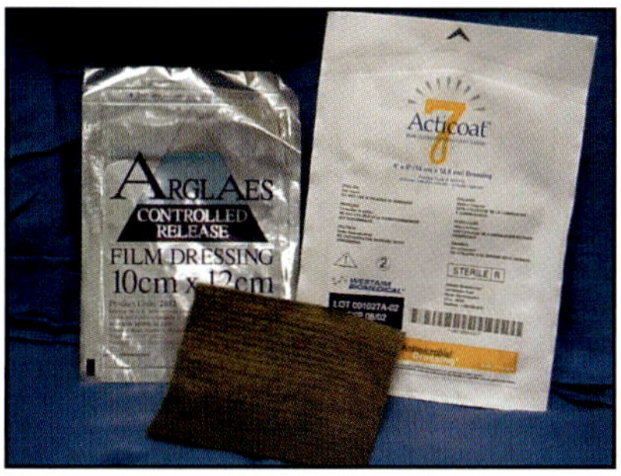

Figure 9. Antimicrobials

Silver

The use of silver has been documented for its broad-spectrum antimicrobial activity and compatibility with humans throughout history. The present recognized antimicrobial properties of silver have been empirically evident for more than 3000 years (12). A plethora of literature has reviewed its historical use, antimicrobial properties and toxicity. In 1881, a German obstetrician named Dr. Crede used a 1% silver nitrate solution to eliminate congenital blindness (Ophthalmia neonatorum) in newborns caused by post-partum infection of Neisseria gonorrhea (13). In 1887, von Behring used the same compound to treat typhoid and anthrax. In 1964, Moyer (14) first used silver for the care of burns. And in 1968, Fox (15) introduced silver sulfadiazine (SSD), still used today.

Silver dressings are some of our most advanced wound care dressings currently on the market. They are effective not only against microbes such as *methicillin resistant Staphylococcus aureus* (MRSA) and *vancomycin-resistant Enterococci* (VRE), but also provide a hostile environment to fungus and viruses, additionally decreasing inflammation (16). Ionic silver kills detrimental gram positive and gram negative bacteria, is safe, and to date has no known clinical resistance (17, 18). This is because of silver's multifaceted mode of action on pathogenic metabolic pathways. Silver ions attack the cell membrane, the membrane transport system, the RNA and DNA function as well as the protein function rendering it nearly impossible for bacterial mutation to occur. With ease it can occur when antibiotics are used. Antibiotic resistant bacteria, for example MRSA and VRE are easily eliminated in dressings that have silver ions present. The longevity of silver ion presence in the dressings, through their controlled release mechanisms, ensures that the wound environment is hostile to bioburden for relatively long periods of time.

While clinical resistance at this time has not occurred, resistance has been created in the laboratory when bacteria have repeatedly been exposed to bacteriostatic levels of silver in place of bactericidal levels (19, 20). In fact, Levy is quoted as saying "The current wide spread and uncontrolled use of silver may result in more bacteria developing resistance, analogous to the emergence of antibiotic- and biocide-resistant bacteria" (21). One of the questions the clinician should ask when choosing a silver dressing is whether the dose of silver is bacteriostatic or bactericidal. We should heed the lessons of the past when making our silver choices. While silver ions are bactericidal at low concentrations in water, when exposed to complex, organic biological fluids, such as wound exudate a higher concentration is needed (22). In complex organic fluids, concentrations greater than 40 ppm and as high as 60.5 ppm are required for the silver to be bactericidal (23).

Currently, there is a plethora of silver products on the market with a wide range of silver delivery. Thomas et al. (24), examined the silver content and antimicrobial activity of 10 common silver dressings on the market. They found significant differences in the activity of the products. There was a clear relationship between the silver content of the dressing and ability of the dressing to be bactericidal, but other factors were also identified. The other factors included: whether the silver was a surface coating or dispersed within the structure of the dressing; what form of silver (ionic, metallic or bound, and the dressing's affinity for moisture. Dressings that had surface silver, silver in ionic form, and those dressings that retained moisture performed the best.

The challenge to clinicians is to critically exam the wide selections of silver products and to choose those that will do the best for the patient.

Polyhexamethylene biguanide (PHMB)

Polyhexamethylene biguanide is a polymeric broad-spectrum cationic antimicrobial agent that is odorless, clear, and colorless (25). PHMB is a membrane-active agent that also impairs the integrity of the outer membrane of gram-positive and gram-negative bacteria, although the membrane may also act as a permeability barrier (26). Recently this agent has been added to dressings as both barriers and active antimicrobials capable of impairing or preventing the growth and penetration from a barrier perspective (27) and actively killing pathogens such as methicillin resistant *Staphylococcus aureus* (MRSA), vancomycin-resistant *Enterococci* (VRE), *Escherichia coli, Pseudomonas aeruginosa, Bacteroides fragilis, Clostridium perfringens* and yeasts such as *Candida albicans* from a sustained antimicrobial activity (28).

PHMB has been safely used in ophthalmic solutions (29), peri-operative cleansing solutions (29) and other consumer products such as mouth wash (30).

The cytotoxicity and hemolysis profile of PHMB containing products is excellent. PHMB is neither a primary skin irritant nor a hypersensitizing agent, which make it particularly well-suited to chronic wound care. There is little or no evidence to suggest that the use of PHMB would lead to the emergence of resistant strains to the agent, or that it may encourage development of cross resistance to antibiotics. The addition of this safe and effective versatile biocide is a positive development in wound management.

Cadexomer iodine

Iodine is a potent broad-spectrum antiseptic agent with a controversial past because it has been shown to impair the function of cells involved in wound healing in vitro (31). Improved formulations of iodophors or "iodine carriers" provide a release of low levels of iodine over a longer period of time. These present the clinician with a viable iodine containing product for wound bioburden management. They have been available for several years in the form of cadexomer iodine. Cadexomer iodine is a slow-release antimicrobial capable of absorbing excess wound exudate while offering a sustained level of iodine in the wound bed (32). Appraisal of its benefits show that it is accepted topically and has demonstrated accelerated healing of chronic leg ulcers (33). Cadexomer iodine also has established effectiveness in vivo against *Staphylococcus aureus* and methicillin-resistant *Staphylococcus aureus* (34). Iodine needs moisture/hydration in order to be activated, similar to silver ion containing products The clinical trend in recent years have been more favorable to silver and PHMB containing products compared to iodine containing products.

Biologics and biosynthetics (Figure 10)

Bioengineered cellulose provides moist wound healing and versatility significantly reducing pain and shortening healing time (35). Other biologics and biosynthetics derived from natural sources provide a healing scaffold or matrix, assisting the granulation and

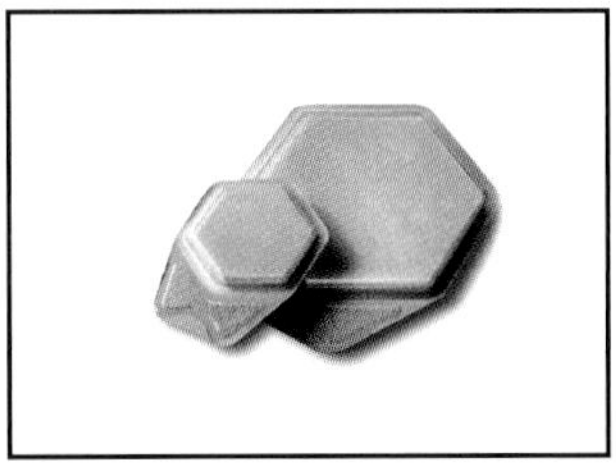

Figure 10. Matrix

epithelialization of partial- and full-thickness wounds. These matrix dressings provide a higher incidence of wound closure in recalcitrant wounds as compared to standard of care (36, 37).

Collagen (Figure 11)

Produced by fibroblasts, collagen represents the most abundant protein in the human body and the skin (38). It is a natural structural protein found in all three phases of the wound healing cascade and stimulates cellular migration and contributes to new tissue development and wound debridement (5). Collagen dressings in the form of sheets, gels, and particles encourage the deposition and organization of newly formed tissue, creating an environment that fosters healing. These materials are known to stimulate and recruit specific cells such as macrophages and fibroblasts to positively enhance and influence wound healing. They can be moisturizing or absorptive, depending on the delivery system, maintaining moist wound healing, are easy to apply and remove and tend to be conformable.

Collagen dressings are usually formulated with Type I bovine (cowhide or cow tendon) or avian collagen (derived from birds) or Type III porcine collagen (derived from pigs). Oxidized regenerated cellulose, a plant material, has been combined with collagen to produce a dressing capable of binding to and protecting growth factors and by binding and inactivating matrix metalloproteinases (MMPs) in the wound environment (39).

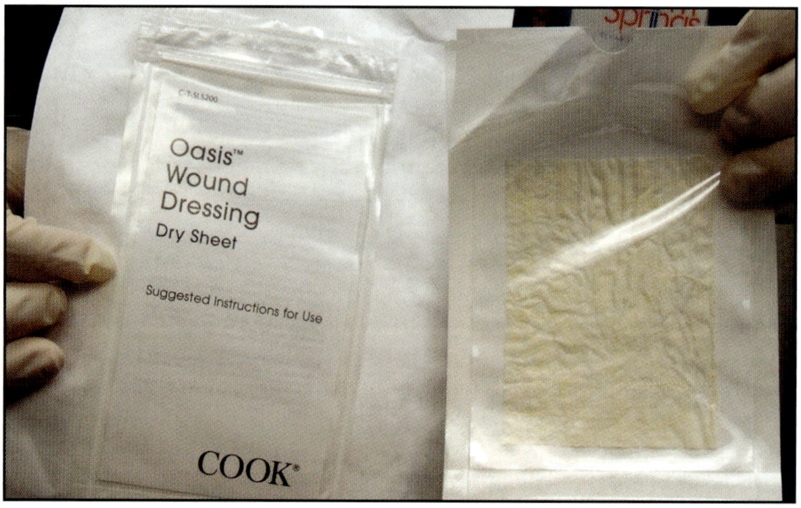

Figure 11. Collagen

Polyacrylates (Figure 12)

This activated absorbent polyacrylate polymer core dressing absorbs large protein molecules (necrotic tissue and bacteria) while irrigating with Ringer's solution, a physiologic fluid, creating a "rinsing effect." The interactive dressing supports both moist wound healing and autolytic debridement, gently removing dead tissue from the wound bed while creating an ideal healing environment. Polyacrylates debride at a mean rate of 38% (40). New research shows that polyacrylate gel absorbents debride just as well as collagenase (41). Recent literature has also shown that the product may be effective in reducing wound bioburden by interfering with biofilm as well (42).

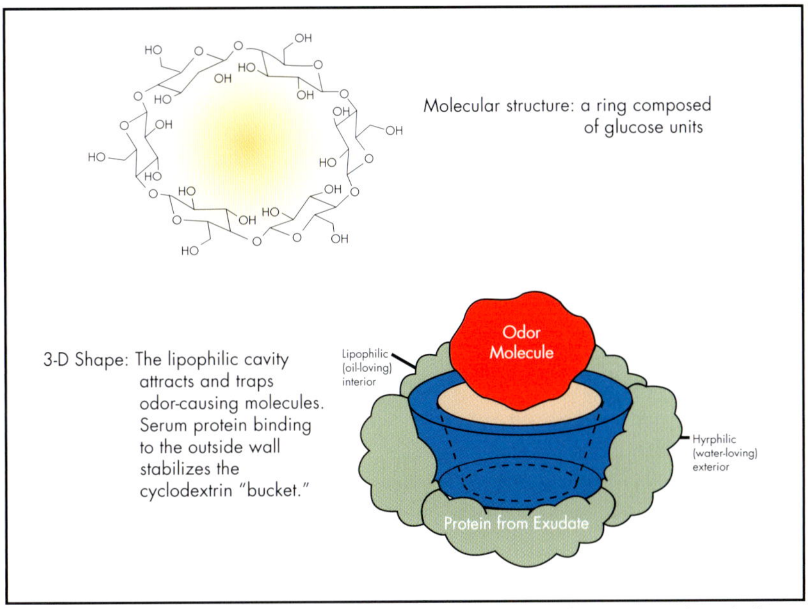

Figure 12. Mollecular structure and bucket-shaped conformaiton of cyclodexrin (starch) molecule capture lipophilic odor molecules, which neutralize the odor

Managing odor with dressings

The use of odor-controlling dressings is one measure to manage wound odor (43). These products are designed to act like filters or traps to absorb odor-causing molecules. Some of these goods incorporate charcoal that absorbs unpleasant smells from wounds. Activated charcoal is a widely used deodorizing agent. It works by absorbing many odor molecules onto the large surface area of the activated charcoal, which prevents the volatile odor molecules from reaching receptors in the nose (44). Charcoal has been incorporated into some modern wound dressing for this purpose.

Most odors are lipophilic. Novel dressings that utilize cyclodextrins (same technology as in Febreze®, Proctor and Gamble, Cincinnati, Ohio) use a bucket-shaped conformation of the hydrated cyclodextrin molecule to capture lipophilic odor molecules, which then neutralize the odor (Figure 12). Cyclodextrins occur naturally and are proven safe to use in modern wound care. How do these newer odor elimination dressings compare to the older technology of charcoal based dressings? Cyclodextrins work optimally in the presence of wound exudate and need humidity to work effectively (45). Charcoal activity decreases in the presence of wound exudate. Additionally, serum proteins inactivate charcoal dressings, while cyclodextrines' odor absorbing function is enhanced by it (45). In addition, cyclodextrins intrinsically have a longer active time of odor absorbing function by nature of their material (45).

Managing pain with dressings

Dressing removal is considered to be the time of most pain (46). Dried dressing and adherent products are most likely to cause pain and trauma at dressing changes. Products designed to be non-traumatic should be used to prevent tissue trauma.

One of the most important things to consider in selecting a dressing to diminish pain in the wound is that the chosen dressing must minimize the degree of sensory stimulus to the sensitized wound area (47). Any dressing that sticks to the wound bed, such as gauze, or dries within the wound bed and is then pulled away sends more sensory information to receptors in the skin than one that is easily rinsed away or slides off the inflamed tissue (47). Dressings, such as sheet and amorphous hydrogels, hydrofibers, alginates, soft silicones (46), cellulose dressings (48) provide beneficial wound healing environments and also offer a virtually pain-free dressing removal while curtailing the pain experience during wearing time.

Be sure to select dressings with absorbency that matches exudate levels (47). Choose dressings that can remain in situ for longer periods of time (46), thus minimizing the chances of wound manipulation and a harmful aggravation of the pain cycle. Contact layers or dressings that remain in close proximity to the wound bed during dressing changes also have proven beneficial in the pain arena (49). Don't neglect pain management during wound cleansing, either. Appropriate non-cytotoxic wound cleansers used at body temperature (~100°F) assist in keeping discomfort lower (50). Avoid cytotoxic solutions, such as povidone iodine or hydrogen peroxide, when cleaning the wound (51) as these can cause discomfort as well as being lethal to fibroblasts and keratinocytes.

Simple measures, such as the use of skin preparations (primarily the no-sting varieties), polymers that adhere to the skin to strengthen and prepare it for the adhesive application, provide less trauma to sensitive periwound skin (52). Use them whenever you dress a wound. When removing a dressing, make every possible effort to avoid unnecessary manipulation of the wound and prevent further damage to the delicate granulation and healing tissue within the wound bed and periwound skin. If the dressing has become dried out, moisten it with an isotonic solution before removing (53). Choose dressings that allow less frequent and, therefore, less painful dressing changes. Also, consider contact layers that stay in place when the dressings are changed; thus, staving off potential wound bed pain.

Another area of concern with regard to the wound care patient and pain is how the dressing is attached. In a study by Dykes et al. some adhesive dressings caused skin stripping upon removal (54). One of the many myths surrounding wound pain is that, "paper tape is the least painful way to secure a dressing". Heightened nerve sensation in a wide area around a wound can make any adhesive tape painful to remove (47). A thorough review of the dressings and tapes that you and your facility use is imperative. Are they gentle on thin, aging epidermis, young immature integument and skin that has endured critical illness, adhering with a low sensitivity adhesive, yet allowing easy removal and repositioning? Careful evaluation of your protocols is a necessary and important first step. State-of-the-art "tapeless" ways of securing a dressing have been around for centuries: Montgomery straps, Kling gauze, elastic netting, "grip" elastic support bandages and tubular dressings that offer a bit of support and compression (7-8 mm Hg) not only provide support to the dressing but further protect from the injury and pain of removal and reapplication of tape (55).

Current Best Practices

Until research proves otherwise, current guidelines for treatment and care of pressure ulcers have supported the use of clean dressings and clean dressing change technique over sterile methods (56). Bergstrom and her colleagues have shown that there is not sufficient evidence that using sterile technique has any significant effect on wound healing outcomes. Expert opinion advocates a no-touch technique that tries to guarantee that the procedure utilized to treat wounds will not increase the ulcer's bioburden. In the case of patients with compromised immune systems (i.e., cancer, HIV, AIDS, organ transplant), sterile dressings and sterile technique is warranted.

Standardization of products and wound treatments generates benefits, primarily when protocols and clinical pathways are established collaboratively based on recent published guidelines, a review of the literature for available research and/or best practice (57).

DRESSING SELECTION

For the clinician today, the job of selecting a dressing can be daunting. The use of the traditional six categories of dressings is no longer adequate as most of the latest dressings do not fit easily in a category and actually manage the tasks of multiple categories. The first step in selection is to understand the four basic goals of wound healing (Table 2).

The first goal is to maintain a moist healing environment. Moist wound healing promotes epithlialization, enhances autolytic debridement, prevents wound desiccation, and decreases pain. The second goal is to remove eschar and debris from the wound bed. This will decrease bioburden, improve epithlialization, and decrease inflammation. The third goal is to control exudate. Increased exudate can cause periwound maceration and contributes to an increased bioburden in the wound. The fourth goal is to prevent further wounding. Patients may unknowingly traumatize their wounds because of neuropathy or a dressing or product may be chosen which actually traumatizes the wound or surrounding skin.

In this chapter we will present two methods of dressing selection. The first is based upon Ovington's methodology (58). Goals, form, and function is combined with a nursing assessment of the wound and the patient prior to

TABLE 2. GOALS OF WOUND MANAGEMENT

Goal #1: Maintain moist healing environment
Goal #2: Remove escar and debris from wound bed
Goal #3: Control exudate
Goal #4: Prevent further wounding

dressing selection. The dressing must match the patient, the wound, and the setting. In Ovington's article 11, she gave an all-purpose performance-based approach to using wound dressings by asking six basic assessment questions when deciding on a wound dressing.

1.) What does the wound need? Determined by a complete assessment of the wound and surrounding tissues. Assessment is performed at each dressing change, including the initial. Apply the goals. Anticipate that the needs of the wound will change as the tissue envelope normalizes and the healing process progresses.

2.) What does the product do? This is the function. Read the product literature and clinical data available.

3.) How well does it do it? Examine clinical studies and laboratory comparisons to other products in the same category. Talk with other clinicians. Evaluate it on your patients. Does the dressing perform how it is stated? Not all dressings are equal.

4.) What does the patient need? Comprehensive assessment of the patient, including psychosocial. Do they need a dressing that doesn't require daily changes? Do they need protection from trauma, or is there a large amount of exudate?

5.) What is available? Health insurance coverage, facility formulary, and reimbursement?

6.) What is practical? Examine the goals of wound management. Does the dressing choice satisfy the goals? Is the dressing easy to apply (patient/family), easy to obtain and cost effective?

Cost effectiveness of the product should be considered during the selection process. This means understanding indirect costs as well as the direct cost involved in wound care. Direct cost examples include, but are not limited to the primary and secondary dressings, pharmacy, caregiver time, and diagnostic procedures. Indirect costs are similar to overhead costs, and include examples such as increased length of stays, treatment complications, and litigation. The clinician should read published studies critically to take cost-per-unit outcome into account to determine if treatment measures are cost effective. Sometimes the most expensive product can be less expensive in the long run because it leads to faster healing with a reduced amount of complications.

The second methodology of dressing selection has been recently published by Fleck and focuses on six simple questions.

1.) Is the wound healing? If the answer is "yes", proceed with current best practice treatment. If the answer is "no", consider other etiologies and care modalities, assess bioburden (bacterial or other microbial overload in the wound), look at intrinsic and extrinsic risk factors such as nutrition, pressure, shear, etiology, debris and devitalized material in the wound bed, temperature of the wound, circulation, maceration, desiccation, chemical stress and medications as well as other co-morbidities. Confer and consult with colleagues if this is outside your scope of knowledge and/or practice (59). You should expect to see progress toward wound healing within 2-4 weeks of initiation of treatment (60).

2.) Is the tissue viable (living) or necrotic (dead)? The single most important parameter in reducing the level of bacterial contamination in the chronic wound is removal of all devitalized material (51). If it is viable, support it and keep it moist. Vital, healthy living tissue is usually red or pink. If it is necrotic, debride it (56). Necrotic tissue can be yellow, gray, black or some combination of these colors (5). It has no function, other than to slow healing, splint the wound open, and provide a breeding ground for critical colonization (61–65).

A dry cell is a dead cell so moist wound healing is the goal with all wounds. Dr. George Winter's studies in the early 1960s proved that moist wound healing provided for better healing outcomes with less pain and scarring (4). The work of Hinman and Maibach further connected these findings in human models just a year later (66).

3.) Is the wound wet or dry? For most favorable outcomes, providing an optimal level of moisture (56, 63) is recommended. If the wound is "wet," apply a product that manages exudate while maintaining an optimal amount of moisture. If the wound is "dry," apply a product that donates or maintains moisture at optimal levels. One of the most important criteria for dressing selection is exudate amount.

Research and clinical experience have identified that in a moist environment, exudate provides the cells involved in wound repair with nutrients, controls infection and provides the best environment for healing. Moreover, revascularization occurs earlier in moist conditions (67). Studies have demonstrated that cells communicate and respond to growth factors and cytokines contained within wound exudate (68).

4.) Is there dead or open space in the wound? If so, and it is deep, it is necessary to fill the space, loosely packing the open area when dressing the wound (56, 69). If there is no dead space, covering the wound, if it is flat, is all that's required (5). Covering the wound provides a physical barrier to microbes, a humid, moist and thermally insulated environment and protection from the outside environment.

5.) Is the wound or surrounding area edematous? Many wounds are accompanied by edema beyond the inflammatory phase. Furthermore, lower limb wounds are often secondary to poor venous return or venous hypertension. Without compression these wounds fail to progress (70, 71). Evaluate lower limb wounds, ascertaining the patient's ankle-brachial index (ABI) and/or toe brachial index before applying compression wraps

6.) What is the condition of the periwound skin or the skin surrounding the wound (including the skin of a recently closed wound)? If the skin surrounding the wound is compromised and/or painful, avoid adhesives or use great caution. Use of a polymer skin preparation, especially the no-sting varieties (72), before attaching any dressing is helpful. This will assist to strengthen and protect the skin without causing pain or discomfort. Also consider using protective products such as barrier creams and adhesive removers to treat this vulnerable skin with care. Soap-free, pH balanced non-cytotoxic cleansers should additionally be used to gently cleanser the area surrounding a wound (73). Remember, this is the skin that will eventually support the wound healing and from where the epithelial cells will migrate (74).

Wet-to-dry and Moist Gauze

In the United States, wet-to-dry and gauze dressings are still the most commonly used primary dressing substance (75). Many reasons for the persistence of gauze and saline used as wound management mainstays include: lack of knowledge from physicians and nurses on advanced dressings and how they work, confusion due to the plethora of advanced products, incorrect view that advanced dressings come with a high price, and gauze is a "one size fits all" modality that is readily available, perceived as inexpensive and the dressings have been used throughout history (6). There is also evidence that they are used inappropriately (6). Recent journal articles, texts, as well as expert opinion support the principle of moist wound healing, but in practice the use of gauze, predominantly as a wet-to-dry dressing, does not guarantee a moist wound environment (76).

Wet-to-dry dressings are described in the literature as a means of mechanical debridement (77). Debridement is the mainstay of wound bed preparation since devitalized material harbors bacteria, delays healing and increases the risk of infection (78). However, it is the opinion of the authors of this chapter that wet-to-dry or moist gauze does not constitute advanced wound caring or advanced therapy. Granted, wet-to-dry gauze is a form of non-selective debridement, however, it is painful if the patient is sensate and can produce negative outcomes. Gauze dressings are not an optimal wound care choice for the patient, the caregiver or the healthcare system and facility. They do not support optimal granulation and healing and are more labor intensive to use than advanced dressings such as polyacrylates, transparent films, hydrocolloids, alginates, hydrogels and foams. Therefore, these archaic regimes should be abandoned since they are not considered standard of care despite The Agency for Healthcare Research and Quality (AHRQ), formerly the Agency for Health Care Policy and Research (AHCPR), Clinical Practice Guidelines for Treatment of Pressure Ulcers (56) have supported the use of wet-to-dry dressing for debridement by maintaining that its use is backed by expert opinion (rated as C on their scale of hierarchy of evidence).

Ovington describes gauze as the most widely used wound care dressing and may be erroneously considered a standard of care (6). Her article comments that 'wet-to-dry' and 'wet-to-moist' are frequently used in clinical practice in a fashion that makes them interchangeable. She describes hampered healing due to local tissue cooling, disruption of angiogenesis by dressing removal, and increased infection risk from frequent dressing changes, strike through, and prolonged inflammation as good reason to abandon this 'traditional' dressing technique (6). Dr. Ovington also offers a cost-effectiveness argument for change. She illustrates the costs of saline and gauze compared with an advanced dressing (Tielle, Johnson & Johnson Wound Management, Somerville, New Jersey), over a four-week period, performed by a home health nurse (6). The largest contribution to cost is nursing time; even with the patient and/or family doing some of his or her care, the cost is decreased with the advanced dressing secondary to fewer dressing changes and better outcomes (less time to closure). Another investigator, Coyne, examined the cost-benefit of wet-to-dry compared to another advanced dressing (TenderWet, Medline Industries, Inc. Advanced Skin and Wound Care, Mundelein, IL) in a nationwide 65 location home care agency (TLC/Staff Builders) realizing a 26% cost-savings alone annually, pointing out that wet-to-dry treatments additionally cause pain, slower healing, and an increased infection rate (79). There are other important considerations when choosing a dressing, such as clinical outcome, quality of life issues, discomfort, disruption of daily routines, and coping with daily activities that can all be addressed by modern products (80).

REIMBURSEMENT

Healthcare is a business and generating revenue is part of a healthy business. Clinicians must consider this when caring for patients. Understanding reimbursement and payment procedures of Medicare and Medicaid, is essential to operating a successful wound care program. Medicare coverage for wound care dressings varies by healthcare setting. Several wound product manufacturers have extensive reimbursement guides located on their websites (Table 3).

Category and HCPCS Codes

Dressings are classified into generic descriptive categories and each category is assigned a HCPCS Code. HCPCS is an acronym for HCFA Common Procedure Coding System. The system is used by Medicare, Medicaid and other insurers. The codes represent non-physician services such as durable medical equipment, prosthetic and orthodic devices, medical supplies, ambulance services, and other health-related products and services. Each code is assigned an allowable fee amount. The fee remains the same regardless of the manufacturer. Fee schedule information is available from each regional carrier.

Utilization Guidelines

Medicare has established utilization guidelines for each dressing category. If a quantity is higher than the guidelines is required, a statement of medical necessity is required from the physician.

Documentation Support

Documentation is necessary to support claim coverage. A physicians order is required specifying dressing type, amount used with each dressing change, dressing change frequency and expected length of need. Documentation needs to contain the diagnosis with a wound description, including the wound stage or grade. Each wound should be described and listed if more than one.

TABLE 3. COMPANIES PROVIDING WOUND DRESSINGS

Company	Telephone/Web Address	Example of Product	
3M Wound Care Products	1-800-228-3957	Tegagen HI Tegasorb	Tegaderm Coban2
AcryMed, Inc	1-88-acrymed *www.acrymed.com*	Silvasorb	
Beiersdorf-Jobst, Inc	1-800-876-3664	Comprilan Artiflex	Gelcast unna boot
BioCore, Inc	1-800-577-4801	Medifill particles, pads and gels	
Carrington Laboratories	1-800-358-5205 *www.carringtonlabs.com*	CarraSmart film, gel, foam dressings	
Coloplast Sween Corp.	1-800-533-0464 *www.coloplast.com*	Seasorb alginate Contreet Silver	Biatain foam
ConvacTec	1-800-631-5244 *www.convatec.com*	Aquacel Aquacel AG	Duoderm Versiva
Derma Science	1-800-825-4325 *www.dermasciences.com*	Dermagran	
DeRoyal	1-800-251-9864 *www.deroyal.com*	CovaDerm Awuasorb	Kalginate Multidex
Dow Hickam Pharmaceuticals	1-800-231-3052	Biobrane Sorbsan	Flexzan Granulex
Ferris Mfg	1-800-765-9636 *www.ferrispolymem.com*	PolyMem	
Gentell	1-800-840-9041 *www.gentell.com*	Dermatell Gentell Hydrogel	Gentel Alginate
Health	1-800-441-8227 *www.healthpoint.com*	Oasis Wound Matrix Panfil	Accuzyme Iodosorb
Hollister	1-800-323-4060	Restore alginate, hydrocolloid and hydrogel	
Hyperion Medical	1-800-743-8111 *www.hyperionmedical.com*	Hyperion alginate, hydrogel and hydrocolloid dressings	
Johnson & Johnson	1-800-255-2500	Progran Tielle	Actisorb Siver Adaptic
Kendall	1-800-962-9888	Curagel Gurofoam	Curasorb Kerlix
Medline Industries	1-800-MEDLINE *www.medline.com/woundcare*	SilvaSorb TenderWet Active	Gentleheal Exuderm
Molinlycke Health Care	1-610-471-0160 *www.molnlyckehc.com*	Mepilex	
Smith & Nephew	1-800-876-1261 *www.snwmd.com*	Profore Acticoat 7	Allevyn Replicare

Description of the wound should include how long the patient has had the wound, progression to healing from onset, and expected healing time. Wound evaluation is required on a regular basis to include type, location, size, drainage amount and any other relevant information.

REFERENCES

1. Zimmerman, LM, Veith I. Great Ideas in the History of Surgery. Baltimore, MD: Williams and Wilkins, 1961.
2. Forrest RD. Early history of wound treatment, Journal of Royal Society Medicine 75: 198-205, 1982.
3. Sinclair RD, Ryan TJ. A great war for antiseptics. Wound Management, 1993; 4(1), 16-18.
4. Winter GD, Scales JT. The effects of air-drying and dressings on the surface of the wound. Nature; 1963; 197:91-92.
5. Ayello EA, Baranoski S, Kerstein MD, et al. Wound treatment options, Chapter 9, in *Wound Care Essentials Practice Principles*, Baranoskin S, Ayello EA, (eds) 2004, Lippincott Williams and Wilkins, Philiadelphia, p. 135.
6. Ovington L. Hanging wet to dry dressings out to dry. *Home Health Nurse*, August 2001, volume 19, number 8, page 477.
7. Ovington LG. The well-dressed wound: an overview of dressing types. *WOUNDS* 1998;10:1A-11A.
8. Turner TD. The development of wound management products. In: Krasner DL, Rodeheaver GT, Sibbald RG (eds). *Chronic Wound Care: A Clinical Source Book for Healthcare Professionals*, Third Edition. Wayne, PA: HMP Communications, 2001:293-310.
9. Baranoski S. Skin tears: The enemy of frail skin. *Advances in Skin and Wound Care*, May/June 2000; 13(3 part 1):123-26.
10. Fleck CA. Ethical wound management for the palliative patient. *ECPN* 2005;100(4):38-46.
11. HPIS Quarterly Market Intelligence Update, 2005.
12. Russell AD, Hugo WB. Antimicrobial activity and action of silver. *Pro in Med. Chem.* 31:351-370, 1994.
13. Crede. Prevention of inflammatory eye disease in the newborn. *Gynaecology Archive*, volume 17, Berlin, 1881, 265-66. Available at: *http://www.who.int/docstore/bulletin/pdf/2001/issue3/vol79.no.3.262-266.pdf#search='Crede%201%25%20silver%20nitrate'* accessed 1-21-06.
14. Moyer CA, Brentono L, Gravens DL, et al. Treatment of large human burns with 0.5% silver nitrate solution. *Arch Surg*. 1965;90:812.
15. Fox CL, Rappole BW, Stanford W. Control of Pseudomonas in burns with silver sulfadiazine. *Surg Gynecol Obstet*. 1969;(14):168.
16. Fleck CA, Paustian C. The use of silver containing dressings: The new "silver bullet" in wound management? *ECPN* 2003;88(4):22-25.
17. Ovington LG. The truth about silver. *Ostomy Wound Management* 2004;50(9A) suppl, 1S-10S.
18. Poon KM, Burd A. In vitro cytotoxity of silver: implication for clincal wound care. *BURNS* 2004;30:140-147.
19. Li, X-Z., Nikaido, H. and Williams, K.E. 1997. Silver-Resistant Mutants of *Escherichia coli* Display Active Efflux of Ag+ and are Deficient in Porins. J Bacteriol. 179(19): 6127-6132.
20. Gupta A, Silver S. Silver as a Biocide:Will resistance become a problem? Nature Biotechnology 1998;16:888.
21. Levy SB, March 1998, Scientific American pp. 32-39
22. Dunn K, Edwards-Jones V. The role of Acticoat with nanocrystalline silver in the management of burns. Burns 2004; 30(Suppl 1): S1-9
23. Maple PA, Hamilton-Miller JM, Brumfitt W. Comparison of the in-vitro activities of the topical antimicrobials azelaic acid, nitrofurazone, silver sulphadiazine and mupirocin against methicillin-resistant Staphylococcus aureus. *J Antimicrob Chemother* 1992; 29: 661-68.

24. Thomas S, McCubbin P. An in vitro analysis of the antimicrobial properties of 10 silver-containing dressings. *J Wound Care* 2003; 12(8): 305-08.

25. Gilbert P. Polyhexamethylene biguanides and infection control. University of Manchester, U.K., available at: *http://www.tycohealthce.com/files/d0004/ty_at2ej8.pdf#search='Polyhexamethylene%20biguanide%20and%20infection%20control%20by%20Peter%20Gilbert'* accessed 1-21-06.

26. McDonnell G, Russell AD. Antiseptic and disinfectants: Activity, action and resistance. *Clinical Microbiology Reviews*, January 1999, 12(1):147-179.

27. Motta GJ, Corbett LQ, Milne CT. Impact of an antimicrobial gauze upon bacterial colonies in wounds that require packing. Tyco Healthcare, 2003, 1-11.

28. Data on file. Xylos Corporation, Longhorne, PA.

29. Kramer A, Behrens-Baumann W. Prophylactic use of topical anti-infectives in ophthalmology. *Ophthalmologica* 1997;211:68-76.

30. Rosin M, Welk A, Kocher T, et al. The effect of a polyhexamethylene biguanide mouthrinse compared to an essential oil rinse and a chlorhexidine rinse on bacterial counts and 4-day plaque regrowth. *J Clin Periodontol* 2002;29:392-399.

31. Fleischer W, Reimer K. Povidone iodine in antisepsis: state of the art. *Dermatology*. 1997:195:3S-9S.

32. Sundberg J, Meller R. A retrospective review of the use of cadexomer iodine in the treatment of chronic wounds. *WOUNDS* 1997;9:68-86.

33. Danielsen L, Cherry GW, Harding K, et al. Cadexomer iodine in ulcers colonized by Pseudomonas aeruginosa. *Journal of Wound Care* 1997:6(4):169-172.

34. Mertz PM, Oliveira-Gandia MF, Davis SC. The evaluation of a cadexomer iodine wound dressing on methicillin resistant Staphylococcus aureus (MRSA) in acute wounds. *Dermatology Surgery* 1999; 25:89-93.

35. Alvarez OM, Patel M, Booker J, et al. Effectiveness of a biocellulose wound dressing for the treatment of chronic venous leg ulcers: results of a single center randomized study involving 24 patients. *WOUNDS* 2004;16(7)224-233.

36. Demling R, Neizgoda J, Haraway D, et al. Small intestinal submucosa wound matrix and full-thickness venous ulcers: preliminary results. *WOUNDS* 2004;16(1):18-22.

37. Etris M, Cutshall WD, Hiles MC. A new biomaterial derived from small intestine submucosa and developed into a wound matrix device. *WOUNDS* 2002;14(4):150-66.

38. Collagen from the Witipedia free encyclopedia available at: http://en.wikipedia.org/wiki/Collagen. Accessed 3-11-06.

39. Cullen B, Smith R, McCulloch E, et al. Mechanism of action of PROMOGRAN, a protease modulating matrix, for the treatment of diabetic foot ulcers. *Wound Rep Reg* 2002;10:16-25.

40. Paustian C, Stegman MR. Preparing the wound bed for healing: The effect of activated polyacrylate dressing on debridement. *Ostomy/Wound Management*, 2003;49(9):34-42.

41. Konig, et al. Enzymatic versus autolytic debridement of chronic leg ulcers; a prospective randomized trial. *J of Wound Care*; 14(7), July 2005.

42. Bruggisser R. Bacterial and fungal absorption properties of a hydrogel dressing with a super absorbent polymer core. *J Wound Care*; 14(9), October 2005.

43. Fleck CA. Fighting odor in wounds. *Advances in Skin and Wound Care*. 19(5):242-245, June 2006.

44. Ovington L. Bacterial toxins and wound healing. *Ostomy Wound Management*, July 2003;49(7A):8-12.

45. Lipman RDA. Avery Dennison Medical, Odour absorbing hydrocolloid dressing for direct wound contact, Poster Number 82, Wound Healing Society (WHS) 15th Annual Meeting, Chicago, May 18-21, 2005.

46. European Wound Management Society Position Document: Pain at Wound Dressing Changes. London, UK: Medical Education Partnership Ltd., 2002:2, 8. Available at *www.aawc1.org*.

47. Briggs M, et al. Minimizing pain at wound dressing-related procedures: A consensus document (A World Union of Wound Healing Societies' Initiative), Medical Education Partnership, Ltd., London, 2004.

48. Alvarez O. Ease the pain of wound care: better choices in debridement and dressing options. Oral presentation at the Symposium on Advances in Skin and Wound Care in San Antonio, TX, 29 April 2006.

49. Reddy M, Kohr R, Queen D, et al. Practical treatment of wound pain and trauma: A patient-centered approach. An Overview. *Ostomy/Wound Management*;49(4A)April 2003:2-15.

50. Van Rijswijk L, Braden BJ. Pressure ulcer patient and wound assessment: An AHCPR clinical practice guideline update. *Ost Wound Manag* 1999; 45(Suppl 1A):56S.

51. Rodeheaver GT. Wound cleansing, wound irrigation, wound disinfection. In: Krasner DL, Rodeheaver GT, Sibbald RG (eds). Chronic Wound Care: A Clinical Sourcebook for Healthcare Professionals, Third Edition. Wayne, PA: HMP Communications, 2001:369–83.

52. Sibbald RG, Campbell K, Coutts P, et al. Intact skin—an integrity not to be lost. Ostomy/Wound Management. 2003;49(6):27-33.

53. Queen, D, Woo K, Shulz VN, Sibbald RG. Ostomy/Wound Management, October 2003;49(10):16-18. October 2003 - Pages: 16 - 18

54. Dykes PJ, Heggie R, Hill SA. Effects of adhesive dressing on the stratum corneum of the skin. *Journal of Wound Care* 2001;10(1):7-10.

55. Fleck CA. Managing Difficult-to-dress wounds. *ECPN*, June 2005:42-49.

56. Bergstrom N, Bennett MA, Carlson, CE, et al. Treatment of Pressure Ulcers. Clinical Practice Guide, Number 15. Rockville, MD: U.S. Department of Health and Human Services, Agency for Health Care Policy and Research. AHCPR Publication No. 95-0653, December 1994.

57. Rolstad BS, Ovington LG. *Principles of Wound Management in Acute and Chronic Wounds Current Management Concepts*, Third Edition, Bryant RA, Nix DP, eds., Mosby/Elsevier, St. Louis, MO, 2007.

58. Ovington LG. Wound Care Products: How to Choose. Advances in Skin & Wound Care: The Journal for Prevention and Healing. September/October 2001 Vol. 14, No. 5 p. 259.

59. Mrdjenovitch DE, Fleck CA. Piecing together wound management. *ECPN*, July/August 2005 30-36.

60. van Rijswijk L, Braden BJ: Pressure ulcer patient and wound assessment: an AHCPR clinical practice guideline update, *Ostomy Wound Management* 45(suppl 1A):56S, 1999.

61. Mulder GD, Vande Berg JS. Cellular senescence and matrix metalloproteinase activity in chronic wounds. *JAMA* 2002;92(1):34–7.

62. O'Meara SO, Cullum N, Majid M, Sheldon T. Systematic reviews of wound care management: (3) antimicrobial agents for chronic wounds; (4) diabetic foot ulceration. *Health Technol Assess* 2000;4(21):1–237.

63. Sibbald R, Williamson D, Orsted H, et al. Preparing the wound bed—debridement, bacterial balance, and moisture balance. *Ost/Wound Manag* 2000;46(11):14–22, 24–8, 30–5.

64. Maklebust J. Using wound care products to promote a healing environment. *Crit Care Nurs Clin North Am* 1996;8(pt 2):141–50.

65. Bucknall T. The effect of local infection upon wound healing: An experimental study. *Br J Surg* 1980;67:851.

66. Hinman CD, Maibach HI. Effect of air exposure and occlusion on experimental human skin wounds. *Nature* 1963;200:377.

67. Dyson M, Young SR, Hart J, et al. Comparison of the effects of moist and dry conditions on the process of angiogenesis during dermal repair. *J Invest Dermatol* 1993;99:729-33.

68. Garrett B, Garrett SB. Cellular communication and the action of growth factors during wound healing. *Journal of Wound Care* 1997;6(6):277-80.

69. Maklebust J, Sieggreen M. *Pressure ulcers: guidelines for prevention and nursing management.* West Dundee, IL, S-N Publications, 1991:212.

70. Fleck CA. Putting the Squeeze on: Understanding venous disease and compression therapy. *ECPN* 2002;82(2):4-9.

71. Fleck CA. Compression and Offloading: Secrets to Healing lower limb wounds. *ECPN* 2004;93(3):14-19.

72. Williams C. (1998) 3M™ Cavilon™ No Sting Barrier Film in the protection of vulnerable skin. *British Journal of Nursing* 7(10): 613-615.

73. Ananthapadmanabhan KP, Moore DJ, Subramanyan K, Misra M, Meyer F. Cleansing without compromise: The impact of cleansers on the skin barrier and the technology of mild cleansing. *Dermatologic Therapy* 2004;17(Suppl 1):16–25.

74. Waldorf H, Fewkes J. *Wound healing, Adv Dermatol* (10):77, 1995.

75. Mc Callon ST, Knight CA, Valiulus P, et al. Vacuum-assisted closure versus saline-moistened gauze in the healing of postoperative diabetic foot wounds. *Ostomy/Wound Management.* 2000;46(8):28-34.

76. Bolton LL, Monte K. Moisture and healing beyond the jargon. *Ostomy Wound Manage* 2000; 46(1A):51S-62S.

77. Bryant RA. Acute and Chronic Wounds, Second Edition. St. Louis, MO:Mosby, 2000:164-5.

78. Kirsner, R. Wound bed preparation. Ostomy/Wound Management;49(2A), February 2003:2-3.

79. Coyne N. Eliminating wet-to-dry treatments. *Reminton Report* September/October 2003 (sup);8-11.

80. Armstrong MH, Price P. Wet-to-Dry Gauze Dressings: Fact and Fiction. *WOUNDS* 16(2):56-62, 2004.

REVIEW QUESTIONS

1.) Impregnated gauze is less adherent to the wound bed and less absorbent than plain gauze.
  a. True
  b. False

2.) Film dressings:
  a. retain moisture in the wound bed
  b. will not tear fragile skin
  c. are used on infected wounds
  d. absorbs exudates

3.) Foam dressings:
  a. adhere to the wound bed
  b. are effective for wounds with dry eschar
  c. never require a secondary dressing
  d. may macerate wound edge if dressing becomes saturated

4.) Alginate dressings:
  a. are used in dry wounds
  b. form moist gel in the wound
  c. are never painful
  d. do not control exudates

5.) Hydrocolloid dressings:
  a. can be used in heavy exudates
  b. can be used in infected wounds
  c. will not adhere to the skin surrounding the wound
  d. facilitates autolytic debridement and reduces pain

Answers: 1a, 2a, 3d, 4b, 5d

CHAPTER 38

Hyperbaric Oxygen Therapy Applications in Wound Care

CHAPTER THIRTY-EIGHT OVERVIEW

NOTES

Hyperbaric Oxygen Therapy Applications in Wound Care

Caroline E. Fife, Robert A. Warriner III

INTRODUCTION

Wounds with inadequate tissue oxygen levels will not heal despite the best wound care. As TK Hunt observed, "The question is not whether increased tissue oxygen is a benefit to healing, but how much." Tissue oxygen levels can be reduced due lack of vascular supply, or due to many other local factors, such as edema, infection, trauma, radiation injury, or reperfusion injury. When tissue oxygen levels fall below the minimum needed for healing, a number of well-described effects occur, including reduced response to infection, defects in host-repair processes, such as fibroblast migration and proliferation, and the arrest of collagen secretion. Collectively these prevent angiogenesis (1).

Oxygen is a drug, with many pharmacological effects. The mechanism by which tissues are supplied with oxygen is via respiration of oxygen, and subsequent delivery by the vasculature. There is no significant topical absorption of oxygen. Therefore, for additional oxygen to be delivered to hypoxic tissues, it must be administered systemically—i.e., it must be breathed. Hyperbaric oxygen therapy (HBO2) is a treatment in which a patient breathes 100% oxygen while inside a treatment chamber at an atmospheric pressure higher than sea level. Monoplace chambers accommodate a single patient and the entire chamber is usually pressurized with 100% oxygen that the patient breathes directly. Multiplace chambers accommodate two or more patients (and usually an attendant or other support personnel), and the chamber is pressurized with compressed air while the patients breathe 100% oxygen via masks, head hoods, or endotracheal tubes. According to the U.S. Food and Drug Administration (FDA), topical oxygen, in which isolated parts of the body are exposed to 100% oxygen, does not constitute hyperbaric oxygen therapy. Topical oxygen should not be equated with hyperbaric oxygen therapy and is not reimbursable by Medicare.

Although the first article describing the therapeutic use of compressed air was written by Fontaine (2) in 1879, the use of oxygen at pressures greater than sea level is a relatively recent development. In the 1950s, the Dutch physician, Ita Boerema, began his animal experiments using HBO2 (3), and first described the adjunctive use of hyperbaric oxygen therapy in the treatment of clostridial myonecrosis (clostridial gas gangrene) in the early 1960s. Since then, the benefits of HBO2 in wound healing have been well described, and HBO2 is often part of the armamentarium of the modern "wound-healing center." Indeed, the American Board of Medical Specialties now recognizes "Undersea and Hyperbaric Medicine" as a subspecialty. Like wound management, the clinical application of both wound care and hyperbaric medicine crosses most specialty boundaries, because no disease process recognizes specialty "niches" in its clinical manifestations. The common thread with all wound-healing clinicians is the concept that natural healing processes can be enhanced by improving or normalizing the wound environment. This chapter will briefly review the physiology of hyperbaric oxygen therapy, its effects on the healing process, and the clinical data to support its use as part of the continuum of wound management.

HOW HBO2 INCREASES TISSUE OXYGEN LEVELS

Under normal circumstances, i.e., breathing air at sea level, the arterial partial pressure of oxygen (pO_2) is about 100 mm Hg. In healthy individuals, the hemoglobin is about 97% saturated under those conditions. Increasing inspired oxygen concentration at sea level (such as breathing 100% oxygen) has little effect on the hemoglobin, because it is already nearly saturated. For example, a gram of fully saturated hemoglobin carries 1.35 ml of oxygen, bound chemically to the hemoglobin molecule. In a healthy person with a normal amount of hemoglobin (about 15 g/dL), the average oxygen-carrying capacity is 20 ml of oxygen for every 100 ml of blood, otherwise defined as 20 volumes percent (20 vol %). In contrast, blood plasma carries only 0.3 ml of oxygen for every 100 ml of blood (0.3 vol %), so blood plasma makes no real contribution to oxygen-carrying capacity when one breathes air at sea level. Therefore, once hemoglobin is fully saturated, the only way to increase oxygen-carrying capacity is to increase plasma-dissolved oxygen.

Breathing pure oxygen at sea level increases the plasma-dissolved oxygen by an additional 2 vol %. As the atmospheric pressure increases, an increasing amount of oxygen is dissolved in blood plasma, as described by Henry's law, which refers to the increased solubility of a gas in liquid based on its partial pressure. Breathing oxygen at twice sea level atmospheric pressure, referred to as 2 ATA, will result in an arterial pO_2 of about 1400 mm Hg—over a 10-fold increase in arterial oxygen tension (4), with soft tissue and muscle pO_2 levels increasing to about 300 mm Hg. Thus, blood oxygen-carrying capacity will have increased from 20 vol % to about 24 vol %, almost entirely due to an increase in plasma oxygen-carrying capacity (see Figure 1).

In general, the blood oxygen-carrying capacity increases approximately 2 vol % for every atmosphere of pressure increase. Indeed, under hyperbaric conditions, enough oxygen can be dissolved in plasma to keep tissues alive in the total absence of hemoglobin. This was elegantly demonstrated by Boerema (3), who showed the potential importance of plasma-dissolved oxygen in his historic study, "Life Without Blood," in which unanesthetized pigs with an average hemoglobin of 0.45 gm/dl behaved normally when kept on pure oxygen at an atmospheric pressure of 3 ATA (3.03 MPa). Although the

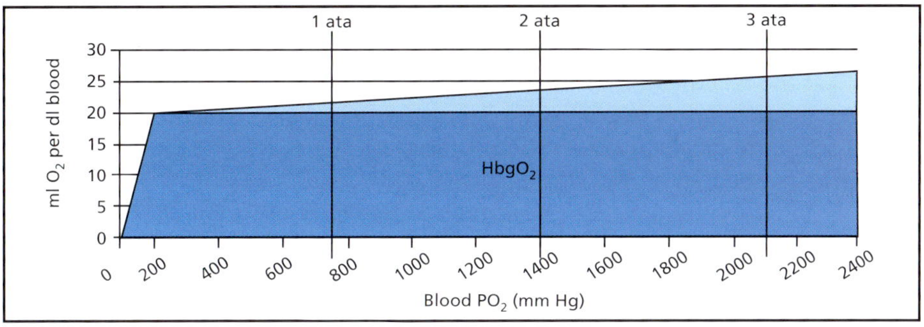

Figure 1. Oxygen carrying capacity of hemoglobin and plasma.
Note: This figure is modified from Sheffield PJ. Smith APS. Physiological and Pharmacological Basis of Hyperbaric Oxygen Therapy. In: DJ Bakker, FS Cramer (Eds), Hyperbaric Surgery: Perioperative Care, Flagstaff, AZ: Best Publishing, 2002; 68.

appropriate treatment for life-threatening anemia continues to be transfusion, there are many case reports in which HBO2 was successfully used to prolong life in patients who refused transfusion on religious grounds. In patients without life threatening anemia who undergo HBO2, the dramatic increase in arterial oxygen levels during treatment also increases the driving force for oxygen diffusion. For example, at 3 ATA (3.03 MPa), the diffusion radius of oxygen into the extravascular compartment is estimated to increase from 64 microns to about 247 microns at the pre-capillary arteriole (see Figure 2). This might allow a small number of capillaries to supply a larger volume of tissue, an effect that might be important in crush injury or threatened flaps.

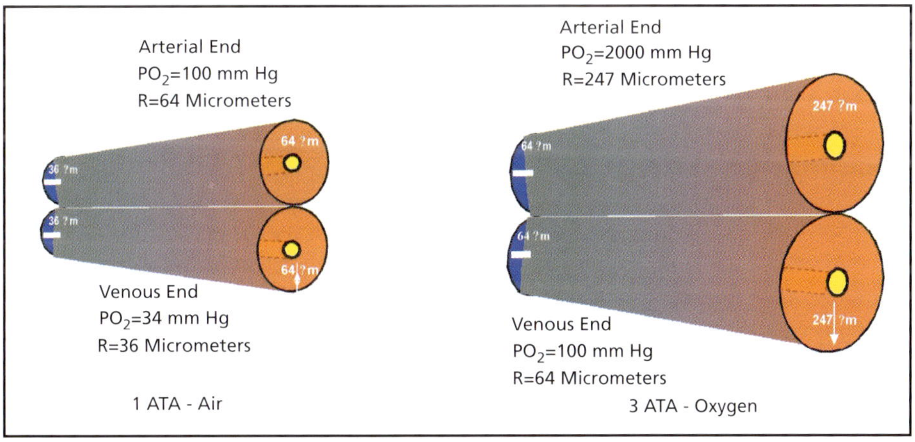

Figure 2. Krogh Erlang model of oxygen diffusion from the capillaries.
Note: This figure is modified from Sheffied PJ, Smith APS. Physiological and Pharmacological Basis of Hyperbaric Oxygen Therapy. In: DJ Bakker, FS Cramer (Eds), Hyperbaric Surgery: Perioperative Care, Flagstaff, AZ: Best Publishing, 2002; 74.

Like any drug, there are overdose and side effects. Pressure itself can cause barotrauma to gas-filled spaces in the body, most commonly the middle ear. Approximately 1–10% of patients experience ear pain from difficulty equalizing pressure in the middle ear through the eustachian tube. At the beginning of the treatment, gases in air-filled cavities contract as the atmospheric pressure in the chamber increases. Rupture of the tympanic membrane is uncommon but possible. Occasionally, tympanostomy tubes are necessary for patients to undergo HBO2. At the termination of the treatment, as the atmospheric pressure of the chamber decreases, gas expands. Thus, air must be able to exit the lungs freely. Rare cases of pneumothorax have been described, and this can lead to arterial gas embolization and death. As a result, patients with severe obstructive lung disease are not candidates for HBO2. Central nervous system oxygen toxicity has been reported at rates ranging from 0.4 per 100 recompressions (5) to 1:80 000 (6) (multiplace chamber with aviator masks). Symptoms can be diverse and range from anxiety to grand mal seizures, with the risk possibly enhanced by hypoglycemia. This is an effect of hyperbaric oxygen on brain neurotransmitters, but there are no long-term negative effects. Due to the rare incidence of this side effect, relative risks of different treatment profiles have been hard to establish. However, Praxis clinical services (now Diversified Clinical Services) recently performed an analysis of clinical data in 48,060 HBO2 treatments administered to 2,450 patients in which each treatment profile provided for similar "air breaks" (periods of breathing hyperbaric air during HBO2 (7). The incidence of seizure in patients treated at 2.0 ATA was 0.039%, compared to 0.212% and 0.168% at 2.4 and 2.5 ATA, respectively. Thus the incidence of oxygen toxicity at 2.0 ATA was significantly less than that observed with the higher treatment pressures. There was also no significant difference between the seizure incidences in the two higher treatment profiles (7). Hyperbaric oxygen also has an effect on the lens of the eye, which, in some patients, causes a transient myopia after a course of therapy. This effect seems to resolve after 3–6 months and does not appear to be linked to cataract development.

THE PHYSIOLOGICAL EFFECTS OF OXYGEN IN WOUND HEALING

The role of oxygen in wound healing has been discussed in detail by APS Smith in the chapter entitled, "Etiology of the Problem Wound." Thus, we will focus on the evidence that HBO2 is an acceptable mechanism for providing adequate oxygen to the wound, and the evidence of its clinical efficacy.

Oxygen has both biochemical and vascular effects, and HBO2 provides intermittent correction of wound hypoxia. The healing of a wound is dependent upon adequate oxygen availability within the vascularized connective tissue of the periwound area. Hyperbaric oxygen therapy increases tissue pO_2 and the driving force for oxygen diffusion in these areas. Whereas oxygen diffuses about 64 microns from a functioning capillary (the thickness of a single sheet of typing paper) under normobaric conditions, it diffuses three times that distance when HBO2 is provided at 3 ATA (3.03 MPa). In addition, HBO2 increases angiogenesis, demonstrating a dose-response relationship between degree of angiogenesis and absolute oxygen pressure (8, 9). One of the ways this is achieved is through stimulation of VEGF (vascular endothelial growth factor). Using an experimental rat model in which animals were randomized to HBO2 or control treatment following wound creation, Sheikh et al. demonstrated that VEGF levels increased 40% by day 5 in the HBO2 group (HBO2 twice daily for 90 min at 2.1 ATA), and decreased to control levels three days after cessation of HBO2 (10).

HBO2 improves wound metabolism. The elevation in tissue pO_2 achieved with HBO2 promotes wound healing by directly enhancing fibroblast replication, collagen synthesis, and the processes of neovascularization and epithelialization (11, 13).

HBO2 also enhances host immune response. Providing oxygen at the cellular level increases leukocyte bactericidal activity (14, 15). In addition, HBO2 promotes leukocyte killing of aerobic Gram-positive organisms, including *Staphylococcus aureus*, and aerobic Gram-negative organisms (16), and is cytotoxic to anaerobes. HBO2 can, therefore, decrease morbidity, mortality, and the need for operative intervention in various necrotizing infections. Further, HBO2 has proved effective as adjunctive therapy in animal models of chronic *S. aureus* and *Pseudomonas aeruginosa* osteomyelitis (17). In addition to enhanced bacterial killing, HBO2 also raises decreased oxygen tensions found in infected bone to normal, or even above normal levels. HBO2 enhances the transport of the aminoglycoside antibiotics (gentamicin, tobramycin, and amikacin) by enhancing transport across the bacterial cell wall, thus increasing the efficacy of these drugs, which can be inhibited in vivo by the local tissue hypoxia common in many patients with severe wounds (18).

HBO2 reduces local tissue edema by arterial vasoconstriction while maintaining higher than normal local oxygen delivery to wounded tissue. In addition to the biochemical effects discussed above, oxygen has direct vascular effects, causing vasoconstriction in both arterial and venous vessels. HBO2has been shown to reduce edema and congestion, effects that contribute to its adjunctive use in threatened replantations (19). While vasoconstriction induced by HBO2 can reduce blood "in-flow" by 20%, the amount of oxygen supplied by the plasma is increased, as described above, so oxygen delivery is maintained (20–22).

HBO2 prevents leukocyte mediated post-ischemic reperfusion injury. The most intriguing aspect of HBO2 is its now well-described ability to mitigate ischemia reperfusion injury, both in musculoskeletal tissue and in the brain. The mechanism operates by preventing the adhesion of leukocytes to the venule wall, thus limiting the production of oxygen free radicals, which cause arteriolar vasoconstriction.

HBO2 has a role in cytokine and cytokine receptor induction, and thus all the benefits of HBO2 in wound healing must be mediated by cytokines. For example, recent data reported by Mustoe's group has demonstrated that HBO2 modulates the signal transduction pathway, which regulates the gene expression for platelet derived growth factor (PDGF)-beta receptor (23). Recent research published by Buras et al. also supports this finding. These investigators used dermal fibroblasts isolated from NIDDM individuals and their non-diabetic siblings, and showed that in the HBO2 treated cell groups (both control and NIDDM; 90 min at 2.5 ATA), both fibroblast proliferation and expression of PDGFR (platelet-derived growth factor receptor) significantly increased. This is an important finding, as it was also demonstrated that the NIDDM fibroblasts proliferated more slowly and had lower expression of PGDFR compared to the non-diabetic counterparts (24). Not only does this suggest a possible synergistic effect between HBO2 and PDGF administration, but suggests another mechanism by which HBO2 enhances angiogenesis. HBO2 also stimulates osteoclast and osteoblast function, which is impaired under hypoxic conditions. Finally, Marx et al. have demonstrated that HBO2 enhances angiogenesis in ischemic-irradiated tissues (25). Histopathological studies have shown that the etiology of delayed radiation injury is endarteritis with tissue hypoxia and secondary fibrosis (26) Dental extractions or surgical reconstructions performed in previously irradiated tissue have high rates of complication and failure unless preoperative HBO2 is performed (27–30). In addition, HBO2 reduces complication rates in patients requiring surgical reconstruction in irradiated fields.

In summary, hyperbaric oxygen therapy has been demonstrated to have the following effects:

- Intermittent correction of wound hypoxia
- Reduction of local tissue edema by arterial vasoconstriction while maintaining higher than normal local oxygen delivery in wounded tissue
- Improved host immune response
    - Improved leukocyte killing of phagocytized bacteria
    - Direct toxic effects on anaerobic bacteria
    - Suppression of exotoxin production
    - Synergism with certain antibiotics.
- Improved wound metabolism:
    - Fibroblast replication and collagen synthesis
    - Epithelialization.
- Prevention of leukocyte mediated post-ischemic reperfusion injury
- Cytokine and cytokine receptor induction
    - Angiogenesis
    - Improved osteoclast and osteoblast function.

AN EVIDENCE-BASED REVIEW OF THE EFFECTS OF HBO2 IN WOUND HEALING

UHMS Accepted Indications for HBO2

Since 1968, the Undersea and Hyperbaric Medical Society (UHMS) has periodically reviewed the available literature on HBO2, and has published a list of indications for which the data support benefit (31). HBO2 is considered the primary treatment for decompression illness, arterial gas embolism, and carbon monoxide poisoning (32). As a result of the beneficial effects detailed above, HBO2 is considered a potentially useful adjunct for a number of other conditions. The following indications are accepted by the UHMS as adjunctive uses of HBO2 in various wound-healing problems:

- Acute thermal burns
- Clostridial myositis and myonecrosis
- Other necrotizing soft tissue infections
- Compromised skin grafts and flaps
- Crush injury, compartment syndrome, and other acute ischemias
- Osteoradionecrosis
- Soft tissue radionecrosis
- Refractory osteomyelitis
- Other wounds with demonstrated periwound hypoxia.

A thorough review of the data for all these conditions is available in Hyperbaric Oxygen 2003, the UHMS Hyperbaric Oxygen Therapy Committee Report. (UHMS, Kensington, MD, *www.uhms.org*) (31).

Although oxygen is a drug, no pharmaceutical companies manufacture it. The current emphasis on evidence-based medicine poses challenges for a modality such as hyperbaric oxygen therapy in which true blinded, randomized trials are technically difficult, and exceedingly expensive. In assessing available data, the hierarchy of evidence-based data is usually considered to be as follows:

- Randomized, controlled trials
- Non-randomized trials
- Cohort studies
- Case-controlled studies
- Case series and registries
- Surveys
- Qualitative, descriptive, studies, case reports
- Professional consensus.

It is not possible to review herein all available data for each hyperbaric indication. The UHMS offers a link to the Cochrane foundation website from which all controlled trials in hyperbaric medicine may be searched (*www.uhms.org*). Furthermore, the 2003 Hyperbaric Oxygen Committee Report, available from the UHMS, provides an evidence-based review of the literature for each indication, and that will not be reproduced here. In the area of HBO2 and wound healing, several exhaustive evidence-based reviews of world literature have been conducted by the following organizations or entities (in reverse chronological order):

- Clinical Evidence Reports, British Medical Journal (2000–2006)
- Cochrane Review group (2004)
- Medical Services Advisory Committee, Australia (2003)
- CMS Coverage Decision for HBO2 in diabetic foot ulcers (2002)
- AHRQ Report to CMS (2001)
- Quebec Ministry of Health (2001)
- Blue Cross/Blue Shield (BCBS) Technology Assessment (1999)
- American Diabetes Association Foot Council (1999)
- Wound Healing Society (1999)
- Alberta Heritage Foundation for Medical Research (1998).

These organizations reviewed the data regarding acute ischemias, acute infections, grafts and flaps, diabetic ulcers, and late effects of radiation and chronic infection (see Table 1). Independently, these organizations concluded that the data for acute ischemia, acute infection, diabetic ulcers, and radiation generally supported the utility of HBO2. The data for chronic infection was less compelling, being older and less well controlled, and that for jeopardized flaps as yet insufficient to review or inconclusive.

With regard to chronic non-healing wounds, the BCBS Technology Assessment concluded, "There is sufficient evidence to support the adjunctive use of HBO2 in the treatment of adequately perfused chronic non-healing wounds of the lower extremity in combination with standard wound care.

Patients who have received standard wound care plus HBO2 have shown better wound healing rates and fewer amputations in comparison to similar patients treated with standard wound care (33)." Similarly, the Wound Healing Society Provision Guidelines for Chronic Wound Care (June 21, 1999) in the Arterial Subcommittee co-chaired by Drs. Harriet Hopf and Judith West determined that "...in communities where accessible, HBO2 should be considered standard of care for wounds that are hypoxic (due to ischemia), and the hypoxia is reversible by hyperbaric oxygenation. The tissue hypoxia, reversibility, and responsiveness to oxygen challenge are measurable by transcutaneous oximetry." Even the conservative report from the Australian Medical Services Advisory Committee concluded, "...as there are no effective alternative therapies and in view of the progress of local data collections and an international trial, funding for HBO2 continue for MBS listed indications at currently eligible sites, for a further three years (34)." (The committee judged that the current clinical evidence was insufficient to judge the applications being considered.)

The American Diabetes Association concluded, "It is reasonable, however, to use this costly modality (hyperbaric oxygen treatment) to treat severe and limb- or life-threatening wounds that have not responded to other treatments, particularly if ischemia that cannot be corrected by vascular procedures is present (35, 36)." Finally, the Agency for Healthcare Research and Quality (AHRQ) made an extensive literature review specifically regarding the issue of hypoxic wounds (all aspects) in preparing a report to Centers for Medicare and Medicaid Services (CMS) in 2001. They reviewed 54 published, peer-reviewed studies, of which 7 were randomized, controlled trials (30, 37–42). In answer to the question "Is there sufficient objective evidence that the use of HBO2, as an adjunctive therapy to standard wound care, aids in wound healing?" posed by CMS, the authors of study answered "Most of the TAs [technology assessments] that we reviewed concluded that HBO2 is a beneficial adjunctive therapy to standard wound care in patients with chronic refractory wounds (progressive necrotizing infections, chronic refractory osteomyelitis). Our assessment of the primary studies on this type of wound concurs with their conclusions."

In examining 13 peer-reviewed studies, including seven RCTs, on the subject of the use of HBO2 in diabetic foot wounds, all classified as Wagner III-IV, Warriner and Fife reported that there were a total of 606 patients in the HBO2 groups with a 71% bipedal limb salvage rate, and in the combined control groups, a total of 463 patients with a 53% bipedal limb salvage rate (43). They compared these results with the Regranex® (becaplermin) clinical trials of diabetic foot ulcer healing (44), which included 922 patients over four trials, and noted that Regranex was given to 478 patients, with healing rates of 43%, compared to control healing rates of 29%. However, these involved only Wagner II, well-vascularized ulcers (44). Thus, it would seem that the hyperbaric oxygen data compares very favorably in the area of efficacy and limb salvage with much more limb-threatening wounds.

The Faglia et al. study (39) was a randomized, controlled trial of 70 diabetic ulcer patients consecutively admitted and randomized to receive HBO2 vs. standardized conventional care. The HBO2 treatment protocol was 2.5 ATA (2.53 MPa) for 90 minutes initially, followed by 2.4 ATA (2.42 MPa) for subsequent treatments. In the HBO2-treated group (mean treatment number 38 ± 8), 3 patients (8.6%) underwent major amputations: 2 below the knee (BKA), and 1 above the knee, (AKA). In the non-HBO2-treated group, 11 patients (33%) underwent major amputations: 7 BKA, and 4 AKA ($P = 0.016$). Of note, the $TcpO_2$ on dorsum of the foot increased significantly in HBO2-treated subjects, but not in the control group (14.0 ± 11.8 mm Hg in the HBO2 group, 5.0 ± 5.4 mm Hg in the non-treated group ($P = 0.0002$). Multivariate analysis of major amputation for all the considered variables confirmed the protective role of HBO2 in diabetic foot ulcers.

Several other notable RCTs that involved the use of HBO2 in the treatment of diabetic foot ulcers include the Doctor et al. study (38), which had 30 patients evenly divided between control and experimental groups, and found significantly less amputation for the experimental group, as well as better infection control. Kalani et al. (45) noted improved healing in their experimental group, although no effect on amputation rate, findings of which were confirmed by the studies of Abidia et al. (46), and Kessler et al. (47) Lin et al. (48) also discovered an improved TCOM when HBO2 was used to treat early diabetic feet. On the basis of all these data, CMS crafted a new coverage policy regarding HBO2 and the diabetic foot ulcer (see section on Medicare Coverage Guidelines).

HYPERBARIC OXYGEN TREATMENT IN WOUND HEALING: MANAGEMENT GUIDELINES

Appropriate use of HBO2 depends on an accurate diagnosis of wound etiology, and an understanding of the mechanism of action of HBO2. A well-vascularized wound might be appropriately treated with HBO2 in the presence of chronic refractory osteomyelitis, but a well-vascularized, neuropathic diabetic foot ulcer would not be an appropriate patient for HBO2, because the treatment for that wound is aggressive off-loading. The benefit of HBO2 in the treatment of compromised flaps was once thought to be limited to correction of hypoxia, but it is now understood that mitigation of ischemia reperfusion injury is an equally important mechanism of action. However, the optimal treatment time for this benefit would be in the immediate post-op period. Thus, recommendations for the clinical use of HBO2 will continue to evolve as our understanding of the physiological mechanisms improves.

Hyperbaric Oxygen Treatment Protocols

Treatment protocols vary depending on the diagnosis and the severity of the wound. Treatments for wound-healing problems are usually delivered at 2.0–2.4 ATA (2.02-2.43 MPa) for between 90 and 120 minutes. There is preliminary data suggesting that, perhaps as a result of vasoconstriction, higher treatment pressures might not always confer a higher tissue pO_2, particularly in patients with large-vessel occlusive disease (49). For example, outcome data failed to show a statistical difference in diabetic wound healing when analyzed by treatment pressure at 2.0 vs. 2.4 ATA (2.02 vs. 2.42 MPa) (50). This is probably because after some minimum threshold is reached, increasing treatment pressure will not confer additional benefit. In the

TABLE 1. SUMMARY OF EVIDENCE-BASED REVIEWS OF HBO2

Report	Authors & Date of Material Reviewed	Primary Source of MAterial Reviewed	Major Findings	Notes
Cochrane Review	Kranke P, Bennett M, Roeckl-Wiedmann I, Debus S. (2004)	Diabetic foot ulcer (4 trials, 147 patients); venous ulcer: (1 trial, 16 patients)	In cases of diabetic foot ulcers, HBO2 significantly reduces risk of major amputation and might improve chance of healing at 1 year.	Report did not recommend HBO2 for any other conditions associated with chronic wounds.
CMS Coverage Decision	Shuren J, Cas RD, Kucken L, Tillman K. (2002)	Wound hypoxia: 8 studies, including 1 RCT; diabetic wounds (lower extremities): 12 studies, including 2 RCTs	Literature inadequately demonstrates that wounds can be primarily classified based on tissue oxygen level, or that $TcPO_2$ can reliably predict wound outcome with HBO2 therapy. Evidence supports use of HBO2 in treatment of lower extremity diabetic wounds that are limb-threatening and ≥Wagner grade III.	With regard to wound hypoxia, since there is no demonstrated evidence for a wound category of hypoxic, the decision to use HBO2 here was denied.
Clinical Evidence Reports (BMJ series)	Hunt D. (2006)	Infected foot ulcers: 1 systematic review, 1 RCT; Noninfected, nonischaemic ulcers: 1 RCT	In cases of severe infected diabetic foot ulcers with full-thickness gangrene or abscess, or with large infected ulcer not healed within 30 days, HBO2 should be considered.	Evidence is updated yearly; series 2000-2006.
AHRQ Report to CMS	Wang C, Lau J. (2001)	ATPI: 1 study; crush injuries: 1 RCT; compromised skin grafts: 2 RCTs; osteo-radionecrosis: 2 RCTs, 1 study; soft tissue radionecrosis: 13 studies; gas gangrene: 17 studies; Progressive necrotizing infections: 9 studies; Chronic refractory osteomyelitis: 2 studies; Chronic non-healing wounds: 2 RCTs, 4 studies	HBO2 is a beneficial adjunctive therapy to standard wound care in patients with chronic refractory wounds (progressive necrotizing infections, and chronic refractory osteomyelitis). HBO2 aids in wound healing for: compromised skin grafts, osteo-radionecrosis, gas gangrene, progressive necrotizing infections, and chronic nonhealing wounds. There is evidence from case series studies suggesting the beneficial effect of HBO2 for soft tissue radionecrosis.	
Medical Services Advisory Committee, Australia	Villanueva E, Harris A, Petherick E, Johnston R, Raulli A, Mitchell A. (2003)	Nonhealing wounds in nondiabetic patients: 2 RCTs, 3 studies; refractory soft tissue radiation injuries: 6 RCTs, 10 studies	Clinical evidence judged inadequate to substantiate claim that HBO2 is cost-effective in treatment of refractory soft tissue radiation injuries or nondiabetic refractory wounds. However, because of lack of effective alternative therapies and in view of progress of local data collections and international trial, funding for HBO2 should continue for another 3 years.	

TABLE 1. (CONTINUED)

Quebec Minstry of Health	Hassen-Khodja RMR, Régnier G. (2001)	No authors listed (1999)	Gas gangrene: HBO2 as an adjuvant treatment in gas gangrene suggested, but RCTs needed; tissue necrosis: same comments as for gas gangrene; osteoradionecrosis: level of evidence supporting the eff cacy of HBO2 in treatment of osteoradionecrosis is fair, whereas for soft tissue necrosis it is lower. Nonetheless, results for soft-tissue necrosis are promising. Diabetic wounds: HBO2 can have a beneficial effect on diabetic wounds; leg ulcers: HBO2 justified in treatment of this chronic condition.	Several other aspects of HBO2 therapy considered not reported here.
BCBS technology study	No authors listed (1999)	Chronic non-healing wounds: 3 RCTs (2 diabetic), 2 studies; split skin grafts: 1 RCT; crush injuries: 1 RCT; chronic refractory osteomyelitis: 1 study; necrotizing soft tissue infections: 4 studies; gas gangrene: 17 studies	Chronic non-healing wounds: beneficial results when HBO2 used; split skin grafts: HBO2 useful when raw creas are extensive; crush injuries: adjunctive HBO2 useful in reducing number of surgical procedures and improving incidence of complete wound healing; chronic refractory osteomyelitis: no benefit; necrotizing soft tissue infections: inconclusive; gas gangrene: possible benefit when HBO2 used.	Several more conditions studied that are not reported here. Study in 3 parts, published in Technological MAP Suppl
American Diabetes Association Foot Concil	No authors cited. (1999)	Consensus multidisciplinary meeting with 8-member panel hearing presentations from 25 experts	Reasonable to use HBO2 in treatment of limb- and life-threatening wounds unresponsive to other treatments, especially if ischemia cannot be corrected by revascularization.	No specific studies used as primary sources.
Alberta Heritage Foundation for Medical research	Mitton C, Hailey D. (1998)	Literature reviewed prior to 1999 for 13 conditions	High level of evidence supporting the use of HBO2 in maxillary osteoradionecrosis and diabetic leg ulcers. Acceptable level of evidence for use of HBO2 in treating gas gangrene. There is a potential role for HBO2 in treatment of soft-tissue radionecrosis and necrotizing soft-tissue infections. Insufficient evidence for use of HBO2 in refractory osteomyelitis, compromised skin grafts, and crush injuries.	Also published in: Int J Technol Assess Health Care 1999;15:661-670.

future, a more precise understanding of the exact tissue pO_2 needed for healing might allow protocols to be individually tailored for each patient. Treatments can be once or twice per day depending on the severity and type of wound. Since HBO2 is adjunctive to appropriate medical and surgical management, concomitant antibiotic administration, diabetes control, debridement, off-loading, edema control, wound care, and other appropriate standards must be maintained.

The number of treatments necessary depends on the rationale for use of HBO2. In a rapidly spreading necrotizing infection, HBO2 might be administered emergently but fewer than ten times until control of infection is achieved. In the case of chronic non-healing wounds, HBO2 might be continued until a confluent granulation tissue bed is achieved. Although specific treatment numbers cannot be recommended, guidelines for institution of peer review are available in the 1999 UHMS Hyperbaric Oxygen Therapy Committee report. Analysis of patient outcomes for those with diabetic foot ulcerations undergoing HBO2 show that the average number of treatments in patients who benefited was 35. However, outcome data also show that diminishing returns are reached at approximately 40 treatments (50). If diabetic patients have not achieved significant improvement by that time, continued treatment with HBO2 is unlikely to yield further benefit.

In this same retrospective analysis, fewer treatments were given to patients who subsequently underwent amputation, because HBO2 was discontinued after a reasonable trial if there was no evidence of benefit. When used as an adjunct for wound healing, evidence of benefit should be apparent after 15–20 HBO2 treatments (51). This mandates continued reassessment of patients undergoing HBO2, to determine whether progress justifies continued treatment. The "prescription" of a specific number of treatments, without regard to patient progress, does not result in cost-effective use of HBO2. Moreover, appropriate use of HBO2 requires the direct and frequent input of a trained hyperbaric physician.

Rationale for HBO2 in Selected Disorders

The physiological basis of HBO2 is provided for the following wound-healing enhancement applications and is not intended to be an exhaustive list.

Uncovered wound conditions: venous stasis ulcers and pressure ulcers

Adequate compression is the standard of care for venous stasis ulceration, and hyperbaric oxygen therapy is only indicated in patients with wound hypoxia and adequate edema control. Usually these are patients with mixed arterial and venous disease. For example, in a double-blind, prospective, randomized study of nondiabetic patients with leg ulcers, hyperbaric oxygen patients had a 35.7% (SD ± 17) reduction in wound size at 6 weeks compared to 2.7% (SD ± 11) in controls (52). Patients who have jeopardized skin grafts or flaps following surgical closure of venous wounds might also benefit from HBO2. However, the Centers for Medicare and Medicaid Services (CMS) has declined to recognize hypoxic wounds as a distinct category. Therefore, patients with stasis ulcers who have failed appropriate treatment with compression and have been demonstrated to have tissue hypoxia with transcutaneous oxygen monitoring (TCOM), would not meet CMS coverage criteria unless they had an acute arterial occlusion or until a skin graft was placed and then failed. The rationale for the benefit of HBO2 in stasis (after edema has been properly controlled) is the correction of tissue hypoxia, and the enhancement of angiogenesis as described above.

The primary treatment for pressure ulceration of the sacrum, ischium, trochanter, and other areas is adequate off-loading. Nutritional support and aggressive wound management are crucial, although for superficial pressure sores, conservative management is usually adequate. For deeper pressure ulcerations, the vacuum assisted device (VAC®) has proven to be highly effective, and surgical treatment, including excision with primary closure, skin grafting, or flap rotation, are often necessary. The role of HBO2 is limited to adjunctive therapy for chronic osteomyelitis, or complications of plastic surgical reconstruction, and is never a primary treatment for pressure ulcer treatment and is not reimbursable by CMS for that indication. One exception would be foot ulcerations that develop due to a combination of pressure and ischemia, which would be treated as part of a limb-salvage protocol.

Arterial insufficiency ulcers

As discussed in the chapter by Boccolandro entitled, "Critical Limb Ischemia and Limb Salvage" the primary treatment of arterial ischemia is revascularization. If revascularization is not feasible, or if tissue hypoxia persists following revascularization, HBO2 can be of benefit. Patients can be screened with TCOM and referred for angiography if their baseline $TcpO_2$ values, or clinical history of rest pain or claudication suggest critical ischemia. After revascularization, TCOM can be repeated, and (if baseline values are improved) patients can be followed with conservative wound care or, if still below healing threshold, an in-chamber TCOM can be performed to determine the likelihood of benefit from HBO2 as described below. Correction of tissue hypoxia with HBO2 results in collagen synthesis, angiogenesis, and thus the production of granulation tissue. Treatment can be given at 2.0 or 2.4 ATA (2.02 or 2.43 MPa). Outcome studies have failed to show a difference between these 2 treatment pressures, probably because the key is not the gauge pressure, but the $TcpO_2$ achieved in the tissue, with values above 200 mm Hg in the chamber being a critical threshold. Despite the documented benefit of HBO2 in ischemic wounds, CMS covers HBO2 only for acute arterial insufficiency (embolization), not for chronic arterial disease.

Thermal burns

HBO2 preserves ischemic tissues by relieving hypoxia, decreasing fluid loss, and limiting burn wound extension and conversion. HBO2 increases the flexibility of red cells, reduces tissue edema, preserves intracellular adenosine triphosphate, and maintains tissue oxygenation in the absence of hemoglobin. Adjunctive HBO2 also appears to stimulate nitric oxide production, ultimately affecting gene expression/suppression. Through these mechanisms, HBO2 might be useful in treating both anaerobic and aerobic infections that are frequently associated with severe burns. HBO2 is also beneficial in facilitating the rapid spread and arborization of new capillaries, as well as stimulating fibroblast growth, enhancing collagen formation, reducing lipid peroxidation, and subsequently improving epithelialization. All these factors are associated with better healing and improved morbidity.

Clostridial myositis and myonecrosis (gas gangrene)

Gas gangrene (Clostridial myonecrosis) is caused by the anaerobic, spore-forming, gram-positive encapsulated bacilli of the genus Clostridium. *C. perfringens* produces a tissue-necrotizing toxin that causes clostridial myositis and myonecrosis, an acute, rapidly progressive, invasive infection of the muscles, characterized by profound toxemia, extensive edema, massive tissue death, and a variable degree of gas production. HBO2 is an adjunct to surgery and antibiotics in treating gas gangrene to halt the spread of infection and toxicity. The alpha-toxin produced by *C. perfringens* contributes to systemic vascular collapse. However, one exposure to oxygen tensions of about 250 mm Hg ceases alpha-toxin production, and at 1500 mm Hg, the dose is bactericidal. Adjunctive HBO2 treatments are usually given at 3 ATA (3.03 MPa) with the patient breathing 100% oxygen for 90 minutes during each treatment. HBO2, surgical, and antibiotic management can be continued over 5–7 treatments during the next 3–5 days. Using HBO2 for treating gas gangrene reduces morbidity and prevents or lowers the level of amputation necessitated by limb gas gangrene (53).

Crush injuries, compartment syndrome, and other acute traumatic peripheral ischemias

Acute traumatic peripheral ischemias (ATPI) include crush injuries, compartment syndromes, thermal burns, frostbite injuries, compromised skin grafts and flaps, and threatened replantations. The immediate threat to surviving injured tissue after an ATPI relates to the sufficiency of vascular perfusion. The primary rationale for using HBO2 is to counteract trauma-related tissue hypoxia and edema, as well as their related consequences. Adjunctive HBO2 increases oxygen delivery in the blood, enhances oxygen availability to the injured tissue, and enhances post-traumatic edema reduction. HBO2 also protects tissue from reperfusion injury for which several actions have been identified. First, HBO2 antagonizes lipid peroxidation of the cell membrane that occurs after toxic oxygen radicals interact with membrane lipids. Second, HBO2 interferes with initiation of reperfusion injury by blocking the sequestration of neutrophils on post-capillary venules, and antagonizing the beta-2 integrin system, which initiates the neutrophil adherence response to the post-capillary venule endothelium. Third, it might also provide sufficient additional oxygen for reperfused tissues to generate oxygen radical scavengers. Using adjunctive HBO2 for ATPI reduces the number of surgeries and improves healing rates (37). In addition, adjunctive HBO2 is widely accepted for use in limb salvage/reattachment to minimize an amputation site. The rationale for using HBO2 in frostbite is to prevent a foot or leg amputation, and help with the reperfusion injury that results from frostbite or other surgical procedures, which reintroduce blood back into a hypoxic area of the body. Treatments are usually given at 2.0–2.5 ATA (2.02–2.53 MPa).

Osteomyelitis (refractory)

Acute osteomyelitis is not a covered indication by CMS for HBO2. Prior to therapy, refractory osteomyelitis must be documented by appropriate studies or bone biopsy. Oxygen tensions in infected bone are usually below 20 mm Hg compared to 30–40 mm Hg in healthy tissue, and HBO2 elevates bone oxygen tensions to near normal levels. The rationale for adjunctive HBO2 to aid the surgical and antibiotic management of chronic osteomyelitis is primarily to stimulate osteogenesis, improve fibroblastic activity, increase collagen production, and stimulate new capillary growth to fill voids. The effect of HBO2 on microorganisms in chronic osteomyelitis appears to be antibiotic enhancement and improved bacterial killing. HBO2 at 2.0–2.5 ATA (2.02–2.53 MPa) is combined with excision of sequestra, and antibiotics. Normally a course of 40 treatments is given for bone infections.

Delayed radiation injury (soft tissue and bony necrosis)

Delayed soft tissue radionecrosis or osteoradionecrosis can occur six months to many years after radiation exposure. The mechanism is an endarteritis with resultant tissue hypoxia, and thus far, hyperbaric oxygen therapy is the only treatment that has been shown to cause neovascularization in the radiated tissue bed. Extensive work by Marx and colleagues (27–30) has demonstrated that preprocedure and postprocedure HBO2 dramatically reduces oral surgical complications in the irradiated field. Prior to the adjunctive use of HBO2, dental extractions and reconstructive procedures performed in irradiated fields often had up to a 70% complication or failure rate. Prophylactic pre-operative HBO2 is also used to reduce the risk of nonhealing when surgery is performed in the irradiated site. The protocol usually consists of 20 pre-extraction treatments followed by ten or more postextraction treatments. Prior to extensive reconstructive surgery, up to 30 treatments can be given, with ten or more postoperative treatments. Soft tissue radionecrosis of the bladder or bowel are significant complications of cancer treatment, and life-threatening hematuria or incapacitating tenesmus can result. HBO2 has been shown in numerous case series to be of benefit, although, it is not uncommon for patients to require as many as 60 HBO2 treatments for this indication. This expense is easily justified in cases in which the bladder is saved (see the 2003 UHMS Hyperbaric Oxygen Therapy Committee report for further information). CMS covers late effects of radiation.

Skin grafts and flaps (compromised)

The ability of hyperbaric oxygen therapy to increase the diffusion distance of oxygen, as well as the blood oxygen-carrying capacity, while simultaneously decreasing edema, makes it an ideal adjunct to acutely compromised flaps. In the past, patients were referred for HBO2 when there was visual evidence of flap necrosis, but recently, it has become apparent that a significant mechanism of HBO2 in flap salvage is its ability to mitigate ischemia reperfusion injury. To benefit optimally from this mechanism, patients should receive HBO2 postoperatively almost immediately for cases in which there is a known significant ischemia reperfusion injury (a long warm ischemia time in a re-implantation, for example). However, if delivered early, only one or two HBO2 treatments might be needed (54). If HBO2 is begun for the purpose of flap salvage, treatment at 2.0–2.4 ATA (2.03–2.52 MPa) is probably adequate, and TCOM or laser Doppler flowmetry can be helpful in determining flap viability. Teamwork with the plastic surgeon is essential to determine the clinical endpoint.

Enhancement of wound healing

Problem wounds are those that have failed to respond to established medical and surgical management. They are usually compromised by tissue hypoperfusion, tissue hypoxia, and infection, and include diabetic foot ulcers, nonhealing, postoperative wounds, nonhealing traumatic wounds, and vascular insufficiency ulcers. In the hypoxic environment of these wounds, healing is halted by decreased fibroblast proliferation, diminished collagen production, impaired capillary angiogenesis, and the inability to control infection. HBO2 directly promotes wound healing by restoring the oxygen tension needed to enhance fibroblast replication, collagen synthesis, capillary budding, granulation tissue formation, epithelialization, and bacterial extermination (55, 56). In so doing, it produces granulation tissue, increases the potential for skin grafting, and decreases the likelihood of amputation. Treatments are usually given at 2.0–2.5 ATA (2.02–2.53 MPa) with diminishing returns reached by 35–40 treatments. The evidence-based data for HBO2 in diabetic foot ulcers has been thoroughly presented above.

Patient Selection for Hyperbaric Oxygen Therapy

This section will focus on the selection of patients with hypoxic wounds. After exhaustive review of the literature, similar themes emerged in the discussion of how patient selection is best approached. Phrases such as, "failure to respond to conservative measures after adequate revascularization (American Diabetes Association)," and "tissue hypoxia reversible with HBO2, demonstrated by TCOM (Wound Healing Society)," provide the backdrop for this discussion. HBO2 is never indicated for well-vascularized neuropathic foot ulcers; the treatment for these wounds is off-loading.

The physician begins with a thorough history and initial evaluation of the systemic and local factors detailed in other chapters, after which there must be an assessment of whether periwound oxygen levels are adequate for spontaneous healing. TCOM represents a simple, non-invasive method for assessing the likelihood of spontaneous healing and a screening tool for vascular disease. Generally, $TcpO_2$ values less than 40 mm Hg are considered inadequate for spontaneous healing. If $TcpO_2$s are adequate, the wound can be treated with conservative management. However, when $TcpO_2$ values and history suggest further vascular testing is warranted, the severity of the wound, the debility of the patient, and the proposed intervention will determine the most appropriate study. We prefer to go directly to magnetic resonance angiography, if possible, to obtain the anatomical information lacking in Doppler studies, avoiding renal-toxic dye, and the risk of bleeding complications inherent in standard angiography. It is then possible to make decisions regarding the feasibility and the advisability of revascularization. After revascularization, we recheck TCOM values again. Values consistent with spontaneous healing might allow conservative management, but if values are still below those expected for spontaneous healing, the next step might be an in-chamber TCOM and perhaps a course of HBO2.

The selection process would be:

- Evaluate $TcpO_2$ for likelihood of spontaneous healing (>40 mm Hg)
- If $TcpO_2$ is low, then determine whether large vessel flow is adequate
- Once large vessel flow is optimized, evaluate $TcpO_2$ in-chamber to determine if HBO2 will be of benefit.

We evaluated the outcome of a series of 29 consecutive limb-threatening lesions in diabetic patients who underwent angioplasty for revascularization. After a mean follow up period of 12 months, 23 patients (79%) experienced progressive healing, with 15 (65%) being discharged from hyperbaric oxygen treatment by the end of the follow-up period. Mean time to wound healing was three months. Six patients (21%) had poor outcomes, two requiring BKA due to osteomyelitis despite technically successful angioplasties, one amputated due to a worsening wound, and three could not be revascularized. The $TcpO_2$ improved in all the patients who were successfully revascularized from 27.8 ±9.9 mm Hg to 54.5 ±14.7 mm Hg ($P < 0.0001$). Patients whose postprocedure $TcpO_2$s remained below 40 mm Hg received HBO2 to assist with wound healing. TCOM performed better than Doppler ABI in predicting the technical success of angioplasty, as well as in screening the patients who were referred for angioplasty, and in determining which patients would receive HBO2 afterward (57).

Simultaneously, there must be an assessment of limb functionality. Hyperbaric oxygen cannot resurrect necrotic tissue. A transmetatarsal amputation is a stable, functional amputation, which allows the patient to walk without a prosthesis, and be easily fitted with a shoe. A patient with two necrotic toes might be best served by having a transmetarsal amputation after revascularization, with hyperbaric oxygen therapy reserved for treatment of the flap postoperatively if there is concern over its viability.

The hyperbaric physician must complete the evaluation of the patient with regard to the safety and the appropriateness of HBO2. As discussed in the section on How Hyperbaric Oxygen Increases Tissue Oxygen Levels, HBO2 is a drug with side effects. Patients with chronic obstructive lung disease must be assessed carefully, and seizure disorders must be controlled. A variety of other underlying disease processes can affect patients in the hyperbaric environment, which is why hyperbaric physicians receive specific training. Patients must then be frequently assessed regarding their response to treatment, and whether continued HBO2 is warranted.

TISSUE OXYGEN MEASUREMENTS

Transcutaneous oximetry ($TcpO_2$ or TCOM), which uses a modified Clark electrode in a heated thermistor, is in common usage at many wound-healing centers. It is a non-invasive and painless method of assessing tissue oxygen availability. However, it has the disadvantage of requiring intact skin for measurement, and thus may be used only in the periwound area. Since this technique relies on the diffusion of oxygen to the heated electrode, highly calloused, edematous, or infected skin decreases the reliability of measurements. Nevertheless, the $TcpO_2$ represents a physiological snapshot of the oxygen tension of the skin surrounding a wound, and has been evaluated as a way of assessing the spontaneous healing potential of wounds (ie, whether patients will heal without HBO2), and of determining which patients might benefit from subsequent HBO2. In a study that did not involve the use of hyperbaric therapy, Wyss et al. reported that in postoperative patients, sea level air $TcpO_2$ readings <20 mm Hg were associated with poor healing, 20–40 mm Hg represented intermediate healing, and > 40 mm Hg readings indicated good healing (58). Pecoraro et al. also found a 39-fold increase in risk of early healing failure in diabetic foot ulcers when the measured $TcpO_2$ was <20 mm Hg (59). Thus, a low $TcpO_2$ is associated with a high risk of amputation while patients with periwound $TcpO_2$ values greater than 40 mm Hg on room air might heal without intervention. As a caveat, we reported a 5-center retrospective study in which 48% of the hyperbaric patients had a baseline $TcpO_2$ below 20 mm Hg, yet demonstrated a failure rate of only 35% (50). This might suggest the effectiveness of HBO2. For this reason, while baseline, sea level, air $TcpO_2$ levels are used to determine whether the wound might heal spontaneously, they are of no value in determining whether HBO2 will be of benefit.

A variety of techniques have been employed to enhance the predictive value of $TcpO_2$. Observing the absolute value and the relative increase in $TcpO_2$ while breathing oxygen at sea level seems to increase the accuracy of $TcpO_2$ in postamputation healing. It has also been shown to be of benefit in predicting the outcome from hyperbaric oxygen therapy (60). In-chamber $TcpO_2$ has previously been demonstrated to have the strongest statistical relationship to benefit from HBO2. The accuracy of $TcpO_2$ was evaluated in a retrospective analysis of over 1000 patients with diabetic foot ulcers, all of whom underwent treatment with HBO2, with an overall success rate of 75.6% (50). An increase in periwound $TcpO_2$ while breathing oxygen at sea level was useful in selecting patients likely to benefit from HBO2: if oxygen-breathing $TcpO_2$ values increased to above 35 mm Hg at sea level, the likelihood of benefiting from subsequent HBO2 was 77%, and the test was 69% accurate with PPVs (positive predictive values) in the ranges 33–42%. The absolute increase (in mm Hg) with oxygen breathing was better than the percent increase (or ratio) over baseline, because many patients with a baseline near zero were not healed if their HBO2 doubled or tripled (ie, increasing 2 mm Hg to 6 mm Hg). However, the most reliable test for benefit from HBO2 was the increase in periwound $TcpO_2$ while breathing oxygen in the hyperbaric chamber. If in-chamber $TcpO_2$ increased to 200 mm Hg or better, the likelihood of benefiting from HBO2 was 94%, and this test was 75% accurate, with PPVs in the range of 40–58%. These data did not directly demonstrate the effectiveness of HBO2, because there was no control group of similar patients who received sham or no therapy. However, for many of these patients with modified Wagner III or IV lesions, HBO2 was the only alternative to amputation. In light of the overall success rate of 75.6% in this large series of patients, the benefit of HBO2 is encouraging. These data confirm those previously reported by Wattel et al. (60), demonstrating that patients with transcutaneous oxygen values of 100 mm Hg in the vicinity of the wound while breathing pure oxygen at 2.5 ATA heal 75% of the time, whereas patients with lower values go on to amputation.

HBO2 treatments usually last only one to two hours, raising the question as to whether this time period is sufficient to affect biological processes. Data confirm that oxygen tension values can remain elevated for up to three hours after the cessation of hyperbaric therapy, and baseline tissue oxygen levels begin to increase as angiogenesis occurs. By measuring transcutaneous oxygen levels near healing diabetic foot wounds, Sheffield demonstrated this improvement in the form of capillary density (56). Moreover, Faglia et al. (39) documented a highly significant and long-lasting increase in transcutaneous oxygen values in diabetic patients who benefited from hyperbaric oxygen therapy. Marx et al. (25) have also demonstrated the same changes in ischemic-irradiated tissues.

If our goal is to screen patients for the most cost-effective use of HBO2, then we wish to screen out patients who are destined to fail. A sea level $TcpO_2$ assessment has an accuracy of about 70%, while the accuracy of in-chamber $TcpO_2$ approaches 75%. Even with these effective screening tools, our prediction would still be incorrect in one out of four cases and patients who might benefit from HBO2 would be deprived of the therapy. Therefore, these "cut-off" scores must serve as guides to therapy. A rational approach might be to provide a trial of therapy and then reassess the patient on the basis of clinical progress or improved $TcpO_2$ values after a reasonable number of treatments (ie, 15 treatments).

If periwound transcutaneous O_2 levels are low and unresponsive to sea level or in-chamber oxygen breathing, patients should undergo vascular assessment (preferably by angiography) to select those patients who might benefit from revascularization (see section on patient selection). In some cases, angioplasty might be an adequate means of revasacularization, for the purpose of wound healing. Data suggest that following cases of technically successful angioplasty, if $TcpO_2$ remains low, HBO2 might then be successfully used for healing of ischemic ulcerations (57). In cases in which $TcpO_2$ level is low and revascularization is not possible, the usefulness of HBO2 is limited. Outcome data showed that some patients with very low in-chamber $TcpO_2$ still benefited from HBO2 (50). Therefore, in these instances, a trial of therapy might be indicated on a case-by-case basis if limb loss is the only alternative. Combining the use of laser Doppler flowmetry (LDF) might be useful in selecting HBO2 candidates.

An additional potential benefit of transcutaneous oxygen measurement might be its use in determining when a patient has obtained maximum benefit from therapy. In the past, HBO2 treatments have been performed until complete granulation of the wound was visible. However, it seems likely that there is some point at which angiogenesis will be sustained in the wound, even if HBO2 is discontinued. As third-party payers increase pressure to reduce health care costs, a reliable method has been sought for determining the earliest point at which HBO2 can be discontinued without sacrificing outcome. Data have suggested that HBO2 might be discontinued when baseline periwound $TcpO_2$ values have normalized. While Faglia et al. (39) have shown a highly significant and durable increase in transcutaneous oxygen values in diabetic patients who benefited from hyperbaric oxygen therapy, further research is needed to determine if HBO2 discontinuation can be recommended solely on the basis of improved $TcpO_2$, prior to the achievement of an adequate, visible granulation tissue base.

Available evidence would support the use of $TcpO_2$ in the following way:

1. An initial baseline $TcpO_2$ breathing air to determine whether tissue hypoxia exists. A high value (perhaps greater than 40 mm Hg) would suggest that the wound has adequate oxygen availability and the etiology of delayed healing is not due to hypoxia.
2. If baseline $TcpO_2$ is low, in-chamber $TcpO_2$ is the most accurate way to determine possible benefit from HBO2. In-chamber $TcpO_2$ of >200 mm Hg suggests that benefit from HBO2 is likely. Patients with in-chamber values of <100mm Hg should be referred for revascularization.
3. In the absence of in-chamber data, a $TcpO_2$ value breathing oxygen at sea level less than 40 mm Hg may be used as an indicator that a course of HBO2 would be beneficial. In a retrospective study of 46 patients, Sheffield et al. showed that a $TcpO_2$ model in which a $TcpO_2$ in air was >0 mm Hg, coupled with an absolute $TcpO_2$ in oxygen >35 mm Hg, and an oxygen challenge increase >50% was useful in predicting healing (61).

For more information about tissue oximetry applications see the chapter entitled "Non-Invasive Wound Assessment Tools" by D Dietz and PJ Sheffield.

LASER DOPPLER FLOWMETRY

Laser Doppler flowmetry (LDF) with heat provocation has promise as a tool for evaluating tissue ischemia and for qualifying patients for HBO2 (61). LDF measures the total blood perfusion in local tissue, including capillaries, arterioles, venules, and shunts. LDF indicates if the tissue is ischemic. With local heat provocation (44°C) vasodilatation is maximized, enabling the use of LDF to assess the tissue reserve capacity and severity of ischemia. Combining LDF and $TcpO_2$ will provide additional information that should be useful for selecting the appropriate treatment to enhance wound healing.

To evaluate the patient, LDF perfusion is assessed for 5 minutes to establish a baseline before the LDF probe is heated to 44°C to create maximum vasodilatation. The percentage change in mean perfusion before and after heat provocation is calculated (LDF % increase) to indicate the degree of ischemia. Perfusion of local tissue is considered normal with an LDF % increase of greater than 500. Values of 150–500 are considered moderately ischemic, and values below 150 are considered severely ischemic. Laser Doppler flowmetry with local heat provocation also appears to be a useful complement to $TcpO_2$ for assessing wounded patients, especially when $TcpO_2$ values are low (61).

For more information about laser Doppler flowmetry applications see the chapter entitled "Non-Invasive Wound Assessment Tools" by D Dietz and PJ Sheffield.

Patient Example (Suboptimal Management)

Patient #1 is a 54-year-old African American female with IDDM and severe peripheral vascular disease on dialysis, deemed inoperable by vascular surgery, status post right great toe amputation for gangrenous changes. Baseline air $TcpO_2$ could not be obtained adjacent to the wound, because of edema and tissue necrosis, but on the dorsal foot near the ankle, the baseline $TcpO_2$ was 30 mm Hg. Her in-chamber $TcpO_2$ was 1,000 mm Hg, suggesting she would be a good HBO2 candidate (see Figure 3A). During the course of HBO2 she received aggressive wound care, including debridement (her insurance company denied the VAC®). However, after 44 treatments, while the wound had granulated to some degree, she infarcted the second toe (See Figure 3B). A transmetatarsal amputation was then required which took six months to heal with conservative care. (Her insurance company denied further HBO2). In retrospect, given the limited response she had demonstrated after 15–20 treatments, despite her encouraging in-chamber $TcpO_2$s, a better management plan would have been to perform the transmetatarsal amputation early on, and use HBO2 to treat the resulting wound healing problems after that amputation. This is also an example of the "diminishing returns" noted in the retrospective data analysis (50). Patients who have not done well after 40 treatments are unlikely to benefit from further treatments.

As a footnote, the same patient returned eight months later with ischemic changes in all five toes on the left foot. Dorsal foot $TcpO_2$ was 24 mm Hg with a poor response to sea level oxygen (62 mm Hg) and she had ischemic rest pain. In-chamber $TcpO_2$ on the dorsal foot was <100 mm Hg. She was deemed inoperable by vascular surgery. $TcpO_2$s at the below the knee were encouraging at 63 and 70 mm Hg. She was not felt to be a candidate for HBO2 since all five toes were necrotic, and she appeared to have no possibility for healing a transmetatarsal amputation. The patient chose to postpone surgery as long as pain could be controlled with medication. She was managed with pain medication and supportive care and continued to live alone. Twelve months later she underwent a left BKA. Compare this to Patient #2.

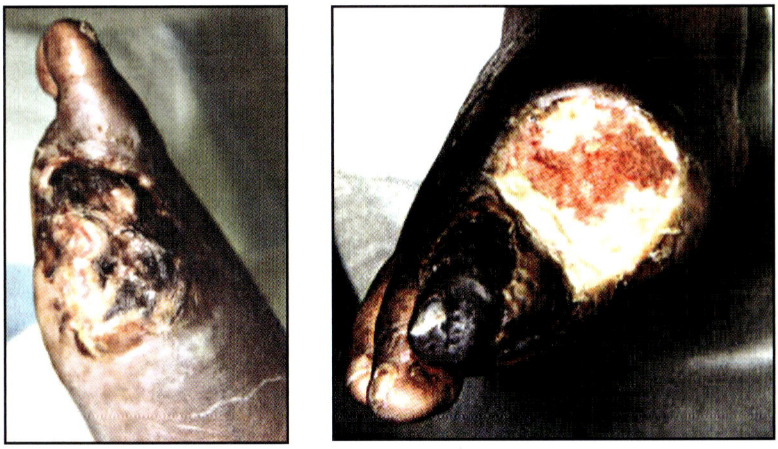

Figure 3. (A) Suboptimal Management Case. Post right great toe amputation for gangrenous changes.
(B) After 44 HBO2 treatments the wound had granulated to some degree, but she infarcted the second toe.

Patient Example (Optimal Management)

Patient #2 is a 40-year-old Latin American male, hypertensive, with IDDM, and end-stage renal disease, status post renal transplant, on prednisone and Rapimmune. His anemia was treated with Epogen. He was status post 5th day amputation for osteomyelitis with subsequent wound dehiscence (Figure 4A). The wound probed to bone and tendon was exposed after debridement. Periwound $TcpO_2$ was 32 mm Hg, but in-chamber oxygen values were 356 mm Hg. The patient underwent aggressive wound care and HBO2, as well as treatment with the VAC® (see Figure 4B). HBO2 was discontinued after 20 treatments when he was noted to have a good granulation tissue bed (Figure 4C), and wound healing continued with conservative care (Figure 4D).

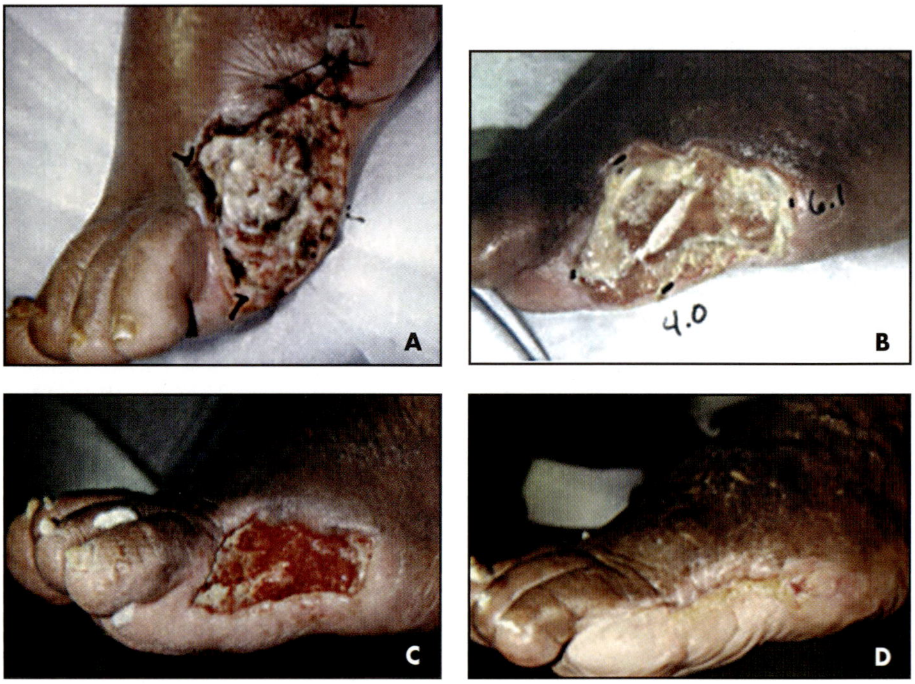

Figure 4 A–D. (A) Optimal Management. Patient has wound dehiscence post 5th day amputation for osteomyelitis.
(B) The patient underwent aggressive wound care and HBO2, as well as treatment with the VAC®.
(C) HBO2 was discontinued after 20 treatments when patient had good granulation tissue bed.
(D) Wound healed with conservative care.

COST IMPACT

Fortunately, soft tissue and bony radiation necrosis occur in only 1–5% of the approximately 600,000 patients who receive therapeutic radiation annually in the U.S. However, when complications do occur, the cost of management is reduced from about $140,000 when HBO2 is not utilized, to about $42,000 when HBO2 and surgery are combined in optimal fashion. Similar cost advantages are anticipated in the treatment of radiation injuries of other tissues, as well.

Complications from acute traumatic peripheral ischemias are costly and limb-threatening. Infection, nonunion, and amputations occur in approximately 50% of severe open fractures and crush injuries. When HBO2 is used during the prefasciotomy, lag phase of the compartment syndrome, the cost of management has been estimated to be one-fourth of that incurred when compartment syndrome is surgically decompressed (62). Moreover, Bouachour confirmed the cost-benefit of HBO2 with fewer surgeries and improved healing rates (37). In patients who develop chronic osteomyelitis, HBO2 is not only clinically effective but also significantly cost effective: 60–85% of patients who failed to respond to years of costly surgery and antibiotics had infections successfully arrested when HBO2 was used in conjunction with intensive surgical and antibiotic therapy (63–66). In addition, in a limited review, cost-effectiveness was five-fold in favor of using HBO2 for refractory osteomyelitis (67).

Of critical interest in light of the new Medicare coverage decision, is the cost-benefit of HBO2 for diabetic foot ulcers. HBO2 demonstrates the most cost-benefit if patients who would have healed anyway are screened out, as well as patients for whom limb salvage is not possible, either because they are not revascularizable, or because of the advanced nature of tissue loss at the time of consultation. For the rest, bipedal limb salvage represents an extraordinary saving in healthcare dollars. Fewer than 50% of elderly diabetics are rehabilitated to walking with prosthesis. Furthermore, the cost of a primary amputation in 1986 was reported to be in excess of $40,000 (68). Clearly, these data show that primary amputation is far from an expeditious solution to the problem of foot wounds in diabetics. In addition, the likelihood of contralateral amputation increases 10% per year, nearly assuring that a diabetic will be a bilateral amputee within ten years of the first below-the-knee amputation. The progression, first to wheelchair dependency, and then to total dependency is an expensive decline for the individual, the society, and the taxpayer. In 1997 dollars the cost of amputation is in excess of $2.7 billion yearly (69).

In 1988, Cianci reported a series of 19 diabetics as a subset of 39 patients with lower limb lesions, for whom a salvage rate of 89% was possible (70). Forty-two percent of these patients had undergone successful revascularization and were referred, because of infection or nonhealing wounds. Salvage was defined as bipedal ambulation (if two limbs were originally present) and wound coverage for at least one year. Hyperbaric oxygen costs were $12,668 and were reflected in total hospital charges of $34,370, with an average stay of 35 days. More recently, he reported a longitudinal outcome study of 41 diabetic patients averaging 63.1 years in age (71). With an average Wagner score of IV, all patients had limb-threatening lesions, of whom 20 (49%) had undergone revascularization. The extremities of 35 patients (85%) were salvaged in this instance. Hyperbaric oxygen charges were $15,000, total hospital charges were $31,264, and the average length of stay was 27 days, which compares favorably with the cost of primary amputation, and certainly the cost of rehabilitation. Follow-up at two points—1991 and 1993—has also demonstrated durability of 32 and 55 months, respectively. Clearly, postponing the initial amputation postpones subsequent amputation. Assuming an average Medicare reimbursement of approximately

$500 per HBO2 treatment, and an average of 36 treatments, a course of HBO2 at $18,000 would still represent a substantial cost savings compared to a below-the-knee amputation, and might keep the patient ambulatory and living independently.

The cost-effectiveness of HBO2 as an adjunct therapy in the treatment of diabetic ulcers has also been studied using a decision-tree model and a hypothetical cohort of 1000 patients aged 60 years and with severe diabetic ulcers. The results showed that at years 1, 5, and 12 following HBO2, the incremental cost per additional quality-adjusted life year (QALY) gained was $27,310, $5,166, and $2,255 respectively (72). This is a cost-effective intervention, as in the USA, interventions that cost less than $50,000–100,000/QALY gained have been considered cost-effective, with those less than or $20,000/QALY especially cost-effective (73–75).

CMS 35-10 MEDICARE COVERAGE GUIDELINES FOR DIABETIC FOOT WOUNDS

In coverage memorandum published December 27, 2002, CMS stated, "The evidence is adequate to conclude that HBO2 therapy is clinically effective and thus reasonable and necessary in the treatment of certain patients with limb threatening diabetic wounds of the lower extremity," (Transmittal AB-01-183). However, CMS determined that the evidence was inadequate to conclude that hypoxic wounds represented a distinct wound type for purposes of Medicare coverage, and thus Medicare decided not to expand coverage to hypoxic wounds. To qualify for HBO2 in the treatment of a diabetic foot ulcer, patients must meet each of the following three criteria:

- Type I or Type II diabetes with a lower extremity wound due to diabetes
- The wound must be a Wagner Grade III or higher
- The patient must have failed an adequate course of standard wound therapy.

Figure 5 is a decision tree showing selection of HBO2 for diabetic wounds of the lower extremities.

The ICM codes to document this include 250.7 and 250.8 (diabetes) and the following wound location codes: 707, 707.1, 707.10, 707.12, 707.13, 707.14, 707.15, and 707.19. (See Bangasser and Bozzuto chapter on Reimbursement). On July 25, 2003, Transmittal AB-03-102, Change Request 2769.1, the code 707.15 was added, which allows the treatment of toes. It is important to note that the code for thigh wounds is not included on this list, so a non-healing above-the-knee amputation would not be covered if it were specifically coded as a wound of the thigh.

Hyperbaric oxygen therapy is covered only after there are no measurable signs of healing after at least 30 days of treatment with standard wound therapy. In the coverage memorandum, CMS clearly defined "standard wound therapy" to include assessment of vascular status and correction, if possible, of vascular problems in the affected limb, optimization of glucose control, debridement of necrotic tissue, maintenance of moist wound bed, appropriate off-loading, and treatment of infection. "Measurable

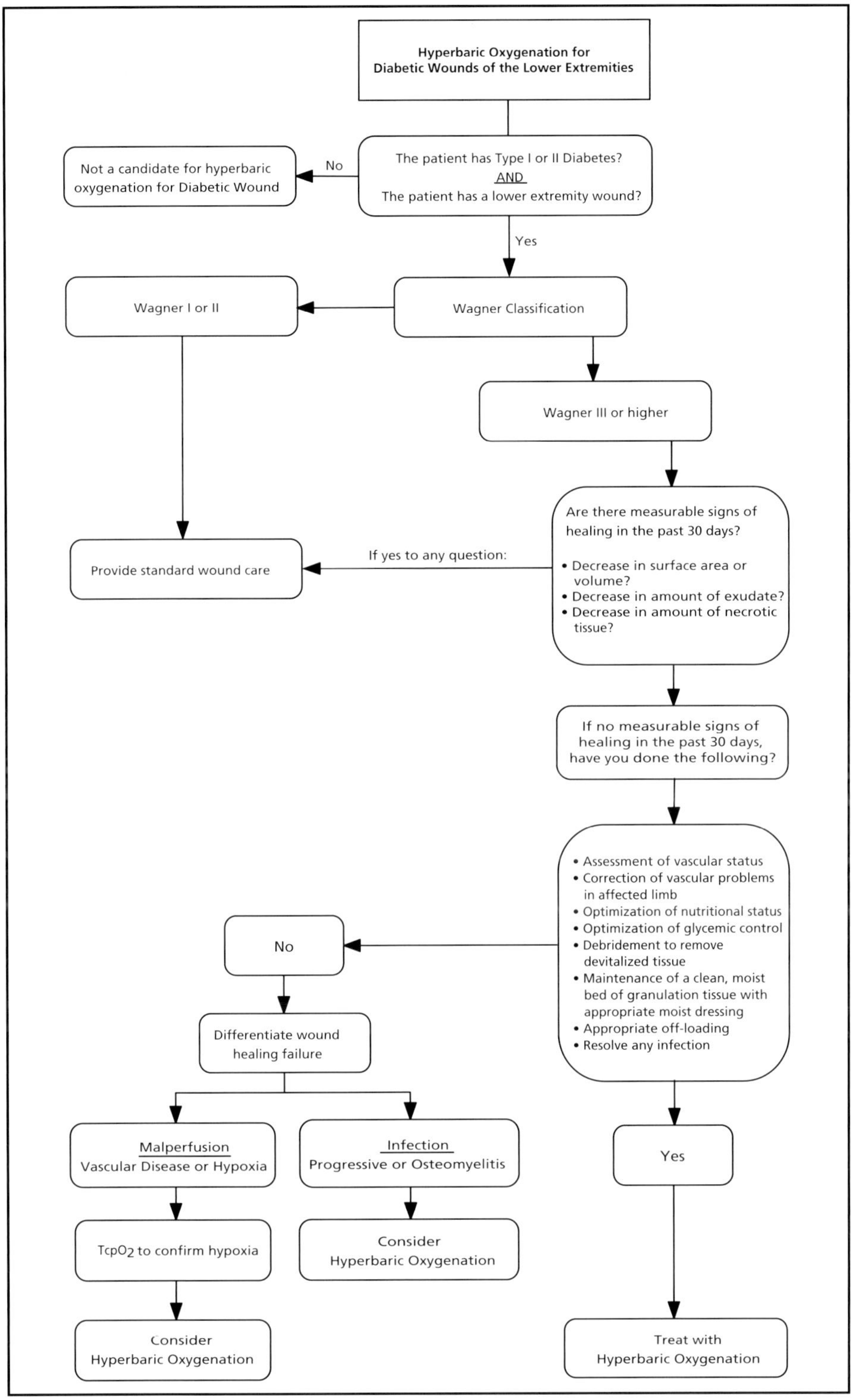

Figure 5. Selection of hyperbaric oxygenation for diabetic wounds of the lower extremities. Courtesy of Robert A. Warriner III, M.D.

signs of healing," is defined as a decrease in wound volume or size, a decrease in exudate, or a decrease in necrotic tissue.

It is clear from reading the CMS memorandum that satisfying these requirements necessitates careful and thorough documentation in the medical records. Documentation would clearly need to include the date of onset, the Wagner score, and the size of the wound, as well as it response to therapy. Wagner III wounds are usually defined as a deep ulcer with abscess, osteomyelitis, or joint sepsis. While it may seem self evident, it is important to state that the wound is a result of the diabetes in order to provide the necessary linkage for billing purposes.

CMS chose not to require TCOM as a criterion for patient selection. However, as discussed in the section on patient selection, TCOM is the most accurate way to determine whether wounds are likely to benefit from HBO2. Once HBO2 is begun, CMS requires that the wound be re-evaluated every 30 days during the HBO2 course. The coverage decision also clearly states that continued HBO2 would not be covered if there were no measurable signs of healing during the 30-day period. Again, the key is documentation. Wound measurements or descriptors must clearly state improvement in the parameters of size, or the presence of drainage or necrotic tissue. As discussed previously, hyperbaric oxygen therapy should be discontinued if there is no evidence of benefit. These criteria are not unreasonable.

CONCLUSION

Hyperbaric oxygen therapy is a treatment provided by a physician with specific expertise and training. When patients are carefully selected, appropriately followed, and treatment discontinued at maximal benefit, HBO2 can reduce the amputation rate in diabetic foot ulcers, and save healthcare dollars. HBO2 can also be usefully employed as an adjunctive therapy in several other wound-care conditions, including radiation-induced necrosis, acute traumatic peripheral ischemia, crush injury, compartment syndrome, and refractive osteomyelitis.

REFERENCES

1. La Van FB, Hunt TK. Oxygen and wound healing. *Clinc Plast Surg* 1990:17:463-472.
2. Fontaine JA. Emploi chirugicale de l'aire comprime. *Un Medic* 1879;28:448.
3. Boerema I, Meijne NG, Brummelkamp WK, et al. Life without blood. A study of the influence of high atmospheric pressure and hypothermia on dilution of the blood. *J Cardiovasc Surg* 1960;1:133-146.
4. Saltzman HA. Rational normobaric and hyperbaric oxygen therapy. *Ann Intern Med* 1967;67:843-852.
5. Smerz RW. Incidence of oxygen toxicity during the treatment of dysbarism. *Undersea Hyperb Med* 2004;31:199-202.
6. Yildiz S, Uzun G, Kiralp MZ. Hyperbaric oxygen therapy in chronic pain management. *Curr Pain Headache Rep* 2006;10:95-100.
7. Beard T, Warriner R III, Pasceri P, et al. Adverse events during hyperbaric oxygen therapy (HBO2), a retrospective analysis from 25 centers. [Abstract] UHMS Annual Meeting, June 2005, Las Vegas, USA.
8. Gibson JJ, Angeles AP, Hunt TK. Increased oxygen tension potentiates angiogenesis. *Surg Forum* 1997;48:696-699.
9. Cianci P. Advances in the treatment of the diabetic foot: Is there a role for adjunctive hyperbaric oxygen therapy? *Wound Repair Regen* 2004;12:2-10.
10. Sheikh AY, Gibson JJ, Rollins MD, et al. Effect of hyperoxia on vascular endothelial growth factor levels in a wound model. *Arch Surg* 2000;135:1293-1297.
11. Knighton D, Silver I, Hunt TK. Regulation of wound healing angiogenesis-effect of oxygen gradients and inspired oxygen concentration. *Surgery* 1981;90:262-270.
12. Davis JC, Buckley CJ, Barr PO. Compromised soft tissue wounds: Correction of wound hypoxia. In: Davis JC, Hunt TK, eds. Problem Wounds: The Role of Oxygen. New York: Elsevier;1988:143-152.
13. Marx RE. Radiation tissue damage. In: Camporesi EM, Barker AC, eds. Hyperbaric Oxygen Therapy: A critical review. Bethesda, MD: Undersea & Hyperbaric Medical Society 1991:95-104.
14. Hohn DC. Oxygen and leukocyte microbial killing. In: Davis JC, Hunt TK, eds. Hyperbaric Oxygen Therapy. Bethesda, MD: Undersea Medical Society, Inc., 1977;101-110.
15. Knighton DR, Fiegel VD. Oxygen as an antibiotic: The effect of inspired oxygen on infection. *Arch Surg* 1990;125:97-100.
16. Mader JT, Adams KR, Wallace WR, et al. Hyperbaric oxygen as adjunctive therapy for osteomyelitis. *Infect Dis Clin N Am* 1990;4:433-44.
17. Mader JT, Brown GL, Guckian JC, et al. A mechanism for the amelioration by hyperbaric oxygen of experimental staphylococcal osteomyelitis in rabbits. *J Infect Dis* 1980;142:915-922.
18. Mader JT, Adams KR, Couch LA, et al. Potentiation of tobramycin by hyperbaric oxygen in experimental Pseudomonas aeruginosa osteomyelitis. Paper presented at: 27th Interscience Conference on Antimicrobial Agents and Chemotherapy; October 4-7, 1987; New York, NY.
19. Chang N, Goodson WH III, Gottrup F, et al. Direct measurement of wound and tissue oxygen tension in postoperative patients. *Ann Surg* 1983;197:470-478.
20. Hunt TK, Pai MP. The effect of varying ambient oxygen tensions on wound metabolism and collagen synthesis. *Surg Gynecol Obstet* 1972;135:561-567.
21. Robson MC, Stenberg BD, Heggers JP. Wound healing alterations caused by infection. *Clin Plast Surg* 1990;17:485-492.

22. Hunt TK. The physiology of wound healing. *Ann Emerg Med* 1988;17:1265-1273.

23. Bonomo SR, Davidson JD, Yu Y, et al. Hyperbaric oxygen as a signal transducer: upregulation of platelet derived growth factor-beta receptor in the presence of HBO2 and PDGF. *Undersea Hyper Med* 1998;25:211-216.

24. Buras JA, Veves A, Orlow D, et al. The effects of hyperbaric oxygen on cellular proliferation and platelet-derived growth factor receptor expression in non-insulin-dependent diabetic fibroblasts. *Acad Emer Med* 2001;8:518-519.

25. Marx RE, Ehler WJ, Tayapongsak P, et al. Relationship of oxygen dose to angiogenesis induction in irradiated tissue. *Am J Surg* 1990;160:519-524.

26. Rubin P. Late effects of chemotherapy and radiation therapy: A new hypothesis. *Int J Radiat Oncol Biol Phys* 1984;10:5-34.

27. Marx RE, Ames JR. The use of hyperbaric oxygen in bony reconstruction of the irradiated and tissue-deficient patient. *J Oral Maxillofac Surg* 1982;40:412-420.

28. Marx RE. A new concept in the treatment of osteoradionecrosis. *J Oral Maxillofac Surg* 1983;41:351-357.

29. Marx RE, Johnson RP. Problem wounds in oral and maxillofacial surgery: The role of hyperbaric oxygen. In: Davis JC, Hunt TK, eds. *Problem Wounds: The Role of Oxygen.* New York: Elsevier; 1988:65-123.

30. Marx RE, Johnson RP, Kline SN. Prevention of osteoradionecrosis: A randomized. prospective clinical trial of hyperbaric oxygen versus penicillin. *J Am Dent Assoc* 1985;111:49-54.

31. Feldmeier JJ (ed). Hyperbaric oxygen 2003: Indications and results. Hyperbaric oxygen therapy Committee Report. Kensington, MD: Undersea and Hyperbaric Medical Society; 2003.

32. Tibbles PM, Edelsberg JS. Hyperbaric oxygen therapy. *New Engl J Med* 1996;334:1642-1648.

33. Blue Cross Blue Shield Association Assessment Program. Hyperbaric Oxygen Therapy for Wound Healing—Parts I, II, III. Blue Cross Blue Shield Association Technology Evaluation Center 1999;14(2), 14(15), 14(16).

34. Medical Services Advisory Committee (MSAC), Department of Health and Aged Care, Australia. *Hyperbaric Oxygen Therapy*, November 2000, MSAC applications 1018-1020 Assessment Report.

35. American Diabetes Association. Consensus Development Conference on Diabetic Foot Wound Care. *Diabetes Care* 1999;22:1354-1360.

36. Consensus Panel: Cavanagh, Buse, Frykberg, Gibbons, Lipsky, Pogach, Reiber, Sheehan. ADA Consensus Development Conference on Diabetic Foot Wound Care. *Diabetes Care* 1999;22:1354.

37. Bouachour G, Cronier P, Gouello JP, et al. Hyperbaric oxygen therapy in the management of crush injuries: A randomized double-blind placebo-controlled clinical trial. *J Trauma* 1996;41:333-339.

38. Doctor N, Pandya S, Supe A. Hyperbaric oxygen therapy in diabetic foot. *J Postgrad Med* 1992;38:112-114.

39. Faglia E, Favales F, Aldeghi A, et al. Adjunctive systemic hyperbaric oxygen therapy in treatment of severe diabetic foot ulcer. A randomized study. *Diabetes Care* 1996;19:1338-1343.

40. Marx RE. Clinical Applications of hyperbaric oxygen. In: Kindwall E, ed. *Hyperbaric Medicine Practice*. Arizona: Best Publishing; 1995:460-462.

41. Perrins DJD. Influence of hyperbaric oxygen on the survival of split skin grafts. *Lancet* 1967;1(7495):868-871.

42. Tobey RE, Kelly JF. Osteoradionecrosis of the jaws. *Otolaryngol Clin North Am* 1979;12:183-186.

43. Warriner RA III, Fife CE. What you should know about using HBO2 in diabetic wounds. *Podiatry Today* 2003;16:14-18.

44. Embil JM, Papp K, Sibbald G, et al. Recombinant human platelet-derived growth factor-BB (becaplermin) for healing chronic lower extremity diabetic ulcers: an open label clinical evaluation of efficacy. *Wound Repair Regen* 2000;8:162-168.

45. Kalani M, Jorneskog G, Naderi N, et al. Hyperbaric oxygen (HBO2) therapy in treatment of diabetic foot ulcers. Long-term follow-up. *J Diabetes Complications* 2002;16:153-158.

46. Abidia A, Laden G, Kuhan G, et al. The role of hyperbaric oxygen therapy in ischaemic diabetic lower extremity ulcers: a double-blind randomised-controlled trial. *Eur J Vasc Endovasc Surg* 2003;25:513-518.

47. Kessler L, Bilbault P, Ortega F, et al. Hyperbaric oxygenation accelerates the healing rate of nonischemic chronic diabetic foot ulcers: a prospective randomized study. *Diabetes Care* 2003;26:2378-2382.

48. Lin TF, Chen SB, Niu KC. The vascular effects of hyperbaric oxygen therapy in treatment of early diabetic foot. *Undersea Hyperb Med* 2001;28(Suppl):67.

49. Hildreth S, Smith L, Sutton T, et al. In-chamber transcutaneous oximetry (TCOM) at 2.0 vs. 2.4 ATA: What is the best treatment pressure? *Undersea Hyperb Med* 1999;26(Suppl) 44.

50. Fife CE, Buyukcakir C, Otto GH, et al. The predictive value of transcutaneous oxygen tension measurement in diabetic lower extremity ulcers treated with hyperbaric oxygen therapy; a retrospective analysis of 1144 patients. *Wound Repair Regen* 2002;10:198-207.

51. Otto GH, Fife CE, Buyukcakir C. Effects of smoking on cost and duration of hyperbaric oxygen therapy for diabetic patients with non-healing wounds. *Undersea Hyperb Med* 2000;27:67-123.

52. Hammarlund C, Sundberg T. Hyperbaric oxygen reduced size of chronic leg ulcers: A randomized double blind study. *Plast Reconstr Surg* 1994;93:829-834.

53. Sheffield PJ, Smith APS. Physiological and Pharmacological Basis of Hyperbaric Oxygen Therapy. In: DJ Bakker, FS Cramer, *Hyperbaric Surgery: Perioperative Care*. Flagstaff, AZ: Best Publishing; 2002:63-109.

54. Zamboni WA. Applications of hyperbaric oxygen therapy in plastic surgery. In: Oriani G, Marroni A, Wattel F, eds. *Handbook on Hyperbaric Oxygen Therapy*. New York: Springer-Verlag; 1996.

55. Davis JC, Hunt TK, eds. Problem Wounds: The Role of Oxygen. New York: Elsevier; 1988.

56. Davis JC, Hunt TK, eds. Hyperbaric Oxygen Therapy. Bethesda, MD: Undersea Medical Society; 1977.

57. Hanna GP, Fujise K, Kjellgren O, et al. Infrapopliteal transcatheter interventions for limb salvage in diabetic patients: Importance of aggressive interventional approach and role of transcutaneous oximetry. *Am J Cardiol* 1997;30:664-669.

58. Wyss CR, Harrington RM, Burgess EM, et al. Transcutaneous oxygen tension as a predictor of success after an amputation. *J Bone Joint Surg* [Am] 1988;70:203-207.

59. Pecoraro RE, Ahroni JH, Boyko EJ, et al. Chronology and determinants of tissue repair in diabetic lower-extremity ulcers. *Diabetes* 1991;40:1305-1313.

60. Wattel FE, Mathieu MD, Fossati P, et al. Hyperbaric oxygen in the treatment of diabetic foot lesions. Search for healing predictive factors. *J Hyperb Med* 1991;6:263-268.

61. Sheffield PJ, Dietz D, Posey KI, et al. Use of transcutaneous oximetry and laser Doppler with local heat provocation to assess patients with problem wounds. In: Petri NM, Andric D, Ropac D, eds. Proceedings, First Congress of Alps-Adria Working Community on Maritime, Undersea, and Hyperbaric Medicine, Split, Croatia. Croatian Maritime, Undersea and Hyperb Med Soc Croatian Med Assoc 2001:341-344.

62. Strauss M. Crush injury, compartment syndrome and other acute traumatic peripheral ischemias. In: Kindwall EP, Whelan HT, eds. *Hyperbaric Medicine Practice*. Flagstaff, AZ: Best Publishing; 1999:753-778.

63. Depenbusch Fl, Thompson RE, Hart GB. Use of hyperbaric oxygen in the treatment of refractory osteomyelitis: A preliminary report. *J Trauma* 1972;12:807-812.

64. Bingham EL, Mullen JE, Winans RG, et al. The treatment of refractory osteomyelitis with hyperbaric oxygen: A progress report. In: Trapp WG, Banister EW, Davison EJ, Trapp PA, eds. Proceedings of the Fifth International Conference on Hyperbaric Medicine. Burnaby, Canada: Fraser University; 1973:264-269.

65. Davis JC. Refractory osteomyelitis of the extremities and axial skeleton. In: Davis JC, Hunt TK, eds. Hyperbaric oxygen therapy. Bethesda, MD: Undersea Medical Society; 1978:217-227.

66. Strauss MB, Hart GB. Cost-effective issues in hyperbaric oxygen therapy complicated fractures. *J Hyperbaric Med* 1988;3:199-205.

67. Strauss MB. Economic considerations in chronic refractory osteomyelitis. Paper presented at: Fifth Annual Conference on Clinical Applications of Hyperbaric Oxygen; June, 1980; Long Beach, CA.

68. Mackey WC, McCullough JL, Conlon TP, et al. The cost of surgery for limb-threatening ischemia. *Surgery* 1986;99:26-35.

69. Levin ME. Diabetic foot lesions: Pathogenesis and management. *J Enterostomal Ther* 1990;17:29-34.

70. Cianci P, Petrone G, Drager S, et al. Salvage of the problem wound and potential amputation with wound care and adjunctive hyperbaric oxygen therapy: An economic analysis. *J Hyperb Med* 1988;3:127-141.

71. Cianci P, Hunt TK. Long term results of aggressive management of diabetic foot ulcers suggest significant cost effectiveness. *Wound Repair Regen* 1997;5:141-146.

72. Guo S, Counte MA, Gillespie KN, et al. Cost-effectiveness of adjunctive hyperbaric oxygen in the treatment of diabetic ulcers. *Int J Technol Assess Health Care* 2003;19:731-737.

73. Laupacis A, Feeny D, Detsky AS, et al. How attractive does a new technology have to be to warrant adoption and utilization? Tentative guidelines for using clinical and economic evaluations. *CMAJ* 1992;146:473-481.

74. Heudebert GR, Centor RM, Klapow JC, et al. What is heartburn worth? A cost-utility analysis of management strategies. *J Gen Intern Med* 2000;15:175-182.

75. Smith AF, Brown GC. Understanding cost-effectiveness: a detailed review. *Br J Ophthalmol* 2000;84:794-798.

REVIEW QUESTIONS

1.) Oxygen is transported to tissues in potentially useful amounts in the following ways:

   a. Chemically bound to hemoglobin
   b. Physically dissolved in plasma
   c. Cutaneously absorbed through the skin
   d. Both A and B

2.) The mechanisms by which hyperbaric oxygen therapy can be of benefit include:

   a. Increasing collagen cross linking
   b. Inhibiting bacterial growth
   c. Activating growth factor receptors
   d. Stimulating angiogenesis
   e. All of the above

3.) Which statements are true about hyperbaric oxygen therapy?

   a. HBO2 should be used rather than revascularization in ischemic patients
   b. Air trapping is not a risk factor for pulmonary barotrauma
   c. Seizures occur less frequently at 2.4 ATA than 2.0 ATA
   d. None of the above are true

4.) According to Medicare, proper use of HBO2 in the diabetic foot ulcer includes (pick all that apply):

   a. A Wagner III ulcer
   b. A wound which has been present for 2 weeks
   c. A patient which has undergone appropriate vascular evaluation
   d. Both A and C

5.) Potential complications of hyperbaric therapy include all except:

   a. Transient myopia
   b. Otic barotrauma
   c. Hyperoxic seizures
   d. Decreased memory

Answers: 1d, 2e, 3d, 4d, 5d

NOTES

CHAPTER 39

ADVANCED THERAPEUTICS: THE BIOCHEMISTRY AND BIOPHYSICAL BASIS OF WOUND PRODUCTS

CHAPTER THIRTY-NINE OVERVIEW

Advanced Therapeutics: the Biochemistry and Biophysical Basis of Wound Products

Adrianne P.S. Smith, Thomas M. Bozzuto

INTRODUCTION TO WOUNDS AND GOALS FOR ADVANCED THERAPEUTICS

Topical and ingested agents have long been used for wound healing. Australian Aborigines crushed and applied tea tree leaves for cuts and skin infections. Topical zinc and honey were used by many cultures including the Egyptians at least as far back as 1500 B.C. Native Americans applied poultices of witch hazel leaves and bark for wounds, and used various anti-infective methods rendering puerperal fever rare while it decimated European women, and avoided the amputations and gangrene that killed hundreds of thousands of Frontier War and Civil War soldiers. Topical aloe vera has been reported in many cultures for decreasing inflammation and promoting cellular repair. Calendula flower applications have been long and widely used to accelerate skin wound healing, inhibit wound infections, and reduce inflammation. Licking wounds, dating from prehistory in many animals, and likely humans too, has been demonstrated to impart lytic, anti-infective and growth agents. The enzyme lysozyme specifically digests bacterial protective coating and has been used in Eastern Europe for over 40 years for surgical wounds. Two more antibacterial and antifungal agents in saliva are cystatins and histatins. Saliva is a major source of epidermal growth factor (EGF) and nerve growth factor (NGF). Thus, there may be some truth to the concept of, "Kiss it and make it better."

A brief "modernization" period in 20th century wound treatment led to sterile, dry dressings and frequent antibiotic scrubs. Providers used wound drying in an attempt to improve wound sterility. Then the original work by Dr. George Winter published in 1962, demonstrated the value of a moist wound environment (3). Wounds created on the backs of pigs healed more quickly if they were kept moist than if they were allowed to dry out and scab over. Recently attention was directed towards "naturalization" of the wound bed. Warm temperature and reduction of devitalized tissue and bacterium became the next focus. Debridement using chemicals, maggots, pulsating water sprays, or surgical excision were directed at decreasing the bioburden. Recognition that biofilms develop in wounds, as occurs with other fluid-surface interfaces, emphasized the need to aggressively "balance" contents at the wound base. Subsequent advances in knowledge concerning the role of various cell types, communication molecules, and surrounding gel matrix have also lead to changes in our approach to wound care. Platelet derived growth factor (PDGF-BB), esters of hyaluronic acid, collagen-granules, powders, and sheets, tissue grafts with fibroblast and keratinocytes were developed in an effort to simulate, replace, or enhance naturally occurring components in the wound. Additional focus has been directed at the biochemical, electrical, and physical environment in the wound bed. Current practice supports a moist environment with enough reduction in the bioburden to favor healing. Advanced modalities are employed to maximize the wound healing processes.

Within the last 5–10 years, we have witnessed a technological explosion in the field of wound healing. With this new knowledge comes the ability to improve the outcomes of patients who previously would have suffered with chronic, non-healing, debilitating wound problems. New wound assessment strategies, such as optimal lavage irrigation systems, more selective debriding agents, bio-engineered tissues, aggressive surgical intervention, hyperbaric oxygen, physical medical interventions and interactive primary and secondary dressings are just a few of the advances available to improve wound healing.

ADVANCES IN STANDARD CARE

The goal for standard therapy in wound care is to promote a normal wound healing environment. Standard wound care involves assuring adequate oxygen and perfusion; nutritional stability with essential proteins, minerals and vitamins; reduction of edema fluid; appropriate off-loading; infection and inflammation reduction; glucose and triglyceride control; pain relief; and balancing local moisture and temperature at the wound site. With standard care, granulation tissue normally grows from the edge towards the center at a rate of approximately 0.2 mm/day.

When healing fails to progress normally despite adequate standard intervention, then advanced modalities are considered. The transition between standard and advanced care is becoming more blurred over time, as many prior advanced treatment modalities are becoming common practice standards. There exists more than several thousand currently marketed products for wound healing which cannot all be reviewed in this forum. This chapter will concentrate upon the various wound healing processes and the use categories of these products that will enhance those efforts.

Nutrition

For optimal wound healing, nutrition may need to be maximized using protein and vitamin supplements, additional minerals; and sometimes medications that promote weight gain. The pneumonic "Pro-BACE with Zinc" is a helpful reminder of common nutrients frequently used for outpatient wound healing nutritional supplementation: **Protein** (specifically L-Arginine and Glutamine), vitamins **B** complex, **A**, **C** and **E**; with **Zinc**.

1. **Protein**
   - **L-arginine,** is a semi-essential amino acid produced at adequate levels in the basal state. However, during episodes of stress or injury its production may become inadequate to meet demand, therefore increased exogenous intake may be required. L-arginine improves the immune response by supporting T-cells from the thymus gland, and supports skin and connective tissue healing through the formation of collagen used for soft tissue, muscle, cartilage, bone, and tendon repair. It also promotes wound healing by supporting perfusion through increased nitric oxide synthesis, which provides vasorelaxation. Usual recommended dosage is two grams per day.
   - **Glutamine,** the most abundant amino acid in the body, acts as the body's "nitrogen shuttle" by accepting free ammonia from the bloodstream for subsequent production of amino acids, amino sugars, nucleotides, and urea. Supplementation may be considered for patients after trauma, major burns or post-operatively. Supplemental glutamine increases protein production, reduces muscle breakdown in response to injury, promotes wound healing, and restores body protein stores. Recommended dose vary greatly from a typical dose of 2–4 grams daily in divided doses for general wound healing and intestinal support, and 10–40 grams per day in divided doses (usually bulk powder form) for critically ill adults. Normal protein intake requires 0.8 g/kg/day, while during wound healing may require 1.2–2.1 g/kg/day.
2. **Micronutrient supplementation** includes vitamin supplementation with B-complex, vitamin A, vitamin C (for hydroxyproline), and vitamin E. (BACE). The antioxidative capability of this combination to prevent ischemic-reperfusion injury and edema during renal transplantation, extremity revascularization operations, hepatic resection, and myocardial infarction has been noted. Recommended vitamin therapy consists of two ampoules of Omnibionta (which contains vitamins B complex A, C, and E) diluted in 500 ml physiological saline solution, that is infused intravenously prior to reperfusion onset.
   - **Vitamin B-complex** consists of a group of similarly structured chemicals to include B-I (thiamine), B-2 (riboflavin), B-3 (niacin), B-5 (pantothenic acid), B-6 (pyridoxine), B-7 (biotin), B-12 (cobalamin), and folic acid (folate or folacin). Para-aminobenzoic acid (PABA), inositol and choline are often included in this group. Vitamins in the B-complex are used for proper cellular formation, particularly in nerve cells. Vitamin B complex products are generally available in two forms: B-50s and B-100s. In a B-50 complex, look for a minimum of the following: 400 mcg folic acid, 50 mcg B-12 and biotin, and at least 50 mg of all the other B vitamins. Generally twice this amount is found in B-100 complexes, except for the folic acid (400 mcg), which remains the same. A B-100 typically contains 100 mcg B-12 and biotin, and 100 mg of all the other B vitamins. Daily recommendations for supplementation usually include one B-100 daily or B-50 twice a day.

- **Vitamin A** (retinal) deficiency is associated with reduced fibronectin, chemotaxis, adhesion, and tissue repair. Seven-day supplementation with Vitamin A causes an increase in collagen synthesis, bursting strength of scar, increased and lymphocyte activation. Replacement with 10,000–20,000 IU is recommended.
- **Vitamin C** (ascorbic acid) is a cofactor required for the function of several hydroxylases and monooxygenases. Its specific importance in wound healing to prolyl-hydroxylase is essential for the production of hydroxyproline necessary for stable triple-helix collagen production. Recommended daily oral dosage is 500–1500 milligrams per day.
- **Vitamin E** (alpha-tocopherol) protects membrane fatty acids from free radical oxidation. Patients with vitamin E deficiency have poor immune functional responses to infection. Vitamin E supplementation decreases scar appearance weakens tissue, scar and tendons, and normalizes the breaking strength in post-radiation skin. Recommended doses are 15 IU per day.

3. **Zinc (Zn)** has a profound influence on wound healing. Cellular proliferation during wound healing requires approximately 200 zinc-dependent enzymes. In patients with nutritional zinc deficiency, newly formed collagen has reduced tensile strength, delaying closure of wounds and ulcers. Factory farming techniques have depleted the soil of zinc in many states. Zinc deficiency is common in the United States, particularly in hospitalized patients. Zinc oxide aids restoration of epithelium during wound repair. Mechanisms of action are not clear. Evidence supports zinc's antioxidant role in protecting against free radical-induced oxidative damage. It is concentrated 5–6 times more in the epidermis than the dermis. Calamine lotion, "pink zinc," is a mixture of zinc oxide powder and a small amount of ferric oxide dissolved in mineral oil. While topical zinc oxide produces beneficial effects, zinc sulfate seems to be ineffective. Oral doses are 15–30 grams per day.
4. **Copper (Cu)** is transported in blood by the plasma protein ceruloplasmin, which increases rapidly following injury and inflammation. Ceruloplasmin oxidizes ascorbate and cysteine, which are important for wound healing. Additionally Cu protects healing tissues from the effect of superoxide radicals produced by phagocytes during the debridement phase of wound healing. Copper is essential for collagen formation, collagen cross-linking, and collagen maturation. Copper is a vital co-factor for the hydroxylation enzyme, lysyl oxidase, and important for strong cross bridging. Copper is usually supplemented orally as a fortified vitamin in combination with other micronutrients. In some formulations, topical copper may be released into the wound as occurs with treatments of Panafil® (Healthpoint, LTD.)

Edema Reduction

1. **Controlling Periwound edema:** Wound fluid drainage onto adjacent tissue causes local periwound tissue damage. A host of absorptive

(drying) and fluid "managing" agents with carbohydrates, cellulose, collagen, calcium alginates obtained from seaweed, cotton, and synthetic materials are available to remove the excessive drainage. Some products act by wicking with hypertonic profiles, like Mesalt® (Mölnlycke Health Care), a hypertonic saline impregnated gauze-like strip that can be packed into a wound to provide unidirectional wicking for removal or redirection of wound fluids away from the periwound tissue. The carbohydrate and cellulose products like Multidex® (DeRoyal Industries, Inc.) provide structure similar to granular substance in the extracellular matrix, while others provide collagen. Products may be biologically active to stimulate tissue growth or inhibit infection. The overall goal of older edema control dressings was to reduce the excessive fluid without over-drying. Current goals are to maintain the moist wound environment and add components that promote healing or remove components that impede healing.

2. **Compression Therapy**. With all the "high tech" interventions available, it is important to mention the low tech, highly effective therapy that must accompany any edema control therapy for venous ulcer therapy in the lower extremity, barring arterial compromise-compression therapy. A Markov model study designed to estimate the expected annual cost per patient treated with a four-layer compression bandaging system, Profore® (Smith & Nephew) versus "usual care" was accomplished by Carr, from the New York Health Economics Consortium (18). In a cohort of 100 patients reviewed for a 52 week period, Profore® associated with a systematic treatment regime is unambiguously more cost-effective. National cost of uncoordinated poor compressive care could waste several million dollars nationally on an annual basis. Other options such as Unna's boots (Gelocast) continue to be useful clinically.

Debridement

1. **Autolytic debridement** occurs while maintaining a moist wound environment. Several products attempt to maximize the moisture available in the wound bed by absorbing excessive fluids into a matrix that contains materials (such as 20% glycerin) to prevent drying out the wound bed. Innovative discoveries in materials that afford a higher level of wound exudate absorption (Hydrofiber® Technology– ConvaTec; Microlattice™ Technology–AcryMed; Biosynthesized Cellulose–Xylos Corporation) enhance regulation, absorption, and maintenance of moisture in the wound bed. Products recognized for superior absorption include: Aquacel®–ConvaTec; Flexigel®– AcryMed, X-Cell®–PDI, Inc. and TenderWet®-Medline. Aquacel® is a hydrophilic non-woven sheet composed of hydrocolloid-sodium carboxymethylcellulose-fibers. These fibers absorb fluids from the wound bed and use it to convert into a moist gel matrix. This prevents the fluid from wicking across the gel in the typical capillary action seen with other compounds. Hydrofibers can absorb 23 times their weight in fluid compared to calcium alginate that absorbs only 5–15 times its weight. Although these products have different compositions, several products have been specifically designed

to donate moisture to the wound bed to prevent over-drying. TenderWet® is a multilayered wound-dressing pad with a core of superabsorbent polyacrylate. It has a higher affinity for protein-containing solutions than for salt-containing solutions. The pad is pre-saturated with lactated Ringers solution (equivalent) and donates moisture and electrolytes (sodium, potassium, and calcium) to the wound bed. The dressing provides 12 hours of continuous wound base "rinsing" and should be removed after 24 hours. X-Cell® is composed of water and biosynthesized cellulose obtained from a bacterium, *Acetobacter xylinum*. The cellulose fibers biosynthesized from this organism are about 200 times smaller than traditional multilayered cellulose obtained from plants, creating an exceptional high surface area to volume ratio. This characteristic affords the biosynthesized cellulose to be 100 times more absorbent. It has a fluid holding capacity up to 700 times its dry weight. The unique nonwoven, multi-layered three-dimensional structure not found in synthetic polymeric materials, attributes better control of porosity, fiber density and fluid absorption/donation capability of the material. X-Cell® can donate up to 80% of the water from the original matrix to a dry wound. It can be formed or cut into virtually any size or shape and left in place for up to seven days.

2. **Mechanical debridement** includes using any method of scrubbing to physically remove debris. The methods used include the use of micropore sponges (similar to surgical sponges), use of wet to dry treatments, immersion hydrotherapy (whirlpool) and showering hydrotherapy, or pulsed lavage therapy (Surgilav Plus, Stryker Instruments). Scrubbing is often done with micropore sponges to remove debris. Wet to dry treatments use moist gauze that is allowed to dry onto the base of the wound. Removing the gauze without pre-wetting is associated with removal of adherent cells, tissue, and debris. Unfortunately, this technique leaves residual gauze fiber in the base of the wound and is associated with pain. Immersion hydrotherapy provides deep tissue warming to increase circulation, decrease pain, and desensitize sensitive areas in rehabilitation for hand injuries, as well as being used for mechanical debridement. If tissues are borderline ischemic the warming can increase metabolic load, and the patient may experience pain. In the past, whirlpool therapy was widely used as an adjunct to treat large burns. Currently the trend towards early debridement and surgical closure was greatly impacted with use of this modality in burn therapy. Whirlpool hydrotherapy was once a mainstay treatment for large wounds; however, maceration of diabetic, elderly, and chronically debilitated patients and the potential for infection has now lead to a more convenient, cost-effective practice of showering hydrotherapy as opposed to immersion hydrotherapy, and this reduces infection risks. Showering hydrotherapy or pulsed-lavage therapy (Surgilav Plus, Stryker Instruments) has improved the convenience of cleansing wounds with less pain in the in-patient, out-patient, and home settings.
3. **Chemical debridement** allows the maintenance of a moist wound environment while at the same time adding proteolytic agents designed to enhance debridement for faster resolution of the biofilm and pro-

inflammatory materials. The papain/urea products Accuzyme® and Panafil® (Healthpoint, Ltd.) obtain their proteolytic enzyme from the papaya fruit. Urea, a denaturing enzyme, aids in chemical proteolysis by breaking the hydrogen sulfide and other disulfide bonds that maintain the protein in a folded position. As the protein unfolds, urea quickly separates from the papain to allow papain to enzymatically denature the devitalized, necrotic tissue in the wound bed. Viable cells rapidly metabolize the urea into ammonia and carbon dioxide, both of which are released from the wound. In combination with the urea, papain, a serine protease, has twice the degradative capacity in the presence of necrotic or non-viable tissue. Papain is active over a pH range of 3–12. Heavy metals in the wound base decrease the activity of the serine protease, therefore mixing this product with other agents like Silvadene®, Betadine® or Zinc is not advisable. Accuzyme® is designed specifically to debride. Panafil® with copper chlorophyllin, while retaining its capability as a debriding agent to promote continuous cleaning of the wound base, is better designed to promote granulation tissue development. The actions of copper and chlorophyllin assist in facilitating granulation tissue development. The copper chlorophyllin components promote of fibroblast proliferation, improve collagen secretion rates, strengthen collagen cross-linking and reduce hemagglutination to support blood flow delivery of oxygen and nutrients to the cells. Collagenase Santyl® Ointment (Smith & Nephew), a sterile enzymatic debriding ointment, contains 250 collagenase units per gram of white petrolatum USP. The collagenase enzyme, derived from Clostridium histolyticum digests collagen in necrotic tissue. It is not as effective against fibrinous eschar, so scoring or excision of the eschar should be undertaken before applying this product to achieve its optimal effectiveness. The optimal pH range of Santyl® is 6–8. Higher or lower pH conditions will decrease the enzyme's activity. Detergents such as acetic acid and heavy metal ions such as Silvadene® and Acticoat® should be avoided.

4. **Biosurgical Debridement** with Larvae Therapy, a common practice in Britain and other portions of Europe, has not been widely accepted in the United States. Maggots have been deliberately used to debride wounds and combat infection for over 150 years, and was a popular treatment in the early twentieth century. Despite the reluctance of American medical providers to adopt their use, sterile live maggots are proven highly effective in treating infected or necrotic wounds of all types. When introduced into a chronic wound, maggots quickly remove slough or necrotic, infected, even malignant tissue, leaving surrounding healthy tissue untouched. Larvae therapy using Lucilia (Phaenicia) sericata larvae is highly efficient and cost effective. Sherman reported the use of maggot therapy to treat foot and leg ulcers in diabetic patients who were failing conventional therapy (41, 42). Maggot therapy hastened the growth of granulation tissue and produced overall greater wound healing rates as compared to conventional therapy. Within two weeks, maggot therapy decreased necrotic tissue by 4.1 cm^2, while conventional therapy produced no significant changes. After five

weeks, conventional therapy produced a one-third reduction in necrotic tissue whereas maggot therapy completely removed the necrotic tissue. Proposed mechanisms of action to enhance granulation tissue healing in addition to digestion of wound debris include: proteolytic enzymatic liquefaction, consumption of necrotic material, alkaline wound pH from NH_4/Ca carbonate excretion, serous exudate "washout" from larvae irritation, bacterial destruction from consumption and anti-bacterial secretions, allantoin and urea secretion promote healing, and mechanical stimulation from crawling. Sterile maggots are readily available in the European and some United States wound treatment centers with demonstrated success in treating necrotic, dry or sloughy, infected, non-healing of wounds, abscesses, burns, cellulitis, gangrene, ulcers, osteomyelitis and mastoiditis. They are effective in infected wounds, including infections from antibiotic resistant strains such as MRSA (methicillin-resistant *S. aureus*). Also, maggots can be used when the patient has impaired host defenses, such as diabetic patients. Growing problems with multi-resistant strains of bacteria, and limitations of other forms of wound debridement, have lead to resurgence in use. Use of maggots is variously called "Larval Therapy," "Maggot Debridement Therapy," and "Biosurgery," perhaps to euphemistically allay initial reticence.

5. **Ultrasonic Debridement** is performed with a probe that emits high frequency sound waves to the wound site, which loosens dead tissue. Ultrasound is non-ionizing radiation. Sound waves are produced by vibration of piezoelectric discs and the resulting mechanical energy that is transferred to tissue causes the molecules to oscillate. There are two non-thermal ultrasound effects: cavitation and acoustic streaming. Cavitation occurs when changes in local pressure produced by ultrasound causes the formation of microsized bubbles or cavities in tissue fluids or in an ultrasound coupling media such as normal saline (0.9% NSS). Acoustic streaming is the time-independent fluid motion generated by a sound field. At sufficiently high ultrasound intensities, bubbles expand then implode which may result in destruction of tissue and the turbulence created by the imploding bubbles is a mechanism by which destruction of fibrin and bacteria occurs. Low frequency ultrasound (25kHz) is provided by the Sonoca 180™ by Söring (Fort Worth, Texas), and Celleration (Eden Prairie, MN) produces a MIST™ non-contact ultrasound system which provides ultrasound at 40 kHZ. Misonix, Inc. (Farmingdale, NY) produces SonicOne™. Ultrasonic debridement has also been shown to be effective in debridement of bone as well as soft tissue. Ultrasonic debridement is contraindicated in the presence of neoplasm, thrombophlebitis, or hemorrhagic conditions or tissue previously treated with radiation or over the spinal cord.
6. **Surgical Debridement** is the gold standard for excising or reducing the bioburden from the wound base. Unfortunately, in the wake of the tremendous wealth of new technology many providers forget to utilize the most effective and efficient method for removing devitalized tissue, debris, biofilm, infected suture material and other foreign

> bodies. More than just removing senescent cells from the margin of the wound as occurs in the wound care center with sharp technique, surgical debridement entails removal of all non-viable tissue to "get back to healthy tissue" where the vascular supply and host defenses will be able to support healing. The overall goal of aggressive surgical debridement is to convert non-healing chronic wounds into actively healing acute wounds.

Piaggesi compared outpatient surgical treatment of non-infected neuropathic diabetic foot ulcers with conventional non-surgical management, where Group A (conservative) received relief of weight-bearing with regular dressing changes and Group B (surgical) received surgical excision of the wound and or removal of bone segments underlying the lesion with surgical closure (40). In the treatment of diabetic non-infected neuropathic foot ulcers, early aggressive surgical intervention produced faster healing times, fewer complications or relapses, and was safely done in an outpatient setting with better patient satisfaction. Many patients with complex, complicated wounds known to be recalcitrant to healing will be better served with a surgical referral as part of a multi-disciplinary treatment team. Milas reported healing calciphylaxis ulcers in five patients with end-stage renal disease utilizing an aggressive approach including early recognition, diligent wound care, frequent debridement, parathyroidectomy, and appropriate skin grafting or revascularization (38). Complete wound healing was observed between three and six months with no recurrences during the follow-up period, averaging nine months. Apelqvist reported significant cost savings associated with multi-disciplinary approach to treat diabetic foot ulcers in 314 consecutively presenting diabetic patients to a University Hospital in Sweden (26). The foot care team consisting of diabetologist, orthopedic surgeon, diabetes nurse, podiatrist and orthotist treated both inpatients and outpatients. When compared to the cost generated without the guidance of a multi-disciplinary team, the cost for inpatient total average cost to heal primarily reduced to 37%; while closure with amputation reduced to 82% of original costs. Savings are noted in the areas of topical treatment, dressing products, visits to the care team, antibiotics and orthopedic appliances.

Topical Antimicrobial Agents

Initial infection and inflammation control should begin with reducing the bioburden to reestablish what Sibbald and others have dubbed a "bacterial balance." This refers to the point where host defenses are capable of conducting a normal healing process in the face of agents that may produce a proinflammatory environment. Even though all chronic wounds are colonized, the goal is to remove enough of the bioburden to overcome the impediment to wound healing. At the wound site, initial intervention should always begin with cleansing and debridement. Advances have been made in the application and availability of all five major types of debridement: autolytic, mechanical, chemical, biosurgical, and surgical. Aside from the situation where invasive infection mandates the use of some form of antibiotic therapy, the use of topical non-antibiotic antimicrobial agents has become the mainstay of current therapy. Acknowledging the inevitable colonization state of both acute and chronic wounds coupled with the increasing number of antibiotic-resistant organisms; revealed the need for safe and effective topical antimicrobial agents that would reduce bacterial colony counts with little collateral damage to host tissue.

Current infection prevention and inflammation treatment strategies focus upon topical intervention with anti-bacterial agents that reduce the bacterial load including multi-drug resistant organisms such as methicillan-resistant Staphylococcus aureus (MRSA) without increasing the probability of generating new resistant organisms.

1. **Povidone-iodine (Betadine®)** provides immediate release of iodine and remains a staple topical antiseptic for treating and preventing wound infection. Concern over the effect povidone-iodine on granulation tissue has led to several studies evaluating the toxicity of povidone-iodine to healthy tissue with contradictory results. In heavily exudative, infected, or critically colonized wounds a brief course of povidone-iodine may be safe and effective. However, the Agency for Health Care Policy and Research (AHCPR) guidelines for pressure ulcer management specifically advise against the use of povidone-iodine. The sterioisomer of povidone does not appear to have the drawbacks of povidone.
2. **Iodosorb®** gel and **Iodoflex®** sheets (Healthpoint, Ltd.) prove to be highly effective in healing exudative wounds. Cadexomer iodine promotes autolytic debridement, absorbs a heavy amount of exudate, controls drainage, protects the skin around the wound from maceration, and helps reduce the foul odor of heavily contaminated wounds. Studies show that concentrations of up to 0.45%, cadexomer iodine is non-toxic to fibroblasts *in vitro*. In additional *in vitro* studies, Zhou found no changes in viability, morphology, cellular proliferation, ability to produce collagen, and cell outgrowth from explants (52). Skin biopsies obtained from chronic exudative wounds being treated with cadexomer iodine demonstrated no evidence of cell necrosis, displayed re-epithelialization, and revealed bacteria within the cadexomer beads, suggesting the cadexomer traps bacterium. With a safe profile, Cadexomer iodine is approved for use in second-degree burns, heavily draining wounds, or wounds producing copious liquid exudate heavily contaminated with bacteria. Proper use requires a secondary covering or wound dressing. Change the dressing when the color of the gel changes from brown to yellow or gray. Contraindications are allergy or sensitivity to iodine. In a cost benefit analysis utilizing cadexomer iodine to treat deep exudative diabetic foot ulcers in a 12-week open, randomized, comparative study, Apelqvist noted no clinical difference in 12 patients treated with cadexomer iodine as compared to 13 patients treated with gentamicin, streptodomase/streptokinase, or dry saline gauze; however, treatment costs for the cadexomer patients were significantly less (26).
3. **Silver** is an excellent heavy metal antimicrobial agent. It was initially applied as silver nitrate with immediate release. Silver is a broad-spectrum antimicrobial agent that controls yeast, molds, and bacteria, including methicillin resistant *Staphylococcus aureus*

(MRSA) and vancomycin resistant *Enterococci* (VRE) when applied at an appropriate concentration. Silver exerts at least three major wound-healing actions without damaging newly forming skin cells: inhibiting cellular respiration, denaturing nucleic acids, and altering cellular membrane permeability. The antimicrobial effect of silver ions is practically instantaneous. Silver also provides anti-inflammatory properties by decreasing excess metalloproteinase (MMP-2 and MMP-9, and TNF--expression) activity by decreasing zinc, essential for MMP activity, and increase wound calcium, conferring a pro-epithelialization effect. Resistance to silver is rare and silver is relatively non-toxic to human cells. Elemental silver must be delivered to the wound as an ion. Carrier mediums used to deliver silver ion include nitrate (0.5% silver nitrate) for immediate release and Sulfadiazine (Silvadene®) for a more sustained release. These delivery systems create the toxicity associated with these agents, not the silver. Silver ions slowly released in an extended fashion use different carriers to avoid potential toxicity. Anti-microbial silver dressing such as Arglaes®, Acticoat® (Smith & Nephew Westaim Biomedical Corp), InteliCoat® (Sun Capital Partners/Rexam), SilvaSorb™ (AcryMed, Inc.), Silverlon® (Argentum/Keomed), ActiSorb® Silver 220 (Johnson & Johnson, Medical, Inc.), Aquacel® AG Silver Hydrofiber (ConvaTec), X-static/SilverCel® (Advanced Medical Solutions group-AMS/Johnson & Johnson, Medical, Inc.) Contreet® hydrocolloid (Coloplast Group) and Calgitrol®Ag (Magnus Products) are some of the many products available. Calgitrol®Ag Plus is a calcium alginate product with maltodextrin and silver in a gel form for treatment of deep penetrating wounds; while, ABA-1 (Trima Ltd.) employs collagen additives to the silver construct. Metallic silver coated on either polyethylene or nylon-Acticoat® and Silverlon®, respectively, requires oxidation for the release of silver ions. Other delivery systems utilized the silvers salts as a means to deliver ionic silvers. The typical salts are silver chloride (SilvaSorb™ and Aquacel™ Ag), silver ammonium complex of Contreet®, silver calcium-phosphate (Arglaes™) and silver carbon (ActiSorb™). Ionic silver salts are more readily available to the wound.

Inhibiting Inflammation

1. **Matrix Metalloproteinases (MMP)** impart a message that supports and promotes new tissue growth and development, in acutely healing wounds. Current literature supports the premise that the matrix modifying molecules are vital for wound healing. In fact, the same molecules generated in excess that can impede wound healing in chronic wounds. These enzymes are an important class of proteases involved in the extracellular matrix remodeling. Currently five major modes of action have been elucidated: collagenase, gelatinase, and stromelysins, membrane-bound, and unclassified MMPs, They perform major steps in the hydrolysis of proteins. Normally, a balance exists between synthesis of active MMP and inhibition by tissue inhibitors of

matrix metalloproteinase (TIMP). In problem wound healing or other disease states, the balance is skewed to degradation and pathogenesis. Inhibiting MMP production should theoretically permit growth factor activity to resume with wound tissue production. Tetracycline derivatives (esp. Doxycycline) and some macrolide antibiotics (esp. Erythromycin) are known to decrease MMP production through a mechanism unrelated to their antimicrobial properties. Non-antimicrobial chemically modified derivatives (CMTs) have been generated and are now undergoing investigation.

2. **Promogran® Collagen Dressing** (Johnson & Johnson Medical) is a sterile, freeze dried composite of 45% oxidized regenerated cellulose (ORC) and 55% collagen. In the presence of wound exudate it transforms into a soft, conforming, biodegradable gel. Proteases (MMPs) are bound to the gel matrix and inactivated while growth factors are bound and subsequently released in an active form as the dressing undergoes biodegradation in situ. Promogran® is contraindicated in patients with known hypersensitivity to either ORC or collagen. If signs of sensitivity develop during therapy, the treatment should be discontinued. Cost benefit evaluation by Ghatnekar compared Promogran® plus good wound care to good wound care alone, in Markov-based health economic model of non-superficial diabetic foot (19). Under this model, Promogran® showed a cost-savings in the treatment of neuropathic foot ulcers with 26% of ulcers healed within 3 months compared to 20.7% healed in the same time frame with good wound care alone. Over a 12 month period, Promogran® users spent an average 3.75 months in the healed state; whereas, good wound care patients spent 3.41 months healed.

INCREASING BLOOD FLOW

Perfusion

Previously, maximizing the delivery of oxygen and nutrients to tissue focused upon surgical correction of large vessel disease to improve flow. Newer endovascular techniques provide less invasive options for peripheral vascular intervention with angioplasty (see the chapter titled, "Chronic Critical Limb Ischemia and Limb Salvage" by Boccolandro), New discoveries suggesting MMP-9 participation in atheroma initiation, progression and rupture suggest a role for MMP inhibition have been studied. Porter reported that the use of Marimastat, an orally active chemically modified derivative, significantly reduced neointimal thickening in an arterial graft mode (23) using a cultured human saphenous vein.

Hyperbaric Oxygen Therapy (HBO2)

Hyperbaric Oxygen Therapy (HBO2) is the use of high dose oxygen inhalation therapy attained from breathing 100% oxygen inside a pressurized hyperbaric chamber. The use of HBO2 is detailed in the chapter "Hyperbaric Oxygen Therapy Applications in Wound Care" by Fife and will not be reiterated here. Oxygen is delivered to the tissues via respiration, not by absorption. Application of topical oxygen cannot be equated with legitimate hyperbaric oxygen therapy. Topical oxygen is not reimbursable by Medicare.

HBO2 exerts its healing effect through physiological and pharmacological pathways. Physiological mechanisms include fully saturating hemoglobin, dissolving in the plasma to be carried to the tissue, and increased oxygen diffusion from the capillary wall approximately 2–3 times the usual distance. The therapeutic effects of HBO2 are related to the ability of oxygen and/or pressure under hyperbaric conditions to:

- Reverse hypoxia,
- Alter ischemic effect,
- Influence vascular reactivity,
- Reduce edema,
- Stimulate nitric oxide changes,
- Modify growth factors and cytokine effect by regulating their levels and/or receptors,
- Induce changes in membrane proteins affecting ion exchange and gating mechanisms,
- Promote cellular proliferation,
- Accelerate collagen deposition,
- Stimulate capillary budding and arborization,
- Accelerate microbial oxidative killing,
- Improve select antibiotic exchange across membranes,
- Interfere with bacterial disease propagation by denaturing toxins,
- Modulate the immune system response, and
- Enhance oxygen radical scavengers thereby decreasing ischemia-reperfusion injury.

Data from numerous controlled trials and studies are detailed in the chapter "Hyperbaric Oxygen Therapy Applications in Wound Care" by Fife and in Hyperbaric Oxygen 2003 edited by Feldmeier (200). HBO2 is reimbursable by Medicare and is cost effective when patients are appropriately selected and monitored. Patients requiring revascularization should have the procedure prior to initiating HBO2 whenever possible. Transcutaneous oximetry may be very useful in patient selection (199). Appropriate use of HBO2 requires the supervision of a trained hyperbaric physician.

Deep Tissue Warming and Radiation

In an attempt to optimize wound healing, Warm-Up® Active Wound Therapy (Augustine Medical, Inc., Eden Prairie, MN), also known as non-contact normothermic wound therapy (NNWT), uses a non-contact radiant-heat bandage to treat chronic venous ulcers when conventional wound-healing therapy fails. The Warm-Up heats the wound to a pre-determined temperature. Kloth completed a prospective randomized controlled trial on 40 inpatients with 43 Stage III and Stage IV chronic full-thickness pressure ulcers using the NNWT device on 21 wounds and moisture-retentive dressings on 22 wounds (56). The NNWT protocol required the sterile dressing to be in place for 24 hours per day, seven days per week (except during the daily wound change). The wound was irrigated daily with normal saline; and exposed to radiant heat for three one-hour periods per 24 hours. NNWT therapy healed wounds at a faster rate than controls, with the healing rate being greatest in larger wounds. Although infrared therapy studies preliminarily suggested potential accelerated wound healing, subsequent studies did not show NNWT to be any more effective than conventional therapy. No comparison evidence with this delivery system is available to suggest infrared light therapy is any more effective than other heat modalities.

Hydrotherapy as a warming tool is discussed above.

Ultraviolet Exposure

Ultraviolet Exposure (from the sun) has long been used to treat a variety of conditions and wounds. The use of ultraviolet light to treat dermatologic conditions is called heliotherapy and has proven effectiveness in many diseases including psoriasis, vitiligo, atopic dermatitis, and uncontrolled itch (pruritus). Within the spectrum of UV light, ultraviolet A (UVA) causes tanning and is generally not recommended. Exceptions are: use in combination with psoralen (PUVA) to treat photodermatoses and use in combination with hydrogen peroxide for the treatment of leprosy. Ultraviolet C (UVC) is the wavelength most commonly recommended for dermatologic therapy. However, the ozone layer filters ultraviolet C, so modern sources of UVC are artificial. Human exposure to ultraviolet C may cause keratoconjunctivitis and erythema and requires protection of the skin and the eyes when exposed to levels above recommended exposure limits. Intact skin epidermis absorbs the majority of UVC rays. In the denuded surface of wounds, energy is absorbed by dermal components with various effects. UV light for infected wounds, like that used in operating rooms, reduces antibiotic resistant strains of bacteria such as methicillin-resistant *S. aureus*, (MRSA). UVC irradiation of chronic wounds seems to stimulate fibronectin and contraction of fibroblast-populated collagen lattices. Other potential mechanisms of increased wound healing by UVC are increased production of transforming growth factor alpha (TGF-α) and a number of epidermal growth factor receptors (EGFR), epidermal hyperplasia with enhanced re-epithelialization at the wound periphery, granulation tissue stimulation, and sloughing of necrotic tissues. The ultraviolet spectra found in old solar lamps used previously in wound care have been measured and found to contain significant amounts of UVC in addition to ultraviolet B (UVB) and UVA irradiances. Their spectra are compared with that of a modern sunbed. Further research to clarify these observations need to be carried out.

TISSUE-RELATED ADVANCED MODALITIES

Several tissue-replacement products have been developed to simulate or replace major components of granulation tissue such as fibroblast, collagen, gel matrix, and blood vessels. Since there currently is no readily available test to determine which specific wound component requires replacement or activation, the replacement is done empirically. Agents are applied singularly or in combination. Some products are used off-label with respect to indication or location of application. However, the overabundance of products and their associated cost makes this practice costly and time-consuming. Growth factors, allografts, autografts, and xenografts may provide tissue or chemical components required for wound healing that the patient does not produce in adequate amounts. Stem cells, growth factors, and gene-therapy are gaining more support for application in the wound-healing arena.

Some treatments employ light, energy, or chemicals to stimulate the patient cells, *in vivo*, to activate and secrete higher amounts of missing factors; while, others involve the extraction of cells or tissue to be treated, *in vitro*, then reapplying to the wound.

Extracellular-Matrix Components

The components of the extracellular matrix (ECM) include: 1) structural proteins-collagen and elastin, 2) specialized "anchoring" protein-fibronectin, laminin, and fibrillin, vitronectin and 3) proteoglycans and glycosaminoglycans (GAGs)hyaluronic acid, chondroitin sulfate, heparan sulfate, heparin, dermatan sulfate, and keratan sulfate. Most wound healing products designed to mimic the naturally occurring components of the extracellular matrix (ECM) are derived from bovine, porcine, or shark. Synthetic or semi-synthetic products are also available for some of the components.

Concerns have been raised over the use of bovine-derived material given the recent Great Britain epidemic outbreak of Bovine Spongiform Encephalopathy (BSE), a degenerative disease, which affects the central nervous system of cattle with an incubation period of 2–8 years. Currently there are no treatments or valid tests to detect the disease in a live animal. Epidemiologic data suggest that the Great Britain BSE epidemic (1986) resulted from feeding cattle meat and bone meal from sheep infected with scrapie, a similar sheep derived spongioform encephalopathy. Great Britain cases of variant Creutzfeldt-Jakob Disease (Variant CJD) appear to be associated with the BSE epidemic but no causality has been proven. Currently the USDA restricts the importation of live ruminants from countries where BSE is known to exist. The FDA recently prohibited protein derived from mammalian tissues to be used in ruminant feed for animals in the U.S. (Federal Register June 5, 1997; 21 CFR Part 589 "Substances Prohibited From Use in Animal Food or Feed; Animal Proteins Prohibited in Ruminant Feed."). The goal in applying these restrictions with dose monitoring is to prevent transmission of currently known and unknown organisms through the use of medical devices.

Hyaluronic Acid Products

Hyaluronic acid is a disaccharide sugar composed of the linear polymer of glucuronic acid-N-acetyl glucosamine. It is the most common component of the cellular matrix in most skin tissue, and controls extracellular hydration and osmoregulation. Cell-to-cell interaction, proliferation, migration, differentiation and adhesion all depend upon hyaluronic acid. Hyaluronic acid facilitates growth factor activation. Intercellular communication depends upon the moisture of the ECM environment. High osmolality affects whether or not receptors will be expressed on the cells, rendering them receptive to communication chemicals sent from other cells. Hyaluronic acid helps determine whether there will be high secretion of collagen leading to scarring, which is the healing process of adult tissue. Diabetes causes decreased hyaluronic acid synthesis into wounds while excessive deposition occurs within the tunica media of larger vessels.

Hyaluronic acid improves the healing rate of corneal lesions and venous stasis ulcers. In tympanic membrane studies one percent hyaluronic acid effectively and rapidly healed central perforations in 100 percent of cases. However, hyaluronic acid also created hypertrophy of the canal.

Repetitive dosages of exogenous hyaluronic acid in a gel form have been found to stimulate fibroblasts, which secrete a lesser amount of better organized, finer collagen bundles. This structurally improved collagen is associated with healthier, "younger" tissue that is more resilient. Repetitive doses of hyaluronic acid generated tissue that more closely resembled tissue formed by regeneration, as opposed to scarring. For dermal wounds, constructs of hyaluronic acid are being employed to promote healing.

1. **Hyaff®** (GonvaTec) was dispensed in the ester form to facilitate processing, storing, and shipping. Esters convert to acids when mixed with water, such that the dry woven sheet becomes a gel of hyaluronic acid mixed with 40% calcium alginate filler. Clinical trials by the Edmond's group in Canada (64) reported improved healing in diabetic foot ulcers and reduced sinus tracts using the benzyl ester of Hyaff-11. Vasquez et al. reviewed a preliminary report of 36 diabetic foot ulcer patients treated with Hyalofill® for 20 weeks or until healed (73). They noted healing in 76% within 6–14 weeks. However, deeper UT 2A wounds were 15 times less likely to heal than the more superficial wounds.
2. **Multidex®** (DeRoyal Industries, Inc.) is also a carbohydrate based product. It is a hydrophyllic maltodextrin powder wound dressing with 1% ascorbic acid. The ascorbic acid (vitamin C) additive provides a vital precursor for collagen hydroxyproline synthesis. Multidex® fills the wound site and mixes with wound exudate to form a protected moist environment that promotes granulation and epithelial proliferation.
3. **Calgitrol®DX** (Magnus™ Bio-Medical Technologies, Inc.) brand calcium alginate wound dressings with maltodextrin are sterile sheets of a calcium alginate foam matrix.

Collagen Products

Whereas hyaluronic acid is the most predominant carbohydrate in the body, collagen is the most abundant protein, accounting for approximately one-third of the total body protein. Of the 20 distinct human collagens encoded by specific genes, Type I, II, and III are the most predominant. Type I collagen found in bone, skin, tendons, and ligaments composes the basis for connective tissue and Type IV comprises the basal lamina that surrounds all tissues and organs. Fibroblasts secrete collagen in the largest quantity. Early in granulation tissue formation, Type III is initially deposited but later replaced by Type I collagen. Collagen production represents a vital component of active wound healing. Initial trauma to blood vessel wall releases collagen degradative products and exposes Type IV basal laminar collagen. This stimulates platelets to aggregate and activate with resultant hemostasis. Endothelial cells, attracted by degradative products migrate towards and cover the defect. Additionally, collagen is chemotactic for macrophages, fibroblast, and keratinocytes, which fill and resurface the wound defect, and secrete vascular endothelial growth factor (VEGF). Collagen affords structural support, flexibility, and capacity to maintain a moist wound environment. Moisture enhances collagen production and heals wounds faster. There are three kinds of collagen products in common use: porcine Type I collagen, bovine Type I collagen, and bovine collagen (mixed types) powder or hydrogel combinations. Knowing the structure of normal collagen is important to choosing collagen products. Because of repetitive amino acid sequencing, collagen is aligned in triple-helical bands. In this sequence, "proline-hydroxyproline-any amino acid," creates linear "notches" in the triple-helix that conveys both physical and chemical information for interaction with cells. Migrating fibroblasts, macrophages, keratinocytes, and endothelial cells use the banded chemical information for directional alignment. Therefore, it is important for the collagen to maintain a proper orientation. Monocytes migrate to an area ten-fold more aggressively when the collagen is organized. In powdered collagen products, whether dry or mixed with a hydrogel, the collagen is fragmented and misaligned. Sheets of native or woven collagen maintain a more natural orientation and provide better directional information for migrating cells. Collagen sheets may prove a better choice for promoting granulation tissue filling and re-epithelialization by guiding migrating fibroblast and keratinocytes, respectively.

On the other hand, even though fragmented collagen particles may not provide appropriate directional information they remain highly absorptive. Collagen particles are more easily concentrated into a hydrogel, which substantially increases the absorptive capability of the gel. Therefore, this form of collagen may be used to improve osmoregulation of the wound bed. Collagen properties, strength, elasticity, and compatibility enhance its use as a medical device.

In wound healing, collagen functions as a cover dressing for burns and wounds; osteogenic and bone filling material; anti-thrombogenic surface for vascular stents; immobilization agent for therapeutic enzymes (MMP); and vehicle for drug delivery. The relative percentage of different types of collagen (Types I, II, III) and the composition of the matrix surrounding them influences these properties. For example, hyaline cartilage with Type II collagen in thin fibrils is soft, gelatinous, and flexible; elastic cartilage with Type II collagen combined with elastic fibers is more solid, flexible, compressible, and resilient; and fibrous cartilage with Type I collagen in layers that interrupt the matrix and oriented parallel to the stress plane is less compressible, less flexible, more tenacious with higher tensile strength. Parallel distinctions clinically may be seen in granulation tissue formed by the addition of collagen in healing wounds. Type I bovine or porcine collagen is the majority type of collagen used in wound healing products.

1. **Oasis**™ (Cook/Healthpoint, Ltd.) is a porcine-derived collagen sheet applied as a single use biologic tissue to enhance dermal wound healing. A sterile, dehydrated acellular collagen results from treating the pig intestine to remove all but the stromal layer collagen. The collagen sheet is fenestrated to allow easy fluid drainage. Collagen can be used on partial thickness wounds or full thickness wounds. It is contraindicated in cases of porcine sensitivity or religious or ethical beliefs precluding use of pork or animal products. It is not recommended in 3rd degree burns because of their lack of vascularity.
2. **Medifil®II** (BioCore™) consists of spherical hydrophilic particles of bovine Type I collagen, 0.1-0.3 mm in diameter, which may be sprinkled directly into the wound or applied in a gel form. A pad form is also available for cavities or deep wounds.

3. **Nu-Gel™** Collagen Wound Gel (Johnson & Johnson Medical, Inc.) consists of bovine Type I collagen sheets, a hydrogel containing collagen that maintains a moist wound environment and encourages autolytic debridement.
4. **SkinTemp®** (BioCore™) is a composite of nylon mesh to which a porous collagen membrane is attached. As blood vessels and cells grow into the graft, the nylon mesh provides structure and strength but can subsequently be easily removed without disturbing the underlying granulation tissue. SkinTemp® may be used as a temporary skin dressing at the burn site or at the partial thickness skin graft donor site.
5. **Integra®** Dermal Regeneration Template (Johnson & Johnson, Medical, Inc.) is a two-layer system where the outer layer is made of a thin silicone protective film and the inner layer is constructed of a complex matrix of cross-linked fibers composed of pure bovine Type I collagen fibers and glycosaminoglycans (GAGs) made from shark cartilage. The silicone layer provides protection from infection, improves fluid management, and reduces heat loss. The collagen/GAG complex promotes vascular and cellular in-growth to aid in dermal "regeneration." The silicone outer layer is removed in 14–21 days and the residual skin defect is then covered with an epidermal auto-graft. The process allows for a thinner, smaller donor graft and the donor site heals faster than traditional split-thickness skin grafts. Integra® received FDA approval for burn treatment in 1996. When compared with traditional split-thickness skin graft therapy, treatment with Integra® produces less hypertrophic scarring, yielding skin that is more supple, more resilient, less skin contracture, and more esthetically pleasing.
6. **Fibracol®** Collagen-Alginate Wound Dressing (Johnson & Johnson, Medical, Inc.) a composite dressing of 90% collagen and 10% calcium alginate combines the structural support of collagen with the gel-forming capability of an alginate.

Fibroblast and Keratinocyte Products

The epidermis of normal skin is avascular and made of keratinocytes (skin cells), both differentiated cells and keratinocyte stem cells. Keratinocytes make up most of the epidermis. The dermis is vascular, and contains glands and follicles. Dermal tissue does not regenerate into normal dermis after serious burns. Instead, scar tissue forms causing various deformities. To replace skin after burns, traumatic wounds, and major operations, autologous skin is often harvested as a graft for wound coverage. Availability of donor sites, further pain, and scarring are problems. Fibroblasts, the major cell type comprising the dermis, secrete the majority of collagen and extracellular matrix, as well as many growth factors. Fibroblasts in bioengineered tissues are cultured to "grow out" the immunogenicity such that the tissues may be applied to patients without engendering a graft-versus-host response. Nonetheless, Badiavas et al., have noted the development of foreign body-like granulomas in the base of bi-layer grafted wounds, (venous and burn) (83). Cultured bilayered allograft cells are of neonatal foreskin origin; therefore, they secrete more hyaluronic acid than adult cells, which persists longer and tends to regenerate more like normal skin without the disadvantages of scarring normally seen in adult healing. Skin substitutes are primarily used as replacement tissues applied to a well-granulated wound base. Increasingly, skin substitutes are being applied to stimulate a variety of nonhealing wounds.

1. **Apligraf®** (Organogenesis, Inc.) is a cultured bilayer dermal-epidermal skin substitute, frequently referred to as a human skin-equivalent (HSE), or Graftskin®. It comes in a circular disk of bovine Type I (tendon) base collagen in lattice form which supports fibroblasts and dermal epithelial cells. Over this is cultured a layer of allogenic keratinocytes forming a stratified epidermis. The result is essentially a full thickness skin equivalent with all growth factors and chemical messengers needed in healing skin. Actual "take" like a split thickness skin graft is rare but may occur. It hypothesized that the bilayered HSE generates its effect by locally synthesizing and releasing multiple growth factors in specific combination and concentrations, which improve the impaired reparative process of chronic wounds. Falanga compared the clinical efficacy of compression therapy vs. combined Graftskin®/compression therapy to treat venous ulcers, with greater than one-year duration (88). He reported Graftskin® combination therapy as being three times more effective at eight weeks and two times more effective at 24 weeks in completing wound closure. Sibbald presented a cost benefit analysis study conducted at the University of Toronto suggesting that the use of Apligraf® in conjunction with a four-layered compression dressing was more effective than the four-layered dressing alone in the treatment of venous leg ulcers (91). The cost of adding Apligraf® to the dressing also increased the cost but provided a projected benefit of 22 ulcer days averted per patient at an incremental cost of $304 (societal). The FDA list of approved indications includes venous ulcers and diabetic ulcers. Case reports and collected series support the effective use of Graftskin® as a skin replacement at excised tumor sites, donor sites, partial-thickness thermal burns, covering meshed skin grafts, arterial insufficiency ulcers, cosmetic surgical sites, areas of contracture, acute partial-and full-thickness excisional wounds, and for epidermolysis bullosa (EB). Apligraf® is delivered in a sealed bag within a temperature controlled Styrofoam packing. The product is shipped overnight with an expiry such that the graft may still be viable for 2–3 days. Once opened, application should occur within two hours. Minimal handling of the graft is advised to avoid damaging the cells. The cells take best to a clean debris-free well-granulated wound base. The graft should be fenestrated to allow fluid generated during the healing process to escape. An environment conducive to warm, moist wound healing should be provided. Bulky secondary dressings that may cause excessive pressure on the wound base should be avoided. Special considerations may preclude its application in patients with religious or ethical beliefs concerning the use of bovine derived products. Apligraf® is also contraindicated for use in individuals with known hypersensitivity to bovine proteins. Patients should be consented prior to application.

2. **Dermagraft®** (Advanced Tissue Sciences, Inc.) is a cryopreserved, bioengineered tissue of human neonatal fibroblast cells seeded on rectangular sheets of biodegradable mesh. Unlike natural skin, Dermagraft® does not contain macrophages, lymphocytes, blood vessels, or hair follicles. The dermal portion is a porous lattice of cross-linked bovine Type I collagen and glycosaminoglycan (chondroitin-6-sulphate). This collagen GAG layer functions as a biodegradable structure until new dermal tissue (neodermis) grows. Fibroblasts, macrophages, lymphocytes, and endothelial cells infiltrate the dermal component, progressively building a neovascular network. As healing progresses, native collagen is deposited by fibroblasts, and the collagenous component biodegrades over the next 30 days. After the neodermis has been generated, the synthetic polysiloxane polymer (silicone) "epidermal" layer is removed and replaced with a thin autograft. In diabetic foot ulcers, the scaffold degrades in approximately one week and removal of the scaffold is done at that time. Eight (8) applications may be needed to achieve complete healing. In venous stasis ulcers, Dermagraft® cells colonize the wound site for at least six months. Perdue et al. reviewed a multi-centered study in the use of Dermagraft®-TC as compared to cadaver allograft for the temporary closure of excised burn wounds with a mean burn size of 44% total body surface (TBS) and 28% TBS full-thickness (100). The study found Dermagraft®-TC to be equivalent or superior to allograft with regard to autograft take at post-treatment day 14. Dermagraft®-TC did not develop epidermal slough, resulted in less bleeding than allograft while maintaining an adequate wound bed, and proved easier to remove. Newton described a laser Doppler measurement increase of seventy-five percent (75%) blood flow at the base of foot ulcers treated with eight (8) Dermagraft® applied weekly in type 2 diabetic patients (98). These changes correlate with improved healing and may represent angiogensis or vasodilation of existing vessels. Browne linked graft-stimulated healing rates in diabetic neurotrophic foot ulcers to the level of colonizing organisms (95). No growth correlated with a wound healing rate of 0.2 cm per week Colony forming of 105–106 units/gram correlates with a healing rate of 0.15 cm per week, and greater than 106 colony forming units/gram correlates with a healing rate of 0.05 cm/per week. Interestingly, Browne also reported that five of the eight patients studied (75%) had greater or equal to 105 colony forming units/gram organisms present despite the absence of clinical signs of infection. Thus, a higher level of "critical colonization" may exist in diabetic patients without good clinical signs of infection, suggesting a need to biopsy or empirically pretreat with topical or oral therapy to reduce the level of bacterial colonization in diabetic neurotrophic wounds prior to the application of a graft. Overall, it appears that when used to treat chronic diabetic foot ulcers of greater than six weeks duration, Dermagraft® proves to be a safe and effective treatment. Marston et al. reported a randomized, controlled, multi-center study with 314 patients enrolled, comparing Dermagraft® to conventional therapy (99),

resulting in thirty percent (30.0%) Dermagraft® patient healed at 12 weeks versus approximately eighteen percent (18.3%) for conventional therapy. The cost effectiveness of using Dermagraft® is well outlined in a French 52-week study by Allenet et al. who applied a Markov model to simulate the health status of a cohort of 100 patients with a diabetic foot ulcer treated either with conventional therapy or with Dermagraft® (94). Dermagraft® healed more ulcers 76.5% (median time 14–15 weeks) versus standard therapy which healed 69.33% (median time 28–29 weeks). Dermagraft® decreased recurrences (14.29 vs. 25.09) within a 52-week period. Because Dermagraft® healed more ulcers, the average cost to heal ulcers using the graft was lower. Dermagraft® is supplied frozen in a clear bag containing one piece [2 in x 3 in (5 cm x 7.5 cm)] for a single-use application after it is thawed. The product should be applied within 30 minutes of thawing to ensure cellular viability. Specific instructions regarding thawing are provided by the vendor and should be followed carefully. The graft may be cut to size. It is then covered with a non-adherent dressing, without packing the wound, and the dressing is usually changed after 72 hours.

3. **Cultured Keratinocytes.** Autogenic keratinocyte sheets are grown from small pieces of the patient's skin and cultured for later replacement. Cultured allogenic keratinocyte sheets can be produced from neonatal foreskin and donor skin in 2–3 weeks. Allogenic keratinocytes are cultured to grow out the immunogenicity. The sheets can be cryopreserved and stored at a tissue bank as long as six months. To make a keratinocyte sheet, a small piece of neonatal foreskin or patient skin is separated into layers with the enzyme dispase. The epidermal layer is minced and keratinocytes are filtered, collected, and cultured in a serum-free medium supplemented with growth factor, hydrocortisone and insulin, and co-cultivated with a non-proliferative feeder layer of T3 fibroblast. The resulting keratinocyte sheet can be lifted from the culture dish in 2–4 weeks for surgical reimplantation to the wound site, sealed with surgical clips, and closed for approximately 30 days. Both autologus and allogenic grafts can be used temporarily or permanently depending on wound condition. Newer bio-engineered constructs are being generated with focus upon meeting certain requirements that may not be completely fulfilled with currently available products. A wound that is devoid of lamina densa and lamina lucida as occurs with burns and in some wounds may have the future benefit of an extracellular matrix (ECM). The ECM is secreted by human umbilical vein endothelial cells (HUVECs) and assembled on gelatin coated plates overlaid by a mixed matrix secreted by human dermal microvascular endothelial cells (HDMECs) and human dermal fibroblasts, which provides a viable acellular scaffold for use in wound healing.
4. **Cadaver skin,** cryopreserved and glycerolized, has been predominately utilized as temporary dressings in burn patients. Recent practice changes in burn care have resulted in earlier burn wound excision and complete coverage with autograft, cadaver skin, synthetic dressings,

and/or amnion. Glycerol preserved allograft skin appears to be preferable to cryopreserved allograft skin where it is used as a temporary wound closure because it is easier to handle and store. Cryopreserved skin appears to be more advantageous in cases where the integration of a dermal component as a permanent part of wound closure is desired since the dermis has an excellent survival rate and keratinocytes may be grafted at a later date. Unfortunately the demand for cadaver skin in the United States has outstripped supply (4–7 fold) and there exists the risk of infectious disease transmission, including HIV, or other yet to be discovered viruses.

Other common products used by some burn centers include: AlloDerm® (LifeCell), and E-Z Derm™ (Brennen Medical, Inc.). AlloDerm® is an acellular freeze-dried dermal graft derived from donated human cadaver skin. It is processed to eliminate the entire epidermis, eradicate dermal cells, inhibit matrix metalloproteinases (MMPs) while maintaining the basement membrane and collagen, elastin, proteoglycans, and vascular structures. AlloDerm® should be used as a biological scaffold for dermal-epidermal regrowth. On the other hand, E-Z Derm™, a biosynthetic wound dressing derived from porcine, is a xenograft in which the collagen has been chemically crosslinked with an aldehyde to provide strength, durability and convenient storage at room temperature. E-Z Derm™ is used as a temporary protective barrier that allows natural healing to continue undisturbed.

In some centers, cultured keratinocytes are still used as a temporary burn dressing. Donor skin obtained from the patient is processed to produce a large sheet of keratinocytes with approximately a 10,000-fold expansion. Unfortunately, this process is fraught with difficulties to include a required 2–3 week delay, survival of less than a week due to full-thickness defects, and the absence of a dermal layer predisposes the wound to contracture and blistering.

GROWTH FACTORS AND GROWTH PROCESSES

Growth factors are proteins that mediate all cellular functions, usually by binding locally to cell receptors. The following growth factors known to exert significant influence in wound healing include: platelet derived growth factor (PDGF), fibroblast growth factor 1 and 2 (FGF), transforming growth factor alpha and beta (TGF), epidermal growth factor (EGF), and insulin-like growth factor (IGF-1). Interleukins, specialized cytokines that facilitate the cross-take specifically between white blood cells are also intimately involved the modulating the cellular message. Within the base of chronic non-healing wounds, the levels of various growth factors are decreased in association with an elevation in the level of MMPs. Rationale for using additional growth factors in an attempt to accelerate wound healing include: 1) abnormal expression of extracellular matrix proteins inhibit growth factors, 2) decreased growth factor receptor expression, and 3) development of senescent phenotypes that may respond to exogenously supplied growth factors.

Specific Growth Factors of Interest:

1. **Platelet-Derived Growth Factor (PDGF)** is chemotactic for neutrophils, fibroblasts, and macrophages by regulating the expression

of integrins, which are proteins that mediate adhesion of neutrophils and macrophages to endothelial cells. Intravascular cells are coated with the selectin adhesion molecules so that they will be recognized by the integrin receptors that line the endothelial wall. The selectin-integrin connection triggers changes in the intravascular cell that allows it to transmigrate through desmosomes in the endothelial wall to enter into the tissue spaces. In this fashion, PDGF released from platelets activates polymorphonuclear cells (PMN) and macrophages. Macrophages also secrete PDGF. In the tissue, fibroblasts exposed to PDGF undergo proliferation and exhibit activation with increased secretion of collagen and extracellular matrix components. Once activated, fibroblasts also secrete PDGF to assist the macrophage in inducing other fibroblasts, endothelial cells, and smooth muscle cells to replicate. The activated macrophages secrete vascular endothelial growth factor, to direct angiogenesis. There are many other key growth factors.

2. **Fibroblast Growth Factors (FGF)** attract and induce replication of fibroblasts, keratinocytes, and other cells.
3. **Transforming Growth Factor-beta (TGF-β)** stimulates angiogenesis and fibroplasia while inhibiting both MMP production and keratinocyte proliferation.
4. **Epidermal Growth Factor (EGF)** stimulates keratinocyte migration and granulation tissue formation.
5. **Insulin-like Growth Factors-1 (IGF-1)** belongs to a family of more than five factors with endocrine effects similar to growth hormone (GH).
6. **Keratinocyte Growth Factor (KGF also called FGF-7)** stimulates keratinocyte migration, proliferation, and differentiation. KGF also stimulates nerve growth factor.
7. **Nerve Growth Factor (NGF)** controls development of sympathetic postganglionic neurons and possibly dorsal root (sensory) ganglion cells in mammals.
8. **Connective Tissue Growth Factor (GTGF)** attracts and induces replication of various connective tissue cells.
9. **Vascular Endothelial Growth Factor (VEGF)** is important for the growth and survival of endothelial cells.

Angiogenesis (neovascularization) is the formation of new capillary blood vessels from pre-existing blood vessels. It is a locally regulated process that occurs over a short duration. The process involves three steps: 1) breakdown of previous existing vessel wall, 2) migration of endothelial cells in response to angiogenic stimulus, 3) formation of new vessels. The process begins with budding of existing endothelial cells, proceeds through elongation, and then finalizes with coalescence. It is regulated by **Interleukin-8 (IL-8), Vascular Endothelial Growth Factor (VEGF)**, as well as, **Basic Fibroblast Growth Factor (FGF-basic)**. Macrophages are recognized as the cell with the greatest influence upon the angiogenic process. To prevent overgrowth of capillary sprouts and promote appropriate vascular differentiation, macrophages also secrete inhibitory factors. **Interleukin-1 (IL-1)** appears to be the link between infection and wound healing. Monocytes/

macrophage cells have a tremendous role in promoting tissue repair. These are the same cells that differentiate into antigen-presenting cells (APC) that provide information to lymphocyte T helper cells to initiate the cellular immunity response for the host protection. **Interleukin-4 (IL-4)** is a cytokine. After migration the cells loose motility and transform into epitheloid cells. They fuse into giant cells and are activated to secrete tissue destructive factors.

Growth Factor Medications

1. **Regranex®** is a form of platelet-derived growth factor, PDGF-*ββ*, developed by Johnson & Johnson. Regranex® is the only single agent growth factor that has been formally released for use to heal dermal wounds. This factor was chosen because of its prominent role in the wound healing process at multiple levels involving multiple cells types. Other growth factor agents have not shown sufficient clinical effectiveness for full development and release at this time. Exogenously applied growth factors may be degraded by matrix metalloproteinases (MMP), or be adsorbed or inactivated by gauze and dressing materials. Senescent cells in the wound bed may not respond to the stimulatory efforts of exogenous growth factors, and since they are live enzymes, they must be temperature controlled to prevent heat inactivation. Regranex® (becaplermin 0.01% gel-Ortho-McNeil Pharmaceutical) is a non-sterile topical gel containing becaplermin, a bio-engineered recombinant human platelet-derived growth factor (PDGF). Regranex® attracts macrophages, which secrete vascular **endothelial growth factor (VEGF)**, initiating angiogenesis. In response to becaplermin, fibroblasts, proliferation begins with increased secretion of gel matrix and collagen. Activated fibroblast and macrophages also release additional growth factors that regulate further granulation tissue development. Saba et al. reported the effects of PDGF on wound healing in both animal and human models, with PDGF-treated wounds healing faster than controls (116). Biopsies taken at 20 days showed PDGF generated granulation tissue with fine collagen fibers deposited throughout the wound site, characteristics consistent with immature granulation tissue and wounds that close by reepithelialization and filling in with scar. The findings suggested that PDGF heals by reepithelialization with the prevention of wound contraction.

   Since Regranex® is an active enzyme, it requires storage and handling within an appropriate refrigerated temperature range, but not frozen. Heating inactivates the enzyme such that prolonged durations of time left without refrigeration may render the medication ineffective. At time of this writing, Regranex® has FDA approval for adequately vascularized, neuropathic lower extremity diabetic ulcers that extend into the subcutaneous tissue that have received standard of care therapy without improvement. Other applications are considered "off-label," even though it is common practice to apply Regranex® to other wounds in diabetic patients, decubitus ulcers, venous ulcers, and slowly healing post-operative wounds. Known contraindications are hypersensitivity to parabens, and neoplasms. Regranex® is also contraindicated for use in wounds that are showing normal progression. Regranex® should be used in conjunction with standard ulcer care practices including initial sharp debridement, pressure relief and infection control. Regranex® use is not recommended for longer than 20 weeks. It is recommended that the dressing be changed within 12 hours but the medication is only applied every 24 hours. In common practice, the dressing is changed once daily instead of twice to reduce dressing costs and for patient convenience.

Kantor and Margolis (113) presented a cost effectiveness estimate based upon four treatment options: 1) standard care (SC), 2) standard treatment in a specialized wound care center (WCC), 3) treatment with becaplermin, or 4) treatment with platelet releasate (PR). Utilizing published data from clinical trials, meta-analyses, and a data base of 26,599 patients, they projected the effectiveness of each treatment, showing treatment with becaplermin to be the most effective; becaplermin (43.0%), platelet releasate (36.8 %), specialty wound center (35.6%), and standard care (30.9%). Cost effectiveness ratios projected incremental cost of increasing the odds of healing by 1% over standard therapy was $414.40 for PR, and $36.59 for becaplermin. As a pharmaceutical, Regranex® is covered by most prescription drug plans.

2. **Colony Stimulating Factors (CSF)** is the principal growth factor regulating maturation, proliferation, and differentiation of the precursor cells of neutrophilic granulocytes. Granulocytes and macrophages are necessary for angiogenesis to occur. Granulocyte influence on angiogenesis is inferior to that of macrophages but the presence of granulocytes is necessary. The colony stimulating factors are most frequently used human recombinant erythropoietin (Epogen®-Amgen, Procrit®-GlaxoSmithKline, rh E-CSF) , Filgrastim-G-CSF (Neupogen® Amgen, Inc.), and Sargramostim GM-CSF (Leukine®, Prokine® Immunex) to mobilize cells from bone marrow, and support the immune system after transplantation and delayed engraftment. Modification of Filgrastim produced a larger molecule, Pegfilgrastim® (Amgen, Inc.). This created a granulocyte colony-stimulating factor (G-CSF) with a long half-life and sustained duration of action, Sargramostim. Combinations of Filgrastim, Sargramostim, and IL-3 are more effective than any agent alone. Edmonds reported "encouraging results" using Filgrastim on diabetic foot ulcers. De Ugarte presented a small case series of three patients treated with GM-CSF with complete healing of their wounds within 1–4 weeks, despite inherited medical disorders associated with leukocyte dysfunction and non-healing wounds (106). Topical application of GM-CSF and subcutaneous (s.c.) infusion pump for the local delivery enhanced healing. In wound healing, local application may be more effective than systemic and IL-3. GM-CSF agents, or Pegfilgrastim® alone or in combination may be more advisable therapeutic interventions. Cost analysis by Whalen (110) was accomplished evaluating Filgrastim with Sargramostim in the treatment of outpatient neutropenic patients receiving myelosuppressive chemotherapy; Filgrastim ($1,036 US) vs. Sargramostim ($1,318 US).

3. **Buffy Coat Derived Mediators:** The Buffy coat is the leukocyte/ platelet-enriched fraction of blood obtained by centrifuge. It contains from 2.5–9 times more DNA material than the same volume of whole blood and accounts for approximately 1% of total blood volume. The Buffy-coat contains the platelets and five types of leukocytes: granulocytes consisting of the eosinophils, basophils, and neutrophils; and the agranulocytes consisting of the lymphocytes and monocytes. Lymphocytes account for 30% of the circulating leukocytes with 90% of those being T-lymphocytes. B-lymphocytes impart humoral-immunity becoming plasma cells and secreting antibodies; while, T lymphocytes impart cellular-immunity through antigen presentation. Monocytes make up only five percent of circulating leukocytes and serve to maintain the body's population of macrophages (histiocytes) and antigen presenting cells. Platelets, ranging from approximately 100,000-400,000 (per microliter of whole blood) arise from myeloid tissue and constitute the major cell type found in the Buffy coat. Buffy coat platelets produce the majority of the growth factors suspended in a fibrin gel base. Buffy coat, wound care derivatives fall into two categories. The first commercially marketed wound repair product was based on platelet releasate, was represented by Procuren®; Platelet Derived Wound Healing Formula (Curative Health Systems, now licensed to Cytomedix, Inc,). While Procuren® is no longer available at this writing, it is important to note that true platelet releasates do not contain any Buffy coat cellular or blood components, but only extracted growth factors. The effective Procuren® protocol designated a 12 hours on, 12 hour off cycle interspersed with moist dressings. The now prevalent procedures are based on autologous Buffy coat gels or Platelet Rich Plasma (PRP). The end result of the procedure is the application of a platelet gel or autologous, blood derived tissue graft in the wound. Like the erythrocytes, leukocytes express a number of antigens on the cell surfaces that are important in transplantation. Because these gels should only be applied to the original donor, antigenic immune issues should not be a factor, but care should be taken to ensure the patient does not have an allergy to bovine derived products. Moreover, since the Buffy coat and the grafts are obtained from and returned to the same patient, FDA approval has not been sought in these procedures. As long as the whole blood, Buffy coat gel or graft materials are not stored, blood-banking rules currently do not affect the use or delivery of this procedure. The use of a bedside or procedure room centrifuge requires local compliance review with Clinical Laboratory Improvement Amendments (CLIA).

   To prepare a Buffy coat fraction, whole blood is centrifuged at a rate of 2,500–4,750 rpm for 8–18 minutes at room temperature. Three distinct component layers will develop with plasma on top, leukocytes and platelets (Buffy coat) in the middle, and erythrocytes on the bottom. Newer more efficient systems can recover platelets from a sample of whole blood at almost twice that recovered using older centrifuge procedures, 70.6%. Once the platelets are recovered, proprietary formulations (usually containing thrombin) are added to stimulate the Buffy-coat cells and proteins. Stimulation of the Buffy coat will lead to several reactions, including conversion of soluble fibrinogen to insoluble fibrin and the degranulation of the platelets to release growth factors into the gel. Platelets and growth factors that are used successfully to heal wounds are concentrated from 2.5 to 9 times baseline levels dependent on centrifuge type and protocol. Applications protocols range from weekly to "as needed," utilize "moist wound care techniques," and may include additional antibiotics, antimicrobial therapy, or vitamins.

Several companies provide equipment, disposables, and support for gel based procedures performed in office, clinic or hospital settings (Safeblood® Technologies, Inc., Little Rock, Arkansas, Cytomedix, Inc., Little Rock Arkansas, and Harvest Technologies).

CELLULAR STIMULATORS (GROWTH PROMOTERS)

Cellular promoters are agents that provoke cellular responses similar to those seen *in vivo*. The agents may illicit chemotaxis with migration, proliferation, differentiation, adherence, morphologic changes or secretory responses. Some stimulators are recombinantly generated to produce agents found normally within the tissue while others are of plant, yeast, or bacterial extraction. Still other chemicals are used to alter receptors or other structures on the cellular membrane to exert their effect. Some of the better-known stimulators will be reviewed below.

Platelet Promoters

Platelets aggregate at areas of exposed Type IV and Type V collagen found in damaged blood vessels. The agents usually considered the primary agonists for platelet activation include: adenosine diphosphate (ADP), thrombin, and collagen. Collagen facilitates platelet activation. Fibrin sealant used as "surgical glue" contains fibrinogen and thrombin. Used primarily for hemostasis, they exhibit varying capacity to promote granulation tissue development.

Macrophage Promoters

1. **Biafine®** (Medix, Pharmaceutical, America, Inc.) is a macrophage cell stimulator. Recruited macrophages remove necrotic tissues and tissue debris, reducing inflammation. Macrophages stimulate fibroblast proliferation, to aid healing. Fibroblast proliferation subsequently promotes epithelial growth. As an oil-in-water emulsion it provides moisture to soften non-viable tissues, aid in autolytic debridement, and reduce irritation. The active ingredient, trolamine, was recently evaluated in an ex vivo skin model by Boisnic, who determined that a "radioprotective" function may be attributed to its ability to reduce capillary alterations, restore CD34 expression, and promote epithelial cell proliferation while decreasing collagen secretion and IL-1 expression. These finding suggest the mechanism of Biafine® is at the dermal level with granulation tissue formation not epidermal resurfacing. Clinical findings of a phase II Study (Szumacher) to delineate the purported radioprotective qualities of Biafine® in breast cancer patients receiving radiation therapy did not show a beneficial radioprotective effect with Biafine®.

2. **Copper-Chlorophyllin Sodium (CCu-Na)** the sodium copper salt and the water-soluble analogue of the sodium copper chlorophyll, exhibit several beneficial qualities: antioxidant, anti-carcinogen, anti-mutagen, anti-inflammatory and wound-healing promoter. Chlorophyllin are derivatives of chlorophyll where the central metal is something other than magnesium as occurs in chlorophyll. As an antioxidant, CCu-Na is more effective than ascorbic acid or glutathione. Chlorophyllin exerts an anti-inflammatory effect by suppressing lipopolysaccharide (LPS) induced nitric oxide (NO) production to down regulate a pro-inflammatory response. Copper chlorophyllin sodium inhibits *Staphylococcus aureus* coagulase and interferences with bacterial respiration to decrease wound bacterial burden. Chlorophyllin stimulates fibroblasts with proven healing capacity in dermal wounds. Additionally the chlorophyllin reduces wound odor. Panafil® (Healthpoint, Ltd.) is the most readily available source of chlorophyllin for wound care. It is the water-soluble analogue and therefore exceptional bioavailability compared to the sodium-copper salt, insoluble form.

MECHANICAL ADJUNCTIVE THERAPIES

Negative Pressure Wound Therapy (NPWT)

The first NPWT product was called Vacuum Assisted Closure (Wound VAC®, Kinetic Concepts, Inc). Recently, a second product has entered the market (BlueSky Versatile 1™ Wound Vacuum System, BlueSky Medical). For purpose of illustration, we will describe the Wound VAC® system since there are more published reports using that system. NPWT affects healing by generating negative pressure in a controlled suction, either continuously or intermittently, at approximately 125 mm Hg to a wound bed through a sterile sponge. Physical modality generically prescribed as "controlled subatmospheric pressure dressing" or "negative pressure wound therapy" (NPWT) is fast becoming a mainstay for chronic wound care therapy. NPWT promotes wound healing by a number of mechanisms. The negative pressure wound environment reduces interstitial edema, decompresses the lymphatics, decreases the bacterial load, promotes granulation tissue, and maintains a moist, insulated environment. Reducing fluid load (edema) increases transcutaneous oxygen levels, as edema impedes oxygen diffusion. As edema fluid is removed, tissue lactate levels correspondingly decrease, along with other potentially inhibitory chemical factors. Negative pressure wound therapy dramatically stimulates angiogenesis. Fibroblasts produce growth factors in response to tissue deformity.

After first cleaning the wound, a sterile open foam dressing is applied into the wound cavity using either a black polyurethane or white polyvinyl alcohol sponge. The open interconnected sponge weave allows pressure to be distributed equally throughout the sponge with the opportunity for pockets, which would predispose to infection. A fenestrated evacuation tube exits the foam and connects to the pump. As suction is applied, the sponge is pulled into the wound bed. Wound fluid continually drains from the wound bed into a disposable container, isolated from both patient and caregiver. Frequency of dressing change is reduced to every other day, increasing comfort and compliance, and reducing costs. The concept of the open foam is to pull the granulation tissue into the open foam cells. The white sponge was created to be used in areas where granulation tissue is not desirable, such as over tendon. Contraindications for NPWT include untreated osteomyelitis and malignant wounds; thin, abraided, erosive skin; in areas where the margin does not accommodate adherence such that vacuum pressure is lost; and in actively bleeding wounds. The NPWT canister shuts down once full, so if bleeding does occur, it should be self-limiting. Anticoagulants are a relative contraindication; consideration should be given to the level of anticoagulation; in many cases NPWT may be judiciously applied. Although there are literature reports of VAC® therapy used in fistula wound care, this practice is considered to be a relative contraindication.

Multiple studies support the use of the NPWT in a variety of wounds for assistance with closing large defects such as infected post-operative sternal sites, decubitus ulcers, residual defects after artificial joints of the hip, or knee have been removed, abdominal wall wounds being treated with open technique, and pelvic surgeries for infection in gynecologic or urologic surgeries. Diabetic lower extremity wounds-neuropathic ulcers, amputation post-operative sites, and areas of breakdown secondary to prosthesis wear have all responded well to this intervention. Heavily exudative wounds or wounds with exposed structures that need protection such as fixation appliances, Dacron mesh and artificial joints have improved from reported use of VAC® therapy. NPWT has been used to immobilize grafts and flaps, prepare graft beds, and close donor sites. It has been applied favorably in the pediatric and geriatric populations to close large defects of the chest or abdomen, which develop from sternal wound infections after cardiac surgery or with abdominal compartment syndrome and uncontrolled intraperitoneal sepsis in the pediatric patient. To manage infected sternal wounds Gustafsson reported using a strategy with C-reactive protein levels to guide subsequent surgical closure of the sternal defect (with a mean of nine days, range 3–34 days) after NPWT had assisted volume reduction and granulation tissue development (140). NPWT facilitates a closing method for the distracted fascia1 edges that avoids the need for skin grafting. In situations where a split-thickness graft is indicated, NPWT provides a safe and effective method for securing STSGs and is associated with improved graft survival as measured by a reduction in number of repeated STSGs. NPWT treatment at flap donor sites has been helpful in closure of these areas. In pressure ulcer care, NPWT speeds the formation of granulation tissue, decreases the amount of localized edema, increases blood flow, and accelerates healing. Treatment for open fracture wounds shows great success. It has also proven effectiveness in developing injuries of the hand and foot. Cro et al. described using NPWT to manage three patients with moderate to high volume output enterocutaneous fistula where conventional therapy had failed (135). Two of the three reported patients progressed to complete closure and all three had improvement in the excoriated periwound. Not all patients are candidates for NPWT; those patients with severe peripheral vascular disease or smaller forefoot wounds may be better treated by other modalities.

Extensive biochemical basis of NPWT has not been fully elucidated. NPWT may exert its effects through a myriad of mechanisms including:

- Removal of pro-inflammatory exudative fluids,
- Reduction in edema fluid and tissue pressures,
- Removal of matrix metalloproteinases which degrade growth factors,
- Stimulation or removal of senescent cells along the wound base,
- Mobilization of reparative cells (macrophages) to the site of deformation,
- Stimulation of angiogenesis through the effect of tissue pressure changes that activate angiogenic growth factors/substances or macrophage and/or fibroblast stimulatory secretion of VEGF,
- Improvement in local oxygenation through edema reduction, angiogenesis induction, or pressure gradient changes,
- Activation and proliferation of fibroblasts in response to the intermittent deformation pressures, and perhaps,
- Changes in the "current of injury" based upon changing the flow gradients of ions in the tissue.

Further research is required to sort out which of these or other mechanisms are responsible of the positive clincial outcomes noted with this therapy.

Cost benefit analyses of stage III and IV pressure ulcers of the trochanteric and trunk region presented by Philbeck et al. in 1999 supported a cost savings of approximately $9,000US for management using NPWT in association with a low air mattress as opposed to a low air mattress alone (142). In this review comparing Medicare home healthcare records of 1,032 patients (1,170 wounds) to a historical control analysis by Ferrell (1993), the addition of negative pressure therapy instead of saline soaked gauze. afforded a faster closure for a larger average wound size, (Ferrell- average wound size 4.3 cm^2 with closure rate of 0.090 cm^2 per day. Philbeck- average wound size 22.3 cm^2 with closure rate of 0.23 cm^2 per day). Additionally the projected duration of open wound would be decreased from 247 days (Ferrell) to 97 days (Philbeck). Evans reviewed the literature in 2001 to assess the overall effectiveness of topical negative pressure (TNP) in treating chronic wounds (136). At that time, NPWT appeared to provide a trend towards promoting faster healing but all of the published studies had small sample sizes. Cost effectiveness, quality of life impact, pain and comfort influence were not reported. An optimum TNP regimen could not be determined. In 2003, Issues in Emerging Health Technologies, Fisher recommended more studies to evaluate the effectiveness of NPWT therapy when the types of dressings are the same for patients in the groups being compared and NPWT therapy is the only differing intervention (138).

Electrical Stimulation Therapy

Electrical stimulation therapy is the use of electrical current as an energy source that is transferred to an open wound and its surrounding tissues. Normal, healthy intact skin has a negative 23 mV potential compared to the underlying tissue because of the salt (NaCl) released onto the skin. As sodium (Na+) is pumped back into cells it leaves an overall negative charge on the skin surface. Inside the tissue local charge differences exist because of the orientation of the positive sodium (Na+) and potassium (K+) ions as balanced by the negative chloride (Cl-) ions and negatively charged proteins across the cell membrane. The bi-layered membrane provides separation distance across which ions may flow, setting up potential local currents. Activation of cell membrane pumps, gates, and pores facilitate ionic movement. When conditions are conducive, the ions flow and generate small currents called local potentials. Injured, open wound tissue exhibits an electropositive charge relative to the surrounding intact skin. This "current of injury" purportedly affects cellular migration and communication. Dry wound environment impedes current flow since dryness increases resistance. On the other hand, moist wound environment supports current flow. Bioelectric currents alter cellular communication to promote healing. Diabetic foot wounds, pressure ulcers, venous insufficiency ulcers, arterial insufficiency ulcers, post-traumatic wounds, and fractures have shown positive improvement with electrical stimulation therapy. The overwhelming majority of tissues in the human body use bioelectrical stimulation to affect biochemical interactions. This may account for the universal utility of this therapy.

In the realm of wound care, electrical stimulation is indicated as adjunctive therapy to control acute and chronic pain, reduce edema, reduce muscle spasms, reduce joint contractures, minimize disuse atrophy, promote tissue repair, strengthen muscle tissue, facilitate fracture healing, and deliver medication locally to deep tissues. Treatments are applied as intermittent therapy given one or more times a day in 45-minute intervals for 40-60 treatment days. Contraindications include: 1) cardiac disability, 2) pacemakers, 3) pregnancy 4) menstruation- when treatments occur over abdomen, lumbar or pelvic region, 5) cancerous lesions, 6) infection sites when not using for medication delivery, 7) exposed metal implants, and 8) nerve sensitivity.

A choice of waveforms and energy patterns are available for application. Monophasic and biphasic waveforms differ in their ability to deliver charge to the tissue immediately surrounding the electrode. Balanced biphasic waves deliver a negative net charge, whereas, monophasic waveforms generate a transferable charge. Voltage, the electromotive driving force propelling the electrons, dictates the depth of energy penetration. High voltage patterns (greater than 100–150 V) or low voltage patterns (less than 100–150 V) can be used in medicine. Various devices generate different waveforms: smooth (sine), spiked, square, or continuous. These different patterns allow for differential activation of the tissue being treated. Pulse frequency is the number of pulses that occur in a unit of time, Hertz (Hz). Applicable pulse frequencies are: 1) low frequency- 1K Hz and below as used in muscle stimulation units, 2) medium frequency-1K to 100K Hz as used in interferential and Russian stimulation LVGS units, and 3) high frequency above l00K Hz as used in TENS, HVGS (HVPC), and diathermies. In applying this therapy, two electrode pads, oriented 180 degrees apart emit energy that is coupled to the patient via a wet conductive medium. Capacitively-coupled pads may be placed in the wound bed and at a distance from the wound. The polarity can be adjusted according to the stage of the wound (inflammation, negative vs. proliferation-positive or alternating between positive and negative). The negative electrode acts as the cathode, an area of high electron concentration and the positive electrode acts as the anode, an area of low electron concentration. Some systems are designed such that the orientation of the pads does not matter because the energy transmitted alternates during the course of the treatment without requiring pad adjustments. Electrodes placed close together will give a superficial stimulation and be of high density, while those placed farther apart penetrate more deeply with less current density. Larger electrode pads provide a more dispersed pattern with a lower density than smaller pads. Depending on the desired treatment pulse rates may also be adjusted. Higher amperage provides deeper penetration but some patients develop discomfort or pain with increased amperage. Therefore, this is adjusted for comfort at the time of therapy. The strongest stimulation is where the current leaves the body (i.e., the anode pad if pads are unidirectional). Currently in wound care, the most commonly recommended treatment modality uses a monophasic twin peaked high voltage pulsed current. Monophasic application requires one negative electrode and one positive electrode to create a circuit with the patient as the conductive medium between the two electrodes. HPVC pulse width ranges from 20–200 microseconds, associated with minimal pH and temperature changes. HPVC is associated with muscle reeducation (requires 150V), nerve stimulation (requires 150V), edema reduction, and pain control.

Electrical stimulation exerts its effect through several mechanisms of action that are categorized as either excitatory or non-excitatory. Excitatory effects include: 1) peripheral nerve stimulation for pain modulation (sensory, motor and pain fiber stimulation), and 2) peripheral circulation improvement (vasodilation and muscle pump function). Non-excitatory (cellular level) effects include: 1) protein synthesis, 2) mobilization of blood proteins, 3) bactericidal effects, 4) edema reduction via resorption of interstitial fluids. Goldman's five-year retrospective study reviewing the success of HVPC in ischemic lower extremity patients is promising, with 90% of HVPC-treated wounds healing in one year compared with 29% of the wounds that received only standard care. The improvement in periwound tissue transcutaneous oxygen pressure ($TcpO_2$) suggests improved reperfusion may play a role. Houghton used HVPC 3 times per week to treat patients with 42 chronic leg ulcers from a variety of etiologies (diabetic, arterial insufficiency, venous insufficiency), in a prospective, randomized fashion (151). Over a four-week treatment period, wounds of all etiologies decreased to approximately one half the initial wound size, healing twice as fast as the sham control.

Pneumatic Compression Therapy

Lower extremity compression therapy with a pneumatic pump is successful at healing ulcerations (diabetic, venous and arterial insufficiency). The addition of oxygen to lower extremity compression has not been compared to compression without oxygenation. Montori (157) completed a Mayo Clinic review of 107 patients with critical limb ischemia and non-healing wounds who received treatment with intermittent compression pumps after presenting to the Mayo Clinic (1998–2000). Of all the wounds, 64% were multi-factorial in etiology, and 60% had associated $TcpO_2$ levels below 20 mm Hg. With a mean of six months treatment, complete wound healing with limb preservation was achieved by 40% of patients even with baseline $TcpO_2$ levels below 20 mm Hg. Patients with osteomyelitis or active wound infection (48%); insulin-dependent diabetic patients (46%); and patients with previous amputation (28%) healed with non-oxygenated compression therapy of the lower extremity. For topical "hyperbaric" oxygen therapy, Edsberg reports a prospective controlled trial in eight (8) geriatric patients using topical "hyperbaric" oxygen versus topical oxygen and electrical stimulation in a long term care facility to treat stage III and IV pressure ulcers (155). Improved healing was noted in the decubitus ulcers, with healing times ranging from 8–49 weeks. The addition of electrical stimulation to topical oxygen in three of the eight patients presented did not improve outcome.

Anodyne (MIRE) Therapy

Monochromatic Infrared Energy (MIRE) therapy uses a low-energy (cold) laser generating light in the infrared spectrum. The light energy is generated by light emitting diodes embedded in pads, which are held on the treatment site by Velcro straps. Anodyne therapy is promoted for various chronic non-healing wound applications, for reversing peripheral diabetic neuropathy, and treating lymphedema. The mechanism for claims of increased circulation and decreased pain may be vasodilation, possibly by increasing release of nitric oxide. Anodyne is FDA approved only for relief of neuropathy but there is anecdotal evidence that it aids in wound healing. There are no known side effects. Leaving pads on longer than recommended can cause superficial burns.

ALTERNATIVE MEDICINE PRODUCTS DISCLAIMER

The Food and Drug Administration (FDA) does not evaluate the safety or efficacy of herbal preparations. Herbal preparations fall under the Dietary Supplement Health and Education Act of 1994 (Public Law 103-417). This act states that dietary supplements (including herbal preparations) may not make any claims as to the cure, mitigation, treatment, or prevention of diseases. They may make structure and functional claims such as "supports healthy bones and joints." Some herbal supplements that are used in the food or cosmetic industry are listed by the FDA as "Generally Recognized as Safe (GRAS)." Some of the alternative products mentioned in this section do not fall into this list. Any practitioner wishing to utilize alternative therapies for use in patient care should be aware of the various laws regarding their use, and the literature regarding the safety and efficacy of these preparations and be aware whether the manufacturer follows accepted Good Manufacturing Practice (GMP) and that their preparations are marked as Standardized Extracts or Guaranteed Extracts which shows that the product contains a stated amount of what is known or suspected to be the main active ingredient in the preparation.

Honey

Honey is produced by bees (Apis mellifera) from the nectar of several varieties of plants. Pharmacological activity can vary depending on the type of plant from which the nectar is obtained. Honey is thought to improve wound healing by promoting the formation of granulation tissue. It promotes the growth of epithelial cells by providing a barrier to moisture which helps keep the wound hydrated. Enzymes and hydrogen peroxide in honey can aid in debridement. Honey inhibits the growth of *Pseudomonas pyocyanea, Pseudomonas aeruginosa, Escherichia coli, Staphylococcus aureus, Proteus mirabilis,* coliform species,

Klebsiella species, *Streptococcus faecalis*, and *Streptococcus pyogenes*. Antibacterial peptides (apidaecins and abaecin) have been isolated in honeybees. The high osmolality, low pH, and hydrogen peroxide in honey also contribute to antimicrobial activity. High osmolality causes shrinkage of microbes, because of intracellular water loss. Hydrogen peroxide is formed by the action of glucose oxidase.

Honey provides more than just "carbohydrate filler" in the ECM. Honey is a source of simple carbohydrates, protein and vitamins. Its composition on average is 17.1% water, 82.4% total carbohydrate and 0.5% proteins, amino acids, vitamins and minerals. Fructose (38.5%) and glucose (31.0%) provide the main carbohydrate constituent with maltose, sucrose and other sugars comprising the remaining 12.9% of carbohydrate. The vitamins found in honey include niacin, riboflavin and pantothenic acid; minerals present include potassium, calcium, copper, iron, magnesium, manganese, phosphorus and zinc. The vitamin, mineral, antioxidant and amino acid content of a particular type of honey varies by floral source. Honeys derived from particular floral sources, "Tea Trees," in Australia and New Zealand (Leptospermum spp) exhibit enhanced antibacterial activity, and these honeys have been approved for marketing as therapeutic honeys (Medihoney and Active Manuka honey). Processing honey by pasteurization may influence the medicinal quality of the product.

Honey applied topically rapidly removes bacteria, including antibiotic-resistant strains, removes odor, has anti-inflammatory action, debrides the wound, creates a moist environment, promotes wound healing by stimulating tissue regeneration and preventing scarring and hypertrophy, reduces need for grafting, provides a protective barrier, and is not adherent. Both honey and sugar have high osmolarity and bind water, inhibiting bacterial growth. Honey's specific bactericidal activity derives from plant phytochemicals and bioflavonoids, and continuous low-grade secretion of hydrogen peroxide by the action of peroxidase on enzymes added by bees to the nectar they collect. Honey in the wound produces a nontoxic level approximately 1,000-times lower than that of rinse solutions. Honey's deodorizing effect in wound dressings is due to antibacterial activity against anaerobes that cause odor, such as *Clostridium* species, and gram-negative rods, such as *Pseudomonas* and *Proteus*.

In a recent study in India, Subrahmanyam made histological and clinical comparisons between 25 patients with fresh partial-thickness burns, group 1, dressed with honey and group 2, dressed with Sulfadiazine (SSD) (196). The honey treated group showed faster re-epithelialization (Honey: 84% day 7 and 100% day 21 vs. SSD: 12% day 7 and 80% day 21). Moreover, honey dressed wounds showed an earlier subsidence of acute inflammatory changes; whereas, the SSD dressed wounds showed a sustained inflammatory reaction even upon epithelialization. Commercial wound honey is available, sterilized by gamma irradiation, and is common for burn therapy in modern Western hospitals. The procedure includes applying approximately 25–35g of active honey to an absorbent pad, and then securing on the wound with a secondary dressing. Increase fluidity, if needed, by warming in lukewarm water. Do not use heat, which destroys the antibacterial ability. There are no adverse effects on wound healing. Tonks reported an investigative study to evaluate the ability of honey to influence the immunocompetent cells using human monocytes and a monocytic cell line (monomac-6) (197). The study evaluated Manuka, pasture, and jelly bush honey with cane sugar syrup (artificial honey) as the control. The levels of all three formulations of honey showed increased response of the tested factors (TNF-α, IL-1β, and IL-6) in response to exposure to the honey and sugar compound. Jelly bush honey produced the most significant elevations of these inflammatory cytokines, which are normally released from monocytes during the healing process.

Aloe

Aloe is a succulent plant (Aloe vera and Aloe barbadensis) with thick leaves. Aloe gel is the clear, jelly-like substance obtained from the thin-walled mucilaginous cells in the center of the leaf. The active constituents include emodin anthrone, dithranol, chrysarobin, and allantoin. The carboxypeptidase and salicylate components of aloe gel can inhibit bradykinin, a pain-producing agent. The magnesium lactate component can inhibit histamine, which may reduce itching. The C-glucosyl chromone component appears to reduce topical inflammation. Aloe gel might inhibit the synthesis of thromboxane A2, a potent vasoconstrictor. By inhibiting thromboxane A2, aloe gel is thought to increase microcirculation and prevent ischemia in wounds, which may speed the healing of burns and frostbite. In animal models, aloe seems to prevent the inhibition of wound contraction caused by silver sulfadiazine (SSD). SSD is often applied to wounds, especially burn wounds, to prevent infection. But SSD seems to slow wound healing by inhibiting contraction and epithelialization. Applying aloe in conjunction with SSD seems to improve the speed of wound healing compared to SSD alone. However, there is also evidence SSD improves the rate of wound healing better than aloe when each product is used alone. This suggests that there might be a synergistic effect when SSD and aloe are used together.

Aloe's effects may also be due to high concentration of amino acids, vitamin E, vitamin C, zinc, and essential fatty acids. If aloe juice is ingested, normal intestinal bacteria metabolize contents of aloe vera to form aglycones, which exert a powerful laxative effect. Purified aloe vera gel extract for wound healing (Carrington Dermal Wound Gel) is available. In a full-thickness burn animal study comparing aloe vera gel extract (Carrington)—group I; sulfadizine (Silvadene®)—group II, salicylic acid cream (aspirin)—group III, and plain gauze—group IV, Rodriguez found that the gel treated animals healed faster with wound bacterial counts being effectively decreased by both Silvadene® and aloe vera. There is one study (Schmidt & Greenspoon, 1991) (192) that shows that aloe vera gel may retard wound healing.

Chamomile

Chamomile is an aromatic perennial herb (Matricaria recutita) with feathery foliage and white and yellow flowers. The applicable part of German chamomile is the flowerhead. Active constituents of German chamomile include quercetin, apigenin, and coumarins, and the essential oils matricin, chamazulene, alpha bisaboloid, and bisaboloid oxides. German chamomile might have anti-inflammatory effects. Preliminary research suggests it can inhibit the enzymes cyclooxygenase and lipoxygenase, which reduces the production of prostaglandins and leukotrienes. Quercetin and apigenin can inhibit histamine release from mast cells that are antigen stimulated.

Topical chamomile has been historically used to speed wound healing. Combined with corticosteroids and antihistamines, chamomile is used for stasis ulcers from inadequate circulation in elderly bedridden patients, and wound healing after tattoo removal.

Calundula

Calundula is a Mediterranean annual herb (Calendula officinalis). Calendula flowers were historically used for wound healing, and controlling inflammation and infection. Calendula is approved in Germany for treating poorly healing wounds. The applicable part of calendula is the flower. Calendula is used for wound healing due to potential anti-inflammatory effects. The faradiol monoester is believed to play an important role in anti-inflammatory activity. Some evidence suggests the water-soluble flavonoids might be responsible for the wound-healing effects. Preliminary data suggests that calendula may inhibit human immunodeficiency virus (HIV) replication. Calendula also shows some evidence of antibacterial and anti-tumor activity. The procedure includes steeping one tablespoon (15 grams) of calendula flowers in hot water for 15 minutes and then applying as a compress for at least 15 minutes, several times a day, tapering as the wound improves.

Tea Tree Oil

Tea tree oil is obtained by the distillation of the leaves of the tea tree. Three different species of flowering trees known as Myrtaceae grown in Australia and New Zealand are known as 'Tea-trees.' The Australian Tea tree (Melaleuca alternifolia), and two New Zealand Tea trees, Manuka (Leptospermum scoparium) and Kanuka (Kunzea ericoides) produce essential oils that are used for medicinal purposes. The oil contains more than 100 monoterpenoid, sesquiterpenoid, and alcohol compounds. Up to 90% consists of terpinen-4-ol, 1,8-cineole, alpha-terpineol, terpinolene, and alpha- and gamma-terpinene. The primary constituent terpinen-4-ol is active against numerous pathogenic bacteria and fungi but seems to spare normal skin flora. The constituents, alpha-terpineol and linalool, may also contribute to its antimicrobial activity. Tea tree oil appears to disrupt the permeability barrier of microbial cell membrane structures, causing loss of chemiosmotic control.

Tea tree oil has been found to inhibit growth of the yeast *Candida albicans*. The oil has in vitro activity against *Enterococcus faecium* and *Enterococcus faecalis*, including vancomycin-resistant strains, *Klebsiella pneumoniae*, including gentamicin-resistant strains, and *Stenotrophomonas maltophilia*. Tea tree oil also has in vitro activity against both methicillin-sensitive *Staphylococcus aureus* and methicillin-resistant *Staphylococcus aureus* (MRSA). The oil seems to have limited activity against *Pseudomonas aeruginosa*. Oils produced with increased concentrations of terpinen-4-ol seem to have greater activity against these organisms.

Tea tree oil has also been found to inhibit in vitro growth of the yeast species *Malassezia*, commonly found on human skin. It is also active against *Propionibacterium acnes*, *Escherichia coli*, *Aspergillus flavus*, *Trichophyton mentagrophytes*, and *Trichophyton rubrum*. Tea tree oil also seems to have in vitro activity against herpes simplex virus.

Tea Tree Oil is obtained from crushed leaves applied directly to cuts and infected skin. Alternatively, tea tree oil concentrate (70–100%) is applied to small wound areas. Tea tree oil should not be use on burns. Ernest completed a four electronic data based review of tea tree oil (167). Four trials suggested tea tree oil might be effective in acne and fungal infections. The data was promising but not compelling. Further studies were suggested.

Trypsin

Trypsin is a proteolytic enzyme formed in the small intestines by the action of enteropeptidase on trypsinogen. Trypsin supplements are derived from fungi or bacterial sources, pancreas of livestock, or from plant sources. It is used to remove dead tissue that remains after trauma, infections such as decubitus ulcers, and surgical procedures. The removal of dead cells allows the growth of healthy tissues. Some topical preparations that are available contain balsam of Peru and castor oil to protect the skin and prevent premature epithelial destruction.

Gotu Kola

The applicable parts of Gotu kola are the above ground parts. The primary constituents responsible for the pharmacological effects are thought to be the saponin-containing triterpene acids, 1–8%; and their sugar esters, including asiatic acid, madecassic acid, asiaticoside A (madecassoside), and asiaticoside B. Gotu kola also contains essential oils; flavonoids; and flavone derivatives including quercetin and kaempferol, sesquiterpenes, stigmasterol, sitosterol, and isothankuniside.

The triterpenoid saponins (e.g., asiaticoside and madecassoside) seem to increase wound healing and decrease venous pressure in venous insufficiency. Asiaticoside and other terpenoids might have anti-inflammatory activity. The terpenoid extract seems to improve connective tissue remodeling by increasing fibroblast activity, stimulating collagen synthesis, increasing epithelial turnover over, and decreasing capillary permeability.

Gotu kola is thought to increase the production of Type I collagen in scar formation over type II. Type II collagen is associated with hypertrophic scarring. The terpenoid extract might help stabilize arterial plaques by increasing collagen within plaques. Plaques with low collagen content are structurally weak and are associated with an increased risk of rupture and embolism. There is also some evidence that asiaticosides may promote wound healing by stimulating collagen and glycosaminoglycan synthesis.

Other Herbs

Several other herbs have various cellular stimulating effects. Comfrey (Symphytum officinale) is so well known as a topical anti-inflammatory that it called "healing herb." Recent literature warns against the use of topical comfrey because it can be systemically absorbed. The major concern about comfrey is the hepatotoxic pyrrolizidine alkaloid (PA) content. These constituents are hepatotoxic, pneumotoxic, carcinogenic, and mutagenic. Witch hazel (Hamamelis virginiana) is used topically to decrease inflammation and stop bleeding. Horsetail (Equisetum arvense) has been recommended for use both internally and topically to decrease inflammation and promote wound healing. Horsetail contains thiaminase, an enzyme that can cause thiamine deficiency. Horsetail contains tiny amounts of nicotine and may cause nicotine allergy or theoretically, nicotine toxicity if taken in large quantities. Topical chaparrals (Larrea divaricata) compresses decrease inflammation and pain, and promote minor wound healing. The applicable part of chaparral is the leaf. Nordihydroguaiaretic acid (NDGA), a constituent of chaparral, may have antioxidant properties and also selectively inhibits lipoxygenases. It is also involved with platelet-derived growth factor receptors and the protein kinase C intracellular signally family, which suggests it might have anticancer activity. Both U.S. Food and Drug Administration and Health Canada have advised consumers against using products containing chaparral due to safety concerns. There are several reports of serious poisoning, acute hepatitis, kidney and liver damage, and irreversible renohepatic failure when taken orally.

SUMMARY

This chapter covers several of the many wound healing approaches. Many modalities exist, with more being developed and others long known are being reemployed. Some are simple, some highly engineered, and all to the same end of enhancing the body's own wound healing ability. Advanced and simple therapeutics will not live up to their effective potential without measures for good patient health and nutrition.

REFERENCES

Introduction

1. Babu M; Wells A. Dermal-epidermal communication in wound healing. *Wounds* 13(5):183-189, 2001.
2. Schultz GS, Sibbald RG, Falanga V, et al. Wound bed preparation: a systematic approach to wound management. *Wound Repair Regen* 2003 Mar; 11 Suppl 1:Sl-S38.
3. Winter GD, Formation of the scab and the rate of epithelialisation of superficial wounds in the skin of a young domestic pig. *Nature* 1962, 193:293-294.

Oxygen and Perfusion

4. Curci JA, Petrinec D, Liao S, et al. Pharmacologic suppression of experimental abdominal aortic aneurysms: a comparison of doxycycline and four chemically modified tetracyclines. *J Vasc Surg* 1998 Dec; 28(6):1082-93.
5. Davies MG, Hagen PO. Pathophysiology of vein graft failure: a review. *Eur J Vasc Endovasc Surg* 1995 Jan; 9(1):7-18.
6. Porter KE, Turner NA. Statins for the prevention of vein graft stenosis: a role for inhibition of matrix metalloproteinase-9. *Biochem Soc Trans* 2002 Apr; 30(2):120-6.

Nutrition

7. Cerwenka H, Bacher H, Werkgartner G, et al. Antioxidant treatment during liver resection for alleviation of ischemia-reperfusion injury. *Hepatogastroenterology* 1998 May-Jun; 45(21):777-82.
8. L-glutamine. *Altern Med Rev* 2001 Aug; 6(4):406-10 PMID: 11578256 [PubMed - indexed for MEDLINE].
9. Nagel E, Meyer zu Vilsendorf A, Bartels M, et al. Antioxidative vitamins in prevention of ischemia/reperfusion injury. *Int J Vitam Nutr Res* 1997; 67(5):298-306.
10. Nusgens BV, Humbert P, Rougier A, et al. Topically applied vitamin C enhances the mRNA level of collagens I and III, their processing enzymes and tissue inhibitor of matrix metalloproteinase 1 in the human dermis. *J Invest Dermatol* 2001 Jun; 116(6):8.
11. Rabl H, Khoschsorur G, Petek W. Antioxidative vitamin treatment: effect on lipid peroxidation and limb swelling after revascularization operations. *World J Surg* 1995 Sep-Oct; 19(5):738-44.
12. Rostan EF, DeBuys HV, Madey DL, et al. Evidence supporting zinc as an important antioxidant for skin. *Int J Dermatol* 2002 Sep; 41 (9) :606-ll.
13. Scolapio JS, McGreevy K, Tennyson GS, et al. Effect of glutamine in short-bowel syndrome. *Clin Nutr* 2001 Aug; 20(4):319-23.
14. Spungen AM, Koehler KM, Modeste-Duncan R, et al. 9 clinical cases of nonhealing pressure ulcers in patients with spinal cord injury treated with an anabolic agent: a therapeutic trial. *Adv Skin Wound Care* 2001 May-Jun; 14(3):139-44.
15. Szkudlarek J, Jeppesen PB, Mortensen PB. Effect of high dose growth hormone with glutamine and no change in diet on intestinal absorption in short bowel patients: a randomized, double blind, crossover, placebo controlled study. *Gut* 2000 Aug; 47(2):199-205.
16. Thomson AB, Keelan M, Thiesen A, et al. Small bowel review: Diseases of the small intestine. *Dig Dis Sci* 2001 Dec; 46(12):2555-2566.

Edema Reduction

17. Axisa B, Loftus IM, Naylor AR et al. Prospective, randomized, double-blind trial investigating the effect of doxycycline on matrix metalloproteinase expression within atherosclerotic carotid plaques. *Stroke* 2002 Dec; 33(12):2858-64.
18. Carr L, Philips Z, Posnett J. Comparative cost-effectiveness of four-layer bandaging in the treatment of venous leg ulceration. *J Wound Care* 1999 May; 8(5):243-8.
19. Ghatnekar O, Willis M, Persson U. Cost-effectiveness of treating deep diabetic foot ulcers with Promogran in four European countries. *J Wound Care* 2002 Feb; 11(2):70-4.

20. Gloviczki P, Bergan JJ, Rhodes JM, et al. Mid-term results of endoscopic perforator vein interruption for chronic venous insufficiency: lessons learned from the North American subfascial endoscopic perforator surgery registry. The North American Study Group. *J Vasc Surg* 1999 Mar;29(3):489-502.

21. Lippmann HI, Fishman LM, Farrar RH, et al. Edema control in the management of disabling chronic venous insufficiency. *Arch Phys Med Rehabil* 1994 Apr; 75(4):436-41.

22. Porter KE, Thompson MM, Loftus IM, et al. Production and inhibition of the gelatinolytic matrix metalloproteinases in a human model of vein graft stenosis. *Eur J Vasc Endovasc Surg* 1999 May; 17(5):404-12.

23. Porter KE, Loftus IM, Peterson M, et al. Marimastat inhibits neointimal thickening in a model of human vein graft stenosis. *Br J Surg* 1998 Oct; 85(10):1373-7.

24. Roach DM, Fitridge RA, Laws PE, et al. Up-regulation of MMP-2 and MMP-9 leads to degradation of type IV collagen during skeletal muscle reperfusion injury; protection by the MMP inhibitor, doxycycline. *Eur J Vasc Endovasc Surg* 2002 Mar; 23(3):360-9.

25. Sybrandy JE, van Gent WB, Pierik EG, et al. Endoscopic versus open subfascial division of incompetent perforating veins in the treatment of venous leg ulceration: long-term follow-up. *J Vasc Surg* 2001 May; 33(5):1028-32.

Debridement

26. Apelqvist J, Ragnarson-Tennvall G, Persson U, et al. Diabetic foot ulcers in a multidisciplinary setting. An economic analysis of primary healing and healing with amputation. *J Intern Med* 1994 May;235(5):463-71.

27. Armstrong DG, Lavery LA, Vazquez JR, et al. How and why to surgically debride neuropathic diabetic foot wounds. *J Am Podiatr Med Assoc* 2002 Jul-Aug; 92(7):402-4.

28. Attinger CE, Bulan EJ. Debridement. The key initial first step in wound healing. *Foot Ankle Clin* 2001 Dec; 6(4):627-60.

29. Bowler PG. Wound pathophysiology, infection and therapeutic options. *Ann Med* 2002; 34(6):419-27.

30. Center for Medicare and Medicaid Services. Coverage Issues Manual Section 60-25, Noncontact Normothermic Wound Therapy (NNWT). Baltimore, MD: CMS; 2002. Center for Medicare and Medicaid Services. Warm-Up Wound Therapy® a/k/a Noncontact Normothermic Wound Therapy Updated (02/13/02) (#CAG-00114N). Baltimore, MD:CMS; 2002. *http://www.hcfa.gov/coverage/8b3-hhh.htm* (accessed March 8, 2002).

31. Chambers L, Woodrow S, Brown AP, et al. Degradation of extracellular matrix components by defined proteinases from the green bottle larva Lucilia sericata used for the clinical debridement of non-healing wounds. *Br J Dermatol* 2003 Jan; 148(1):14-23.

32. Dow G, Browne A, Sibbald RG. Infection in chronic wounds: controversies in diagnosis and treatment. *Ostomy Wound Manage* 1999 Aug; 45(8):23-7, 29-40; quiz 41-2.

33. Ennis WJ, Formann P, Mozen N, et al. Ultrasound therapy for recalcitrant diabetic foot ulcers: results of a randomized, double-blind, controlled, multicenter study. *Ostomy/Wound Management* August 2005;51(8): 24 - 39

34. Khare M, Keady D. Antimicrobial therapy of methicillin resistant Staphylococcus aureus infection. *Expert Opin Pharmacother* 2003 Feb; 4(2):165-77.

35. Mayhall CG. The epidemiology of burn wound infections: then and now: *Clin Infect Dis* 2003 Aug 15; 37(4):543-50. Epub 2003 Jul 30.

36. McCarty Stanisic M, Provo BJ, Larson DL, et al. Wound debridement with 25kHz ultrasound. Advances in skin and wound care Nov/Dec 2005; 18 (9):484-490.

37. McGuckin M, Goldman R, Bolton L, et al. The clinical relevance of microbiology in acute and chronic wounds. *Adv Skin Wound Care* 2003 Jan-Feb; 16(1):12-23; quiz 24-5.

38. Milas M, Bush RL, Lin P, et al. Calciphylaxis and nonhealing wounds: the role of the vascular surgeon in a multidisciplinary treatment. *Vasc Surg* 2003 Mar; 37(3) :501-7.

39. Parks WC. Interstitial collagenase in the healing epidermis. In: Abatangelo S, Donati L, Van Scheidt W, editors. *Proteolysis in Wound Repair* Berlin: Springer, 1996: 21.

40. Piaggesi A, Schipani E, Campi F, et al. Conservative surgical approach versus non-surgical management for diabetic neuropathic foot ulcers: a randomized trial. *Diabet Med* 1998 May; 15(5):412-7.

41. Sherman RA. Maggot therapy for treating diabetic foot ulcers unresponsive to conventional therapy. *Diabetes Care* 2003 Feb;26(2):446-51.

42. Sherman RA. Maggot Debridement Therapy (MDT). http://biotherapy.md.huji.ac.il/maggot.debridement.htm

43. Thai TP, Houghton PE, Campbell KE, et al. Ultraviolet light C in the treatment of chronic wounds with MRSA: a case study. *Ostomy Wound Manage* 2002 Nov; 48(11):52-60.

44. Vetra H, Whittaker D. Hydrotherapy and topical collagenase for decubitus ulcers. *Geriatrics* 1975;30:53.

45. West BR, Nichter LS, Halpern DE, et al. Ultrasound debridement of trabeculated bone: effective and atraumatic. *Plast Reconstr Surg* 1994 Mar;93(3):561-6.

46. Young S. Ultrasound Therapy. In: Kitchen S, ed. *Electrotherapy: evidence-based practice* 11th ed. New York, NY. Churchill Livingstone; 2002:211-30.

Topical Antimicrobial Agents

47. Bianchi J. Iodoflex and Iodosorb in the treatment of venous leg ulcers. *Br J Nurs* 2001 Mar 8- 21; 10(5):342-6.

48. Flynn J. Povidone-iodine as a topical antiseptic for treating and preventing wound infection: a literature review. *Br J Community Nurs* 2003 Jun; 8 (6 Suppl):S 36-42.

49. Fumal I, Braham C, Paquet P, et al. The beneficial toxicity paradox of antimicrobials in leg ulcer healing impaired by a polymicrobial flora: a proof-of-concept study. *Dermatology* 2002; 204 Suppl 1:70-4.

50. Hawkins-Bradley B, Walden M. Treatment of a nonhealing wound with hypergranulation tissue and rolled edges. *J Wound Ostomy Continence Nurs* 2002 Nov; 29(6):3204.

51. Mertz PM, Oliveira-Gandia MF, Davis SC. The evaluation of a cadexomer iodine wound dressing on methicillin resistant Staphylococcus aureus (MRSA) in acute wounds. *Dermatol Surg* 1999 Feb; 25(2):89-93.

52. Zhou LH, Nahm WK, Badiavas E, et al. Slow release iodine preparation and wound healing: in vitro effects consistent with lack of in vivo toxicity in human chronic wounds. *Br J Dermatol* 2002 Mar; 146 (3):365-74.

53. Paddock HN, Schultz GS, Perrin KJ, et al. Clinical assessment of silver-coated antimicrobial dressings on MMPs and cytokine levels in non-healing wounds. Annual meeting presentation, *Wound Healing Society* Baltimore, MD, May 28-June 1, 2002.

Thermoregulation Therapy

54. Ahmad SI. Control of skin infections by a combined action of ultraviolet A (from sun or UVA lamp) and hydrogen peroxide (HUVA therapy), with special emphasis on leprosy. *Med Hypotheses* 2001 Oct; 57(4):484-6.

55. Hambidge A. Reviewing efficacy of alternative water treatment techniques. *Health Estate* 2001 Jun; 55 (6) :23-5.

56. Kloth LC, Berman JE, Nett M et al. A randomized controlled clinical trial to evaluate the effects of noncontact normothermic wound therapy on chronic full thickness pressure ulcers. *Adv Skin Wound Care* 2002 Nov-Dec; 15 (6):270-6.

57. Nussbaum EL, Biemann I, Mustard B. Comparison of ultrasound/ultraviolet-C and laser for treatment of pressure ulcers in patients with spinal cord injury. *Phys Ther* 1994 Sep; 74(9):812-23; discussion 824-5.

58. Svenoe T, Falk ES, Henriksen K. Irradiances and health risks associated with the use of UV lamps and sunbeds. *Rev Eur Sci Med Farmacol* 1995 Mar-Jun; l7 (2-3):53-62.

Tissue-Related Modalities

59. U.S. Department of Health and Human Services. Guidance for FDA Reviewers and Industry Medical Devices Containing Materials Derived from Animal Sources (Except for In Vitro Diagnostic Devices) U.S. Department of Health and Human Services, Food and Drug Administration Center for Devices and Radiological Health CDRH BSE Working Group Document Issued on: 11/6/98. CDRH Facts on Demand at 1-800- 899-0381 or 301-827-0111, specify number 2206 when prompted for the document shelf number.

60. Hunt TK, Hopf H, Hussain Z. Physiology of wound healing. *Adv Skin Wound Care* 2000 May- Jun; 13 (2 Suppl):6-11.

61. Micheels P. Human anti-hyaluronic acid antibodies: is it possible? *Dermatol Surg* 2001 Feb; 27(2):185-91.

Hyaluronic Acid Products

62. Abatangelo G. Marelli M. Healing of hyaluronic acid-enriched wounds: histological observations. *J Surg Res* 1983 Nov; 35(5):410-6.

63. Chen WYJ, Abatangelo G. Functions of hyaluronan in wound repair. *Wound Rep Reg* 7(2) 79- 89, 1999-review.

64. Edmonds M, Bates M, Doxford M, et al. New treatments in ulcer healing and wound infection *Diabetes Metab Res Rev* 2000 Sep-Oct; 16 Suppl 1:S51-4.

65. Gandolfi SA, Massari A, Orsoni JG. Low-molecular-weight sodium hyaluronate in the treatment of bacterial corneal ulcers. *Graefes Arch Clin Exp Ophthalmol* 1992; 230(1):20-3.

66. Galosso U. Use of hyaluronic acid in the therapy of varicose ulcers of the lower limbs. *Minerva Chir* 1978 Nov 15; 33(21):1581-96. (Italian)

67. Iocono JA. Repeated additions of hyaluronan alters granulation tissue deposition in sponge implants in mice. *Wound Rep Reg* 1998 Sept-Oct; 6(5):442-8.

68. Longaker MT, Chiu ES. Studies in fetal wound healing. V. A prolonged presence of hyaluronic acid characterizes fetal wound fluid. *Ann Surg*, 1991Apr; 213 (4) :293-6.

69. Maguen E, Nesburn AB, Macy JI. Combined use of sodium hyaluronate and tissue adhesive in penetrating keratoplasty of corneal perforations. *Ophthalmic Surg* 1984 Jan; 15 (1):55-7.

70. Marshall KW. Intra-articular hyaluronan therapy. *Foot Ankle Clin* 2003 Jun; 8(2):221-32.

71. Strachan RK, Smith P, Gardner DL. Hyaluronate in rheumatology and orthopaedics: is there a role? *Ann Rheum Dis* 1990 Nov; 49(11):949-52. Review.

72. Tonello C, Zavan B, Cortivo R, et al. In vitro reconstruction of human dermal equivalent enriched with endothelial cells. *Biomaterials* 2003 Mar; 24(7):1205-11.

73. Vazquez JR, Short B, Findlow AH, et al. Outcomes of hyaluronan therapy in diabetic foot wounds. *Diabetes Res Clin Pract* 2003 Feb; 59(2):123-7.

Collagen Products

74. Abatangelo G, Brun P, Cortivo R. Collagen metabolism and wound contraction. In: Altmeyer P, Hoffmann K, el Gammal S, et al. editors. *Wound healing and skin physiology* Berlin: Springer, 1995: 71.

75. Diegelmann RF. Collagen metabolism. *Wounds* 2001; 13(5):177-182.

76. Doillon CJ, Silver FH. Collagen-based wound dressing: effects of hyaluronic acid and fibronectin on wound healing. *Biomaterials* 1986 Jan; 7(1):3-8.

77. Jeffrey JJ. Collagen degradation. In: Cohen IK, Diegelmann RF, Lindblad WJ, editors. Wound healing: biochemical and clinical aspects. Philadelphia: WB Saunders, 1992.

78. Leibovich SJ. Mesenchymal cell proliferation in wound repair: the role of macrophages. In: Hunt TK, Heppenstall BR, Pines E, RoveeD, editors. Soft and hard tissue repair. Biological and clinical aspects. Westport, CT: Praeger Publishers, 1984: 329.

79. Pachence JM. Collagen-based devices for soft tissue repair. *J Biomed Mater Res* 1996 Spring; 33 (1):35-40.

80. Patino MG, Neiders ME, Andreana S, et al. Collagen as an implantable material in medicine and dentistry. *J Oral Implantol* 2003; 28(5):220-5

81. Postlethwaite AE, Kang AH. Collagen- and collagen peptide-induced chemotaxis of human blood monocytes. *J Exp Med* 1976; 143: 1299-307.

82. Postlethwaite AE, Seyer JM, Kang AH. Chemotactic attraction of human fibroblasts to type I, II, and III collagens and collagen- derived peptides. *Proc Natl Acad Sci* USA 1978; 75: 871.

Fibroblast and Keratinocytes

83. Badiavas EV, Paquette D, Carson P, et al. Human chronic wounds treated with bioengineered skin: histologic evidence of host-graft interactions. *J Am Acad Dermatol* 2002 Apr; 46 (4):524-30.

84. Sabolinski ML, Alvarez O, Auletta M, et al. Cultured skin as a 'smart material' for healing wounds: experience in venous ulcers. *Biomaterials* 1996 Feb; 17(3):311-20.

Apligraf

85. Brem H, Young J, Yomic-Canic M, et al. Equivalent (HSE) in treatment of diabetic foot ulcers. clinical efficacy and mechanism of bilayered living human skin. *Surg Technol Int* 2003 Jun; 11:23-31.

86. Eaglstein WH, Alvarez OM, Auletta M, et al. Acute excisional wounds treated with a tissue-engineered skin (Apligraf). *Dermatol Surg* 1999 Mar; 25 (3):195-201.

87. Fivenson DP, Scherschun L, Chourair M, et al. Graftskin therapy in epidermolysis bullosa. *J Am Acad Dermatol* 2003 Jun; 48(6):886-92.

88. Falanga VJ. Tissue engineering in wound repair. *Adv Skin Wound Care* 2000 May-Jun; 13(2 Suppl): 15-9.

89. Gohari S, Gambla C, Healey M, et al. Evaluation of tissue-engineered skin (human skin substitute) and secondary intention healing in the treatment of full thickness wounds after Mohs micrographic or excisional surgery. *Dermatol Surg* 2002 Dec; 28(12):1107-14; discussion 1114.

90. Ozerdem OR, Wolfe SA, Marshall D. Use of skin substitutes in pediatric patients. *J Craniofac Surg* 2003 Jul; 14(4):517-20.

91. Sibbald RG, Torrance GW, Walker V, et al. Cost-effectiveness of Apligraf in the treatment of venous leg ulcers. *Ostomy Wound Manage* 2001 Aug; 47(8):36-46.

92. Shen JT, Falanga V. Innovative therapies in wound healing. *J Cutan Med Surg* 2003; 7(1):217-24.

93. Waymack P, Duff RG, Sabolinski M. The effect of a tissue engineered bilayered living skin analog, over meshed split-thickness autografts on the healing of excised burn wounds. The Apligraf Burn Study Group. *Burns* 2000 Nov; 26(7):609-19.

Dermagraft

94. Allenet B, Paree F, Lebrun T, et al. Cost-effectiveness modeling of Dermagraft for the treatment of diabetic foot ulcers in the French context. *Diabetes Metab* 2000 Apr; 26(2):125-32.

95. Browne AC, Vearncombe M, Sibbald RG. High bacterial load in asymptomatic diabetic patients with neurotrophic ulcers retards wound healing after application of Dermagraft. *Ostomy Wound Manage* 2001 Oct; 47(10):44-9.

96. Economou TP, Rosenquist MD, Lewis RW 2nd, et al. An experimental study to determine the effects of Dermagraft on skin graft viability in the presence of bacterial wound contamination. *J Burn Care Rehabil* 1995 Jan-Feb; 16(1):27-30.

97. Gentzkow GD, Iwasaki SD, Hershon KS, et al. Use of Dermagraft, a cultured human dermis, to treat diabetic foot ulcers. *Diabetes Care* 1996 Apr; 19 (4):350-4.

98. Newton DJ, Khan F, Belch JJ, et al. Blood flow changes in diabetic foot ulcers treated with dermal replacement therapy. *J Foot Ankle Surg* 2002 Jul-Aug; 41 (4):233-7.

99. Marston WA, Hanft J, Norwood P, et al. The efficacy and safety of Dermagraft in improving the healing of chronic diabetic foot ulcers: Results of a prospective randomized trial. *Diabetes Care* 2003 Jun; 26(6):1701-5,

100. Perdue GF, Hunt JL, Still JM Jr, et al. A multicenter clinical trial of a biosynthetic skin replacement, Dermagraft-TC, compared with cryopreserved human cadaver skin for temporary coverage of excised burn wounds. *J Burn Care Rehabil* 1997 Jan-Feb; 18(1 Pt 1):52-7.

101. Sacks MS, Chuong CJ, Petroll WM, et al. Collagen fiber architecture of a cultured dermal tissue. *J Biomech Eng* 1997 Feb; 119(1):124-7.

Cultured Keratinocytes

102. Boyce ST, Warden GD Principles and practices for treatment of cutaneous wounds with cultured skin substitutes. *Am J Surg* 2002 Apr; 183(4):445-56.

103. Schaefer BM, Wallich R, Schmolke K, et al. Immunohistochemical and molecular characterization of cultured keratinocytes after dispasemediated detachment from the growth substratum. *Exp Dermatol* 2000 Feb; 9(1):58-64.

104. Lariviere B, Rouleau M, Picard S, et al. Human plasma fibronectin potentiates the mitogenic activity of platelet-derived growth factor and complements its wound healing effects. *Wound Repair Regen* 2003 Jan-Feb; 11 (1):79-89.

105. Solomon DE, An in vitro examination of an extracellular matrix scaffold for use in wound healing. *Int J Exp Pathol* 2002 Oct; 83(5):209-16.

Growth Factors

106. De Ugarte DA, Roberts RL, Lerdluedeeporn P, et al. Growth factor medications. *Pediatr Surg Int* 2002 Sep; 18(5-6):517-20. Epub 2002 Jun 15.

107. Dube PH, Revell PA, Chaplin DD, et al. A role for IL-1 alpha in inducing pathologic inflammation during bacterial infection. *Proc Natl Acad Sci U S A* 2001 Sep 11; 98(19):10880-5. Epub 2001 Aug 28.

108. Edmonds M, Bates M, Doxford M, et al. New treatments in ulcer healing and wound infection. *Diabetes Metab Res Rev* 2000 Sep-Oct; 16 Suppl l:S3l4.

109. Stull DM. Colony-stimulating factors: beyond the effects on hematopoiesis. *Am J Health Syst Pharm* 2002 Apr 1; 59(7 Suppl2):S12-20.

110. Whalen CR, Watson TL, Baize T, et al. Formulary management of colony-stimulating factors. *Am J Health Syst Pharm* 2002 Apr 1; 59(7 Suppl2):S21-7.

Growth Factor Medications

111. Ghatnekar O, Persson U, Willis M, et al. Cost effectiveness of Becaplermin in the treatment of diabetic foot ulcers in four European countries. *Pharmacoeconomics* 2001; 19(7):767-78.

112. Glover JL, Weingarten MS, Buchbinder DS, et al. A 4year outcome-based retrospective study of wound healing and limb salvage in patients with chronic wounds. *Adv Wound Care* 1997; 10: 33- 38.

113. Kantor J, Margolis DJ. Treatment options for diabetic neuropathic foot ulcers: a cost-effectiveness analysis. *Dermatol Surg* 2001 Apr; 27(4):347-51.

114. Margolis DJ, Kantor J, Santana J, et al. Effectiveness of platelet releasate for the treatment of diabetic neuropathic foot ulcers. *Diabetes Care* 2001; 24: 483-488.

115. Richard S, Schuster MW. Stem cell transplantation and hematopoietic growth factors. *Curr Hematol Rep* 2002 Nov; 1 (2) :l03-9.

116. Saba AA, Freedman BM, Gaffield JW, et al. Topical platelet-derived growth factor enhances wound closure in the absence of wound contraction: an experimental and clinical study. *Ann Plast Surg* 2002 Jul; 49 (1) :62-6; discussion 66.

117. Stacey MC, Mata SD, Trengove NJ, et al. Randomized double-blind placebo controlled trial of topical autologous platelet lysate in venous ulcer healing. *Eur J Vasc Endovasc Surg* 2000; 20: 296-301.

114. Wagner S, Coerper S, Fricke J, et al. Comparison of inflammatory and systemic sources of growth factors in acute and chronic human wounds. *Wound Repair Regen* 2003 Jul-Aug;11 (4):253-60.

Chemical Stimulators (Growth Promoters)

119. Albala DM. Fibrin sealants in clinical practice. *Cardiovasc Surg* 2003 Aug; 11 (4 Pt 2) :5-11.

120. Babbush CA, Kevy SV, Jacobson MS. An in vitro and in vivo evaluation of autologous platelet concentrate in oral reconstruction. *Implant Dent* 2003; 12 (1):24-34.

121. Boisnic S, Branchet -Gumila MC, Nizri D, et al. Histochemical and biochemical modifications induced by experimental irradiation of human skin maintained in survival conditions and modulation by application of an emulsion containing trolamine. *Int J Tissue React* 2003; 25(1):9-18.

122. Chandra RK, Conley DB, Kern RC. The effect of FloSeal on mucosal healing after endoscopic sinus surgery: a comparison with thrombin-soaked gelatin foam. *Am J Rhinol* 2003 Jan- Feb; 17(1):51-5.

123. Constant JS, Feng JJ, Zabel DD, et al. Lactate elicits vascular endothelial growth factor from macrophages: a possible alternative to hypoxia. *Wound Repair Regen* 2000 Sep-Oct; 8(5) :353-60

124. Chernomorsky SA, Segelman AB. Biological activities of chlorophyll derivatives. *N J Med* 1988 Aug; 85 (8) 669-73.

125. Coulomb B, Friteau L, Dubertret L. Biafine applied on human epidermal wounds is chemotactic for macrophages and increases the IL-l/IL-6 ratio. *Skin Pharmacol* 1997; 10(5-6):281-7.

126. Egner PA, Wang JB, Zhu YR, et al. Chlorophyllin intervention reduces aflatoxin-DNA adducts in individuals at high risk for liver cancer. *Proc Natl Acad Sci USA* 2001 Dec 4; 98(25):14601-6. Epub 2001 Nov

127. el-Nakeeb MA, Yousef RT. Antimicrobial activity of sodium copper chlorophyllin. *Pharmazie* 1974 Jan;29 (l):48-50.

128. Gear AR, Camerini D. Platelet chemokines and chemokine receptors: linking hemostasis, inflammation, and host defense. *Microcirculation* 2003 Jun; 10(3-4):335-50.

129. Hojo M, Inokuchi S, Kidokoro M, et al. Induction of vascular endothelial growth factor by fibrin as a dermal substrate for cultured skin substitute. *Plast Reconstr Surg* 2003 Apr 15;111(5) :1638-45.

130. Kamat JP, Boloor KK, Devasagayam TP. Chlorophyllin as an effective antioxidant against membrane damage in vitro and ex vivo. *Biochim Biophys Acta* 2000 Sep 27; 1487(2-3):113-27

131. Larato DC, Pfau FR. Effects of a water-soluble chlorophyllin ointment on gingival inflammation. *N Y State Dent J* 1970 May; 36(5):291-3.

132. Unemori EN, Lewis M, Constant J, et al. Relaxin induces vascular endothelial growth factor expression and angiogenesis selectively at wound sites. *Wound Repair Regen* 2000 Sep- Oct; 8(5) :361-70

Mechanical (Physical Modalities)

133. Hess CL, Howard MA, Attinger CE. A review of mechanical adjuncts in wound healing: hydrotherapy, ultrasound, negative pressure therapy, hyperbaric oxygen, and electrostimulation. *Ann Plast Surg* 2003 Aug; 51 (2):210-8.

Negative Pressure Wound Therapy (NPWT)

134. Clare MP, Fitzgibbons TC, McMullen ST, et al. Experience with the vacuum assisted closure negative pressure technique in the treatment of non-healing diabetic and dysvascular wounds. *Foot Ankle Int* 2002 Oct; 23(10):896-901.

135. Cro C, George KJ, Donnelly J, et al. Vacuum assisted closure system in the management of enterocutaneous fistulae. *Postgrad Med J* 2002 Jun; 78(920):364-5.

136. Evans D, Land L. Topical negative pressure for treating chronic wounds: a systematic review. *Br J Plast Surg* 2001 Apr; 54(3):238-42.

137. Fabian TS, Kaufman HJ, Lett ED, et al. The evaluation of subatmospheric pressure and hyperbaric oxygen in ischemic full-thickness wound healing. *Am Surg* 2000 Dec; 66(12):1136-43.

138. Fisher A, Brady B. Vacuum assisted wound closure therapy. *Issues Emerg Health Technol* 2003 Mar; (44): 1-6.

139. Fleck TM, Fleck M, Moidl R, et al. The vacuum-assisted closure system for the treatment of deep sternal wound infections after cardiac surgery. *Ann Thorac Surg* 2002 Nov; 74(5):1596-600; discussion 1600.

140. Gustafsson R, Johnsson P, Algotsson L, et al. Vacuum-assisted closure therapy guided by C-reactive protein level in patients with deep sternal wound infection. *J Thorac Cardiovasc Surg* 2002 May; 123 (5):895-900.

141. Isago T, Nozaki M, Kikuchi Y, et al. Negative-pressure dressings in the treatment of pressure ulcers *J Dermatol* 2003 Apr; 30(4):299-305.

142. Philbeck TE Jr, Whittington KT, Millsap MH, et al. The clinical and cost effectiveness of externally applied negative pressure wound therapy in the treatment of wounds in home healthcare Medicare patients. *Ostomy Wound Manage* 1999 Nov; 45(11):41-50.

143. Prokuski L. Negative pressure dressings for open fracture wounds. *Iowa Orthop J* 2002; 22:20-4.

144. Markley MA, Mantor PC, Letton RW, et al. Pediatric vacuum packing wound closure for damage-control laparotomy. *Pediatr Surg* 2002 Mar; 37(3):512-4.

145. Scherer LA, Shiver S, Chang M, et al. The vacuum assisted closure device: a method of securing skin grafts and improving graft survival. *Arch Surg* 2002 Aug; 137 (8):930-3; discussion 933-4.

146. Yuan-Innes MJ, Temple CL, Lacey MS. Vacuum-assisted wound closure: a new approach to spinal wounds with exposed hardware. *Spine* 2001 Feb 1; 26(3):E30-3.

Electrical Stimulation Therapy

147. Agency for Health Care Policy and Research (AHCPR). AHCPR Treatment Guidelines for Pressure Ulcers. U.S. Government Printing Office 1994. Treatment of Pressure Ulcers Clinical Guideline Number 15 AHCPR Publication No. 95-0652: December 1994. A printable copy of this resource is available free of charge online at: *http://hstat.nlm.nih.gov/hq/Hquest/db/local.ahcpr.clin.putc/screen/TocDisplay/s/61076/action/Toc.*

148. Centers for Medicare and Medicaid Services (CMS). Decision concerning reimbursement for electrical stimulation therapy for wound care. *http://www.aptasce.com/news/cms_decision_regarding_electrica.htm.*

149. Sussman C. Electrical stimulation for wound healing. In: Wound Care: A Collaborative Practice Manual for Physical Therapists and Nurses, Edited by C Sussman, and B Bates Jensen. Gaithersburg, MD: Aspen Publications, 1997. Excerpt may be found online at: http://woundcare.org/newsvol1n3/ar10.htm.

150. Goldman R, Brewley B, Zhou L, et al. Electrotherapy reverses inframalleolar ischemia: a retrospective, observational study. *Adv Skin Wound Care* 2003 Mar-Apr; 16(2):79-89.

151. Houghton PE, Kincaid CB, Lovell M, et al. Effect of electrical stimulation on chronic leg ulcer size and appearance. *Phys Ther* 2003 Jan; 83(1):17-28.

152. Sussman C. The role of physical therapy in wound care. In: Chronic Wound Care: A Source book for Health Care Professionals. Krasner D. Wayne, PA: Health Management Publications, 1990.

153. Gogia PP. Clinical Wound Management, In: Wound Healing: Alternatives in Management, LC Kloth, JM McCulloch, *JA Feedar* 2nd Ed. Thorofare, NJ: Slack, Inc; 1994

Other Chronic Wound Therapies

154. Burghart K. The topical hyperbaric oxygen therapy debate. *Ostomy Wound Manage* 2003 Apr; 49 (4) :8; author reply 8.

155. Edsberg LE, Brogan MS, Jaynes CD, et al. Topical hyperbaric oxygen and electrical stimulation: exploring potential synergy. *Ostomy Wound Manage* 2002 Nov; 48(11):42-50.

156. Goodson W, Hohn D, Hunt TK, et al. Augmentation of some aspects of wound healing by a "skin respiratory factor." *J Surg Res* 1976 Aug; 21 (2):125-9.

157. Montori VM, Kavros SJ, Walsh EE, et al. Intermittent compression pump for nonhealing wounds in patients with limb ischemia, The Mayo Clinic experience (1998-2000). *Int Angiol* 2002 Dec; 21 (4) :360-6.

158. Sen CK, Khanna S, Gordillo G, et al. Oxygen, oxidants, and antioxidants in wound healing: an emerging paradigm. *Ann NY Acad Sci* 2002 May; 957:239-49.

Alternative Medicines

159. Allen P. Tea tree oil: the science behind the antimicrobial hype. *Lancet* 2001; 358:1245.

160. Belcaro GV, Rulo A, Grimaldi R. Capillary filtration and ankle edema in patients with venous hypertension treated with TTFCA. *Angiology* 1990; 41:12-8.

161. Brinkhaus B, Lindner M, Schuppan D, et al. Chemical, pharmacological and clinical profile of the east Asian medical plant Centella asiatica. *Phytomedicine* 2000;7:427-48.

162. Carson CF, Cookson BD, Farrelly HD, et al. Susceptibility of methicillin-resistant Staphylococcus aureus to the essential oil of Melaleuca alternifolia. *J Antimicrob Chemother* 1995; 35:421-4.

163. Chan CH, Loudon KW. Activity of tea tree oil on methicillin-resistant Staphylococcus aureus (MRSA). *J Hosp Infect* 1998; 39:244-5.

164. Cox SD, Mann CM, Markham JL, et al. The mode of antimicrobial action of the essential oil of Melaleuca alternifolia (tea tree oil). *J Appl Microbiol* 2000; 88:170-5.

165. Dutta T, Basu UP. Crude extract of Centella asiatica and products derived from its glycosides as oral antifertility agents. *Indian J Exp Biol* 1968;6:181-2.

166. Efem SE. Clinical observations on the wound healing properties of honey. *Br J Surg* 1988; 75:679-81.

167. Ernst E, Huntley A. Tea tree oil: a systematic review of randomized clinical trials. *Forsch Komplementarmed Klass Naturheilkd* 2000 Feb; 7(1):17-20.

168. Foster S, Tyler VE. *Tyler's Honest Herbal* 4th ed., Binghamton, NY: Haworth Herbal Press, 1999.

169. Food and Drug Administration. FDA Advises Dietary Supplement Manufacturers to Remove Comfrey Products From the Market. July 6, 2001. *http://www.cfsan.fda.gov/~dms/dspltr06.html*

170. Hammer KA, Carson CF, Riley TV. Susceptibility of transient and commensal skin flora to the essential oil of Melaleuca alternifolia (tea tree oil). *Am J Infect Control* 1996; 24:186-9.

171. Hormann HP, Korting HC. Evidence for the efficacy and safety of topical herbal drugs in dermatology: part I: anti-inflammatory agents. *Phytomedicine* 1994;1:161-71

172. Hutter JA, Salman M, Stavinoha WB, et al. Antiinflammatory C-glucosyl chromone from Aloe barbadensis. *J Nat Prod* 1996; 59:541-3.

173. Incandela L, Belcaro G, Nicolaides AN, et al. Modification of the echogenicity of femoral plaques after treatment with total triterpenic fraction of Centella asiatica: a prospective, randomized, placebo-controlled trial. *Angiology* 2001; 52 Suppl 2:S69-73.

174. Incandela L, Belcaro G, De Sanctis MT, et al. Total triterpenic fraction of Centella asiatica in the treatment of venous hypertension: a clinical, prospective, randomized trial using a combined microcirculatory model. *Angiology* 2001; 52 Suppl 2:S61-7.

175. Incandela L, Cesarone MR, Cacchio M, et al. Total triterpenic fraction of Centella asiatica in chronic venous insufficiency and in high-perfusion microangiopathy. *Angiology* 2001; 52 Suppl 2:S9-13.

176. Kalvatchev Z, Walder R, Garzaro D. Anti-HIV activity of extracts from Calendula officinalis flowers. *Biomed Pharmacother* 1997;51:176-80.

177. Kaufman T, Kalderon N, Ullmann Y, et al. Aloe vera gel hindered wound healing of experimental second-degree burns: a quantitative controlled study. *J Burn Care Rehabil* 1988;9:156-9.

178. Klein AD, Penneys NS. Aloe vera. *J Am Acad Dermatol* 1988; 18:714-20.

179. Lis-Balchin M, Hart SL, Deans SG. Pharmacological and antimicrobial studies on different tea-tree oils (Melaleuca alternifolia, Leptospermum scoparium or Manuka and Kunzea ericoides or Kanuka), originating in Australia and New Zealand. *Phytother Res* 2000 Dec; 14(8):623-9.

180. Lusby PE, Coombes A, Wilkinson JM Honey: a potent agent for wound healing? *J Wound Ostomy Continence Nurs* 2002 Nov; 29 (6):295-300.

181. Maquart FX, Chastang F, Simeon A, et al. Triterpenes from Centella asiatica stimulate extracellular matrix accumulation in rat experimental wounds. *Eur J Dermatol* 1999;9:289-96.

182. May J, Chan CH, King A, et al. Time-kill studies of tea tree oils on clinical isolates. *J Antimicrob Chemother* 2000; 45:639-43.

183. Miller MB, Koltai PJ. Treatment of experimental frostbite with pentoxifylline and aloe vera cream. *Arch Otolaryngol Head Neck Surg* 1995;121:678-80.

184. Morykwas MJ, Mark MW. Effects of Ultraviolet Light on Fibroblast Fibronectin Production and Lattice Contraction. *Wounds* 1998 10(4):111-117.

185. Newall CA, Anderson LA, Philpson JD. *Herbal Medicine: A Guide for Healthcare Professionals* London, UK: The Pharmaceutical Press, 1996.

186. Oliva B, Piccirilli E, Ceddia T, et al. Antimycotic activity of Melaleuca alternifolia essential oil and its major components. *Lett Appl Microbiol* 2003; 37(2):185-7.

187. Pointel JP, Boccalon H, Cloarec M, et al. Titrated extract of Centella asiatica (TECA) in the treatment of venous insufficiency of the lower limbs. *Angiol* 1987; 38:46-50.

188. Postmes T, van den Bogaard AE, Hazen M. Honey for wounds, ulcers, and skin graft preservation. *Lancet* 1993;341:756-7.

189. Reynolds T, Dweck AC. Aloe vera leaf gel: a review update. *J Ethnopharmacol* 1999;68:3-37.

190. Robbers JE, Speedie MK, Tyler VE. *Pharmacognosy and Pharmacobiotechnology* Baltimore, MD: Williams & Wilkins, 1996.

191. Rodriguez-Bigas M, Cruz NI, Suarez A. Comparative evaluation of aloe vera in the management of burn wounds in guinea pigs. *Plast Reconstr Surg* 1988 Mar; 81 (3):386-9.

192. Schmidt JM, Greenspoon JS. Aloe vera dermal wound gel is associated with a delay in wound healing. *Obstet Gynecol* 1991;78:115-7.

193. Sheikh NM, Philen RM, Love LA. Chaparral-associated hepatotoxicity. *Arch Intern Med* 1997; 157:913-9.

194. Shukla A, Rasik AM, Jain GK, et al. In vitro and in vivo wound healing activity of asiaticoside isolated from Centella asiatica. *J Ethnopharmacol* 1999;65:1-11.

195. Stickel F, Seitz HK. The efficacy and safety of comfrey. *Public Health Nutr* 2000; 3:501-8.

196. Subrahmanyam M. A prospective randomised clinical and histological study of superficial burn wound healing with honey and silver Sulfadiazine. *Burns* 1998 Mar; 24(2):157-61.

197. Tonks AJ, Cooper RA, Jones KP, et al. Honey stimulates inflammatory cytokine production from monocytes, *Cytokine* 2003 Mar 7; 21 (5):242-7.

198. Widgerow AD, Chait LA, Stals R, et al. New innovations in scar management. *Aesthetic Plast Surg* 2000;24:227-34.

Hyperbaric Oxygen Therapy

199. Fife C.E. Hyperbaric oxygen therapy applications in wound care. In: Wound Care Practice, Sheffield PJ, Fife C.E, Smith APS (eds) Flagstaff, AZ: Best Publishing 2004; 661-684.

200. Feldmeier JJ. Hyperbaric Oxygen 2003. Kingston, MD: UHMS, 2003

REVIEW QUESTIONS

1.) The supplemental metal required by most by enzyme systems with regard to wound healing is
   a. Copper
   b. Zinc
   c. Iron
   d. Silver

2.) The most highly effective therapy in control of venous edema of the lower extremities is
   a. hydrocolloid dressings
   b. bioengineered grafts
   c. compression therapy
   d. diuretics

3.) With regard to enzymatic debridement agents, which of the following statements are/is true
   a. Heavy metals (Zn Cu, Ag) decrease enzymatic activity in the wound
   b. Copper and chloroplyllin assist in granulation tissue development
   c. collagenase is not as effective as papain/urea against fibrinous eschar so scoring or excision of the eschar is necessary
   d. all of the above

4.) Matrix metalloproteinases
   a. are important in the degradation of bacteria, necrotic tissue, and old extracellular matrix
   b. may be harmful to growing tissue and growth factors if produced in excess
   c. may be reduced in chronic wounds by judicious use of certain bio-active dressings
   d. all of the above

5). The only growth factor currently available commercially for use in non-healing wounds is
   a. VEGF
   b. PDGF
   c. KGF
   d. none of the above

Answers: 1b, 2c, 3d, 4d, 5b.

NOTES

Section 5
Communication and Trust

CHAPTER 40

Comforting the Patient

CHAPTER FORTY OVERVIEW

NOTES

COMFORTING THE PATIENT

Lena L. Soto, Kimberly M. Sheffield

"I have found it of enormous value when I can permit myself to understand another person." Carl R. Rogers

INTRODUCTION

In accomplishing successful wound care the healthcare providers' most important partner is the patient. Establishing communication, trust and mutual respect can ensure a successful partnership. With information from the field of Behavioral Health, this chapter offers a guide for medical staff that can implement skills for comforting patients who have difficult wounds.

UNDERSTANDING THE PATIENT

Trauma and Grief

Trauma. In addition to the wound, our patient could have experienced any of a number of traumatic events that influence their response to treatment.

- Being notified of the sudden or untimely death of a close friend or relative (and perhaps being a survivor of this same event)
- Being diagnosed with a life-threatening illness
- Surviving a natural disaster
- Being in a serious accident
- Recalling physical or emotional abuse in childhood or in adult relationships. This abuse may cause difficulty in dealing with reality or, if in the past, could affect how the patient deals with this new experience
- Being a victim of crime
- Seeing the effects of violence in their home or neighborhood
- Experiencing a significant financial loss
- Seeing the end to a career, secondary to institutional collapse or health changes affecting the patient or a family member
- Loosing the home and all personal belongings to a fire or flood
- Fighting a perpetual battle with an illness requiring dependence on others
- Experiencing loss of a body part or its function, or the need for a lifestyle change

At some time in our lives, it is inevitable that we will experience trauma. The patient could have recently experienced a traumatic event, or could have had past trauma that might impact behavior. Judith Herman, MD (1) explains the impact of trauma:

> "Traumatic events are extraordinary, not because they occur rarely, but rather because they overwhelm the ordinary adaptations to life. Unlike commonplace misfortunes, traumatic events generally involve threats to life or bodily integrity, or a close personal encounter with violence or death. They confront human beings with the extremities of helplessness and terror, and evoke the responses of catastrophe. The common denominator of trauma is a feeling of intense fear, helplessness, loss of control, and threat of annihilation."

The wound center treats patients who have difficult, problem wounds. Some have already been counseled by their primary physician that a major surgical procedure or amputation of a limb might be necessary if their wound care is unsuccessful. This adds anxiety to an already traumatic experience. To improve the healing potential in these patients, many wound centers offer hyperbaric oxygen (HBO2) as adjunctive therapy in patients with hypoxic wounds.

Case 1

Charlie (a pseudonym) had undergone rectal cancer treatment over five years ago and was given a clean bill of health. Yearly he had received a colonoscopy exam and all was well until this time. Charlie and his wife, Marge, were told he had developed radionecrosis. Both knew this was a possibility but neither thought it would happen, especially with each passing year. Dejected, Charlie and Marge decided to attack this setback head on. His physician had prescribed hyperbaric oxygen therapy as an adjunct to his wound care.

Arriving at the scheduled appointment time, Charlie was apprehensive and not sure if he could complete the proposed hyperbaric oxygen treatments. Marge stood by his side through the interview and exam. Both learned this treatment would require extensive commitment on their part as they would have to be there five days a week for about three hours each weekday morning for 40 to 60 treatments. Then Charlie heard the worst news: he would be confined inside a large chamber for two of those hours and, worse yet, he would have to wear an oxygen hood on his head for thirty-minute intervals. As an alternative, he was also offered treatment in the monoplace chamber but that, to him, would be even worse. During the hyperbaric unit tour, Charlie was reminded of a past military experience that had resulted in his profound claustrophobia, and found that he could barely look inside. However, he said he would give it a try.

The next morning, Marge drove Charlie to the wound treatment center. His anxiety increased exponentially as he changed into his cotton scrubs and checked in. The rectal bleeding had made him quite weak so he decided a wheelchair might be better than a regular chair. (He couldn't bring himself to walk into the chamber, even though the other five patients seemed to be just fine with what was about to happen.) Two staff members placed a neck ring on him and wheeled him into the chamber. He began to fidget and he felt his pulse increasing as he waited for the others to take their places. As soon as he heard the door close, Charlie had to get out. Staying was beyond his level of tolerance. The inside observer had Charlie removed from the chamber and the treatment proceeded without him. The hyperbaric physician told Charlie he could try again tomorrow. Thinking he could do this on his own, Charlie refused the Ativan offered to him. Marge offered her support and took him home.

There were several days with similar outcomes. Sometimes Charlie could remain for half or more of the treatment before he needed to get out of the chamber. There were other days when his bleeding and rectal pain were more than he could tolerate, even sitting reclined in a wheelchair, and Charlie would stay home. Some days were plagued with diarrhea. During this time, Charlie's rectal follow-ups showed improvement, though slow, and the pain was not completely gone. After completing 56 treatments, with Marge by his side every day, he was finally finished. With congratulations from the other patients and the staff, Charlie left with a healed wound.

Reaction to trauma is as unique as the individual being treated. Table 1 contains some common reactions to trauma. Whether internal or external, wounds are a type of trauma. The patient's reaction depends on some of the following.

- Developmental stage: A five year-old child will be very different in the wound care process than a thirty year old patient.

TABLE 1. COMMON REACTIONS TO TRAUMA

Physical Reactions	Mental Reactions	Emotional Reactions	Behavioral Reactions
Nervous energy, jitters, anxious	Changes in the way you think about yourself	Fear, inability to feel safe	Becoming withdrawn or isolated from others
Upset stomach, diarrhea	Changes in the way you think about the world	Sadness, grief, depression	Easily startled
Rapid heart rate	Changes in the way you think about other people	Guilt	Avoiding places or situations
Dizziness	Hyper vigilance	Anger, irritability	Becoming confrontational and aggressive
Lack of energy fatigue	Less aware, dissociation	Numbness, lack of feelings	Change in eating habits
Teeth grinding	Difficulty concentrating	Inability to enjoy anything	Loss or gain in weight
Skin blanches or pales	Poor attention or memory problems	Loss of trust	Restlessness
Muscle tension, rigidity	Difficulty making decisions	Loss of self esteem	Increase or decrease in sexual activity
Increased respiration rate and depth	Intrusive images	Feeling helpless	Decreased attention span
Mentrual flow shifts	Nightmares	Emotional distance from others	Decreased ability to follow directions
Decreased appetite	Constantly seeks reassurance	Intense or extreme feelings	Over focus on work as way of avoidance
Increased perspiration, clammy skin	Avoids focusing on feelings	Feeling chronically empty	Describes fears as helplessness
Tetany or paralysis, probably most severe reaction	Persistent worry	Blunted, then extreme feelings	Shifts topic of conversation often

- Personal history: Typically a person is more profoundly affected by his or her first life-changing event than by subsequent experiences.
- Social, economic, and cultural perspectives: What might the patient believe about the wound and the subsequent treatment process?

Awareness of a patient's traumatic experiences is useful in developing a treatment approach that will comfort the patient.

Case 2

Carmel (a pseudonym) was approximately 50 years of age when she suffered from a chronic non-healing ulcer on the dorsum of her foot. Following a failed graft, her physician prescribed hyperbaric oxygen (HBO2) therapy as an adjunct to her wound care in an attempt to correct the underlying hypoxia and prepare the wound bed for another graft. Her surgeon had told her that she was not a candidate for revascularization and that this treatment would be her best hope for preventing amputation of the foot. Carmel was thoroughly briefed by the nurses. On her informed consent, she indicated that she understood the risks and benefits of HBO2 for her wound.

When Carmel underwent her first treatment in the hyperbaric chamber she was very upset. She arrived at the wound center in silence. She started crying when the HBO2 treatment began and sobbed intermittently during the entire time she was inside the chamber. Nothing could stop the sobbing. She did not speak, but would nod in response to a question. She did not want to be made more comfortable. She did not want refreshments. She did not want to leave the chamber. The attending doctor decided to continue the treatment with close observation. The staff had provided hyperbaric chamber treatments to hundreds of patients in varying degrees of illness and had never encountered anything like this. On completion of the treatment, Carmel was asked if she could share what was making her so sad. She shook her head "no" and started crying again. The staff took pride in lifting the spirits of patients in their care but, with this patient, they thought they had failed and would not see her again.

The next day Carmel returned for her second treatment. She thanked the staff for their kindness and explained that she was the only member of her family to survive the Holocaust during WWII. The rest of her family had died after being forced into the gas chambers, but she was spared. The term "chamber" had revived an image of the horror she had mentally suppressed for many years. Knowing her sensitivity to the word, the staff was careful to avoid making any reference to the "chamber" in her presence. She finished the course of HBO2 therapy, was successfully grafted, and her foot was saved.

If only we could plan our trauma to occur at a more convenient time:

"...If only I could have had this accident before my wedding."

"...If only I had exercised in a daily regimen like my doctor told me."

"...If only I hadn't cancelled my medical insurance or could have afforded a policy."

"...If only I had taken better care of my diabetes (or other disease process)."

"...If only I could do it over again!"

Patients are on a social clock during which life events should occur in a logical sequence. They have jobs waiting for them to return, children or grandchildren needing rides to school, and pets waiting to be fed. Going for daily wound care for weeks on end places a huge burden on their time and impedes their commitment to family needs. Serious non-healing wounds can completely change a lifestyle. These changes are on a continuum from "...he may walk with a slight limp" to "...he won't ever again be able to walk without an assistive device." In partnership with traumatic events, comes grief.

Grief

According to Elizabeth Kubler-Ross (2), "Grief is the normal, intense, emotional state associated with the loss of someone (or something) with whom (or which) one has had a deep emotional bond. Loss refers to many kinds of deprivation." Dr Kubler-Ross notes many kinds of deprivation to remind us that we not only deal with the psychological affects of death, but grief is also experienced following divorce, bankruptcy, loss of a career, loss of a limb, or loss of a life style. She identifies five common stages in the grieving process beginning with denial.

- Denial
- Anger
- Bargaining
- Depression
- Acceptance

In most wound care situations, time is not going to "stand still" while the patient moves through the stages of grieving to finally accept impaired function or the loss of a limb. The wound requires prompt attention for healing, but the wound care is likely to have a very different schedule than the patient's emotional healing. When a patient is still in denial regarding his diagnosis of diabetes and he is bargaining about medication, diet, and lifestyle changes, he might become depressed when his condition advances to the need for chronic wound care or amputation. A loss of any part of the body constitutes a significant loss, and it might take considerable time before the patient is willing to accept the loss.

To simply acknowledge and be aware of the conundrum that our patient is experiencing is the first step in developing trust and comforting the patient.

Diversity Stressors

In addition to medical and emotional stressors, healthcare providers daily encounter the issue of diversity: Gender, race, age, language, and varied views and ways of thinking. It might be helpful to establish a relationship with a local university and other community experts to help with meeting the diversity needs of children, senior citizens, language and literacy, faith, spirituality, and other socio-economic issues.

Age

Eric Erikson's Theory of Psychosocial Development (3) has eight distinct stages, each with two possible outcomes. The stages are:

- Trust versus mistrust
- Autonomy versus shame and doubt

- Initiative versus guilt
- Industry versus inferiority
- Identity versus role confusion
- Intimacy versus isolation
- Generativity versus stagnation
- Dignity versus despair

According to the theory, successful completion of each stage results in a healthy personality and successful interactions with others. Failure results in a more unhealthy personality and sense of self.

Children

In his chapter, "Wound Care in Pediatric Patients," Dr. Melvin D. Smith, a pediatric surgeon, reminds us that the child is not "just a little adult" (4). Age, size, associated injuries, and other pre-existing concerns correlate to a child's developmental stage. In addition, the child probably has a far more limited perspective of the entire wound care process and medical treatment because, in general, he has had fewer life experiences. In a personal communication, Dr. Smith offered these suggestions on how to comfort pediatric patients.

> "The following maneuvers/steps have been used by me for the past 35 years of operation/caring for patients in the pediatric age group, ranging from 6 months to 16 years of age:
> - *Establish initially a non-physical contact in a soft, non-threatening voice.*
> - *Discuss topics of interest to the patient, directly with the patient, disregarding the presence of the parent; acknowledge the parent, put him/her secondary.*
> - *Discuss play topics, school topics, favorite toy objects, etc.*
> - *Establish physical contact in a non-threatening manner; first shake hands with the parent, then shake hands with the patient; touch non-wounded areas of the body, clothing, etc; "listen" to the heart and lungs of the parent, then let the patient "listen" to the parent. Finally, listen to the heart and lungs of the patient.*
> - *Lastly, look at/ examine / treat the presenting wound."* (4)

To develop trust or to comfort pediatric patients, it is important to approach their treatment at a developmental level that helps them to better understand what is happening to them. A child's coping ability is directly related to his past medical care, if any, and to his past growth and developmental experiences. The child is in a tremendously vulnerable state and our attempts at comforting him/ her (or lack thereof) could be either a positive learning experience or destroy any trust for future health/medical experiences. A child's health care needs will affect him perceptually, cognitively, socially, and emotionally.

The child is also completely vulnerable to the caregiver, the caregiver's perspective of the wound, and the subsequent care the wound will require. The wound care "partnership," has now grown from just patient and medical professionals, to include caregivers (often parents) who are devoted to alleviating their child's affliction.

Case 3

Eric (a pseudonym) is an eleven year old male who was born with spina bifida with the defect extending from mid thorax (T-7) to sacrum. He has been wheelchair bound all his life. Over time, he developed progressive kyphoscoliosis which resulted in a worsening of the ability to carry out his routine daily care with ease. To improve on this, he underwent correction of the kyphoscoliosis in the form of a procedure via a posterior spinal fusion with bone grafts and metal instrumentation. Twelve days postoperatively seropurulent drainage was expressible from the incision. The wound was opened and debrided by the primary surgeon, followed by referral to the wound care service for ongoing care. In consultation with the primary surgeon, it was determined that Eric might be a candidate for negative pressure wound therapy (Wound VAC, KCI, San Antonio, TX).

At the first meeting in our department, all who were involved were "perfect strangers," so the patient, at 11 years old, was apprehensive. The doctor spent a lot of time talking to Eric about what he was doing in school, how he got around in his wheelchair, whether he did "wheelies" with his chair, and what he did to pass the time away when he was not in school. Then, the doctor "examined" his mother and father first and let him listen to their heart beats and let the parents listen to their own heart beats. This is not a hurried-up process, as one can imagine. The doctor talked about what might be seen in the wound before looking at it. They looked at the Wound VAC system and let everyone "touch" it before any attempt at application, and finally, the doctor showed him that he had nothing in his hand that should inflict a lot of pain. Even children with spinal bifida, can/will have spotty sensations which, in fact, can sometimes be increased sensations, but still with total lack of muscle control. In this manner the patient, and his parents, were put at ease so that the assessment could be completed and the Wound VAC therapy could be initiated. Eric tolerated the treatment well. Details and photos of the course of Eric's wound care are at Figures 24-30 at the chapter by ME Smith entitled "Wound Care in Pediatric Patients."

Where children are treated in the wound care service, there should be practice guidelines appropriate for children. Within a hospital setting, the Child Life Program is still relatively new as a mental health service for children. The Association for the Care of Children's Health (ACCH) is growing with the support of the National Child Life Council, Inc (NCLC). The NCLC consists of over 500 programs in hospitals throughout the United States, as well as Canada, Israel, Japan, Romania, and the United Kingdom. These programs help children and their families through the hospital experience by providing family-centered care, developmental support, play opportunities, preparation for procedures, procedural support, advocacy, and other related services.

Frequently, a serious wound can limit a child's mobility or other developmental skills to the point that he/she will require intervention to regain or "catch up" in the affected developmental areas. If a Child Life Program is not already available at the hospital, it might be possible to contact a local university or child development specialist to consult and provide supportive therapy.

Seniors

The final two stages of Erickson's Psychosocial Development refer to middle and late adulthood. Generativity is focused on assisting the younger generation in developing and leading useful lives, whereas stagnation is the feeling of having done nothing to help the next generation. The final stage refers to dignity versus despair. Seniors need a feeling of dignity during their wound care regardless of the situation.

In their chapter, "Wound Healing in the Geriatric Patient," Mouton and Parker (5) outline the unique and complex challenges for wounds in our elderly population. Consulting with specialists in aging/geriatrics will be very useful for comforting senior patients. The elderly frequently have very complex responsibilities and many years of life experience that will affect their response to treatment.

There is a high incidence of wound care needed in the elderly population. The intake interview with the patient (as they begin their treatment) should be comprehensive, to include exploring issues such as how they are presently taking their meals, how they plan to come to their appointments, and who might assist them with dressing changes at home. It is not unusual for elderly patients to rely on public transportation that runs on a strict "drop off" and "pick-up" schedule. If such a patient is late finishing with his appointment, he could quite possibly not have a way home or must wait for hours for the next pick-up, missing a nutritional meal, which subsequently impedes wound healing. Many patients are uncomfortable or embarrassed to let us know that they need to eat, or that they cannot afford the lotion needed for their fragile skin.

Case 4

"Lilly," in her 70's, was in the process of preparing for a hysterectomy. She was living an independent and active life. The only hospitalizations she had experienced were for the birth her three daughters. The most recent hospitalization was about thirty years ago. Lilly commented about all of the admission paperwork and the potential risks that surgery posed. After the surgery, upon opening her eyes, Lilly said quite seriously, "Oh, thank God! I'm still alive!" Her comment expresses the differences in our histories and experiences. She had no previous experience with the statements on the Informed Consent Form that she had to sign that indicated she might not survive the surgery. For those who have worked in a hospital or have recently received medical procedures, such paperwork is standard and sundry. Sometimes it is difficult to understand why a patient is so concerned. "Lilly's" trust level was limited to her minimal medical treatment history. Those who still find meaning in life may have a strong desire to receive the treatment, but may also need more reassurance.

Case 5

TS, an elderly client who had been very healthy until recently, came to the clinic for wound care and adjunctive HBO2 treatment. The admission packet issued at the front sign-in desk included information about patient wishes about Do Not Resuscitate (DNR) status. She did not appear to be anxious about the questions that were asked of her; however, when she saw the hyperbaric chamber, she became visibly anxious and stated that she changed her mind about the treatment. When asked what was the matter, she was hesitant to say. After much questioning she was finally asked if she was frightened of the chamber. She asked if many people had died in there. She had not been to the hospital in quite some time and did not realize that it is now standard practice to ask patients their wishes about DNR status. Since she had been asked about DNR status, she was under the impression that it was common for people to have episodes in the chamber which caused their death. After she was reassured that being in the chamber would not increase her risk of dying, she relaxed and agreed to go ahead with the plan of care.

Language and Literacy

Exploring the patient's learning style, first language, communication, and coping abilities will likely comfort him or her and facilitate wound healing.

- Learning style – Patients must be informed about their wound and "best practices" for wound healing, and this information should be offered in a variety of media. Suggestions include using videos, written instruction/ information, and return demonstration. Include any social support during the learning process, such as a family member who may be available to help with the wound care process.
- First-language – Each community has a unique mix of culture and language. In San Antonio, Texas, the population is approximately 60% Hispanic and 40% Anglo. The patient might speak English, but might be more comfortable speaking Spanish if that is the language of origin. When instructions are presented only in English, a patient might nod that he or she understands, when, in fact, he does not fully understand. Awareness of a patient's heritage (even if we have to ask) and subsequent planning that supports cultural needs will help the patient become a partner in wound healing.
- Communication abilities – Providing written educational materials and instructions to someone who cannot read is like pushing someone into a pool who cannot swim! We should respectfully explore this with our patient, even though he or she may not readily admit it. Audio visual aids can help reinforce written and verbal instructions.
- Coping skills –The patient should be asked what has helped him make it through stressful or life-changing events in the past. Patients who have difficulty dealing with their stressful situation will become frustrated. If healthcare providers cannot alleviate the patient's frustration in coping, they will fail to comfort the patient.

Teaching patients a way to manage their stress reactions and providing them information about resources, comforts them and helps them to cope with their wound care.

It is important that patient education materials and information are delivered in their first language, if possible, and in a media that best meets the patient's literacy needs. Utilizing university students and volunteers to develop, edit, review, and translate materials is a possible way to develop trust and cultural sensitivity. Students and volunteers are sometimes available from language departments, business management, and public relations studies.

Developing a small library (something as simple as a few shelves in the waiting room) with materials that are informative regarding wound care can assist in educating patients about their condition. This may include a video that periodically plays quietly in an area of the waiting room.

Typically, patients who need translation into a language that is unusual for the region will be accompanied by a family member or friend. If they are unaccompanied, it might be fruitful to seek a volunteer translator through neighborhood associations, churches, or schools.

Faith

Faith can be a system of religious belief, or it might be confidence or trust in a person or thing. Patients often accept reports of their medical status based on a confidence or faith in the doctor's honesty in reporting and the laboratory studies that confirm the truth.

The staff must utilize their communication skills and observations when considering what a patient might need in this area. The intake process can respectfully inquire of a patient's needs with questions like:

- "...Is there anything you would like your healthcare providers to know about your faith or denomination that will be helpful in treating your wound?"
- "...Is there anything else you would like for us to know while treating you that will make you more comfortable?"

Healthcare providers treat the wounds, but are also aware that the patients are not simply the sum of their wounds. Each person is made up of life experiences and developmental events. Being aware will go a long way in assisting the patient and developing trust.

In the Spiro et al. book, Empathy and the Practice of Medicine, Dr Joanne Lynn (6) wrote a chapter entitled "Travels in the valley of the shadow" in which she presented a case study on faith and religion.

Case 6

Miss Kauwalski (a pseudonym) was a fifty-six-year old disabled single woman who had extensive local spread of breast cancer with erosive and fungating lesions from chin to groin. The patient required palliative care with twice daily wound dressing changes that were very painful to her. The patient refused any pain medication and would not tell the nurses why. After about two weeks in the wound care setting, the doctor sat alongside her bed and said, "Doing this to you twice a day is so hard for us. Is there anything you could tell me that would make it easier to understand?" The patient replied: "What would we think of Christ on the cross if he had been given your medicines?" She was identifying her suffering with Christ's, and within her religious faith her suffering during life would have value after her passing. Dr Lynn pointed out that within the patient's tradition and understanding, her choice was the only one that made sense. Her beliefs surpassed her painful wound treatment and her death would be with dignity and on her own terms. Once she shared her religious beliefs about suffering with the nurses, they were able to endure with her and to honor her commitment.

[Modified from Lynn J. Travels in the valley of the shadow. In Spiro HM, McCrea MG, Peschel E, et al. (eds): Empathy and the Practice of Medicine:

Beyond Pills and the Scalpel. Prepared under the auspices of The Program for Humanities in Medicine, Yale University School of Medicine 1993] (6).

Spirituality

The central defining characteristic of spirituality is a sense of connection to a much greater being which includes an emotional experience of religious awe and reverence. Moody and Arcangel (7) explain spirituality.

> "Spirituality is our birthright – we come to earth as spiritual beings. Spirituality is remembering that something greater than self exists. Those who are spiritually enlightened conduct their lives with compassion, reverence, conscientiousness, serenity, and joy. They trust that the world is evolving, as it should; thus, they feel at peace with the world, others, and self. Life, death, and mourning, for them, take place at a different level..."

Faith and spirituality for most patients are already established, and they are very uncomfortable when they get the impression that a healthcare provider might be trying to impose his or her faith or spirituality upon them.

Culture

Culture is unique to communities, and includes customary beliefs, social forms, and material traits of a racial, religious, or social group. A unique culture can exist in something as small as a four-member family, or can be as large as an entire branch of the military.

We might receive a patient who has had very little experience or belief in traditional, "Western" medicine, but is now in need of our wound care expertise. It helps to explore with the patient his personal approach to past health care. If his culture calls for home treatment of his burn with various substances such as raw eggs, gentian violet, cassava, engine oil, or kerosene, that might explain why his wound is failing to heal (8).

Humanistic Needs

Once we have established what our patient's past experiences have been, the next consideration in comforting the patient is to determine what he or she will need to enable us to guide them toward healing.

In 1954, Abraham Maslow (9) formulated his theory of personality based upon a hierarchy of humanistic needs. His theory holds that individuals seek fulfillment of desires ranging from the simplest to the most complex needs. He laid out five broad layers of needs in the following order:

- *The physiological needs for basic survival:* air, water, food, shelter, and sex. These basic needs (oxygen, water, protein, salt, sugar, calcium, minerals and vitamins) are all essential for wound healing.
- *The need for safety and security:* safe circumstances, stability, protection, structure, order, and some limits. Vulnerable patients include children, senior citizens, those who find themselves in abusive situations, and those who are disabled. If the patient does not have a secure place to live, he is unlikely to be concerned about keeping his wound sanitarily dressed. Rosenbloom and Williams (10) explain:

  > "... If you believe that nothing you do would insure your safety, you would be unlikely to take steps to protect yourself.

On the other hand, if you believe that you can increase your level of safety and minimize the risk of harm, you are likely to take the necessary steps to do so."

- *The need for love and belonging:* friends, a sweetheart, children, affectionate relationships in general, even a sense of community. Belongingness and love, or intimacy makes us think of emotional warmth, closeness, caring, and support from and with other people. Looked at negatively, some long-term care patients become increasing susceptible to loneliness and social anxieties. Factitious wounds occur when patients intentionally wound themselves in an effort to maintain a social relationship with their healthcare providers.
- *The need for esteem:* One level is the need for the respect of others, the need for status, fame, glory, recognition, attention, reputation, appreciation, dignity, and even dominance. A second level is the need for self-respect, including such feelings as confidence, competence, achievement, mastery, independence, and freedom. The negative version of this need is low self-esteem and inferiority complexes, which is believed to be the root of many psychological problems that warrant special counseling. Depression is known to negatively affect wound healing.
- *The need to actualize the self:* Self-actualization is achieved by reaching one's own greatest potential, becoming the best person one can be, and achieving one's personal life goals. Those who are truly self-actualizing must have the lower needs called "deficit needs" met, at least to a considerable extent. This makes sense. If a person is hungry, he scrambles for food. If he is unsafe, he has to be continuously on guard. If he is isolated and unloved, he has to satisfy that need. If he has low self-esteem, he has to be defensive or compensate. When lower needs are unmet, he can't fully devote himself to fulfilling his potentials, including his potential to heal.

Maslow's hierarchy of needs laid the foundation for the five basic psychological needs outlined by the Traumatic Stress Institute/Center for Adult & Adolescent Psychotherapy in South Windsor, Connecticut: Safety, Trust, Control, Esteem, and Intimacy. Wound specialists can address these needs during the treatment process, and be of great comfort to the patient.

Case 7

J. B. was a gentleman in his late 30's. He had been fully informed of the treatment plan and presented for treatment, but refused to let anyone actually perform wound care. When he was taken to the treatment room, he said he wasn't ready. The nurse said, "That's OK," and sat down next to him. They started talking about where he was from and some other general information. When he was asked where he worked, he got a funny look on his face and said "Promise you won't hold it against me?" The nurse told him, "You can tell me anything. I'm a nurse and we are supposed to be impartial." Then he said that he worked as a claim agent for a health maintenance organization (HMO) that was well known for denying medical reimbursement. Jokingly, she told him there was a special torture room for people like him who work for that dreaded company. They both had a good laugh after which he relaxed and was amenable to treatment.

COMMUNICATION AND TRUST

Effective Communication

Communication skills are essential for successful wound care in partnership with the patient.

Sometimes the patient's needs cannot be met and it is important to acknowledge this fact. However, before giving up, possible options should be explored with the patient. We must have respect for their control and ability to decide what is best for them. We must be prepared to provide referrals to other resources if the patient or practice decides it is best to go elsewhere. The referral process should offer choices of at least three options if that many are available. Referrals should be up-to-date and the patient should be assisted in making the transition.

If a patient is referred elsewhere, he/she deserves a fresh start. The medical staff should be cautious in sharing information with the receiver that is not useful or negative. Both the patient and the receiver deserve an opportunity to develop their own relationship.

For those patients who need ancillary services, a strict protocol should be developed to ensure that the patient gets the services he/ she needs for a positive outcome. There should be a follow-up process inquiring on the success of the referral and how the patient is doing.

Patients should be given the opportunity to directly or anonymously evaluate the care that they received. Evaluations can be offered in written and call form (by neutral callers). Evaluations are only useful if the practice has a way of disseminating the information gained and then improving what has been identified as a problem.

Attending and Interviewing

Skillful interviewers use three basic skills to understand the needs of the interviewee: listening, questioning, and empathy.

Listening

On the most basic level, when in doubt, listen! The patient might be telling us something that will aid in his or her wound care. Helpful hints for listening:

- Maintain eye contact. It is an effective way to communicate that we have a genuine interest in what the patient is saying. Continually glancing away gives the appearance of disinterest. Staring at the patient in an attempt to maintain good eye contact can appear unfriendly, scornful, and aloof.
- Present attentive body language. Patients know we are interested if we face them squarely, lean slightly forward, have an expressive face, and use facilitative, encouraging gestures.
- Pay attention to vocal qualities. The vocal tone and speech rate indicate clearly how we feel about another person. There are many

ways that we can say, "I am really interested in what you have to say" just by altering the vocal tone and speech rate.
- Focus on verbal tracking. The patient has come to us with a topic of concern; whenever possible we should keep with the topic indicated by the patient.

There are several benefits of skilled listening. As we listen, we become aware of how well the patient is listening to us. Since patients from different cultures listen differently, we can modify our attending skills to develop rapport. When we get lost or confused in the consult, we can return to listening. Finally, when the patient moves to a topic that is destructive or nonproductive, we can redirect the conversation.

Questioning

Questioning opens the communication and directs the consult to where we need it to go. In response to our questions, the patient will most likely talk within our frame of reference. There are two types of questions: Open questions and closed questions.

Open questions

One cannot answer an open question with "yes" or "no," so the burden of the consult remains with the patient. Usually, an open question begins with what, how, why, or could.
- "Sam, tell me **what** brings you here today?"
- "**Could** you tell me the different things you have tried so far?"
- "I'm wondering **why** you are experiencing more pain today. Any ideas?"
- "**How** will you know when you are feeling better?"

Closed questions

Closed questions are easily answered with "yes", "no", or a very short sentence, so the burden of the consult will remain with the interviewer. Usually, a closed question leads with is, are, or do.
- "**Do** you have an appointment today, Sam?"
- "**Are** you using the ointment we prescribed for you?"
- "**Is** the pain worse today?"

There are several extra benefits of skilled questioning. It will help gain needed specifics about the patient's world. Open questioning helps the patient explore his own feelings and thoughts about his unique situation. Open questions are especially helpful with pediatric patients, or any patient who is unfamiliar with the medical process.

Developing Respect and Trust

Respect

Respect is an attitude of acknowledging the feelings and interests of another. A respectful attitude rules out unconsidered selfish behavior. Respect for the patient requires consideration, honesty, and tact. A helpful way to address respect issues is to ask oneself:
- "What if this were me? How would I wish to be cared for?"
- "What if this were my Mom? How would I want her to be treated?"

Respect offers dignity to the patient. Taking a hard look at how accessible the restrooms and necessary personal care items are, and making sure the patient never has to ask more than once. Respect also includes protecting the dignity of the patient with proper covering and physical comfort. Respect offers the "least restrictive environment" for the patient by considering ways the patient can have the most control. This is especially important to a patient who has been traumatized. One of the most comforting things for patients is the feeling of respect and trust that they have for the doctor and staff. If members of the wound care staff show respect for each other, it will be observed by patients and will foster trust.

Trust

Trust in our co-workers is the basis of a strong relationship and sets the stage for the patient to trust us. From the minute the patient walks in the door of the practice, he / she begins to develop a sense of trust or mistrust. Trust and safety go together, and mean something different to each individual. Once it is violated, trust can rarely be regained.

Avoid gossip. If the staff members are gossiping and talking about each other, patients can assume that they, too, are being discussed and gossiped about.

Be reliable. Patients need to see that our practice is doing what we say and saying what we mean. If we tell a patient that we are going to go get him a blanket to make him more comfortable, we should do it quickly. If we state to a patient that we are going to have special information for her when she comes to the next appointment, we should make sure that we do it. Reliability can secure trust.

Adhere to strict confidentiality and privacy standards. It doesn't make sense to have a client sign a "Patient's Bill of Rights" promising to protect personal information, only to proceed through intake gathering private information in an open area where others can hear. The patient's blood pressure, blood glucose values, or other health concerns should not be discussed in an open forum where other patients can hear the information.

Empathy

Among the many authorities regarding empathy and its related dimensions or qualities is Dr Carl R. Rogers, the "father" of the "Person Centered" approach (11), who described the related dimensions of empathy.

- Congruence or Genuineness. "Congruence," is derived from the Latin "congruere", meaning to meet together or to agree. It is sometimes called genuineness. Discrepancies and mixed messages are the opposites of congruence. To avoid sending mixed messages, it is important for our body language, facial expression, and tone of voice to be congruent. It is difficult for a patient to trust and feel safe if they do not sense congruence or genuineness.
- Unconditional Positive Regard. This is the most basic aspect of true empathy. With positive regard, we are able to identify what the patient is doing well or correctly. We can selectively attend to what is positive about the patient's statements or experience.
- Accurate Empathetic Understanding. Empathy is the ability to recognize, perceive, and directly experientially feel the emotion of another. Empathy is often characterized as the ability to "put oneself

into another's shoes," or "viewing the world from our patient's frame of reference."

- Respect and Warmth. Warmth means acceptance of and caring about the patient. Respect means believing and expecting that they can do what is needful to make their life work. We show these qualities by posture, smile, and vocal qualities.
- Nonjudgmental Attitude. Adopting a nonjudgmental attitude is difficult, but absolutely necessary to comfort the patient. By accepting the patient's perspective (their feelings and view), being judgmental is less likely. Patients who are dealing with trauma, grief, and wound care, do not desire to be judged.

Comforting the patient offers acceptance for where the patient is in the healing process and the belief that he can take the active stance to assume responsibility for his condition.

Case 8

Tommy (a pseudonym) was a 17 year-old, physically fit male high school athlete being treated for soft tissue crush wounds and fractures in both tibias. He had been lying under his new car when another auto drove over his legs, crushing them at mid tibia. An extended hospital course, and now wound care, was taking its toll. Tommy would not be playing football or getting the planned athletic scholarship for college. Wheelchair bound, angry and in despair, he would not respond to the usual kindness that the nursing staff exuded. On his second day at the Wound Center, the nurses were arguing over who had the duty to care for him. On his first day he had been especially hateful with cruel remarks and throwing paper at them. Now he was yelling at the nurses in the treatment room. A senior staffer at the wound center decided to resolve the problem, entered the treatment room, dismissed the nurses, and then proceeded to "chew him out" for his inappropriate behavior. Tommy was told that he must apologize to each of the nurses. He left the wound center in silence and never came back. He checked out of the hospital and was lost to follow-up.

In retrospect, the situation had been handled poorly, regrettably failing to show any empathy or compassion to this patient. If only we could do it over again!

SUMMARY

Wound care is effective only if the patient is willing to accept the care. Each patient presents with a problem wound and with a unique life. Communication and trust between patient and healthcare providers facilitate the healing process. A cooperative patient keeps his or her regular, frequent appointments and aids in the process of daily wound care. When it is over, the patient, doctor, and wound care staff appreciate the partnership in quality medical care.

ACKNOWLEDGEMENT

The authors thank Leah Garza, Paul J. Sheffield, and Melvin D. Smith for contributing additional cases presented in this chapter.

REFERENCES

1. Herman J. Trauma and Recovery, *The Aftermath of Violence-from Domestic Abuse to Political Terror*, Basic Books, 1992.
2. Kubler-Ross E. *On Death and Dying*. New York, NY: Macmillan, 1969.
3. Erikson, E.H. *Childhood and Society*. New York: Norton. 1950.
4. Smith MD, Wound care in pediatric patients, In: Sheffield PJ, Fife CE (Eds) *Wound Care Practice*. Flagstaff, AZ: Best Publishing, 2007.
5. Mouton CP, Parker R. Wound healing in the geriatric patient. In: Sheffield, PJ, Fife CE. (Eds) *Wound Care Practice*. Flagstaff, AZ: Best Publishing, 2007.
6. Lynn J. Travels in the valley of the shadow. In Spiro HM, McCrea MG, Peschel E, et al. (eds): Empathy and the Practice of Medicine: Beyond Pills and the Scalpel. Prepared under the auspices of The Program for Humanities in Medicine, Yale University School of Medicine. 1993.
7. Moody R Jr, Arcangel D. *Life After Loss: Conquering Grief and Finding Hope*. San Francisco, CA: Harper-San Francisco, A Division of Harper Collins Publishers Inc, 2001
8. Olaitan PB, Iyidobi EC, Olaitan JO, et al. Burns and scalds: First-aid home treatment and implications at Enugu, Nigeria. *Annals of Burns and Fire Disasters*, vol XVII(2), June 2004.
9. Maslow AH., *Motivation and Personality*, New York, NY: Harper and Brothers, 1954.
10. Rosenbloom D, Williams MB, Watkins BE. *Life After Trauma: A Workbook for Healing*. New York, NY: Guilford Press, 1999.
11. Rogers CR. *On Becoming a Person: A Therapist's View of Psychotherapy*. Boston, MA: Houghton Mifflin Company, 1961.

Additional references that were not specifically cited

12. Lerner H. *The Dance of Intimacy: A Woman's Guide to Courageous Acts of Change in Key Relationships*. New York, NY: Harper & Row, 1989.
13. Corey G. *Theory and Practice of Counseling and Psychotherapy*. Pacific Grove, CA: Brooks/Cole Publishing Company. 4th Ed. 1997.
14. Ivey AE. *Intentional Interviewing and Counseling: Facilitating Client Development*. Pacific Grove, CA: Brooks/Cole Publishing Co, 2nd Ed, 1988.
15. Superior Physicians. A quarterly publication for participating physicians of Superior Health Plan. *Seven Steps to Improve Work Relationships in Your Practice*. Summer 2006.
16. Vilas, Deborah. *Learning How To Play: The Development of a Course on Play Techniques for Child Life Specialists*. Play Therapy is published by the Association for Play Therapy. Volume 1, Issue 2- June 2006.

REVIEW QUESTIONS

1.) Kubler-Ross identified the five stages of grief as:
   a. Afraid, anger, sadness, guilt, despair
   b. Denial, anger, bargaining, depression, acceptance
   c. Sadness, gloominess, misery, hopelessness, anguish
   d. Melancholy, dejection, desolation, despondency, anguish

2.) In comforting the patient what are the areas that should be taken into consideration?
   a. Age and developmental stage of the patient
   b. Language and literacy of the patient
   c. Faith and spiritual needs of the patient
   d. All of the above

3.) The most important partner in successful wound care is:
   a. The nurse on duty
   b. The psychiatrist on duty
   c. The patient
   d. The payer

4.) Important attending skills include all EXCEPT:
   a. Eye contact
   b. Attentive body language
   c. Closed questioning
   d. Vocal qualities
   e. Verbal tracking

5.) Open questions cannot be answered with "yes" or "no" so when they are used in the interviewing process, they:
   a. Usually open with "is," "are," or "do."
   b. Put the burden of the consult on the interviewer.
   c. Are not helpful with pediatric patients
   d. Are helpful with any patient who is unfamiliar with the medical process.

Answers: 1b, 2d, 3c, 4c, 5d

CHAPTER 41

Ethics in Wound Care and Hyperbaric Medicine

CHAPTER FORTY-ONE OVERVIEW

NOTES

Ethics in Wound Care and Hyperbaric Medicine

Caroline E. Fife

Physicians are problem solvers. They make diagnoses, weigh the risks and benefits of various options, and initiate treatment. In general, physicians are uncomfortable with the concept that there might not be a "right" answer to a problem. Unlike scientific or medical questions, however, ethical questions rarely have well-defined "right" answers, although there are often "best answers." Medical ethics, when used properly, provide the physician with a structured approach to the resolution of the challenging ethical dilemmas facing the modern clinician.

WHAT IS "ETHICS"?

In philosophy, ethical behavior is that which is "good" or "right." But how can the attending physician(s) know what is right in a given situation or for a given patient? It is useful to begin with an understanding of the components of the "Doctor-Patient Relationship" which is, fundamentally, an unequal one. Patients are vulnerable because they are ill, and the relative education and knowledge of the physician places him or her in a position of power in relation to the patient. Just as society has changed over time, so has the nature of the doctor-patient relationship. In the past, a paternalistic approach was expected and even encouraged, but such an attitude is poorly tolerated by today's society. Nevertheless, the majority of patients expect their physician to give them the best advice possible.

In much the same way that society has changed, medicine itself has changed and evolved. For thousands of years, interventions such as purging, blistering, bleeding, the use of arsenic and numerous other "treatments" were considered the norm. It is a wonder that patients survived the ministrations of their physicians, and in fact, many did not.

By the early 20th century, science began to take hold of medicine. To quote ethicist Eugine Bousaubin, "At some point in the 1900s, an American patient entered a doctor's office and for the first time had more than a 50-50% chance of being helped by the encounter." It is for this reason that the first duty of the doctor to the patient is often considered that of "*nonmaleficence*"—in other words, "first do no harm." Preventing harm is more important philosophically, morally, and legally than "doing good."

The next goal of this relationship is *beneficence*. Beneficence is always acting in the patient's best interest. This is required because patients often cannot act on their own, whether out of ignorance, fear, illness, or vulnerability. The doctor-patient relationship is also *fiduciary*, meaning it is based upon trust and reliance. That depends on the attribute of *altruism* on the part of the physician.

MODERN MEDICINE

The past 100 to 150 years has seen exponential growth in science and technology that has greatly benefited patients and patient care, but trade-offs still exist. Although the modern patient might be safer in his doctor's office than he was in the 18th century, there are risks to modern medicine as well. Many therapies remain unproven (i.e., have not been subjected to a randomized controlled trial), marginal technologies flourish, and patients can have allergic and idiosyncratic reactions to even the most carefully tested pharmaceuticals. Furthermore, patient expectations have never been higher.

Modern technology provides more options than ever and permits more aggressive interventions. Thus, there is a risk of over-using technology to meet those high patient expectations, and high technology does not come cheap: someone must pay for its cost. Therefore, economics tends to be a dominant theme and has the potential to drive therapeutic decisions in all specialties.

These conditions of expectancy, lack of controlled trials, and personal patient cost are particularly true in the field of wound care and hyperbaric medicine, where there has been an explosion of technological advances in the past ten years. Several decades from now, evidence-based medicine in the form of the cost-effectiveness of medical procedures, based on perceived value to the patient and precise costs might routinely assist the physician in decision-making. But until that day arrives, medical professionals working in the field of HBO2 and wound care will continue to face ethical treatment dilemmas on a daily basis.

ETHICAL ISSUES RELATING TO WOUND CARE

A dilemma of modern medicine is that its reimbursement strategy has become procedurally based. Clinicians are paid for what they do for patients, not for what they refrain from doing. Thus the system, by its very nature, encourages intervention. When added to the modern patient's high expectations, the availability of technology, the economic pressures for medical professionals and facilities to generate revenue for economic survival, and the litigious nature of society, which apportions blame if maximal investigation and treatment are not undertaken, the result is a higher probability of expensive medical interventions. This is true for all medical specialties, but as noted is especially true for those medical interventions that are the newest.

The presence of this textbook is evidence that these technological advances have caused "wound care" to evolve into a *de facto* specialty. The logarithmic increase in patients with wound-related problems because of the national epidemics of diabetes and peripheral vascular disease in an aging population has made "wound centers" nearly a requirement for most hospitals. Initiating such programs *de novo* is a daunting task, and many hospitals depend on the services of management companies to assist them in organizing such a service, training staff in the use of these complex technologies, and providing the methods of documenting and billing for these services. In exchange for providing this expertise, these companies usually take a share of the revenue generated by the wound center. However, economic pressures are reducing the size of the "pie" that can be shared among these interests. Medicare reimbursement is diminishing universally, and the percentage of Americans, now at an estimated 44 million, (1) who are uninsured or underinsured is increasing. All of these factors are putting pressure on wound centers to increase their revenue if they are to remain economically viable operations.

As an example, in the wound-healing arena it might be tempting for financial managers to mandate wound debridement at specific intervals because debridement has been scientifically documented to be of benefit in wound healing. However, mandating that patients undergo an invasive procedure at specific intervals, perhaps with less regard to wound status than to generated revenue, is a policy that cannot be condoned from an ethical standpoint.

Clinic visit frequency is another highly debated area across many primary care specialties. Just how frequently do patients need to be followed once a treatment plan has been established? Patients whose treatment plan requires their frequent attendance in a clinic to change a negative-pressure wound dressing or compression bandage three times a week, do not usually require a physician evaluation with similar frequency in the absence of a change in their status. Yet, when a physician tries to minimize the frequency of follow-up visits, he or she might be constrained by the policies of the hospital or clinic. Patients who might travel great distances at considerable effort due to illness, and who are followed by a home-nursing agency that communicates regularly with the physician, might wish to be seen less often than monthly, but clinic policies, economic pressures (and occasionally even third party payors) might demand more frequent visits. These competing pressures make it difficult for the clinician to keep what is "best for the patient" foremost in his mind when deciding on the frequency of follow up visits.

The same is true for diagnostic testing. Some clinics include "spin-off" dollars in the calculation of the economic value of their services. This means that the number of diagnostic studies and procedures, which are generated in the course of treating many types of patients, are considered part of the economic argument for continuing to provide what otherwise might be an economically nonviable service. Such record keeping also might discourage the creation of more efficient methods of evaluation. For this reason, Medicare and other payors are experimenting with "Pay for Performance," "carve-outs," capitated systems, and other unique payment strategies (2). These systems would reward cost-effective thinking, and reward physicians for knowing when advanced technology is really necessary, and when high-quality conservative care is sufficient. The challenge is to create a system that does not reward clinicians for withholding care, which is a charge often levied against "managed-care" plans.

The determination of when to use technology is a difficult one. Hyperbaric oxygen therapy (HBO2) is an intervention that can be life-and-limb saving. It also generates revenue for the hospital, as well as the physician. The cost-benefit of HBO2 is increased when patients who were going to get well anyway or whose limbs would be lost despite HBO2, are excluded from treatment. However, careful selection of HBO2 patients reduces revenue for the hospital and physician, since it likely means that fewer patients will be treated; although it might preserve Medicare reimbursement for this technology for future generations since CMS (the Centers for Medicare and Medicaid Services) continues to evaluate the cost-benefit of all the technology it covers.

WHAT WOULD YOU DO?

Because this is a book on wound care, the following example is used. It is, of course, indicative of the same questions that her stroke doctor, eye doctor, and heart specialist must also consider in deciding how much intervention they should ethically do at this time.

Imagine the following scenario: A 78-year-old Latin American female with adult onset diabetes mellitus is in hospice care because of advanced cardiac disease. You have followed her for years with her various wound-care problems. Her complex medical history includes a stroke, which left her paralyzed on the left, and unable to ambulate, as well as advanced severe peripheral vascular disease. She has a recurrent, right, first metatarsal head lesion, and osteomyelitis appears likely based on the X-ray. Upon examination, the joint space is visible, but there is some granulation tissue in the wound. Transcutaneous oximetry shows that she would likely require a below-the-knee amputation if she underwent any surgery. Her pain is quite manageable with oral medication, and she is still able to make decisions for herself. Her life expectancy is less than 6 months because of her cardiac disease. What would you recommend?

You could order advanced testing to confirm her osteomyelitis (MRI, or bone scans), or angiography to further evaluate her vascular status. These would increase the "spin-off" revenue for your clinic. You could perform regular debridements that would enhance clinic revenue, and she would qualify for HBO2 based on her diagnosis of osteomyelitis. However, it is likely that the best treatment plan for her, after a thorough explanation of her situation, with warnings to her family to watch for systemic infection, is to treat her with antibiotics as needed, and manage her conservatively with a minimum of intervention and testing. Unfortunately, the design of the current healthcare system does not "reward" the clinician or the facility for taking this conservative and perhaps more humane approach.

This case also illustrates the challenges in approaching the topic of amputation in the chronically ill. Issues such as pain control, functionality (i.e., Can the patient ambulate as is or could they ever be expected to ambulate?), life expectancy, and the risk-benefit of the procedure must be determined. A detailed discussion of this topic is beyond the scope of this chapter. However, a well-known tenant of surgery is, "the technical feasibility of a procedure is not sufficient justification for doing it." In other words, just because a procedure can be done does not mean that it *ought* to be done.

As with all medical care and procedures, technological advances in the wound-care industry are likely to continue at a rapid pace. Currently, the wound care physician has access to semi-synthetic human skin, gene-cloned growth factors, numerous biosynthetic substances, advanced types of dressings, and equipment, such as negative-pressure wound therapy. Physicians must weigh the cost of these sophisticated products versus the need or value of them for a particular patient without placing undue consideration on the issue of financial gain for the doctor or facility, or undue hardship on the patient. To repeat: these considerations are not unique to wound care. Technological advances continue in all areas of medicine and all physicians must weigh the same issues.

ETHICAL ISSUES IN HYPERBARIC MEDICINE

HBO2 is the primary medical treatment for decompression sickness, arterial gas embolism, and serious carbon monoxide poisoning. It is also an adjunct treatment for chronic refractory osteomyelitis, clostridial myonecrosis (gas gangrene), crush injury, and other acute traumatic ischemias, selected wounds, severe anemia, necrotizing soft tissue infections, radiation tissue damage, compromised skin grafts and flaps, thermal burns, and some types of intracranial abscesses (3, 4). These comprise the UHMS 13 "approved" indications that the Food and Drug Administration (FDA) recognizes (Reimers, 1997, available at: *www.hyperbaric-clearinghouse.com/techtalk/techtalkfda.doc*). The FDA calls all other indications "off-label."

HBO2 as been reported as useful for over 130 other clinical conditions and the list increases almost weekly (HOC Hyperbaric Care & Wellness Centers, 2006, available at *http://www.hochealth.com/services HBOT.htm*). Hyperbaric chambers now appear not only in hospitals and freestanding facilities, but also in private homes (5). Some parents have even installed chambers in homes or garages and have been reportedly treating their own and other children. Literally thousands of web sites are devoted to the use of HBO2 for these 130 indications, of which HBO2 might appear potentially therapeutic for some, though most to many seem to lack a scientific rationale. Is it ethical for a physician to use HBO2 for any clinical condition in which the benefit is unproven?

Oxygen is not made by a pharmaceutical company making funding for large clinical trials limited and research in all areas of hyperbaric medicine slow. Consequently, until appropriate studies have been performed, physicians need guidelines on how to respond to patients requesting the use of HBO2 for an off-label indication.

THE CALL FOR AN ETHICS REVIEW

In the fall of 1998, the Undersea and Hyperbaric Medical Society (UHMS) invited the major nonprofit professional organizations in hyperbaric medicine to designate representatives to work with professional ethicists (Drs. Evelyn Chan and Baruch Brody) and contribute to a grant fund administered by the Office of Special Projects and Development at the University of Texas, Houston Health Science Center. The purpose of the grant fund was to reimburse the authors for their time. All invited organizations (see Acknowledgements) responded, and their representatives became part of the Working Group on Ethics in Hyperbaric Medicine. After reviewing the published literature on currently accepted indications for HBO2, the FDA regulations regarding the advertising of hyperbaric chambers, and the extensive information available on the Internet, recommendations were created for "off-label" use of HBO2 (6).

Is it Ethical To Use HBO2 for an Indication for which its Benefit Is Unproven?

This question is not unique to HBO2. It is common for physicians to use other drugs and therapies on an off-label basis, but there is clearly some ethical decision that prohibits physicians from prescribing HBO2 for every conceivable unproven indication. Deciding where to draw the line for a particular case will depend on the combination of a physician's individual clinical judgment, an evaluation of the available scientific data, and patient-informed consent. A physician and patient considering an off-label indication must weigh the type and level of scientific data, as well as the potential benefits and risks to the patient, and then determine where the line ought to be drawn for this particular patient through informed consent (7).

As an example, a potentially distressing case appeared on the Internet in which an elderly man discussed the use of HBO2 for his failing memory, and suggested it had also benefited his emphysema. One wonders if the risk of pneumothorax and potentially fatal arterial gas embolism were discussed with this patient before he decided to undergo HBO2 for his failing memory, an indication for which no scientific data exists. The risk-benefit assessment of using HBO2 for failing memory in a man with emphysema would seem to be different than that for an otherwise healthy patient who wishes to undergo HBO2 for a complex migraine, an indication for which some encouraging (albeit limited) data exist.

Applying general ethical guidelines to the field of hyperbaric medicine, it is possible to offer HBO2 on a case-by-case basis for an unproven indication, assuming the above analysis has been performed and consent has been obtained, just as all physicians who use off-label medical procedures or treatments must do.

What Are the Components of Informed Consent?

Physicians have a duty to disclose the risks and benefits of HBO2 treatment, regardless of whether the indication is approved or off-label, so that patients can make an informed decision about whether to undergo a specific treatment. To be legitimate, informed consent can be obtained in oral or written form, but documentation of the key elements of informed consent as well as when it took place must appear in the medical record. A physician should discuss six main issues with a patient considering "off-label" HBO2 as part of informed consent:

1. Are there any other alternative medical treatments that are cost-efficient and successful for the proposed indication?
2. What is the level and type of scientific data supporting the potentially therapeutic use of HBO2?
3. Are the risks of HBO2 acceptable relative to the potential benefit? (The physician should also review the ability of the facility to handle complications arising from HBO2 or the primary disease, the risks and side effects of HBO2 in general, and more specifically in light of a patient's co-morbid condition.)
4. Does the patient understand that he/she will be responsible for the cost of a therapy that might offer no benefit?
5. Is there a research protocol or registry available? If a registry exists for an indication (see below), the physician could offer the patient the opportunity to participate in it. Separate informed consent for registry participation would be required.
6. Informed consent should include physician disclosure of any financial issues that might affect the physician-patient relationship.

Physicians routinely charge for the management (and sometimes for the provision) of the off-label use of drugs, and charging for the off-label use of HBO2 is no different.Because physicians have the potential to receive immediate financial benefit to their facilities or themselves when they administer HBO2 for an off-label indication, particularly since patients often pay in cash and might be desperate, this represents a potential conflict of interest that should be disclosed (8).

The expense of administering the therapy should be reasonable. Patients might pay for unproven treatments that conform to ethical standards and might even pay to participate in research trials if they are informed of their financial obligations, and accept the fact that they are research subjects.

What Is Research?

As detailed in the Chan & Brody's article (6), when physicians repeatedly using HBO2 on an off-label basis for a particular indication and collect information about it in a systematic fashion with the intent to apply the principles of treatment to *other* patients, they move from practicing medicine to performing research. Early on, when information is incomplete, the benefits of an intervention might not be sufficient to justify running a trial. As information accumulates, a window of opportunity appears during which an intervention, such as HBO2, can be tested in a prospective concurrently controlled clinical trial. As more information is systematically collected, evidence supporting the potential benefit of an intervention can arise and justify initiating such a trial. However, if a preponderance of information has already been collected and clearly establishes the benefits of an intervention, a clinical trial might not be needed (9).

It is possible to collect data in a systematic fashion through the creation of registries. These are particularly useful for rare conditions, such as central retinal artery occlusion, for which HBO2 has been shown to be of benefit in a small case series but no one facility can accrue a large number of cases. Registries can serve two functions: 1) collect specific pilot data for use toward designing a prospective, controlled clinical trial; and 2) collect general data, a preponderance of which might obviate the need for such a trial in circumstances where a trial is not feasible.

Drs. Chan and Brody offered the example of extracorporeal membrane oxygenation (ECMO) in the management of neonatal respiratory insufficiency. Because of early reports in the 1970s that neonates receiving ECMO improved significantly compared with historical controls, ECMO increasingly became a standard therapeutic intervention without the results of a controlled clinical trial. By 1992, an International ECMO Registry had demonstrated the overwhelmingly beneficial effect of ECMO. Similar findings were found when a randomized, controlled clinical trial of ECMO in 1993 was aborted two years later. Some have considered that by then, in light of the registry data, it might have been too late to run a trial (9-13).

Suggestions for the creation of a registry can be found in the Chan & Brody's paper (6).

A critical point, however, is that if data are being collected, patients are participating in research, and a written protocol, reviewed by an Institutional Review Board (IRB) is required for this activity.

HEARING WHAT WE WANT TO HEAR

The presence of unsubstantiated information on the Internet produces an extraordinary opportunity to view the interpretation of research through the eyes of the public. There are many instances of this happening in all fields of medicine, but an excellent example of this is demonstrated in the following case:

A randomized, controlled trial of HBO2 in the treatment of cerebral palsy (CP) published by a Canadian group in 2002 (14) showed no difference between the HBO2 group and the group treated with air under pressure. Both groups of children improved somewhat during the study period, presumably due to the physical therapy that the interventions offered, though other psychological effects could have been in play. However, the interpretation of these data on the Internet was that "oxygen works." One quote from a web site expounded, "...the results are really incredible! 23 of the 25 children have great results. Twenty-three have amelioration with their spasticity and may have amelioration with speech and cognitive function." The author apparently did not understand the concept that in a "controlled trial," if there is no difference *between* the groups, then the treatment in question has not been proven to work. We hear what we want to hear.

Desperate patients will grasp at the slimmest of straws. The physicians' duty is to explain in the simplest possible terms the facts as they are known.

THE FDA AND ETHICAL ADVERTISING

Although the Federal Food, Drug, and Cosmetic (FDC) Act does not authorize the FDA to regulate the practice of medicine, it specifically directs the FDA to regulate the promotion of drugs and devices. Promotional materials are unlawful if they promote an unapproved use for the product. While it might seem reasonable that a web site could list the approved indications and the "unapproved" ones separately, or indicate that their facility is engaged in clinical research in certain areas, these distinctions are not acceptable to the FDA. Any promotional materials, which list unapproved uses of HBO2, even if they are designated as unapproved or "in research," are still considered to be encouraging the use of the modality for unproven indications, and such advertisements are not permissible under current FDA regulations. Yet, one can spend literally hours on the Internet, reading examples of facilities and clinicians who are not in compliance with this policy.

As an example, research with hyperbaric chambers has raise another unique issue having to do with the use of a medical device. Hyperbaric chambers are Class II medical devices, (they do not support or sustain human life as in the case of Class III medical devices) but they are not as innocuous as tongue depressors. Chambers developed after 1976 are split into two groups: those that are substantially equivalent to pre-1976 devices, and those that are genuinely new products. Manufacturers of new chambers must notify the FDA with a pre-market notification system, referred to as the 510(k). Devices that are determined to be equivalent to a pre-1976 device must *be marketed with the same restrictions as their pre-1976 predecessor*. Since 1978, the UHMS Hyperbaric Oxygen Therapy Committee report (3) has been recognized by the FDA as a guide in establishing the "indications of use" for hyperbaric chambers in a manufacturer's claim of substantial equivalency for the 510(k). This means that all hyperbaric chambers are cleared for marketing *only* for those conditions that are listed as approved in the UHMS Hyperbaric Oxygen Therapy Committee Report. A chamber could be approved to treat an indication not on this list, but this would require that data to support the use of HBO2 in that condition be submitted to the FDA for review.

The FDA has the legal authority to shut down facilities that fail to comply with its advertising requirement (15). In practice, the FDA lacks the resources to police such breaches, now common on the Internet. Therefore, it seems unlikely that misleading advertising regarding HBO2 can be controlled in the near future because; the FDA does not have the staff to pursue all of these illegal advertising claims. However, physicians should know that their medical license could be revoked for producing such advertising, and hospital-based facilities could suffer severe penalties.

Although regulatory oversight to ensure safety at hospital facilities is strict, there is less oversight at freestanding hyperbaric facilities and no oversight of chambers in homes and garages. Hospital hyperbaric facilities must comply with all hospital regulations plus those of the Joint Commission for Accreditation of Healthcare Organizations and National Fire Protection Association, of which the latter are enforceable by the local fire marshal or other authority having jurisdiction. In addition, hospital facilities are expected to use equipment that conforms to the ASME Pressure Vessel for Human Occupancy standards or equivalent. Freestanding facilities and chambers in private homes are not subject to the same rigid oversight.

Another issue is that of expert supervision at hyperbaric facilities. In the United States, physicians who operate facilities or supervise patients undergoing hyperbaric treatments must be licensed and are accountable to their state licensing board. State boards are sensitive to physician activities involving unproven therapies and interventions that might be considered experimental.

Many freestanding facilities have no physician involvement, thus removing a powerful type of oversight from program operation. The UHMS Guidelines for Hyperbaric Facility Operations (formerly UHMS Operations Committee Report) (16) outlines in detail the requirements for staffing and training personnel in hospital facilities.

At the beginning of the chapter we emphasized that, at the very least, physicians are expected to maintain compliance with appropriate Federal and State regulations governing the practice of medicine. In the case of HBO2, physicians who bill under Medicare are expected to be physically present for the duration of the hyperbaric treatment.

IN SUMMARY

The American Medical Association (AMA) has adopted standards of conduct that define the essentials of honorable behavior for the physician (available at *http://www.ama-assn.org/ama/pub/category/2512.html*). The physician is expected to act with compassion and respect for human rights, uphold standards of professionalism, be honest and competent, respect the law, respect the rights of patients and other health care professionals, support access to care for all patients, and continue to study and advance his or her knowledge. Not only are physicians expected to follow the laws that govern the practice of medicine, they are expected to act in the patient's best interest at all times.

How do you force people to act "rightly?" The answer is you cannot—one cannot legislate morality. The Harvard business school presented an ethics seminar following the Enron debacle, which one attendee summarized by saying, "Don't do anything that will get you in the papers."

The problem with this approach is that what is acceptable behavior will change as society changes, an excuse used by Nazi physicians to justify their heinous crimes. Early physicians understood this dilemma and for this reason created the Hippocratic Oath which begins: "I swear by Apollo Physician and Asclepius and Hygieia and Panaceia and all the gods and goddesses, making them my witnesses, that I will fulfill according to my ability and judgment this oath and this covenant. . ." While the ethics of health care might be described as "contractural," the ethics of patient care are, indeed, "covenantal." The obligation of the clinician to the patient is not merely to do what is legal, but what is right from the standpoint of universal justice. Transcendence has been considered a critical part of medicine since its inception; that a physician is held to a universal standard of right and wrong and not merely to the code of the day.

This is a viewpoint which is becoming increasingly difficult as fewer individuals subscribe to the concept of universal truth or justice. Dr. Edmund Pellegrino, the Founder of The Center for Clinical Bioethics at Georgetown University, summarized it this way, "Ethics requires that the physician be a person who can be expected to habitually act in the patient's interests when no one is watching." The question then becomes, "Who are you when no one is watching?"

ACKNOWLEDGEMENTS

The ethics report was funded through a grant administered by the Office of Special Projects and Development at the University of Texas-Houston Health Science Center with contributions to it from the following organizations: The Baromedical Nurses Association; Sechrist Industries; The Undersea and Hyperbaric Medical Society; National Baromedical Services; The Hermann Center for Environmental, Aerospace and Industrial Medicine; The American College of Hyperbaric Medicine; Reimers Systems, Inc.; Alternative Medicine Research Foundation of Texas; The Association of Diving and Hyperbaric Medical Technicians. The contents of this report represent only the opinion of Dr. Chan and Dr. Brody.

The following individuals were representatives of organizations participating in the Working Group on Ethics in Hyperbaric Medicine: Wayne Evans, MD, Hyperbarics Department, The Toronto Hospital; Caroline Fife, MD, President, UHMS, Director, Hermann Center for Hyperbaric Medicine, the University of Texas Health Science Center, Houston; Eric P. Kindwall, MD, Chairman, Quality Assurance Committee, UHMS; Ms. Carol Noel King, the Alternative Medicine Research Foundation of Texas; Valerie Larson-Lohr, RN, the Baromedical Nurses Association; William Maxfield, MD, Representative of the American College of Hyperbaric Medicine; Lee B. Palmer, B.S.M., C.H.T, Representative of the Certified Hyperbaric Oxygen Technicians; William P. Fife, Ph.D, Professor Emeritus, Texas A&M University; Ms. Trish Planck, The Hyperbaric Oxygen Clinic of Nevada; Ralph Potkin, M.D., UHMS; Ron Sechrist, Chairman and manufacturing representative, Sechrist Industries, Inc.; Keith VanMeter, MD, Representative of the American College of Hyperbaric Medicine; Lindell (Len) K. Weaver, MD, Representative of the Hyperbaric Oxygen Therapy Committee of the UHMS.

REFERENCES

1. Niescierenko ML, Cadzow RB, Fox CH. Insuring the uninsured: a student-run initiative to improve access to care in an urban community. *J Natl Med Assoc* 2006;98:906-911.
2. Grossbart SR. What's the return? Assessing the effect of "pay-for-performance" initiatives on the quality of care delivery. *Med Care Res Rev* 2006;63(1 Suppl):29S-48S.
3. Gabb G, Robin ED. Hyperbaric oxygen. A therapy in search of diseases. *Chest* 1987; 92:1074-1082.
4. Feldmeier JJ (ed). Hyperbaric Oxygen 2003—Indications and Results. The UHMS Hyperbaric Oxygen Therapy Committee Report, Kensington, MD: Undersea & Hyperbaric Medical Society, 2003.
5. National Parent-to-Parent Network. Mothers United for Moral Support, Inc., Newsletters #70-73, Aug.- Oct. 1997, Feb.-Apr. 1998.
6. Chan EC, Brody B. Ethical dilemmas in hyperbaric medicine. *Undersea Hyperb Med* 2001 Fall;28(3):123-30.
7. Shaneyfelt TM, Mayo-Smith MF, Rothwangl J. Are Guidelines Following Guidelines? The methodological quality of clinical practice guidelines in the peer-reviewed medical literature. *JAMA* 1999;281(20):1900-1903.
8. American Medical Association Council on Ethical and Judicial Affairs. Code of medical ethics 1998-1999. Chicago, Illinois: American Medical Association, 1998: 107-113, 118-155.
10. Brody B. The ethics of biomedical research: An international perspective. New York, New York: Oxford University Press, Inc., 1998:31-54, 139-160, 281-288.
11. Lantos J, Frader J. Extracorporeal membrane oxygenation and the ethics of clinical research in pediatrics. *N Eng J Med* 1990;323:409-413.
12. Elliott SJ. Neonatal extracorporeal membrane oxygenation: how not to assess novel technologies. *Lancet* 1991;337:75-82.
13. UK Collaborative ECMO Trial Group. UK collaborative randomized trial of neonatal extracorporeal membrane oxygenation. *Lancet* 1996;348:75-82.
14. Soll R. Neonatal extracorporeal membrane oxygenation: a bridging technique. *Lancet* 1996;348:70-71
15. Hardy P, Collet JP, Goldberg J, et al. Neuropsychological effects of hyperbaric oxygen therapy in cerebral palsy. *Dev Med Child Neurol.* 2002 Jul; 44(7):436-46.x
16. Foreman C, Weitershausen J. Regulation of hyperbaric chambers as medical devices. In: Hyperbaric Facility Safety - A Practical Guide, Workman, WT, ed. Flagstaff, Arizona: Best Publishing Company, 1999: 39-51.
17. Workman WT (ed). Guidelines for hyperbaric facility operations (formerly UHMS Operations Committee Report). Kensington, MD: Undersea & Hyperbaric Medical Society, 2005.

REVIEW QUESTIONS

1.) Medical ethics is:
   a. A way to determine the absolute right answer for any ethical dilemma
   b. A structured approach to finding the best answer for ethical dilemmas
   c. A way to justify a paternalistic approach to caring for patients
   d. A way to help clinicians use their power over patients to get them to do what the clinician wants

2.) By today's ethical standards, "nonmaleficence" that is, "first do no harm," is more important philosophically, morally, and legally than "doing good."
   a. True
   b. False:

3.) In discussing the possibility of HBO2 for an unproven indication, which of the following ought to be covered as part of informed consent?
   a. Whether there are alternative medical treatments that are cost-efficient and successful for the proposed indication
   b. What is the level and type of scientific data supporting the potentially therapeutic use of HBO2
   c. Whether the risks of HBO2 are acceptable relative to the potential benefit
   d. That the patient understands he/she will be responsible for the cost of a therapy that might offer no benefit
   e. The disclosure of any financial issues that might affect the physician-patient relationship.
   f. All of the above

4.) All of the following statements about FDA jurisdiction over hyperbaric chambers are true EXCEPT:
   a. Manufacturers of new chambers must notify the FDA with a pre-market notification system, referred to as the 510(k).
   b. The marketing of chambers is restricted to the indications considered "accepted" in the UHMS Hyperbaric Oxygen Therapy Committee Report.
   c. A chamber could be approved for marketing an indication not on the UHMS if supporting data is submitted to the FDA for review and acceptance.
   d. It is acceptable to state on your website that you have an IRB approved research study for a specific unapproved indication
   e. The FDA can seize your chamber, close your facility, or assess monetary fines if your website advertises HBO2 for unproven uses.

5.) The following things are TRUE regarding HBO2 for unproven indications:
   a. In the U.S., patients can pay to participate in research trials
   b. It is not unethical for physicians to use unproven therapies outside of an IRB if they are making case by case treatment decisions.

c. If a clinician is collecting data with the intention of applying it to other patients, he or she is performing research and needs an IRB.
d. Patients can receive HBO2 for unproven indications if they undergo full consent regarding, among other issues, the unproven nature of the treatment.
e. Physicians can charge for treating patients for unproven indications, as long as the charges are fair, the patient is informed of them in advance, and other consent issues are addressed.
f. All of the above

Answers: 1b, 2a, 3f, 4d, 5f

CHAPTER 42

Legal Aspects of Wound Care and Hyperbaric Medicine

CHAPTER FORTY-TWO OVERVIEW

NOTES

Legal Aspects of Wound Care and Hyperbaric Medicine

Harvey Ferguson, Jr., Nicolyn Garza Harris

INTRODUCTION

Despite the common perception, patients are not generally successful in a malpractice claim against their health care providers. Only a small fraction of patients with a potentially viable claim will actually file a malpractice lawsuit (1). Certain studies suggest that sixty to seventy percent of claims made against physicians are concluded without a finding of liability and without the payment of a monetary damage award. When a medical malpractice case reaches a trial, juries tend to rule in favor of the health care provider a large percentage of the time (2). However, in the continuing tort reform debate, oft-cited figures suggest that medical negligence accounts for 80,000 deaths and 300,000 injuries annually (3). According to the 2004 numbers from the National Practitioner Data Bank (NPDB), the most recent year information is available, 17,696 malpractice payments were reported and the average malpractice payment was $298,460 (4).

These numbers are daunting. Medical malpractice actions remain a part of the medical profession. Too often, patients or their families believe that a bad result (real or perceived) means liability. Claims for medical malpractice have increased in recent history. Before 1960, only one in seven doctors was ever sued during their entire professional career (5). Presently, approximately one in seven doctors is sued for malpractice in any given year (6). Today, it may be the exception that a physician can complete a medical career without a malpractice lawsuit.

Given this legal backdrop, how does a health care provider reduce exposure to malpractice claims? In brief terms, a health care provider is required to conform his behavior to that of a reasonably prudent, ordinary, competent provider. For the physician, the inquiry is commonly whether a diagnosis was missed or whether an inappropriate procedure was performed. In providing its services, a hospital has a similar responsibility to exercise ordinary skill and care that would be exercised by a reasonably competent hospital in the same or similar circumstance. This duty would include an obligation to furnish a patient the care, attention, and protection reasonably required for the patient's condition.

In addition to general principals of legal liability that are applicable to the medical field, wound care treatment and hyperbaric medicine present unique circumstances for exposure to liability. This chapter will provide an overview of the most common issues confronted in a malpractice suit, and will outline affirmative steps a physician can take to minimize exposure to a lawsuit and to aid in a defense if, in fact, a lawsuit is initiated. This chapter also will focus on opportunities to limit exposure and suggest specific means by which wound care policy and procedure can work in favor of health care professionals and facilities. Ultimately, liability exposure is about understanding the risks and taking measures to control and contain them.

MEDICAL MALPRACTICE THEORIES OF LIABILITY

Standard of Care for Medical Malpractice Lawsuits: An Overview

A lawsuit against a health care provider is usually based on the legal concept of negligence (7). Proving that a provider was negligent in his actions or omissions involves showing that there was a breach of the applicable standard of care that caused injuries and damages to a patient. Medical malpractice (8) is a form of a negligence action tailored to the practice of medicine. Medical malpractice arises when a provider does not apply "to the practice of medicine that degree of care and skill which is ordinarily employed by the profession generally, under similar conditions and in like surrounding circumstances (9)." A jury deciding the fate of the parties to a medical malpractice lawsuit is typically asked a relatively simple question: Did the provider fail to do that which a similar provider of ordinary prudence would have done under the same or similar circumstances? As noted earlier, a bad result, by itself, does not furnish a basis for holding a health care provider liable nor does it, alone, support a finding that the provider was negligent with respect to his diagnosis or treatment. Bad results, however, are often the reason a patient or family will pursue a malpractice claim.

Broken down, there are four (4) essential elements of a cause of action in a medical malpractice case:

1. A legally-cognizable duty requiring the health care provider to conform to a certain standard of conduct for protection of another against an unreasonable risk;
2. The failure by the provider to conform to the required standards;
3. Resulting actual injury to the patient; and,
4. A causal connection between the provider's conduct and the patient's injury.

In a medical malpractice lawsuit, the plaintiff/patient must prove by competent testimony that the treatment complained of was negligent. To do so, it is generally necessary for the patient to establish through medical expert testimony the professional standard of care so that a jury can determine whether the treatment by the health care provider/defendant deviated from that standard. If it did, the jury may find that the defendant's actions constituted negligence or malpractice.

There are limitations on how long a provider may be sued for alleged malpractice. The general time-frame in which a plaintiff has to bring a medical malpractice lawsuit is two years from the date of injury, or in special cases, two years from the date the injury is discovered or should have been discovered.

In a medical malpractice case, the plaintiff typically has the burden to prove that the physician failed to use ordinary care and skill. In other words, it is the part of the patient's case to establish through competent evidence and testimony the four elements listed above. It is not the health care provider's burden to prove compliance with the standard of care; yet, part of a proper defense strategy typically includes such evidence. Expert witnesses must generally be used both by the plaintiff and the defendant physician. In legal terms, expert testimony is required whenever a concept is outside of the layman's common sense and practical experience (10), and as medical care is specialized, most laymen need an expert witness to define the parameters of the applicable standard of care. Typically, expert witness testimony is used to establish the standard of care, a breach of duty, and causation (i.e. the physician's negligent conduct caused or contributed to the plaintiff's injury). For example, it would not be within the province of a jury to judge a physician's decision to select between two distinct and recognized courses of treatment. A patient complaining that his physician chose one course over another to the patient's alleged detriment would need an expert medical witness to prove the physician made an error amounting to a deviation in the standard of care. There are exceptions to the typical need for an expert in a medical malpractice case. An obvious example is a surgeon leaving behind a foreign object in his patient's body. Expert witness testimony to prove a deviation from the standard of care under these circumstances is generally not necessary. Whenever an expert witness is utilized, the expert witness must be qualified to testify on the particular topic through his knowledge, education, training, or experience. It is a function of the court to ensure that an expert witness is providing reliable testimony on an issue relevant to the case.

To prevail in a medical malpractice action, a plaintiff/patient must establish each of the four elements of negligence through competent evidence. The failure to prove all elements will result in a ruling in favor of the defendant/provider. Each element of a medical malpractice cause of action is explored in further detail below.

Elements of a Malpractice Action

Duty of care

Generally, a physician cannot be liable to a patient unless the physician has a physician-patient relationship with the patient. It is this relationship which gives rise to the duty of care. The physician-patient relationship typically arises out of the consensual and fiduciary relationship between the patient and physician (11). A physician is generally free to refuse to treat a patient. But this general freedom can have limits. For example, a physician's duty to treat some patients may be created by contract, as is the case in the common scenario where a physician has contracted with a managed care health plan to provide medical care. Here, the physician has agreed to treat qualified patients through the Health Maintenance Organization (HMO). In that situation, the physician-patient relationship is created as a function of the parties' participation in the HMO. In addition, a physician may not refuse treatment for discriminatory reasons, such as the sex or race of the patient. In the typical setting, the physician-patient relationship is based on a patient seeking out the services of a physician and the physician agreeing—either expressly or impliedly—to accept the person as his patient. Until that consensual relationship is made, the physician is not obligated to provide care (12). The physician's duty to his patient translates into a duty of the physician to use reasonable care and skill in his diagnosis, care, and treatment of his patients. In sum, a legal duty arises when the health care provider undertakes the care and treatment of a patient.

In some instances, the formation of the physician-patient relationship is more difficult to determine. For example, if a physician is "on-call" for a hospital emergency room, a question may arise as to whether the E.R. physician is obligated to treat all patients who present to the emergency room for treatment. Related to this scenario, another common area of uncertainty is whether a physician-patient relationship is created through physician-to-physician consultation. Typically, the answer to these questions turns on an examination of the particular facts. Most often, the on-call physician has a duty to care for the hospital's patient through the physician's agreement to provide emergency treatment to the hospital's patients. Again, this obligation is a function of the physician's prior arrangements with the hospital. In the consultation scenario, a physician who simply provides advice and consultation to a colleague, without more, has not obligated himself to provide further care or treatment to the patient. An agreement to be on-call does not in and of itself establish the doctor-patient relationship.

Once the physician-patient relationship has been created, it cannot be unilaterally severed by the physician. A physician is under a duty, in the absence of an agreement limiting services, to continue to provide care after treatment is initiated so long as the patient requires attention. The obligation to continue treatment can be terminated only 1) by the cessation of the necessity which gave rise to the relationship, 2) by the discharge of the physician by the patient, or 3) by the withdrawal of the physician after giving the patient reasonable notice so as to enable the patient to secure another medical provider. Obviously, the patient is free to terminate the physician-patient relationship at any time. However, if further medical care is needed, the physician should advise his former patient to seek additional care. Provided that adequate notice is given and withdrawal does not leave the patient without medical care, a physician is free to terminate his relationship with his patient. A physician's unilateral severance of the professional relationship between the physician and the patient without reasonable notice, at a time when there is still the necessity of continuing medical attention may result in a claim of "patient abandonment."

The same general rules apply to hospitals with some additional exceptions. For example, a hospital providing emergency services is obligated to treat and stabilize patients who present with an emergency medical condition (13). Other federal, state, or local policies may require hospitals to provide a certain percentage of care to indigent patients.

Breach of the duty of care

A malpractice cause of action requires proof of a breach of the applicable standard of care. Again, the breach of duty refers to the failure of the health care provider to act as a reasonably competent physician. To avoid liability, the physician must practice medicine with the care and skill of the average, prudent practitioner of the relevant medical specialty, considering advances in the profession and the state of the given medical profession at the time of treatment (14). An objective standard is used to measure a physician's conduct; thus when breach of the physician's duty of care is analyzed, a physician's "good faith" belief or motivation is typically irrelevant to determining liability (15).

Injury

Injury is the third element necessary to establish a medical malpractice cause of action. In the absence of extreme circumstances, a physician does not typically warrant that her treatment will be successful. What she does warrant, though, is that she possesses and will carefully apply the level of professional skill and care possessed by medical practitioners practicing in the same field (16). Similarly, professional liability does not turn on the finding of a mistake; instead, it turns on whether or not the physician used ordinary care (17).

Injury in a medical malpractice claim can be complicated because most patients seek a health care provider's services when they are already sick. Accordingly, it is not uncommon that even with a breach of the standard of care by the physician, the patient may be in the same condition that she would have been had the physician treated the patient appropriately and in line with the standard of care or that the patient would be in the same condition had a particular course of treatment been withheld. Rather than barring a finding of liability under these facts, the nature and extent of the outcome is considered a factor in the plaintiff/patient's damages. The law recognizes a distinction between a breach in the standard of care and the success or failure of treatment. Similarly, the fact that a particular course of treatment is unsuccessful does not, automatically, mean that a physician committed malpractice, absent a showing that treatment was not done with the ordinary skill and care that the average medical provider would have used in the same or similar circumstances. Accordingly, a physician will not be liable to a patient when an unsuccessful result occurs if he employs the proper treatment (18).

The practice of medicine is dynamic, and new methods of treatment are constantly being created. Using new and experimental methods of treatment on a patient requires a delicate balancing of risk and potential benefits. On the one hand, it is the duty of a physician to keep abreast of her field of practice and use appropriate advancements in her field. Yet, on the other hand, unproven courses of treatment can potentially lead to a malpractice claim. A physician should carefully balance the benefits and risks of any experimental treatment and fully disclose the risks and potential benefits to the patient to avoid a claim of malpractice.

In U.S. jurisprudence, patient injuries pursued through the courts are compensated through monetary damages. Broadly, there are two categories of damages which a plaintiff can be awarded: compensatory damages and punitive damages. Compensatory damages are designed to compensate the plaintiff for her injury, while punitive damages are awarded to punish the defendant for his medical negligence and aim to deter him and others from future malpractice. Punitive damages are a severe award, and most of the time, punitive damages are not awarded (19).

Causation

In addition to proving that the plaintiff was injured and that the defendant is at fault, the final element of a medical malpractice case requires that the plaintiff prove that there is a causal connection between the plaintiff's injury and the defendant's error. Proof of causation requires that other alternative causes for the plaintiff's injuries be reasonably ruled out (20).

Because of the technical and specialized nature of the practice of medicine, proof of causation, except in the most obvious cases, will require expert testimony. Proof of causation requires proof of a probable connection between injury and error, as opposed to mere possibility (21). Although there are variances from state to state, generally there are two components of causation: 1) cause-in-fact and 2) "legal cause (22)." The first component of causation is "cause-in-fact" (also referred to as "but-for causation") and requires a showing that the wrongful act complained of was "a substantial factor in bringing about the injury and without which no harm would have been incurred (23)." Stated another way, cause-in-fact asks the question, "but for the defendant's conduct, would the injury have resulted?" The second component of causation is "legal cause" (also called "proximate cause") and is a limitation the law places on a finding of liability. Proximate cause requires that an act be of the nature for which the law assigns responsibility for the harm suffered by the plaintiff (24). In most jurisdictions, a showing of proximate cause requires a showing that the plaintiff's injury was or should have been foreseeable.

Most medical malpractice claims are based on the health care provider's course of treatment, lack of treatment, or other alleged departure from accepted standards of medical or health care. In the medical malpractice context, proof of the first element of causation, or cause-in-fact, can be particularly challenging because, in most instances, the patient is already sick when he seeks a health care provider's services. The doctrine of "loss of chance" often comes into play in proving the element of causation. This doctrine, which has subtle variances in the various jurisdictions, is best explained by way of example (25). Suppose a patient comes to a doctor with Stage II cancer. The doctor overlooks the cancer, and the cancer is diagnosed a year later by a different doctor, and the patient now has progressed to Stage IV cancer. At the time the patient saw the first doctor that missed the cancer diagnosis, she had a 45% chance of survival. By the time the cancer is actually detected by the second physician, the patient has a 15% chance of survival. The patient's medical malpractice action would be based on a loss-of-chance theory, essentially asserting that although she might not have survived anyway, the physician's negligence caused her to suffer a loss of chance at surviving. The action is based on the provider's alleged breach of an accepted standard of medical care. In sum, causation, at its core, requires a causal connection between the health care provider's act and the patient's alleged injury.

Defenses to a Plaintiff's Medical Malpractice Suit

There are numerous defenses that a health care provider can assert that may operate to bar a plaintiff's recovery or reduce the amount a plaintiff is entitled to recover. Each situation is unique and will require the expertise of an attorney to review and analyze. Further, each jurisdiction has particular nuances in their law that dictate what must be proven and the effect of a successful defense. Note that not all of the defenses described below are available in every jurisdiction. What follows is a general explanation of the most common defenses in a medical malpractice lawsuit with a brief explanation of how each defense operates. In all of the following explanations, keep in mind that the defendant in the medical malpractice case bears the burden of proof with respect to any defense she asserts (26).

Assumption of the risk

Assumption of the risk, contributory negligence, and comparative negligence are similar affirmative defenses, each of which has a different effect in what the defendant is required to prove to be successful in the defense. "Assumption of the risk" is a defense which will totally bar a plaintiff's right to recovery if it is proven. "Assumption of the risk" essentially states that a plaintiff "who voluntarily consents, either expressly or impliedly, to exposure to a known risk cannot later sue for damages incurred from exposure to that risk (27)." An example of express assumption of the risk is a waiver form for sky diving, which fully explains the danger which the plaintiff is agreeing to waive; while an example of an implied danger which the plaintiff assumes the risk of is when a person attempts to lift an obviously heavy object (28). Assumption of the risk is a harsh legal doctrine which has been modified by most states and it is rarely applicable in a medical malpractice case. As detailed below, great care should be taken in explaining the risks and benefits of a medical treatment, and the health care provider should be careful not to assume that the defense of assumption of the risk will foreclose a finding of legal liability when a patient consents to a proposed course of treatment.

Contributory negligence

Closely related to assumption of the risk is the defense of "contributory negligence." "Contributory negligence," at its core, is "that degree of reasonable and ordinary care that a plaintiff fails to undertake in the face of an appreciable risk which cooperates with the defendant's negligence in bringing about the plaintiff's harm (29)." In other words, contributory negligence occurs when the plaintiff fails to exercise reasonable care for his own safety, which contributes to his injury (30). In most jurisdictions, contributory negligence, like assumption of the risk, operates to completely bar a plaintiff's recovery, essentially imposing an "all or nothing" situation on the plaintiff. Note that assumption of the risk, unlike contributory negligence, does not require that the plaintiff was negligent (31).

Comparative negligence

Because of the harsh results of the defense of contributory negligence, many jurisdictions have abolished the doctrine in favor of a principle known as "comparative negligence." "Comparative negligence" reduces the amount a plaintiff can recover in proportion to his own negligence. Proof of "comparative negligence" involves two questions: 1) were both the plaintiff and the defendant negligent; and 2) if both were negligent, what percentage of negligence or responsibility should be assigned to each party (32)? Stated differently, a successful defense of comparative fault requires adequate proof that the plaintiff was negligent. If the plantiff is found to have been negligent, then the plaintiff's recovery of damages is apportioned according to the plaintiff's and defendant's respective fault or responsibility. To find that the plaintiff shares in the responsibility for negligence, comparative negligence asks not whether the plaintiff took a risk, but whether, objectively, the plaintiff's risk was reasonable under the circumstances (33).

Other defenses

A defense that is allowed in some jurisdictions, which mimics a comparative fault scheme, is called "sole proximate cause." Asserting a defense of sole proximate cause requires a showing that the plaintiff's negligence was the sole or only proximate cause of the injury (34). The basic principles of proximate cause, explained above, apply in the context of comparative fault.

When asserted by a defendant as a defense, the doctrine of "last clear chance," while largely replaced by comparative negligence in most jurisdictions, is appropriate when the plaintiff had the last opportunity to avoid injury (35). Essentially, the doctrine functions to examine who had the superior opportunity to avoid the incident that brought about the injury (36).

Another defense that may be applicable when a plaintiff waits too long, according to the law, to bring a lawsuit is the defense of "statute of limitations." This defense operates to bar the plaintiff's right to recover, even if the health care provider was obviously negligent. As discussed above, typically a plaintiff has two years from the date of injury or, in special cases involving latent injuries, two years from the date the injury was or should have been discovered to bring a medical malpractice lawsuit.

Related to defenses that a health care provider can assert when sued is the concept of a counter-claim, where a health care provider asserts an independent cause of action complaining of the plaintiff's conduct. While not relatively common, a counter-claim relevant to when a plaintiff maliciously sues a health care provider without justification is called "abuse of process" or "malicious prosecution (37)." Essentially this is a claim that the health care provider assets against the plaintiff's lawyer or the plaintiff, or both, complaining that the plaintiff did not have a good faith basis for bringing suit against the health care provider. Note that success on this claim typically requires a favorable termination of the original malpractice suit (38).

Other Potential Causes of Action and Forms of Liability

The section above explored the nuts and bolts of a medical malpractice claim against a health care provider. There are, of course, other potential claims that a patient can bring against a provider. These additional claims can be based on other recognized causes of legal action, such as breach of contract or battery. Finally, legal liability can flow indirectly to others who participate in the health care process through, for example, the employer-employee relationship under the doctrine known as vicarious liability. These other forms of liability are reviewed below.

Hospital's potential liability for a physician's negligence

There are two theories in which a hospital or other institution such as an insurer could be liable for a physician's malpractice—direct liability and vicarious liability. Direct liability, the first theory, typically requires some malfeasance on the part of the institution's management regarding patient care or physician competence (39).

As to the second theory, a hospital, as an employer of a physician, may be vicariously liable for the physician's negligence under a legal doctrine called "respondeat superior." This liability is typically limited to negligent acts by the physician performed within the scope of the physician's employment or done at the hospital's direction. Conversely, a hospital is not typically liable for the negligent acts of an independent contractor (40). There are several recognized exceptions to the rule of non-liability for an independent contractor's acts which include: 1) where the hospital "holds out" to the patient or the public that the hospital itself is the provider of medical services or that the physicians associated with the hospital are the hospital's employees, which, in theory, causes patients to rely on the hospital for medical care and treatment; 2) where the independent contractor through whom a hospital sought to discharge its responsibilities is under a contract with a third party to provide medical services; and 3) where the physician's negligence was foreseeable by the hospital (41).

Whether or not a hospital is liable for the actions of a physician turns on the character of the relationship between the physician and the hospital. If the physician is an employee, servant, or agent, then the hospital is generally liable for the physician's acts. As explained, generally, if the physician is an independent contractor, then the hospital is generally not liable. The determination of liability does not turn on labels or method of pay, but instead, turns on the actual interactions between the hospital and physician.

Physician's liability for staff member's negligence

In appropriate circumstances, a physician may be liable for the negligent acts of his staff, such as nurses who assist the physician in his practice, through a doctrine called the "borrowed servant rule" which is a legal concept under the umbrella of vicarious liability. The "borrowed servant rule" states that when a person borrows a servant from another (such as may be the case when an independent contractor surgeon borrows an anesthesia nurse that is a hospital employee, if the nurse commits negligence while under the direct supervision and control of the physician, the physician may be vicariously liable (as opposed to directly liable) for the nurse's negligent acts. Similar to the inquiry into whether a hospital is vicariously liable for the negligent acts of another, the focus in a borrowed servant analysis is on whether the physician had or exercised the right to control details of the nurse's work or conduct.

Products liability litigation

As more fully detailed below, a hyperbaric chamber is a medical device. As a device, it is a "product" and if legally defective, a patient may have a claim against all those in the chain of supply of the chamber, including the manufacturer, distributor, wholesaler, the marketer, and the seller (42). It is conceivable that the prescribing physician of a medical device (a product) could find himself in litigation involving the prescribed device as products liability typically involves all entities in the supply chain of a product.

Products liability litigation borrows its concepts from various different and distinct areas of law. The concept of products liability grew out of a public policy judgment that people need greater protection against dangerous products than was typically recognized by then existing law (43). Products liability law generally covers "any liability of a manufacturer or seller of a product, where personal injury or damage to some other property is caused by a defect in the product (44)." Various theories of recovery under products liability litigation are possible and include: strict liability in tort, negligence, defective design, defective manufacturing, defective marketing, breach of warranty, fraud, and misrepresentation (45). Many states have statutes that deal specifically with products liability, and, if ever faced with a potential products liability claim, it is important to consult with an experienced attorney.

Whatever the particular products liability theory asserted, all products liability cases require a showing that a product is defective and that the defect caused injury (46). Each theory of products liability is briefly explored below.

In a negligence-based products liability case, the plaintiff must prove that "the product was defective, that the defect caused the plaintiff's injury, and that the manufacturer or seller failed to exercise due care in the design, manufacturing, or marketing of the product (47)." Some states have their own negligent products liability statutes that may vary the foregoing, and the development of strict tort liability and breach of warranty have "reduced the utility of negligence as a theory in products liability…(48)"

Strict liability is a legal concept which holds a product manufacturer, supplier, distributor, retailer, and all others involved in the stream of commerce for a product "strictly liable" when a defect in a product is proven, without regard to fault or wrongdoing. The general concept is based on the public policy that those in the supply chain who make a profit are in a better position to absorb the costs of an injury and resulting damages than the innocent plaintiff who is injured by a defective product. Admittedly, this can result in what at times can seem to be a harsh result. Strict liability can be based on a theory of defective manufacturing, defective design, or failure to warn of a danger related to the use of a product. Strict liability generally requires proof that a person in the business of selling a product in the stream of commerce places that product into the stream of commerce and that product 1) had a defective and unreasonably dangerous condition and 2) caused plaintiff's injuries (49). As with negligence in the products liability context, the same basic principals of causation that apply to general negligence apply in the strict products liability context (50). There are three theories in which an entity may be liable for strict products liability. First, a design defect theory of strict products liability requires that a product be defectively designed. Second, a manufacturing defect theory requires that, although a product is properly designed, it is manufactured in such a manner as to have a defect. Finally, a failure to warn theory explores whether or not a manufacturer or seller adequately warned the product user of the dangers associated with a product.

Breach of warranty is another theory of recovery and is typically governed by common law or statutes. Its application can vary widely from state to state. Breach of warranty claims are asserted as either a breach of an express warranty or as breach of an implied warranty (51). Generally, "express warranties" are "those for which the buyer bargained," while "implied warranties" are those which arise by operation of law (as opposed to by agreement between the parties) (52).

Generally speaking, the majority of courts that have examined the issue of whether or not a hospital or medical practitioner can be liable for strict liability in tort or for breach of warranty when a patient is allegedly injured by a medical device have answered this question in the negative (53). The reasoning for this, most often, is that the defendant in such a case was rendering professional services, and is not in the business of selling, disturbing, or supplying products (54). Flowing under these decisions is the theory in which strict liability and breach of warranty are grounded, as both seek to hold the entity or entities liable that are in the business of selling, disturbing, and supplying defective products (55). Nevertheless, products liability law is, in many respects, still developing and changing. Under certain facts, an injured patient may attempt to pursue a products liability case against a health care provider.

A plaintiff in a products liability cause of action based on fraud essentially is asserting that the defendant's fraud caused the plaintiff injury. To recover, the plaintiff must prove the following elements: " 1) false representation made by the defendant; 2) "scienter" or knowledge of the false representation; 3) an intention to induce the plaintiff to act or to refrain from action in reliance on the representation; 4) justifiable reliance by the plaintiff; and 5) damage to the plaintiff (56)." As would be expected, a plaintiff has advantages and disadvantages when bringing a products liability suit grounded in fraud. Advantages include a longer statute of limitations and the possibility to recover punitive damages, while disadvantages include a higher burden of proof with respect to knowledge and intent (57).

Similar to fraud, misrepresentation as to the character or quality of a product can impose strict liability on a seller or other person in the stream of commerce (58). The elements of a strict liability cause of action for misrepresentation are: "1) a misrepresentation of a material fact concerning the character or quality of [property]; 2) the misrepresentation...is made to the public; and 3) physical harm...result[s] to a consumer from justifiable reliance upon the misrepresentation (59)."

There are very few reported cases involving a hyperbaric chamber. The first case is *Vause v. Bay Medical Center*, which was a wrongful death action where a nurse, approximately two hours after exiting a hyperbaric chamber where she was assisting a patient in the chamber, died from nitrogen emoblization due to decompression sickness (60). The nurses' estate sued the hospital supervisor, the supervisor of the hyperbaric chamber, and the operator of the hyperbaric chamber alleging that the chamber was negligently operated. Although the case, in large part, focuses on areas of law unrelated to medical malpractice, a health care provider can take from this case that she should have a competent and properly trained staff operating and supervising the hyperbaric chamber, and the health care provider should examine the staff that works inside the chamber, as well as the patient, for signs of decompression sickness after a session of treatment is completed.

A second case is *Friedl v. Airsource, Inc.*, which involved claims against the distributors of a portable topical hyperbaric chamber for in-home use that caused burns to the patient's feet (61). The Plaintiff claimed that the Defendants failed to instruct her to put water into the machine in order to humidify the oxygen. The court agreed with the Plaintiff, finding that the distributor failed to provide proper operating instructions for the chamber (62). The court noted that manufacturer of a medical device has a duty to warn physicians of a device's dangerous propensities so that the physician can convey relevant warnings to his patient (63). Although this case involves a device that is different from a typical hyperbaric chamber, a practitioner can take from this case that it is imperative that proper warnings and instructions be effectively communicated to the patient.

Should a physician be sued in a products liability suit, many states have laws, whether by common law or statute, that allow a physician to seek indemnity and contribution from an upstream entity in the chain of supply. For example, the physician may be entitled to indemnity and contribution from the manufacturer of a defective device. To reduce exposure to liability, as the *Friedl* case hints, a physician has a duty to pass on warnings and instructions he deems necessary to the patient that he receives from the manufacturer (64). With that addition, the same suggestions regarding limiting liability exposure in a medical malpractice case apply with equal force to causes of action grounded in any of the many forms of products liability litigation.

Other potential causes of action

When a plaintiff brings a medical malpractice lawsuit, rarely does he solely assert only a claim that the provider's care was negligent. Instead, it is common practice for a plaintiff to assert every conceivable cause of action, even though many of the causes of action will ultimately fail. Accordingly, it is important to have an understanding of other common causes of action that may be joined with a medical malpractice action. Reasons for this practice include considerations of different statutes of limitations, varying monetary damage availability (including, for example, punitive damages and attorney's fees), and different proof requirements.

Briefly listed, other common causes of action that an aggrieved patient may pursue include breach of contract, battery, and non-disclosure claims (failure to obtain informed consent). If the core of the plaintiff's complaints against a health care provider is a breach of the provider's professional judgment, absent extraordinary facts, most courts will disallow the above-listed peripheral claims. For the health care provider, nevertheless, it is important to understand potential causes of action so as to implement effective risk management techniques to reduce exposure to liability. As with all causes of action, each state has its own particularities. The following review of these causes of action does not take into account particular variations of a state's applicable law. Finally, many of these claims may overlap, and depending on the state, may or may not be mutually exclusive.

Breach of contract involves the existence of a contract between the patient and the health care provider, that one party offered and the other party accepted for goods or services. Contracts can be oral or written, and to be valid, must also involve a "meeting of the minds" (i.e. each party understood and assented to what was being agreed to) and the exchange of some form of "consideration." Contract law rarely is applicable to a medical malpractice claim. A physician does not agree or promise in advance to deliver a particular outcome to his patients. Therefore, absent a special contract, doctors do not insure or guarantee results or that surgical procedure will be beneficial to the patient (65).

Battery, which is a form of an intentional tort, requires the defendant to intentionally make contact with the plaintiff in a manner that is considered offensive or harmful (66). It is a form of trespass to the person. Stated differently, a battery is the voluntarily touching another person without lawful excuse or justification. For example, say a patient gives consent to have surgery performed on his left shoulder. During the operation, the surgeon concludes that the patient does not need surgery to the left shoulder, but could benefit from surgery to the right shoulder. Operating on the patient's right shoulder without consent is a form of battery. Administering medication to a patient without the patient's knowledge or consent can also constitute a battery.

A non-disclosure claim or a failure to obtain informed consent claim is explained in greater detail below. Essentially, a health care provider must have a patient's permission before a particular course of treatment can begin. The example above regarding the shoulder surgery can also be couched in terms of a lack of consent.

One final subject to discuss is the doctrine of *res ipsa loquitur*. Some jurisdictions allow for the limited application of this concept in medical malpractice cases which allows for an inference that the defendant was negligent. *Res ipsa loquitur* translates into "the thing speaks for itself." It is a circumstantial evidence doctrine and applies when the facts of a particular injury may themselves establish that breach of a duty has occurred. A plaintiff, when attempting to rely on the doctrine of *res ipsa loquitur*, must show that the incident causing the injury is of a type that would not normally occur unless someone was negligent. An example of this would be when surgical instruments are left behind in the patient's body. As noted before, a finding of negligence may not be based solely on evidence of a bad result, but when the evidentiary concept of *res ipsa loquitur* applies, a bad result may indeed be considered as evidence on the issue of negligence.

This review of other causes of action is intentionally brief and is not intended to be comprehensive. Depending on the jurisdiction, these causes of action may be barred when medical malpractice is asserted or may be alternative or supplemental causes of action to a medical malpractice case.

OVERVIEW OF MEDICAL DEVICE LAW AND THE ROLE OF THE GOVERNMENT (67)

A hyperbaric chamber is considered a "medical device (68)." The Federal Food and Drug Administration (FDA) regulates the labeling of all medical devices.

The FDA's authority is found in the Food, Drug and Cosmetic Act of 1938 (FDCA). This Act requires the FDA to ensure that drugs and devices are safe and effective for their intended uses (69). Since the passage of the FDCA, the federal government has passed other laws related to medical devices including (70):

- The Federal Food, Drug, and Cosmetic Act (FDCA), originally enacted in 1938 (71).
- The Medical Device Amendments (MDA), 1976 (72).
- The Safe Medical Devices Act (SMDA), 1990 (73).
- The Food and Drug Administration Modernization Act (FDAMA), 1997 (74).
- The Medical Device User Fee and Modernization Act, 2002 (75).

The federal government regulates the manufacture and marketing of medical devices (76). The federal government does not regulate the practice of medicine (77). Combined, this premise is the foundation of the "practice of medicine doctrine" which maintains that "the FDA lacks authority under the FDCA to regulate patient treatment decisions made by licensed physicians (78)." Applied to a medical device, the practice of medicine doctrine holds that a physician may use a properly marketed device for any indication appropriate in the medical opinion of the treating physician, even if that indication is "off-label (79)." The prudence of "off-label" use is discussed in further detail later in this chapter.

Medical device law is an intricate area and applies primarily to the manufacture, preparation, and assembly of devices (80). A medical practitioner that does not manufacture or market a medical device need not be overly concerned about FDA regulation. The MDA of 1976 created three regulatory classes for medical devices, which are based on the "degree of control necessary to assure that the various types of devices are safe and effective (81)." The degree of regulation increases in proportion to the device's classification—Class I devices are subject to the least regulatory control, Class II devices are subject to special controls, and Class III devices receive the most stringent regulatory control (82). A hyperbaric chamber is classified as a Class II device under the category of "Anesthesiology (83)." Class II medical devices are generally subject to special labeling requirements, mandatory performance standards, and post-market surveillance (84). Other examples of Class II devices are powered wheelchairs and surgical drapes (85).

AREAS OF POTENTIAL LEGAL LIABILITY AND OPPORTUNITIES TO LIMIT LIABILITY EXPOSURE

Introduction

As in the practice of all types of medicine, the health care professional providing wound care must meet the accepted standard of care. Again, the standard of care is defined by an objective assessment of the actions and conduct of the provider. A physician's actions and inactions will be judged through a comparison to the reasonable, prudent physician in the same or similar circumstances.

As an illustration, assume a nursing home resident is transferred to a local hospital for treatment of a recently developed pressure sore to the sacrum. At the time of admission, the ulcer is documented as a Stage I wound. However, since pressure sores form from the inside out, after several days, the full extent of tissue injury becomes apparent, and the ulcer evolves to a Stage III wound, open to the fascia. Despite continued treatment, the wound is eventually documented as Stage IV, extending down to bone. For reasons that may or may not be related to the pressure sore, the patient expires two months after the hospital admission.

In this example, in assessing the propriety of the team's treatment from a legal prospective, the first task is to define what, under the facts presented, was the accepted (i.e. expected) course of treatment. After defining the standard of care, the providers' actions, decisions, and conduct are compared to that objective standard. As noted before, the applicable standards for judging the health care provider's conduct will typically involve a fact-specific review of the nature and circumstances surrounding the patient's care and typically require the expertise of others to help define. From the example above, an obvious question that arises is why did the wound fail to respond to treatment? The ensuing questions asked from that point forward are delineated by the facts and circumstances of the case. As discussed in the theories of liability section, as bad outcome or an error in judgment that results in injury to a patient does not equate to negligence or liability. Instead, if in the example, the estate of the expired patient sues, the estate must establish that the health care providers' conduct fell below the generally accepted standard of medical care.

In the area of wound care, the issues that would help define the applicable standard of care would include:

- Performing an initial assessment of the patient to identify actual and potential risks of treatment and to establish a baseline of the patient's health.
- Making the appropriate diagnoses.
- Developing a comprehensive plan of care setting forth identified problem areas, setting short and long term goals and outlining specific interventions designed to prevent adverse outcomes.
- Informing the patient of the risks, benefits, and anticipated outcomes.
- Implementing the plan of care.
- Evaluating the patient's response to the plan of care with periodic assessments.
- Updating the plan of care consistent with the patient's response.
- Discharging the patient at the appropriate time with appropriate after-care instructions.

The American College of Hyperbaric Medicine has a policy on wound care which focuses on the actual care given to the wound. This policy states that it is a physician's duty when caring for a wound to:

> Evaluate the wound, with respect to changes, either beneficial or adverse, in perimeter size or area, depth, presence or absence of necrotic material or drainage, development of granulation tissue (particularly over exposed tendinous structures or bone), odor,

capillary refilling, swelling, presence of arterial pulses, security of suture or staple lines, development of lines of demarcation of ischemic areas, viability of affected areas, successful take of skin grafts or flaps, development of new lesions, and the proper use of dressing materials, as ordered (86).

Accordingly, compliance with the standard of care would encompass all of the foregoing. And for hyperbaric treatment, additional obligations would include:

- Providing a safe hyperbaric chamber with adequately trained staff.
- Developing a proper safety plan.
- Taking measures to reduce and eliminate fire risk.
- Protecting staff and attendants from harm (i.e. avoiding decompression sickness).
- Monitoring the patient after treatment to respond to any adverse reactions to the treatment.

Returning to the example above, a list of questions in evaluating the patient's response to treatment (or lack thereof) could include:

- Was the patient properly assessed, taking into account complicating health issues and diseases?
- Was the patient's nutritional status evaluated, monitored, and maintained?
- Was the appropriate plan of action chosen based on the patient's condition?
- Did the wound care team follow the selected course of treatment or were there unacceptable lapses or deviations?
- Was the patient's continued deterioration properly monitored to allow for a timely re-assessment of the care plan?
- After further evaluation, did the medical team adequately update the plan of care?
- Did the wound fail to improve despite the best efforts of the wound care team?

The truth is that lawsuits happen. Indeed, it is an extraordinary feat in today's climate to complete a medical career without being sued. In the example outlined above, a lawsuit may very well follow after the death of the patient even if a fair assessment of the facts suggests no wrongdoing. Nonetheless, the use of good medical practices and common sense are remarkable tools to reducing legal liability. Most malpractice claims come from carelessness, inattentiveness, and systematic failures of established policies and procedures.

This section will explore ways that will help limit exposure and aid in the defense of a medical malpractice claim. Separate from the standard of care analysis, five themes for reducing liability claims are outlined as follows:

- Proper documentation
- Adequate training
- Effective communication
- Patient privacy
- Informed consent

Documentation

In a lawsuit, the patient's entire medical record generally becomes evidence. It can thereafter be a sword or a shield. It is important that a patient's medical record be accurate and legible, and that it properly document the course of treatment received by the patient. In whatever form the records are organized and maintained, the patient's medical chart should tell a story, and this story should include:

1. The history and symptoms of the patient;
2. The diagnosis;
3. The clinical findings, observations, test results and treatment plan;
4. The treatments rendered;
5. The treatment alternatives and options;
6. The communications with consultants and staff;
7. The communications with the patient and family;
8. The patient's informed consent to treatment;
9. The reasoning for the course of treatment selected;
10. The outcomes and reasoning for changes in course of treatment;
11. The patient's noncompliance and failed appointments; and
12. The advice and instructions given to the patient (87).

Any missing parts in this story could potentially leave the health care provider without a complete explanation of the patient's course of treatment. Additionally, thorough medical records documenting each step of this story will help the physician defend himself in a malpractice action. The documentation in a patient's medical chart reveals the interaction between the health care provider and the patient so that a permanent record of what was done and said is generated. It also shows the course of interactions between members of the health care team and the ongoing progress of patient care. The quality of medical record documentation is a critical factor in the efforts to prevent and control patient injuries, malpractice claims, and malpractice claim losses.

Deficiencies in documentation can have significant consequences. First, patient injuries can occur because of documentation errors and omissions, and illegible entries that preclude physicians and other health care providers from rendering appropriate treatment. Second, in determining whether or not to file a malpractice claim, the patient's attorney will likely scrutinize the medical records for evidence of any inappropriately rendered care. If the records are incomplete, inaccurate, or cannot be deciphered, the attorney may be more likely to pursue a claim. Third, medical records are one of the primary sources of evidence used in deciding whether a physician is liable for malpractice. Incomplete and inaccurate records can be detrimental to the defense of a medical malpractice claim. Sloppy or inappropriate entries can create the impression that the medical care rendered was less than professional.

From a clinical standpoint, missing, illegible, or incomplete records can cause patient care to suffer amid wasted time and resources. Illegible orders can and do lead to treatment errors, such as giving the wrong medication to the patient (88). A lack of correct and timely information can result in poor choices in clinical practice, medication errors, inappropriate repeating of tests, unnecessary referrals, and over-all poor patient outcomes. Referencing back to the earlier discussion, the standard of care requires a physician to record in a patient's medical record all physical examinations performed on that patient, as well as the results and findings from each examination. In defending against a claim of malpractice, the absence of a notation is assumed to mean that the given procedure or examination did not occur. Further, the absence of detailed notes regarding the outcome and findings of an examination makes it more difficult to prove that a subsequently chosen treatment for the patient was justified. The physician is left to describe to the jury, without the benefit of complete documentation, his treatment choices for the patient based on a general and oftentimes vague recollection. Because most medical malpractice lawsuits are filed well after the actual treatment, it is the medical chart that the parties look to for an objective description of facts and events.

Additionally, when dealing with the care of wounds, documentation must be done at regular intervals and should include:

- An accurate assessment of the risk and benefits of treatment;
- A thorough and proper skin evaluation;
- A list of therapies designed to maintain or treat wounds;
- The patient's response to treatment and therapy;
- The rational for the alterations in treatment;
- The outcome of the plan of care.

Thorough and legible documentation is crucial to the defense of a malpractice action as most malpractice actions will necessitate that the physician provide his treatment records. It is also imperative that the physician have an effective document management system that generates and maintains a consistent, legible, accurate, timely, and objective record of events.

Training of Personnel

Wound care and prevention is typically a team effort with responsibilities shared by physicians, nurses, physical and occupational therapists, nutritionists, pharmacists, administrators, patients, and the patient's family. The education and training of these groups is an important aspect of providing safe and effective medical care. In almost every malpractice lawsuit where the patient's treatment involved the interaction of superiors and subordinates, the patient will allege a failure to properly train and supervise. Toward that end, appropriate educational programs that provide current research-based information should be offered at periodic intervals. Of course, it is essential that the nursing and professional staff be properly trained in wound care assessment techniques and wound care.

Establishing minimum qualification requirements, requiring certification and licensure where appropriate, and providing continuing education and periodic in-service presentations are a few examples of acceptable methods of achieving a high level of patient safety. Adopting formal policies and procedures can provide some structure to ensuring compliance with the established expectations. Finally, documentation of educational courses and training seminars will aid in the defense of a claim alleging that the health care team was inadequately trained.

Effective Communications

Effective communications means that the dialog between the patient (and the patient's family) and the health care team is clear, concise, complete, and sincere.

Patients and their families are often struggling with medical treatment decisions. Obviously, many people feel intimidated by their physician and anxious about the clinic environment. It is a given that good communication is crucial to effective patient care. Not only is communication part of good medical practice, it is part of a physician's ethical obligations. The Code of Medical Ethics of the American Medical Association (AMA) at section E-8.12 reads:

> *It is a fundamental ethical requirement that a physician should at all times deal honestly and openly with patients. Patients have a right to know their past and present medical status and to be free of any mistaken beliefs concerning their conditions. Situations occasionally occur in which a patient suffers significant medical complications that may have resulted from the physician's mistake or judgment. In these situations, the physician is ethically required to inform the patient of all the facts necessary to ensure understanding of what has occurred. Only through full disclosure is a patient able to make informed decisions regarding future medical care.*
>
> *Ethical responsibility includes informing patients of changes in their diagnoses resulting from retrospective review of test results or any other information. This obligation holds even though the patient's medical treatment or therapeutic options may not be altered by the new information.*
>
> *Concern regarding legal liability which might result following truthful disclosure should not affect the physician's honesty with a patient (89).*

Additionally, in 2001, Joint Commission on Accreditation of Healthcare Organizations (JCAHO) adopted patient safety standards as part of its National Patient's Safety Goals. One of the enacted patient safety standards requires a hospital to tell a patient about the outcome of care provided to the patient, whether the outcome is good or bad. The health care industry is moving towards health care where communication with patients is necessary and this open communication is being used as a solution to improving patient care, quality, and safety. As this movement continues, at least to some extent, the law and the courts will follow, holding health care providers to their own standards.

It is essential to listen and understand the patient's expectations. Frank and open dialogue is the most important step to properly informing the patient of the risks, benefits, and possible outcomes of a medical procedure. Health care providers have an obligation to fully inform a patient about his condition and his treatment so that the patient can participate in the choices about his/her health care (i.e. informed consent).

The Code of Medical Ethics of the American Medical Association provides that patients have the right to be informed. Section E-8.08 reads:

> *The patient's right of self-decision can be effectively exercised only if the patient possesses enough information to enable an intelligent choice. The patient should make his or her own determination on treatment. The physician's obligation is to present the medical facts accurately to the patient or to the individual responsible for the patient's care and to make recommendations for management*

in accordance with good medical practice. The physician has an ethical obligation to help the patient make choices from among the therapeutic alternatives consistent with good medical practice. Informed consent is a basic social policy for which exceptions are permitted: 1) where the patient is unconscious or otherwise incapable of consenting and harm from failure to treat is imminent or 2) when risk disclosure poses such a serious psychological threat of detriment to the patient as to be medically contraindicated. Social policy does not accept the paternalistic view that the physician may remain silent because divulgence might prompt the patient to forego needed therapy. Rational, informed patients should not be expected to act uniformly, even under similar circumstances, in agreeing to or refusing treatment (90).

The communication process is both an ethical obligation and a legal requirement governed by state law. It also provides an opportunity for physicians to establish rapport and engage patients in making decisions about their own care. It can also protect the provider from potential malpractice claims.

Protection of Patient Privacy

The information disclosed to a physician and other members of the health care team during the course of treatment is confidential and must always be recognized as such. While providers clearly appreciate the importance of patient confidentiality, this principal is sometimes forgotten in the lunchroom or around the water cooler. Speaking from an uninformed position can be devastating to a patient or family members and can lead to unfounded claims of malpractice.

The patient should feel free to make a full disclosure of information to the health care team. However, gossip, unfounded information, and unconfirmed comments about a patient's care and treatment are inappropriate.

Hospitals and other health care providers are required to maintain the privacy of a patient's health information ("protected health information" or "PHI"). In addition to certain state laws and facility policies, the privacy rules of the Health Insurance Portability and Accountability Act of 1996 ("HIPAA") (91) impose an obligation on certain "covered entities" to maintain the confidentiality of individually identifiable health information. PHI includes information that relates to a patient's past, present, or future condition and includes mental health.

Generally, under HIPAA, a "covered entity" may not release a person's PHI without a patient's express written authorization (92). HIPAA allows for either the patient or a "personal representative," or a person legally authorized to make health care decisions on behalf of the patient, to authorize the release of information (93).

In addition to the HIPAA rules and penalties for violations, the majority of states allow for a private cause of action against a health care provider who impermissibly discloses confidential health information (94). Although it varies from state to state, a claim for such a cause of action is typically couched as an action for breach of contract, malpractice, breach of fiduciary duty, fraud or misrepresentation, or as a breach of an applicable civil statute providing for damages (95). Lastly, the impermissible disclosure of a patient's health information may result in professional disciplinary action.

Informed Consent to Treat

Informed consent is a medical-legal principle that is defined as the consent to treatment obtained after adequate disclosure. The concept of informed consent is simple in theory but complex in actual practice. In broad terms, providing sufficient information to allow the patient to make an informed decision should include the following items: 1) the differential diagnosis; 2) a description of the purpose and nature of the proposed treatment or procedure; 3) the risks associated with the treatment; 4) the benefits and expected outcomes of the proposed treatment; 5) any reasonable alternatives and their associated risks and benefits; and 6) the risks and consequences of no treatment (96). Informed consent is thus the process by which a fully informed patient can participate in choices about his or her health care. The obligation to obtain informed consent originates from both the legal and ethical right the patient has to direct what happens to his or her body and from the ethical duty of the physician to involve the patient in his or her health care. Informed consent is thus more than simply getting a patient to sign a written consent form. It is a process of communication between a patient and physician that results in the patient's authorization or agreement to undergo a specific medical intervention.

The American Medical Association's policy on informed consent (Policy E-8.08 Informed Consent) states:

> *The patient's right of self-decision can be effectively exercised only if the patient possesses enough information to enable an intelligent choice. The patient should make his or her own determination on treatment. The physician's obligation is to present the medical facts accurately to the patient or to the individual responsible for the patient's care and to make recommendations for management in accordance with good medical practice. The physician has an ethical obligation to help the patient make choices from among the therapeutic alternatives consistent with good medical practice. Informed consent is a basic social policy for which exceptions are permitted: 1) where the patient is unconscious or otherwise incapable of consenting and harm from failure to treat is imminent or 2) when risk disclosure poses such a serious psychological threat of detriment to the patient as to be medically contraindicated. Social policy does not accept the paternalistic view that the physician may remain silent because divulgence might prompt the patient to forego needed therapy. Rational, informed patients should not be expected to act uniformly, even under similar circumstances, in agreeing to or refusing treatment. (I, II, III, IV, V) (97).*

Notwithstanding this policy, there are limits on the need and the ability to obtain informed consent. Of course, consent may only be obtained by someone who has capacity. Each jurisdiction has a surrogate or alternate decision making scheme, either by statute or adopted by courts that explains who else, other than the patient, may consent to treatment when the patient lacks the ability to consent (98). Other common limitations to the requirement to obtain informed consent are: when the information is reasonably within the patient's common knowledge; when the patient already is aware of the withheld fact; when an emergency situation arises where immediate treatment is required; where disclosure would "foreclose rational decision" or "pose psychological damage" to the patient (the "therapeutic privilege"); and theoretically, at least, where the patient has waived the right to consent or has refused information (99).

To minimize liability, although not necessarily dispositive on the issue of failure to inform, the physician should ensure that the patient's medical records contain a properly executed informed consent form. As one scholar noted, "...a [signed consent] form is powerful evidence of a physician's compliance with the duty to disclose, but is irrelevant to an ordinary malpractice action brought against a physician for delivering substandard care (100)."

The theory on which legal malpractice recovery may be obtained in a failure to obtain informed consent scenario is that of negligence in failing to disclose the risks or hazards that could have influenced a reasonable person in making a decision to give or withhold consent. In some jurisdictions, the failure to obtain the consent to treat a patient may be considered a civil assault. States vary in their requirements of informed consent, and in some states common law governs while in others the requirements are codified by statute. A common inquiry in a suit alleging failure to obtain informed consent is: by what standard is the information given or withheld to be judged? The prevailing rule is the "reasonable person standard." Here, the adequacy of the consent is measured by the disclosure of information which would influence a reasonable person in deciding whether to consent to a recommended medical procedure. A small majority of states employ a "professional standard" where the standard is governed by what a reasonable physician would have disclosed under the circumstances, while a few states use a "patient standard" of informed consent, which ask subjectively: what would the particular patient need to know and understand in order to make an informed decision (101)?

A frank and open dialogue with the patient is the most important step in the informed consent process, providing an opportunity for the physician to establish rapport and engage the patient in making decisions about his or her own care. The discussion should emphasize that the physician-patient relationship operates as a team in the decision-making process. Additionally it is worth noting that effective discussions with the patient should take place before the patient is admitted to the hospital, when time and opportunity permit. Also, patients are typically in a heightened emotional state. In addition to not feeling well, they probably are experiencing a great deal of anxiety about an upcoming procedure. The physician who sits down with patients to discuss the patient's treatment plan displays a caring and concerned attitude and shows a willingness to spend adequate time to ensure that the patient's questions and concerns are addressed. The physician should use descriptive, unsophisticated terminology to ensure the patient understands complicated medical procedures. Repetition of key phrases and then asking the patient to repeat the key information is an effective way to ensure effective understanding. Drawing diagrams is effective, when appropriate.

When a recommended course of treatment is rejected by a patient, the medical chart should so reflect. In this circumstance it is crucial that the chart document the fact that the patient has received adequate information stressing the importance of compliance. In most instances, clinical institutions have adopted specific consent forms that provide written information to help patients remember the risks, benefits, and alternatives that have been discussed with them. These forms serve as a statement of the disclosure to the patient should the treating physician ever need to establish a defense against an allegation of medical malpractice based on lack of consent to treat. As is the case with all patient interactions, the informed consent process should also be documented in the patient's medical record. Separate from the use of any pre-printed forms, physicians should consider making a notation in the medical chart confirming their discussion and disclosures to the patient. A sample notation in the chart might read:

> Advised patient of need for ________ due to ________. Discussed risks, benefits, and alternatives. Gave _______ handout. Patient stated he/she understood, signed consent, and agreed to proceed. It is my judgment that the patient understands the treatment plan.

ACCEPTED INDICATIONS AND OFF-LABEL USE OF HYPERBARIC CHAMBERS

Using a hyperbaric chamber for a non-approved indication, while prudent in some cases, may increase liability exposure. The Committee on Hyperbaric Oxygen Therapy of the Undersea and Hyperbaric Medical Society has published approved indications for hyperbaric chambers. Those are:

- Air or gas embolism
- Carbon monoxide poisoning and smoke inhalation; Carbon monoxide poisoning complicated by cyanide poisoning
- Clostridial myositis and myonecrosis (Gas gangrene)
- Crush injury, compartment syndrome, and other acute traumatic ischemia
- Decompression sickness
- Exceptional blood loss (anemia)
- Intracranial abscess, Actinomycosis
- Necrotizing soft tissue infections
- Osteomyelitis (refractory)
- Delayed radiation injury (soft tissue and bony necrosis)
- Skin grafts and flaps (compromised)
- Thermal burns (103)

There is a corresponding list of absolute and relative contraindications, published by Merck in "The Merck Manual of Diagnosis and Therapy, § 21, Ch. 292 (104). The Federal Drug Administration (the "FDA") is the organization in the government that approves drugs and devices and which approves indications of use for a given drug or device. A hyperbaric chamber is a medical device. When a medical device is used for a condition that is outside the FDA's approved uses and not set forth in the product's labeling materials, this is known as "off-label use (105)." Much controversy surrounds the prudence of off-label use. Courts and the public at large may view off-label use of a medical device as risky, and accordingly, it may open the door to liability (106). On the other hand, the very means by which a device comes to have a list of indicated uses is not the end of what a physician should use a given device for, as it is implicit in "the practice of medicine" that a physician has discretion regarding what drug or device to use to treat a given condition (107). Off-label use is widespread, and at times, may actually control the standard of care as being an essential treatment (108).

Lastly, off-label uses have become standard in many instances, compromising mainstream, legitimate medical practice (109).

Like the off-label use of any medical device, the off-label use of a hyperbaric chamber is a matter of medical judgment, and accordingly, opens a physician up to professional liability for the exercise of her professional judgment (110). Informed consent, as discussed, can validate a departure from customary practice (111). Under common law, off-label use is not per se negligent, and the standard of care of off-label use is typically shown by evidence of relevant medical standards (112). The American Medical Association, via a trustee, stated at a U.S. Senate Committee meeting its policy on off-label use: "In some instances, prescribing a product off-label is the most appropriate therapy based on the latest, best scientific evidence - and, in some patient populations, it may be the only treatment option (113)." And, the AMA's policy statement on Patient Access to Treatments Prescribed by Their Physicians incorporates off-label use, stating: "The AMA confirms its strong support for the autonomous clinical decision-making authority of a physician and that a physician may lawfully use an FDA approved drug product or medical device for an unlabeled indication when such use is based upon sound scientific evidence and sound medical opinion (114)."

When a physician contemplates a truly novel use for a hyperbaric chamber, thus rendering the risk of such treatment and potential benefits uncertain, ethics and law require that the patient be informed of the novel use for the hyperbaric chamber (115). A leading ethical scholar notes, "If the protocol involves innovative therapy, the physician-investigator may be held liable for failure to negotiate informed consent merely by virtue of having failed to explain that the procedure used represented a departure from customary practice (116)." Conversely, general principals of informed consent do not require a physician to explain all known risks, and in most states, disclosure of risks is governed by their "materiality to the patient's decision (117)." And, it is generally not required that a physician explain the regulatory status of a medical device to his patient, as this is considered disclosure of non-medical information (118).

Off-label use gives rise to the delicate balance between two competing forces—the regulatory objective of protecting patients from unsafe or ineffective medical devices and the physician's right to use professional judgment in treating patients (119). In the midst of this delicate balance, a few certainties about the law related to off-label use exist. First, off-label use of a medical device does not violate FDA Law (120). Second, the mere fact that a physician is using a medical device off-label does not, by itself, constitute malpractice (121). In fact, as a Tennessee court of appeals observed, "Because the pace of medical discovery runs ahead of the FDA's regulatory machinery, the off-label use of some drugs is frequently considered to be 'state-of-the-art' treatment. In some circumstances, an off-label use of a particular...device may even define the standard of care (122)." In this conundrum, it follows that off-label prescribing bears an inherent liability risk (123).

Strategies for minimizing liability exposure when using a hyperbaric chamber for an off-label use include:

- Fully disclosure the benefits and risks to the patient (124); and

- Using a hyperbaric chamber for an off label indication when the potential benefit to the patient outweighs the unapproved status of a particular use (125).

Although most courts that have addressed this issue have held that physicians are not required to inform the patient that a particular treatment is off-label as it relates to informed consent, the better practice is to disclose when a treatment is off-label, explaining why it is the physician's belief that the benefits of the treatment outweigh any potential risks (126).

CONCLUSION

It is vitally important for health care providers to timely recognize and identify problems and risks to the patient. As with any other aspect of patient care, the key to reducing liability is to practice competent medicine, understand where risks are likely to arise, and be proactive in reducing or eliminating those risks where possible. These rules apply to all of the health care facilities' policies and practices, from administration to direct patient care. With respect to wound care, an institution should first establish proper procedures for wound assessment, prevention, and treatment. Next, the health care provider should ensure that its staff knows and follows the policies and procedures. Finally, the providers of care must thoroughly document treatment and properly communicate with a patient regarding treatment. Honest, open, and competent approaches to medical care will reduce liability and assist with a successful defense if a lawsuit is filed.

REFERENCES

1. Only one in eight preventable medical errors that occur in hospitals results in a malpractice claim. Harvard Medical Practice Study, 324 *N Engl Med J* 370, 370-396 (1991).
2. Jury Verdict Research averaged jury verdicts for the past six years and determined that patients won 34% of the time in actions against health care providers. *www.justaskourdoctors.com/statistics-detail.asp?id=15*, last visited on July 18, 2006.
3. Rice Berkeley, Do Doctors Kill 80,000 Patients a Year? Medical Economics. 1994; 71:46-56. See also "To Err is Human: Building a Super Health System" which estimates that the number of American deaths due to medical error is much higher, at 98,000, Linda T. Kohn, et al., Committee on Quality of Health Care in America, Institute of Medicine, 2000.
4. The National Practitioner Data Bank, an organization created by the Health Care Quality Improvement Act of 1986, records malpractice payments made by individual practitioners and provides statistics on these payments. *http://www.npdb-hipdb.com/pubs/stats/2004_NPDB_Annual_Report.pdf*, accessed on July 21, 2006.
5. Hall, Mark A., et al., *Health Care Law and Ethics* 6d, § 267.
6. I.D.
7. As discuss, infra, health care providers can be sued under different theories of liability including battery, breach of contract, or misrepresentation. Actions that question the professional judgment of the provider is usually defined in terms of negligent conduct.
8. The term "medical malpractice" comes from mala praxis which was a legal concept defined as "neglect or unskillful management" in violation of the trust placed in that practitioner. Mohr James C. "American Medical Malpractice Litigation in Historical Perspective." *JAMA* 2000;283:1731-1737.
9. Dietz, Lasura Hunter, et al., American Jurisprudence, 61 Am.Jr. 2d Physicians, Surgeons, Etc. §189 (May 2006).
10. Dietz, Lasura Hunter, et al., American Jurisprudence, 61 Am.Jr. 2d Physicians, Surgeons, Etc. §318 (May 2006).
11. Dietz, Lasura Hunter, et al., American Jurisprudence, 61 Am.Jr. 2d Physicians, Surgeons, Etc. §185 (May 2006).
12. Dietz, Lasura Hunter, et al., American Jurisprudence, 61 Am.Jr. 2d Physicians, Surgeons, Etc. §186 (May 2006).
13. Emergency Medical Treatment and Active Labor Act (EMTALA), 42 U.S.C. § 1395dd.
14. Dietz, Lasura Hunter, et al., American Jurisprudence, 61 Am.Jr. 2d Physicians, Surgeons, Etc. §189 (May 2006).
15. Dietz, Lasura Hunter, et al., American Jurisprudence, 61 Am.Jr. 2d Physicians, Surgeons, Etc. §189 (May 2006).
16. Dietz, Lasura Hunter, et al., American Jurisprudence, 61 Am.Jr. 2d Physicians, Surgeons, Etc. §191 (May 2006).
17. Dietz, Lasura Hunter, et al., American Jurisprudence, 61 Am.Jr. 2d Physicians, Surgeons, Etc. §192 (May 2006).
18. Dietz, Lasura Hunter, et al., American Jurisprudence, 61 Am.Jr. 2d Physicians, Surgeons, Etc. §191 (May 2006).
19. The Bureau of Justice Statistics report that punitive damages are awarded in less than 1 percent of medical malpractice cases. (1996).
20. Shipley, W.E., 13 A.L.R.2d 11.
21. Shipley, W.E., 13 A.L.R.2d 11.
22. Dietz, Laura Hunter, et al., 57A Am Jur. 2d Negligence §415 (May 2006).

23. Dietz, Laura Hunter, et al., 57A Am Jur. 2d Negligence §415 (May 2006).
24. Dietz, Laura Hunter, et al., 57A Am Jur. 2d Negligence §412 (May 2006).
25. For cases similar which discuss the "loss of chance" theory of causation, see *Herskovits v. Group Health Coopratíve of Puget Sound*, 664 P.2d 474 (Waxh. 1983); and *Hicks v. United States*, 368 F.2d 626 (4th Cir. 1966).
26. Dietz, Laura Hunter, et al., 61 Am. Jur. 2d Physicians, Surgeons, Etc., §308 (May 2006).
27. Dietz, Laura Hunter, et al., 61 Am. Jur. 2d Physicians, Surgeons, Etc., §759 (May 2006).
28. Dietz, Laura Hunter, et al., 61 Am. Jur. 2d Physicians, Surgeons, Etc., §777 (May 2006).
29. Dietz, Laura Hunter, et al., 61 Am. Jur. 2d Physicians, Surgeons, Etc., §797 (May 2006).
30. Dietz, Laura Hunter, et al., 61 Am. Jur. 2d Physicians, Surgeons, Etc., §797 (May 2006).
31. Dietz, Laura Hunter, et al., 61 Am. Jur. 2d Physicians, Surgeons, Etc., §769 (May 2006).
32. Dietz, Laura Hunter, et al., 61 Am. Jur. 2d Physicians, Surgeons, Etc., §806 (May 2006).
33. Dietz, Laura Hunter, et al., 61 Am. Jur. 2d Physicians, Surgeons, Etc., §810 (May 2006).
34. Dietz, Laura Hunter, et al., 61 Am. Jur. 2d Physicians, Surgeons, Etc., §994 (May 2006).
35. Dietz, Laura Hunter, et al., 61 Am. Jur. 2d Physicians, Surgeons, Etc., §891-892, 895 (May 2006).
36. Dietz, Laura Hunter, et al., 61 Am. Jur. 2d Physicians, Surgeons, Etc., §890 (May 2006).
37. Dietz, Laura Hunter, et al., 61 Am. Jur. 2d Physicians, Surgeons, Etc., §284 (May 2006).
38. Dietz, Laura Hunter, et al., 61 Am. Jur. 2d Physicians, Surgeons, Etc., §284 (May 2006).
39. Hall, Mark A., et al., *Health Care Law and Ethics* 6d, at 418.
40. Hodson, John D., 51 A.L.R.4th 235 (2006).
41. Hodson, John D., 51 A.L.R.4th 235 (2006).
42. Castelaz, Kimberly, et al., 63 Am. Jur. 2d Product Liaibility §77 (May 2006).
43. Castelaz, Kimberly, et al., 63 Am. Jur. 2d Product Liaibility §3 (May 2006).
44. Castelaz, Kimberly, et al., 63 Am. Jur. 2d Product Liaibility §1 (May 2006).
45. E.g. Castelaz, Kimberly, et al., 63 Am. Jur. 2d Product Liaibility §3 (May 2006).
46. Catelaz, Kimberly, et al., 63 Am. Jur. 2d §4, 19 (May 2006).
47. Castelaz, Kimberly, et al., 63 Am. Jur. 2d Product Liaibility §204 (May 2006).
48. Castelaz, Kimberly, et al., 63 Am. Jur. 2d Product Liaibility §205 (May 2006).
49. Castelaz, Kimberly, et al., 63 Am. Jur. 2d Product Liaibility §558 (May 2006).
50. Castelaz, Kimberly, et al., 63 Am. Jur. 2d Product Liaibility §559 (May 2006).
51. Castelaz, Kimberly, et al., 63 Am. Jur. 2d Product Liaibility §659 (May 2006).
52. Castelaz, Kimberly, et al., 63 Am. Jur. 2d Product Liaibility §659 (May 2006).
53. Sharp, Linda A., 65 A.L.R. 357 (1999). As of date of this publication, there are no reported cases on a finding of liablity based on strict products liablity with respect to a medical instrument, and the majority of courts that have exmaponed liablity for a breach of warranty case have found that a breacy of warrantly cause of action is not applicable. See Id.
54. Sharp, Linda A., 65 A.L.R. 357 (1999).
55. Sharp, Linda A., 65 A.L.R. 357 (1999).
56. Castelaz, Kimberly, et al., 63 Am. Jur. 2d Product Liaibility §885 (May 2006), internal citations ommitted.
57. Castelaz, Kimberly, et al., 63 Am. Jur. 2d Product Liaibility §886 (May 2006).
58. Castelaz, Kimberly, et al., 63 Am. Jur. 2d Product Liaibility §900 (May 2006).
59. Castelaz, Kimberly, et al., 63 Am. Jur. 2d Product Liaibility §905 (May 2006), internal citation ommited.

60. 687 So.2d 258 (Fl.Dist. Ct. of App.—1st Dist. 1997).
61. Note that a topical hyperbaric chamber for in-home use is a wholly separate and different medical device from a "hyperbaric chamber." It is included in this chapter as an illustration because there are so few reported cases involving "hyperbaric chambers."
62. 753 N.E.2d 1085 (Ill. Ct. App—5th Dist., 2001).
63. Id.
64. Id.
65. *Hood v. Phillips* (Tex. Civ. App. 1976) 537 S.W.2d 291, error granted, affirmed 554 S.W.2d 160.
66. Rosson v. Coburn, 876 P.2d 731, 734 n.6 (Okla. Ct. App. 1994), quoting Black's Law Dictionary at 153 (6th ed. 1990).
67. For a more comprehensive overview of medical device law, including labeling, advertising, and reporting requirements, see *http://www.usdoj.gov/usao/eousa/foia_reading_room/usam/title4/civ00110.htm*, last visited August 8, 2006; see generally *http://www.fda.gov/cdrh/*, last visited August 8, 2006.
68. A medical device is: an instrument, apparatus, implement, machine, contrivance, implant, in vitro reagent, or other similar or related article, including any component, part, or accessory, which is -

    1) recognized in the official National Formulary, or the United States Pharmacopeia, or any supplement to them,

    2) intended for use in the diagnosis of disease or other conditions, or in the cure, mitigation, treatment, or prevention of disease in man or other animals, or

    3) intended to affect the structure or any function of the body of man or other animals, and which does not achieve its primary intended purposes through chemical action within or on the body of man or other animals and which is not dependent upon being metabolized for the achievement of its primary intended purposes. FDCA, 21 U.S.C. §321(h).
69. The definition of "device" is similar to the definition of "drug," the key distinction being that devices do not work primarily through chemical action or by being metabolized. See Federal Food, Drug, and Cosmetic Act; 21 U.S.C. §321(h).
70. Edward M. Basile, et al., *Medical device Labeling and Advertising: An Overview*, 54 Food Drug L.J. 519 (1999).
71. For a detailed discussion of the laws regulating medical devices see Edward M. Basile, et al., *Medical device Labeling and Advertising: An Overview* 54 Food Drug L.J. 519 (1999).
72. Pub. L. No. 87-781, 76 Stat. 780 (codified as amended 21 U.S.C. §§ 301 et seq. (1994)).
73. Pub. L. No. 94-295, 90 Stat. 539 (codified at 15 U.S.C. § 55 (1994); 21 U.S.C. §§ 31, 331, 334, 351, 352, 358, 360, 360c-k, 374m 379, 379a, 381).
74. Pub. L. No. 101-629, 104 Stat. 4511 (codified at 21 U.S.C. §§ 301 note, 321, 331, 334, 346a, 352-353, 360, 360c, 360c note, 360d-I, 360i note, 360j, 360j note, 360l, 360gg-hh note, 360ii-ss, 383, 383 note, 42 U.S.C. §§ 263b-n (1994)).
75. Pub. L. No. 101-629, 104 Stat. 4511 (codified at 21 U.S.C. §§ 301 note, 321, 333, 333 note, 351, 353, 360, 360c, 360c note, 360d-I, 360 note, 360j, 360j note, 360l, 360gg-hh, 360 hh note, 360ii-ss, 383, 383 note; 42 U.S.C. §§ 263b-n (1994)).
76. Pub. L. 107-250, 116 Sat. 1588 (codified at 21 U.S.C. § § 301 note, 379i and 379j, 352 note, 360e note, 360j note, 360l note, 379i note, 379j, note (2002).
77. Smith, John J., *Physician Modification of Legally Marked Medical Devices: Regulatory Implications Under the Federal Food, Drug, and Cosmetic Act*, 55 Food Drug L.J. 245, 245 (2000).
78. Smith, John J., *Physician Modification of Legally Marked Medical Devices: Regulatory Implications Under the Federal Food, Drug, and Cosmetic Act*, 55 Food Drug L.J. 245, 245 (2000). Although the FDA lacks authority to regulate the practice of medicine, it does regulate the manufacturing and marketing of products.

79. Smith, John J., *Physician Modification of Legally Marked Medical Devices: Regulatory Implications Under the Federal Food, Drug, and Cosmetic Act*, 55 Food Drug L.J. 245, 251 (2000). The doctrine is codified in the FDCA and in relevant part states, "Nothing in this Chapter shall be construed to limit or interfere with the authority of a health care practitioner to prescribe or administer any legally marketed device to a patient for any condition or disease within a legitimate health are practitioner-patient relationship." 21 U.S.C. § 396.

80. Smith, John J., *Physician Modification of Legally Marked Medical Devices: Regulatory Implications Under the Federal Food, Drug, and Cosmetic Act*, 55 Food Drug L.J. 245, 251 (2000).

81. More information can be obtained at the Department of Justice's website at *http://www.usdoj.gov/usao/eousa/foia_reading_room/usam/title4/civ00110.htm*. Last visited August 8, 2006. A hyperbaric chamber is classified as a ""Class II" device and is considered an anesthesiology and therapeutic device. 21 C.F.R. 868.5470.

82. Information on Premarket Approval Applications, *https://www.fda.gov/cdrh/pmapage.html*, last visitied August 10, 2006.

83. Device Advice, *http://www.fda.gov.cdrh/devadvice/3132.html*, last visited August 10, 2006.

84. Product classification Database, *http://accessdata.fda.gov/scripts/cdrh/cfdocs/cfPCD/classificaiton.cfm?ID=98*, last visitied August 10, 2006.

85. Device Advice, *http://www.fda.gov.cdrh/devadvice/3132.html*, last visited August 10, 2006.

86. Device Advice, *http://www.fda.gov.cdrh/devadvice/3132.html*, last visited August 10, 2006.

87. Available at *http://www.hyperbaricmedicine.org/cpt%2099183.htm*, last visited August 8, 2006.

88. Hall, Mark A., et al., *Health Care Law and Ethics* 6d, page 326.

89. A Texas cardiologist was held liable for a fatal medication mix-up caused by the enduring problem of bad handwriting. A jury found Ramachandra Kolluru, MD, responsible for the death of Ramon Vasquez, who died from an apparent heart attack after taking the wrong medication at eight times the recommended dosage. (Vasquez v. Albertson's, Inc., No. A-103,042 (Tex., Ector County Dist. Ct, Oct. 19, 1999).)

90. AMA Opinions on Practice Matters; E-8.12 Patient Information; issued March 1981; updated June 1994.

91. AMA Opinions on Practice Matters; E-8.08 Informed Consent; issued March 1981.

92. 45 CFR §164.500 et seq.

93. Id.

94. 45 C.F.R. 164.502(g); OCR Privacy Brief / Summary of the HIPAA Privacy Rule, HIPAA Compliance Assistance, United Stated Department of Health and Human Services, page 16, available at *http://www.hhs.gov/ocr/privacysummary.pdf*, last visited August 8, 2006.

95. Hall, Mark A., et al., *Health Care Law and Ethics* 6d, page 168.

96. Hall, Mark A., et al., *Health Care Law and Ethics* 6d, page 169.

97. Beck, James M and Azari, Elizabeth D, *FDA, Off-Label Use, and Informed Consent: Debunking Myths and Misconceptions*, 33 Food Drug L.J. 71, 88 (1998); Lars, Noah, et al., *Informed Consent and the Elusive Dichotomy Between Standard and Experimental Therapy*, 28 Am J. L. and Med. 361, 365 (2002).

98. Issued March 1981. Available at *http://www.ama-ssn.org*, last visited August 8, 2006.

99. Hall, Mark A., et al., *Health Care Law and Ethics* 6d, at 207.

100. Hall, Mark A., et al., *Health Care Law and Ethics* 6d, at 207-208.

101. Hall, Mark A., et al., *Health Care Law and Ethics* 6d, at 209.

102. Lars, Noah, et al., *Informed Consent and the Elusive Dichotomy Between Standard and Experimental Therapy*, 28 Am J. L. and Med. 361, 366-367(2002).

103. The American College of Hyperbaric Medicine's website contains a compensative list of a physician's duty in hyperbaric medicine, which is available at *http://www.hyperbaricmedicine.org/cpt%2099183.htm*, last visited August 8, 2006.

104. Hyperbaric Oxygen 2003: Indications and Results - Hyperbaric Oxygen Therapy Committee Report (June 2003), in relevant part, available at: *http://www.uhms.org/Indications/indications.htm*, last visited August 8, 2006; see also American College of Hyperbaric Medicine, *http://www.hyperbaricmedicine.org/Preferred%20Protocols.htm*, last visited August 7, 2006; see also The Merck Manual of Diagnosis and Therapy, § 21 Special Subjects, Ch. 292. Hyperbaric Oxygen Therapy, available at *http://www.merck.com/mrkshared/mmanual/section21/chapter292/292b.jsp* last visited August 7, 2006.

105. Available at *http://www.merck.com/mrkshared/mmanual/section21/chapter292/292c.jsp*

106. Device Labeling Guidance, FDA Guidance Doc. No. G-91-1. pt III May 8, 1991, available at *http://www.fda.gov/cdrh/g91-1.html*, last visited August 10, 2006; *Washington Legal Foundation v. Kessler*, 880 F.Supp. 26 (D.D.C. 1995). The characterization of a use as "off-label" signifies a regulatory description and is not a legal status or a medical fact; e.g., Beck, James M and Azari, Elizabeth D, *FDA, Off-Label Use, and Informed Consent: Debunking Myths and Misconceptions*, 33 Food Drug L.J. 71 (1998).

107. Beck, James M and Azari, Elizabeth D, *FDA, Off-Label Use, and Informed Consent: Debunking Myths and Misconceptions*, 33 Food Drug L.J. 71, 83 (1998). Certain scholars have indicated that the designation of "off-label use" simply means that the FDA is silent on a given indication. Id.

108. Id.

109. Id.

110. Henry, Veronica, *Off-Label Prescribing: Legal Implications*, J. Legal Med. 20: 365-384 (Sept. 1999).

111. Beck, James M and Azari, Elizabeth D, *FDA, Off-Label Use, and Informed Consent: Debunking Myths and Misconceptions*, 33 Food Drug L.J. 71, 88.

112. Hall, Mark A., et al., *Health Care Law and Ethics* 6d, at 209.

113. Henry, Veronica, *Off-Label Prescribing: Legal Implications*, J. Legal Med. 20: 365-384 (Sept. 1999).

114. AMA Trustee Cecil B. Wilson, MD, March 3, 2005, U.S. Senate Committee on Health, Education, Labor and Pensions, available at *http://www.ama-assn.org/ama/pub/category/14777.html*, last visited August 7, 2006, entitled *AMA Testifies at Senate Drug Safety Hearing*.

115. Policy H-120.988, available at *http://www.ama-assn.org*, last visited August 7, 2006.

116. Beck, James M and Azari, Elizabeth D, *FDA, Off-Label Use, and Informed Consent: Debunking Myths and Misconceptions*, 33 Food Drug L.J. 71, 89 (1998).

117. Levine, Robert, Ethics and Regulation of Clinical Research 241 (2d ed. 1986); see also Beck, James M and Azari, Elizabeth D, *FDA, Off-Label Use, and Informed Consent: Debunking Myths and Misconceptions*, 33 Food Drug L.J. 71, 89.

118. Beck, James M and Azari, Elizabeth D, *FDA, Off-Label Use, and Informed Consent: Debunking Myths and Misconceptions*, 33 Food Drug L.J. 71, 90 (1998). Mr. Beck writes, "A patient's interest in informed consent 'does not place upon the physician duty to elucidate upon all of the possible risks, but only those of a serious nature...The law does not contemplate that a doctor need conduct a short course in anatomy, medicine, surgery, and therapeutics.'" at 90

119. Beck, James M and Azari, Elizabeth D, *FDA, Off-Label Use, and Informed Consent: Debunking Myths and Misconceptions*, 33 Food Drug L.J. 71, 90 (1998).

120. Maxwell, Mehlman, J., Off Label Prescribing, May, 2005, available at *http://www.thedoctorwillseeyounow.com/articles/bioethics/offlabel_11/*, last visited August 8, 2006.

121. Maxwell, Mehlman, J., Off Label Prescribing, May, 2005, available at *http://www.thedoctorwillseeyounow.com/articles/bioethics/offlabel_11/*, last visited August 8, 2006, citing Buckman Co. v. Plaintiffs' Legal Comm., 531 U.S. 341, 350 (2001), stating that "off-label usage of medical devices (use of a device for some other purpose than that for which it has been approved by the FDA) is an accepted and necessary corollary of the FDA's mission to regulate in this area without directly interfering with the practice of medicine."

122. Maxwell, Mehlman, J., *Off Label Prescribing*, May, 2005, available at *http://www.thedoctorwillseeyounow.com/articles/bioethics/offlabel_11/* last visited August 8, 2006, citing Fernite v. Abbot Northwester Hospital, 568, N.W.2d 535, 542 (Minn. Ct. App. 1997.

123. Maxwell, Mehlman, J., Off Label Prescribing, May, 2005, available at *http://www.thedoctorwillseeyounow.com/articles/bioethics/offlabel_11/* last visited August 8, 2006, citing Richardson v. Miller, 44 S.W.3d 1, 13, N.11 (Tenn. Ct. App. 2000),

124. Maxwell, Mehlman, J., Off Label Prescribing, May, 2005, available at *http://www.thedoctorwillseeyounow.com/articles/bioethics/offlabel_11/* last visited August 8, 2006.

125. An overview of adverse effects of HBO2 is available at The Merck Manual of Diagnosis and Therapy, § 21, Ch. 292, available at *http://www.merck.com/mrkshared/mmanual/section21/chapter292/292c.jsp* last visited August 8, 2006.

126. Maxwell, Mehlman, J., Off Label Prescribing, May, 2005, available at *http://www.thedoctorwillseeyounow.com/articles/bioethics/offlabel_11/* last visited August 8, 2006.

127. Maxwell, Mehlman, J., Off Label Prescribing, May, 2005, available at *http://www.thedoctorwillseeyounow.com/articles/bioethics/offlabel_11/* last visited August 8, 2006.

REVIEW QUESTIONS

1.) All of the following statements concerning a medical malpractice lawsuit are true EXCEPT:
   a. A malpractice claim is based on the legal concept of negligence.
   b. To prevail, the plaintiff must prove that the health care provider's treatment deviated from the accepted standard of care.
   c. There are five (5) essential elements of a cause of action in a medical malpractice case.
   d. It is typically necessary for the plaintiff to establish negligence through a medical expert.

2.) Proper medical documentation should be done at regular intervals and should at a minimum include which of the following:
   a. A risk assessment and skin evaluation.
   b. The patient's response to the treatment and therapy.
   c. The rationale for the alterations in treatment.
   d. All of the above.

3.) All of the following are opportunities to limit exposure to legal liability EXCEPT:
   a. Fully disclosing risks and benefits of treatment with the patient.
   b. Utilizing a hyperbaric chamber for a novel, untested, or experimental procedure without the patient's consent.
   c. Thoroughly examining and documenting the patient's wound.
   d. Closely monitoring treatment and making appropriate and timely adjustments to treatment.

4.) Using a hyperbaric chamber for an "off-label" purpose will always result in a finding of medical malpractice.
   a. True.
   b. False.

5.) Which of the following statements is TRUE:
   a. A plaintiff has five (5) years from the date of injury in which to bring a medical malpractice action.
   b. Expert testimony is generally required to prove or to defend against a medical malpractice case
   c. The obligation to obtain the consent to treat a patient is satisfied by simply having the patient sign the appropriate written consent form at the hospital.
   d. Once the staff has been trained, it is not necessary to re-evaluate staff members or to have comprehensive safety controls in place.

Answers: 1c, 2d, 3b, 4b, 5b.

Section 6
Healthcare Delivery

CHAPTER 43

DEVELOPMENT OF A COMPREHENSIVE WOUND CARE CENTER

CHAPTER FORTY-THREE OVERVIEW

NOTES

Development of a Comprehensive Wound Care Center

Rudy C. Pruneda, Paul J. Sheffield

INTRODUCTION

The American population is shifting dramatically to increase the number of persons over the age of 65. Today there are over 34 million Americans age 65 and over, or 13% of all Americans. By the year 2030, 69 million Americans, or 20% of all Americans will be age 65 and over (1). The epidemiology of aging has demonstrated that the elderly become compromised in their healing ability due to lack of proper nutrition, circulation, immunity, diabetes, and the side effects of certain medical treatments such as irradiation for carcinoma. Ageing changes the overall wound healing potential for elders and creates a major problem for those who suffer from pressure ulcers, venous stasis ulcers, and skin tears (2). These wounds are difficult to manage for both patients and clinicians.

Diabetes has become a global healthcare problem with November 15 being designated as World Diabetes Day. In 2003 the global prevalence of diabetes was estimated at 194 million (3). In the United States, there are currently an estimated 16 million diagnosed diabetics, or 6% of the U.S. adult population (4). Many experts feel this number represents only one third of the actual number. Approximately 15% of all diabetics will develop a foot ulcer in their lifetime. Minorities, especially Afro-Americans, Hispanics, and Native Americans, suffer more serious consequences from diabetes, including loss of vision, kidney function, and amputations (5). Cost to the American health care system has been estimated to be $1.5 billion per year.

Most of the amputations start from a diabetic foot ulcer. The incidence of lower leg amputation is estimated to be 5-25/100,000 inhabitants/year, but in diabetics it is 6-8/1,000 inhabitants/year (3). The direct cost of an amputation associated with the diabetic foot is estimated to be between $30,000 and $60,000. The estimated cost for three years of subsequent care ranges from $43,000 to $63,000, mainly due to the increased need for home care and social services (3). Many of the amputations can be prevented through education of people with diabetes and aggressive management of diabetic foot ulcers in the Comprehensive Wound Center.

In addition, another half million patients suffer from venous stasis ulcers, an affliction that arises from edema to the lower legs as a result of faulty circulation of the veins (6).

These painful ulcers prevent patients from enjoying a normal lifestyle and result in a loss of over 2 million workdays. In 1991, the US Department of Health and Human Services set a goal of reducing amputations by 40% by the year 2001. The CDC's MMWR report, published Nov. 2, 2001 stated: "One of the national health objectives for 2000 was to reduce the lower extremity amputation (LEA) from a 1991 baseline of approximately eight per 1000 persons with diabetes to a target of approximately five per 1000. Review of the 1996 data indicated an LEA rate of approximately 11." Thus, we have not come close to reaching this goal.

This chapter addresses the questions that must be answered by administrators and medical staff before making the decision to create a Comprehensive Wound Center.

1. Should the hospital have an organized Wound Center?
2. How does one get it done?
3. What services should be included?
4. Who should participate?
5. What kind of documentation systems should be included?
6. Should hyperbaric oxygen therapy be included?
7. What marketing strategy should be used?

SHOULD THE HOSPITAL HAVE AN ORGANIZED WOUND CENTER?

Hospital Mission. Administrators and medical staff must first decide if an organized Wound Center is congruent with the mission of the hospital.

Demographic Study. Population demographics must be conducted to determine the prevalence of various types of wounds in the hospital's patient population so as to determine whether there is a need for the service. There are several sources of patient demographic information. For example, certain areas of the country have a larger prevalence of diabetes and diabetic foot wounds. Certain ethnic groups (Hispanics, Blacks, and American Indians) suffer more severely from the effects of diabetes than other ethnic groups (5). Demographic studies by the Center for Disease Control (CDC) can be used to identify the prevalence of diabetes in various states. States such as Texas, Arizona, New Mexico, and California have large Hispanic and American Indian groups, while states such as Alabama, Mississippi, Louisiana, Georgia, and the Carolinas have large black populations (4). Information on diabetic prevalence in various states can be obtained by calling the CDC at 404-639-3311 or visiting their website at *www.CDC.gov/nccdphp/ddt/ddthome.htm*.

Other agencies that may have prevalence data on diabetics or chronic wounds include the American Diabetes Association (ADA) (both national and local chapters) and the state and county health departments. Associations such as the American Association for Retired Persons (AARP) can help identify areas of the country that have large elderly populations.

Financial Pro-forma. Space to house the service must be identified and a financial pro-forma must be completed to determine whether it is economically feasible to provide the service.

The logarithmic increase in patients with wound-related problems due to national epidemics of diabetes and peripheral vascular disease in an aging population have made "wound centers" a near requirement for most hospitals (7). This is often a unique service that the hospital can provide the local community and local physicians. Many physicians and podiatrists do not possess all the diagnostic equipment, dressings, surgical techniques, or protocols that can successfully heal recalcitrant ulcers. In addition, the time spent performing wound care in the doctor's office, plus the cost of supplies and nursing salaries, makes it very difficult for the doctor's office to be profitable. Fortunately, the hospital can create a profitable wound care service because of the patient volume, ancillary services, and efficiency with which the service can be managed. If the hospital does not provide the service, the patients must go elsewhere for their wound care, which is often to a competing organization.

Ancillary services must be factored into the financial pro-forma. The challenge of chronic ulcers and other problem wounds is complex and involves multi-factorial solutions. A complete assessment of the patient by physicians and nurses, using laboratory and other diagnostic tests, is required to confirm clinical judgment options and to form appropriate treatment plans. The treatment plan may call for surgical intervention, nutritional assistance, off-loading of affected limbs, compression therapy, antibiotics, hyperbaric oxygen therapy, or other treatment options. All of these services can be coordinated through a Comprehensive Wound Center.

HOW DOES ONE GET IT DONE?

Do It Yourself Versus Contract Services.

The hospital has several options when developing a Comprehensive Wound Center. It can develop the Center alone, hire a consultant to set up the Center, or contract with a wound center management company.

Do It Yourself. One option is for the hospital to do it alone. If local expertise is available, this might be a viable option. However, without local expertise, there is a steep learning curve with considerable investment of time to establish the Wound Center. The hospital must have the expertise to develop appropriate policies, procedure manuals, and forms. Staff training must be budgeted into the overall set up costs. There is also a considerable up-front investment in equipment, including exam chairs, procedure lamps, diagnostic equipment, testing equipment, debridement instruments, computers, and therapeutic tools. Salaries for the nursing, technical, and clerical personnel must be included.

Hire a Consultant. A second option is for the hospital to pay a consultant to assist in setting up the Wound Center. The consultant eliminates the steep learning curve and should accelerate the time line for establishing the Center. The consultant should be able to provide all the information needed to establish the Center. The consultant could also train the doctors and nurses working in the Wound Center. The hospital would usually still be responsible for all the equipment and furniture that exists in the Center.

Contract for Management Services. A third option is for the hospital to contract with a wound care management company to manage the Wound Center.

The cost of construction, equipment and staffing are all negotiating points when dealing with a contractor. Depending on the contract, the wound care management company could provide all the equipment and furniture that exists in the Wound Center, plus they could hire all the management staff and medical directors that run the day-to-day operations. In most instances, the wound care management company would set up a fee-for-service arrangement with the hospital in which they charge for certain procedures done in the Wound Center, such as diagnostic tests, debridements, therapeutic procedures, wound visits, etc. The contract can also be set up so that the wound care company would charge the hospital a monthly management fee to operate the Wound Center or charge a combination of fee for service and management fee.

Working with a consultant or a management services contractor may open the opportunity for staff training and on-going clinical support.

Hospital administration should set up a financial pro-forma using the local economic wage index in which the various scenarios are inserted to determine the financial impact on the bottom line to the hospital. Beside financial considerations, the hospital should ask the question: "What is the impact of having new doctors and nurses run a Wound Center on a day-to-day basis, taking into consideration the medical and legal implications of the activities in the center?" In some cases, it is better for a hospital to contract with a management company that has the experience and is aware of the medical, legal, and day-to-day operational issues that arise.

Location of the Wound Center

A Comprehensive Wound Center should contain the wound care specialists and the appropriate diagnostic and therapeutic equipment to perform the majority of wound care inside the premises; thus allowing patients to confine their visits to one area. In most cases, it is best to locate the Wound Center on the premises of a hospital, especially if the community has a large population of Medicare patients. Close proximity allows better coordination of patient transportation, diagnostic testing, dietician support, and other services such as physical therapy, surgery, and laboratory support. Easy access to the hospital parking lot is important, especially for wheel chair patients.

Hospital space is usually at a premium or occupied with other services, so the Wound Center is sometimes located in a professional building adjacent to the hospital. In these cases, transportation becomes an important consideration. Covered hallways to the hospital should be considered to help minimize exposure of patients to inclement weather. Wheel chair and stretcher access, with doors having a minimum space clearance, must be considered when developing the program.

WHAT KIND OF SERVICES SHOULD BE PROVIDED AND WHO SHOULD PARTICIPATE?

Role of Wound Care Specialists

This type of treatment is best undertaken in a center that incorporates various physician specialties (orthopedic, plastic surgeons, vascular surgeons, infectious disease specialists, podiatrists, endocrinologists) and nurses and technicians trained in wound care. Formal training in hyperbaric oxygen therapy is also required if that capability exists in the Wound Center. Chronic wounds contain fibronectins and other inhibitors of wound healing which prevent successful wound closure; therefore, treatment protocols are designed with the understanding that a chronic wound should be converted to an acute wound via a surgical debridement, when appropriate (8). If infected, the wound is treated with antibiotics until no visible signs of infection are present. The wound is kept moist to facilitate fibroblast function; therefore wound dressings are applied that allow the proper moist environment to exist. Edema is removed from wounds with compression wraps, stockings, and pumps (6).

Protocols are agreed upon by the wound care team, and forms are designed to record visit activities, wound measurements, and any other diagnostic or therapeutic activities. In selected cases, the patient will need hyperbaric oxygen therapy. If that capability does not exist within the Wound Center, arrangements must be made to refer the patient to a hyperbaricist who specializes in wound care. Periodically, wound care staff formally review treatment plans to determine appropriateness, and when needed, make changes or add therapeutic modalities that will enhance healing.

Identifying Team Members

Physicians. Most communities will have physicians and podiatrists who are known as the "wound care experts" and their colleagues will usually refer difficult-to-heal wounds to these individuals. These doctors will usually welcome the opportunity to join a center that is organized to support their efforts. Reimbursement for supplies is usually negligible in a physician's office, plus the doctor has to pay staff to support his/her medical and billing functions. The Wound Center can make staff and supplies available to the doctor's patients.

As an outpatient center of the hospital, the supplies are provided and the staff belongs to the hospital or the contractor of the wound care service, thus, the doctor is spared these expenses. In addition, the Wound Center provides forms that allow the doctors to keep track of their professional activities and billing.

Multi-disciplinary Wound Care Team. It is important to establish a multi-disciplinary team of doctors and other healthcare professionals who can support wound healing activities (9). This can be done by having a number of specialists practice within the Wound Center, or referrals can be made to the specialists to their offices outside the Center. Initially, wounds that are infected, contain necrotic tissue, or contain wound fluids that inhibit healing will benefit from a surgeon who understands the importance of debridement to fresh, bleeding tissue or cancellous bone (9). A vascular surgeon might be needed for revascularization procedures. A plastic surgeon might be needed to perform flaps or skin grafts. Since diabetic patients must keep their blood glucose under control to prevent the harmful effects of compromised white blood cells and restricted blood flow (10, 11), internal medicine, endocrinology, and diabetic education specialists are needed to help develop appropriate treatment plans. A simple injury to the diabetic foot can lead to gangrene or osteomyelitis, so infectious disease specialists are needed for antibiotic management of patients.

Nurses, Physical Therapists, Technical Staff. Nurses with specialty training in wound care are often difficult to recruit. Enterostomal nurses have the background and experience in wounds; unfortunately these nurses are usually only found working in large hospitals or university hospitals. Physical therapists also have wound care experience, but they are usually committed to the Physical Therapy Department. As a general rule, inexperienced RN's and LVN's can be adequately trained at available wound care courses.

If the Center offers hyperbaric oxygen therapy as part of its wound care service, a nursing/technical staff must be hired to support the chambers. Trained hyperbaric technicians may be very difficult to recruit, so individuals with EMT backgrounds or previous military hyperbaric training are hired and trained. These individuals help with wound care, perform non-invasive wound assessments, operate and perform maintenance on the hyperbaric chambers.

Training and Certification in Wound Care

It is important that all team members receive formal training in wound care and there are a number of courses available. The Undersea and Hyperbaric Medical Society (UHMS) is a sponsor of continuing medical education for wound care courses. More information on the courses can be obtained on the UHMS website at *www.uhms.org*

Doctors and nurses can become certified in wound care by the American Academy of Wound Management (AAWM) and other agencies. Before applicants can sit the AAWM exam they have to complete a certain number of years of clinical experience in wound care. For more information, contact the AAWM at +1 (202) 521-0368 or at their web site, *www.aawm.org*. Passing the exam allows wound care specialists to use the initials CWS (certified wound specialist) in their credentials.

Physician/Practitioner Privileges. The Hospital will need to establish criteria for credentialing physicians/practitioners who will participate in the Wound Center. Specific procedures (e.g., debridement, biopsy, hyperbaric oxygen therapy) should be addressed.

LOGISTICAL CONSIDERATIONS

Designing the Center.

Resources that can be helpful in designing the Center include the state department of health and the American Institute of Architects (AIA) and the National Fire Protection Association (NFPA).

The Life Safety Code (NFPA 101) contains information (12) on life safety requirements for the design of new hospitals, nursing homes, limited care facilities, and new ambulatory health care centers. The following points are discussed and highlighted:

1. Minimum construction requirements.
2. Means of egress requirements: door size and construction, stairs, smoke-proof enclosures, ramps, size of hallways, number of exits, arrangement of door exits, emergency lighting.
3. Fire protection requirements.
4. Construction of corridor walls.

5. Subdivision of building spaces.
6. Special protection features.
7. Ventilation, heating, and air conditioning requirements.
8. Emergency lighting and essential electrical systems.

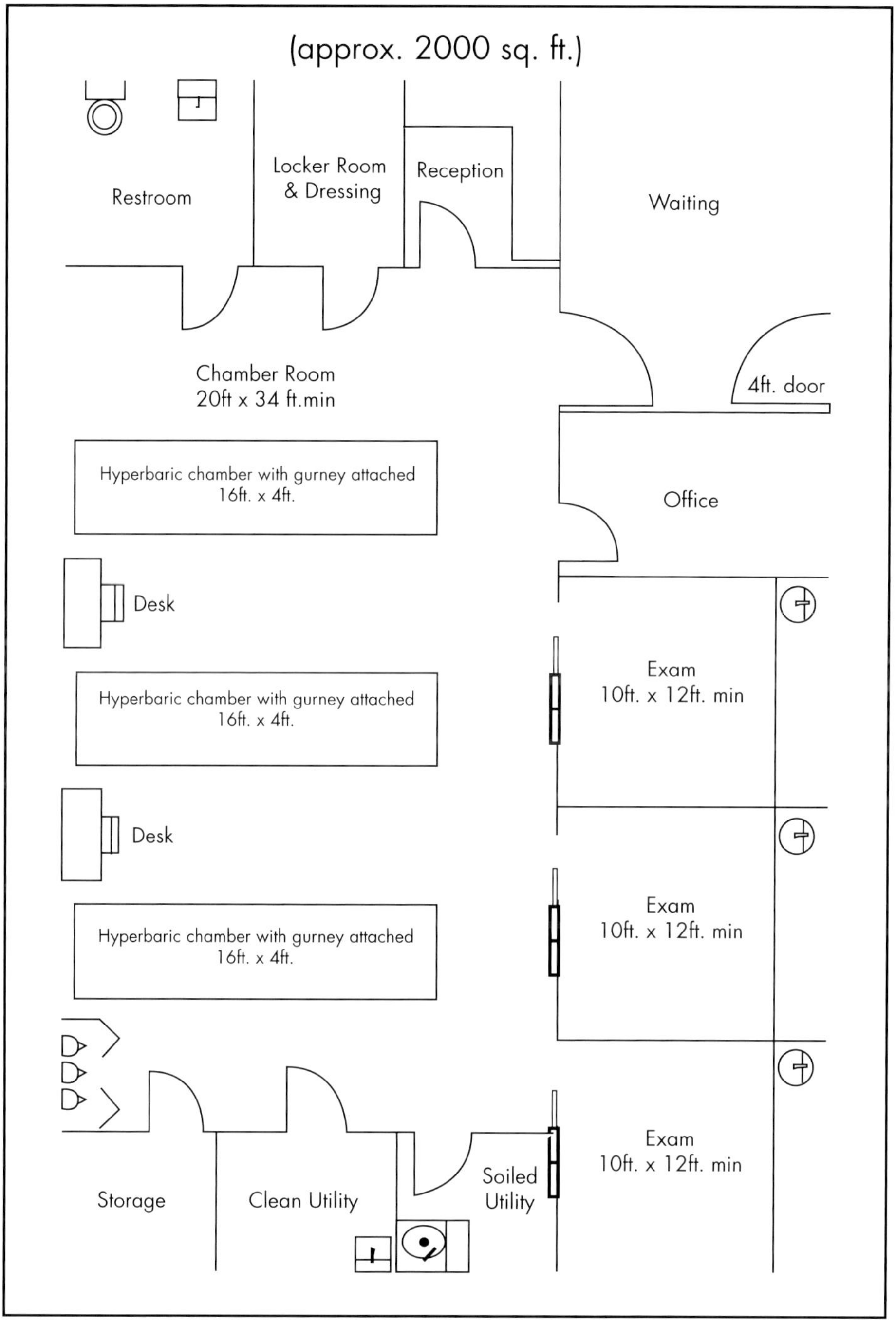

Figure 1. Suggested Layout of Comprehensive Wound Center that Includes HBO2 Capability.

Flow of Patients in the Center

Consideration should be given to establishing a traffic flow that avoids bottlenecks throughout the day. There will usually be three types of patients in the Center: new patients for evaluation, patients for wound care only, and, if the capability exists, patients for wound care and hyperbaric oxygen therapy. Space should be organized so that patient flow is in one direction: from entrance to exit, thus minimizing patients crowding in hallways, waiting for evaluation or wound care procedures.

Time Table for Establishing the Wound Center

In general, once the space has been allocated, the time table for opening the Wound Center is about 2-3 months. It can take longer depending on approval by state and local agencies, architect plans, administration approvals, or when a hyperbaric medicine capability is included (see hyperbaric facility below). The following steps must be accomplished to help expedite final construction and patient treatments:

Construction

1. Architectural drawings completed
2. Approval by the state agency to begin construction
3. Local building permits obtained
4. Approval of a contractor to begin construction
5. Completion of construction and approval for occupancy by local fire marshal
6. Final inspection by state agency to begin patient treatments

Equipment

1. Procedure chair/table
2. Procedure light
3. Patient assessment equipment (e.g., sensory testing, Doppler, $TcpO_2$ monitoring, segmental pulse pressure monitor, laser Doppler, etc)
4. Surgical supplies for debridement procedures
5. Digital camera for wound photos
6. Computer to record wound care activities and schedule patients
7. Hospital grade televisions with VCR capability (for entertainment of hyperbaric oxygen patients)
8. Stretchers with guard rails
9. Wheel chairs for patients

Supplies (through hospital central supply and pharmacy)

1. Curlex rolls
2. Saline
3. Specialty dressings
4. Gels
5. Tape
6. Gauze
7. Scissors
8. Compression wraps
9. Debridement tools

Attach 2 WOUND ASSESSMENT/WOUND CARE

DATE ______________________

WOUND LOCATIONS

Wound #1	Wound #3
Wound #2	Wound #4

Wound Number

#1	#2	#3	#4	SHAPE
☐	☐	☐	☐	Irregular
☐	☐	☐	☐	Round/Oval
☐	☐	☐	☐	Square/Rectangle
☐	☐	☐	☐	Linear/Elongated
☐	☐	☐	☐	Butterfly

#1	#2	#3	#4	UNDERMINING
☐	☐	☐	☐	< 2 cm in any area
☐	☐	☐	☐	2 to 4 cm involving < 50% wound margins
☐	☐	☐	☐	2 to 4 cm involving > 50% wound margins
☐	☐	☐	☐	> 4 cm in any area
☐	☐	☐	☐	Tunneling and/or sinus tract formation

#1	#2	#3	#4	EXUDATE TYPE
☐	☐	☐	☐	None
☐	☐	☐	☐	Serosangulneous: thin, watery, pale red/pink
☐	☐	☐	☐	Serous: thin, watery, clear
☐	☐	☐	☐	Purutenl: think or thick, opeque, tan/yellow
☐	☐	☐	☐	Foul purulent: thick, opaque, yellow/green wth odor

#1	#2	#3	#4	PERPHERAL TISSUE EDEMA
☐	☐	☐	☐	Minimal firmness around wound
☐	☐	☐	☐	Non-pitting edema extends < 4 cm around wound
☐	☐	☐	☐	Non-pitting edema extends > 4 cm around wound
☐	☐	☐	☐	Pitting edema extends < 4 cm around wound
☐	☐	☐	☐	Crepitus and/or pitting edema extends > 4 cm

#1	#2	#3	#4	TYPE OF DEBRIDEMENT PERFORMED
☐	☐	☐	☐	None
☐	☐	☐	☐	Mechanical
☐	☐	☐	☐	Sharp

#1	#2	#3	#4	MATERIAL DEBRIDED
☐	☐	☐	☐	Necrotic
☐	☐	☐	☐	Eschar
☐	☐	☐	☐	Fibrous
☐	☐	☐	☐	Exudate
☐	☐	☐	☐	Clot
☐	☐	☐	☐	Callous
☐	☐	☐	☐	Other:

#1	#2	#3	#4	AREA CLEANSED WITH
☐	☐	☐	☐	Antiseptic cleanser
☐	☐	☐	☐	Surgical soap
☐	☐	☐	☐	Saline
☐	☐	☐	☐	Other:

Wound Number

#1	#2	#3	#4	TISSUE INVOLVED
☐	☐	☐	☐	Non-blanchable erythema on Intact skin
☐	☐	☐	☐	Part-thick skin loss involving epidermis/dermis
☐	☐	☐	☐	Full-thick skin loss involving subcutaneous tissue
☐	☐	☐	☐	Obscurred by necrosis
☐	☐	☐	☐	Full-thick skin loss and/or deeper tissue involved

#1	#2	#3	#4	NECROTIC TISSUE TYPE
☐	☐	☐	☐	Non visible
☐	☐	☐	☐	White/gray non-inviable tissue and/or yellow slough
☐	☐	☐	☐	loosely adherent yellow slough
☐	☐	☐	☐	Adherent, sofft black eschar
☐	☐	☐	☐	Firmly adherent, hard black eschar

#1	#2	#3	#4	EXUDATE AMOUNT
☐	☐	☐	☐	None
☐	☐	☐	☐	Scant
☐	☐	☐	☐	Small
☐	☐	☐	☐	Moderate
☐	☐	☐	☐	Large

#1	#2	#3	#4	GRANULATION TISSUE
☐	☐	☐	☐	Skin intact or partial-thickness wound
☐	☐	☐	☐	Bright, befy red; 75% to 100% of wound filled
☐	☐	☐	☐	Bright, beefy red; < 75% and >25% of wound bled
☐	☐	☐	☐	Pink/dull, dusky red and/or fills < 25% of wound
☐	☐	☐	☐	No granulation tissue present

#1	#2	#3	#4	WOUND IRRIGATION
☐	☐	☐	☐	None
☐	☐	☐	☐	Saline ____________ CC
☐	☐	☐	☐	Other:

#1	#2	#3	#4	NEW DRESSING APPLIED
☐	☐	☐	☐	Enzyme debrider
☐	☐	☐	☐	Hydrating gel
☐	☐	☐	☐	Saline
☐	☐	☐	☐	Packing strip
☐	☐	☐	☐	Alginate
☐	☐	☐	☐	Hydrocolloid
☐	☐	☐	☐	Transparent occlusive
☐	☐	☐	☐	4 x 4
☐	☐	☐	☐	Roll gauze
☐	☐	☐	☐	Compression wrap
☐	☐	☐	☐	Skin cream/Lotion
☐	☐	☐	☐	other (see notes)

NOTES/SIGNATURE:

-------- PATIENT INDENTIFICATION ---------

Figure 2. Sample Wound Assessment Form

WHAT KIND OF DOCUMENTATION SYSTEMS SHOULD BE INCLUDED?

The old saying which states, "If it's not in writing, it didn't happen," applies even more to wound care documentation. Not only is it important for nurses and doctors to have a written record of their activities, but reimbursement agencies frequently ask for documentation to approve payments for evaluation and management services, and procedures.

Forms need to be developed that describe the initial presentation of a patient's wound (wound description, size, exudates, color, smell, etc.), but also all the co-morbidities that may play a part in the patient developing a chronic or problem wound. In addition, follow up visits must also be documented that record wound progress, e.g., wound size (length, width, depth), granulation, color, debridements done, etc. An example of initial documentation form can be seen in Figure 2.

Benchmarking. A method of tracking outcomes should be established as part of the quality assurance program.

Photography. An important part of tracking wound progress is taking photographs of the initial wound appearance and follow up photos at least weekly.

Billing. The hospital is allowed to bill a technical charge for most of the Wound Center activities. The nursing staff will normally follow the orders of the physicians working in the Wound Center; therefore evaluation and management (E & M) codes and procedure codes are used to bill the activities that occur. Table 1 lists the common procedures in a Wound Center that are billed by the hospital for technical fees, along with their corresponding HCPCS/CPT code, APC code, and revenue code (13).

The physicians who work in the Wound Center are also allowed to bill for their professional activity. Table 1 lists some typical physician activities that can occur in a Wound Center. It is important to note that when E & M services are billed, physician and hospital technical activities may not match exactly; however, most reimbursement agencies, especially Medicare, recognize this, and will still pay both parties for their activities.

These codes should be verified with the local Medicare intermediary. Commercial insurance companies and state Medicaid programs sometimes have their own billing codes.

For more details on coding, charging, billing, and collecting for wound care and hyperbaric medicine services, see the chapter by RP Bangasser and TM Bozzuto entitled "Coding, Charging, Billing and Collecting for Wound Care and Hyperbaric Services."

Electronic Documentation Systems

The term "paperless chart" has come into voque in recent years and it conjures up visions of hospitals doing away with all paper charts. At this point, however, the goal has yet to be accomplished in most hospitals. When it is employed, a paperless system should satisfy at least the following:

a). Allow computer entry of patient treatments from initial assessment to final discharge;

b). Allow the record to be printed in order to submit to reimbursement agencies; and

TABLE 1. HOSPITAL TECHNICAL AND PHYSICIAN PROFESSIONAL CODES FOR WOUND CARE & HYPERBARIC OXYGEN PROCEDURES

Procedure Name	Hospital HCPCS/ CPT	Hospital APC	Hospital Rev Code**	Physician CPT	Physician Global Period
Debridement					
Debridement, Partial Thickness	11040	0015	361 or 761	11040	0
Debridement, Full Thickness	11041	0015	361 or 761	11041	0
Debridement, Subcutaneous	11042	0016	361 or 761	11042	0
Debridement, Tissue & Muscle	11043	0016	361 or 761	11043	10
Debridement, Muscle & Bone	11044	0682	361 or 761	11044	10
Debridement of Nails; 1 to 5	11720	0009		11720	0
Debridement of Nails; 6 or more*	11721	0009		11721	0
Avulsion of Nail Plate, Single*	11730	0013		11730	0
Avulsion of Nail Plate, Ea. Additional Nail*	11732	0012		11732	0
Excision of Nail, Partial or complete*	11765	0015		11750	0
Other Surgical Procedures					
I & D, Abscess, Simple or Single	10060	0006	361 or 761	10060	10
I & D, Complicated or Multiple	10061	0007	361 or 761	10061	10
Incision & Removal of Foreign Body	10120	0006		10120	10
I & D, Hematoma, Seroma or Fluid	10140	0007		10140	10
Excision/Biopsy, Level I	11100	0019	361 or 761	11100	0
Excision/Biopsy, Level II	11101	0020	361 or 761	11101	0
Excision/Biopsy, Level III	11102	0021	361 or 761	11102	
Excision/Biopsy, Level IV	11103	0022	361 or 761	11103	
Paring or cutting of callous, single	11055	0012		11055	1 every 60 days
Paring or cutting of callous, 2 to 4*	11056	0012		11056	1 every 60 days
Paring or cutting of Callous, > 4*	11057	0012		11057	1 every 60 days
New Patient Visit					
Limited (10 min ave)	99201	0600	761 or 361	99201	0
Expanded (20 min ave)	99202	0600	761 or 361	99202	0
Detailed (30 min ave)	99203	0601	761 or 361	99203	0
Comprehensive (45 min ave)	99204	0602	761 or 361	99204	0
Extended (60 min ave)	99205	0602	761 or 361	99205	0

TABLE 1. (CONTINUED)

Procedure Name	Hospital HCPCS/ CPT	Hospital APC	Hospital Rev Code**	Physician CPT	Physician Global Period
Established Patient Visit					
Minimal (5 min ave)	99211	0600	761	99211	0
Limited (10 min ave)	99212	0600	761	99212	0
Expanded (15 min ave)	99213	0601	761	99213	0
Detailed (25 min ave)	99214	0602	761	99214	0
Comprehensive (40 min ave)	99215	0602	761	99215	0
Outpatient Consultation, New pt, Limited				99241	0
Outpatient Consultation, New pt, Intermediate				99242	0
Outpatient Consultation, New pt, Expanded				99242	0
Outpatient Consultation, New pt, Comprehensive				99243	0
Outpatient Consultation, New pt, Complex				99244	0
Initial Consult, Inpatient, Limited (30 min ave)				99251	0
Initial Consult, Inpatient, Intermediate (40 min ave)				99252	0
Initial Consult, Inpatient, Expanded (55 min ave)				99253	0
Initial Consult, Inpatient, Comprehensive (80 min ave)				99254	0
Initial Consult, Inpatient, Complex (110 min ave)				99255	0
Follow-up Inpatient Consult, Minimal (10 min ave)				99261	0
Follow-up Inpatient Consult, Minimal (20 min ave)				99262	0
Follow-up Inpatient Consult, Minimal (30 min ave)				99263	0
Tympanometry	92567	0364		92567	0
TCOM (Single Site)	93922	0096	921	93922	2 in 60 days
TCOM (Multiple Sites)	93923	0096	921	93922	2 in 60 days
HBO2 Tx / per 30 minutes	C1300	0971	413		0
Physician attendance & supervision of HBO2, per session				99183	0
Surgical prep of recipient site by excision				15000	90
Skin graft application / Xenograft	15100			15100	90
STSG, face, scalp, eyelids, mouth, neck, ears, orbits, genitalia, hands, feet and/ or multiple digits, first 100 cm^2 or less	15120			15120	90

TABLE 1. (CONTINUED)

Procedure Name	Hospital HCPCS/ CPT	Hospital APC	Hospital Rev Code**	Physician CPT	Physician Global Period
Application of Bilaminate Skin Substitute, *First 25 cm^2 (i.e., Apligraf)	15342		761	15342	10
Application of Bilaminate Skin Substitute, each additional 25 cm^2*	15343			15343	10
Application of Allograft, Skin; 100 cm^2 or less (i.e., Gamma Graft)	15350	0686	761	15350	90
Application of Allograft, Skin; each additional cm^2	15351	0686	761	15351	90
Application of Xenograft, Skin; 100 cm^2 or less (i.e., Porcine graft)	15400	0025	761	15400	90
Application of Xenograft, Skin; each additional 100 cm^2	15401	0025	761	15401	90
Unna Boot Application	29580	0058	761	29580	0

* Services or procedures with an asterisk beside them have specific LMRP requirements that must be met in order to qualify for reimbursement.
** Hospital Revenue Codes vary based on the judgment of Hospital Billing Department. Check with the Medicare intermediary/carrier and private insurance to verify billing codes.
(American Medical Association. Current Procedural Terminology cpt 2006. Chicago, IL; American Medical Association, 2005.)

c). Allow analysis of the data to detect any trends that may affect patient treatment.

The "Healthcare Information and Management Systems Society" (HIMSS) provides leadership for healthcare public policy and industry practices. HIMSS has listed the following as essential attributes for an electronic system to be considered an Electronic Health Record, or EHR:

- It must provide secure, reliable, real-time access to patient health record information.
- It must function as clinicians' primary information resource (i.e., it is THE medical record rather than the paper chart)
- It must assist with delivering evidence-based care
- It must capture data used for continuous quality improvement, utilization review, & risk management
- It must capture the information needed for reimbursement
- It must be able to support clinical research, public health reporting, and population health initiatives.
- It must be able to support clinical trials and other research.

Data are entered by clinicians at the point of service in discrete, machine interpretable fields which allow data exchange and computer analysis, as well as the creation of a central data repository. These discrete fields allow the calculation of both the facility and the physician level of service and thus are directly linked to billing processes. Furthermore, the EHR is the legal medical chart. Paper charts are optional.

At this time, security requirements for hospital medical records departments usually preclude web-based systems from being the legal medical chart, although that may change in the future. In addition, while the World Wide Web is relatively reliable, down time does occur, and these two issues (security and reliability) require EHRs to be run either from a hospital "intranet" or server based. Furthermore, if a paper chart must continue to be kept, or if legal documents are distributed in more than one system (photo files, hospital EHR, or web based system), then the automated system does not meet the definition of being the physician's primary resource. When adopting any electronic system, it is crucial to define what will represent the LEGAL chart and to define the total patient record wherever it may be distributed.

It is anticipated that all documentation will be electronic in the next 10 years, and it may be necessary to use an EHR if the wound care physician wishes to participate in "Pay for Performance" projects by Medicare. Paper charts are rapidly becoming a thing of the past, and the question is not WHETHER to adopt an automated system, but WHICH one will meet the needs of the facility, the physicians and the management. Depending on the system used, it is relatively easy to demonstrate that the financial investment in an EHR is recuperated in the form of increased reimbursement for both the physician and the facility.

EHR Evaluation Tool:

An AHR may be sufficient for many practitioners, so just because a program does not meet the requirements of an EHR does not mean that it will not be useful. It may be necessary to determine what the needs really are. The more sophisticated the system, the more training is required to use it, and, thus, the more challenging it will be to implement.

Following are features of EHRs. When evaluating a system, one should ask if the program can perform these functions:

Functionality. Does the system:

- Record ALL patient clinical data and not specific metrics of interest
- Substitute for the paper chart so that a paper chart is no longer necessary
- Allow its use for POINT OF SERVICE DOCUMENTATION (not retrospective data collection)
- Meet hospital security standards for EMRs

Data Capture. Does the system:

- Allow recording of lab, radiology and other test results
- Allow recording and review of progress notes
- Allow recording and monitoring of current and past meds and med refills

Documentation functions. Does the system:

- Create the Review of Systems (ROS) using only "point and click technology" (no typing, transcription or voice recognition)
- Allow for the creation of "free-form" notes if the doctor wishes
- Give one the ability to customize templates without relying on vendor

- Allow one to create and maintain problem lists
- Allow one to create and maintain medication lists
- Allow one to identify allergies
- Document over-all patient care

Wound care documentation. Does the system:

- Record wound measurements
- Select wound care products with "point and click" technology
- Allow one to update a product list without support from the vendor
- Automatically archive digital photos labeled by location (i.e. there are no manual steps in archiving the photos)
- Automatically graph wound measurements over time

Hyperbaric oxygen documentation. If hyperbaric oxygen is available, does the system:

- Record hyperbaric treatments administered at different levels of pressure
- Provide profiles to record treatments such as carbon monoxide poisoning, decompression sickness, soft and hard tissue radionecrosis, osteomyelitis, etc
- Provide details of patient care during a hyperbaric oxygen treatment, i.e. medications given, blood sugar levels before and after treatment, blood pressure, etc

Transcutaneous oxygen monitoring documentation. If non-invasive vascular testing is available, does the system:

- Record tests results that are administered at different pressures (e.g., 1 ATA, HBO2) and with different challenges (e.g., oxygen challenge, leg elevation results)
- Allow comparison of the various parameters with certain patient populations

Perform correspondence function. Does the system allow one to:

- Automatically generate consultation letter to the referring physician with copies to other health care providers
- Automatically generate treatment updates to the referring physician
- Automatically attach the initial photo and a follow up photo of the wound to correspondence

Perform *security* function. Does the system allow one to:

- Maintain security related to patient information (e.g., password protection, audit trails)

Perform coding and charge-capture functions. Does the system allow one to:

- Receive E&M coding advice for the physician
- Capture appropriate charges automatically from the notes
- Provide an internal "Acuity Scoring System" to determine facility level of service
- Guide correct coding of the wound or ulcer
- Link any procedures to the wound code

Perform practice analysis functions. Does the system allow one to:

- Perform ones own analyses of patient outcomes (without vendor support), such as time to healing of stasis ulcers, etc.
- Find patients with certain characteristics
- Create reports of clinic functions (e.g., levels of service over a time period, patient acuity score by staff)

Track inventory. Does the system allow one to:

- Track inventory
- Automate supply ordering
- Automate DME ordering of wound care supplies

Ease of Operation. Does the system:

- Interface with the hospital EHR (via HL7 interface)
- Minimize data input (i.e, does one have to enter data more than once, either on paper or in the EMR)

SHOULD HYPERBARIC OXYGEN THERAPY BE INCLUDED?

Role of Hyperbaric Oxygen (HBO2) In Wound Healing And Infection Control

Studies by Pai and Hunt (14) revealed that oxygen plays a critical role in wound healing. Their studies revealed that wound healing is oxygen dependent. Knighton (15) showed that oxygen improved white blood cell function to form oxygen radicals that destroy bacterial cell walls. Other researchers have been able to show that oxygen and certain antibiotics act synergistically to destroy bacteria (16). Sheffield (17) demonstrated the benefit of hyperbaric oxygen by measuring oxygen in chronic wounds and noting that hyper-oxygenation corrected the severe hypoxia and enhanced angiogenesis in human wounds, with subsequent healing. Zhao and colleagues (18) demonstrated that receptor sites in a hypoxic wound are opened up with hyperbaric oxygen, thus allowing growth factors to attach and initiate the healing process. Mader and colleagues (19) demonstrated the advantages of using hyperbaric oxygen to treat osteomyelitis in an animal model. Cianci (20) demonstrated that limb salvage with wound care and hyperbaric oxygen is less expensive to the health care system than amputation. Although the diagnoses may vary from center to center, clinical experience has shown that about 25% of the patients referred to the Wound Center suffer from soft tissue hypoxic wounds that might be candidates for HBO2 therapy. Severely hypoxic wound beds render ineffective certain treatments such as skin grafting, growth factor treatments, or living tissue replacements, e.g., fibroblasts, keratinocytes, and dermal composites. Salvage of limbs that have severely hypoxic wound beds require treatment options that correct the hypoxia (revascularization and/or HBO2). Thus, it would be prudent for a Comprehensive Wound Center to have access to HBO2 therapy.

Training and Certification in Hyperbaric Medicine

The Centers for Medicare and Medicaid Services (CMS) encourages physicians who perform hyperbaric therapy to obtain adequate training in the use of hyperbaric therapy by credible professional organizations and in advanced cardiac life support. Several professional societies sponsor continuing medical education for wound care courses.

The Undersea and Hyperbaric Medical Society (UHMS) is a sponsor of continuing medical education for both wound care and hyperbaric medicine courses. Information about the UHMS-sponsored courses can be obtained at the UHMS website at *www.uhms.org*. Some of the other options for course listings are at *www.hyperbaricmedicine.com*, *www.woundcarehbo.com*, and *www.baromedical.com*

Board Certification in Hyperbaric Medicine

Physician Certification in Undersea & Hyperbaric Medicine. Physicians wanting to become board certified in the subspecialty of undersea and hyperbaric medicine through the American Board of Medical Specialties can obtain more information by contacting the American Board of Preventative Medicine (ABPM) or the American Board of Emergency Medicine (ABEM). As of this writing, board certification involves a 12-month fulltime fellowship, at least 25% of which must be in HBO2. A practice pathway is also available until 2010 when it will be closed. As of this writing, there are fewer than 300 physicians who are board certified in undersea and hyperbaric medicine.

Physician Certificate of Special Competency in Undersea and Hyperbaric Medicine. The American College of Hyperbaric Medicine (ACHM) offers a certificate of special competency in undersea and hyperbaric medicine through a practice pathway. It requires an approved 40-hour introductory course in hyperbaric medicine and supervision of 1000 hyperbaric treatments. The ACHM certificate is not recognized as being "board certified"; however, it does help the physician show his or her overall experience in hyperbaric medicine. These certifications are currently not required by Medicare for a doctor to bill for hyperbaric medicine supervision; however, it does give doctors recognition by their peers that a certain knowledge base has been attained. A few hospitals with wound care centers containing hyperbaric chambers require their Medical Director to be certified in Undersea and Hyperbaric Medicine.

Certified Hyperbaric Registered Nurse. Nurses are eligible to take the Certified Hyperbaric Registered Nurse (CHRN) exam after one year hyperbaric nurse experience with a minimum of 480 hours in the past 12 months. This exam is sponsored by the Baromedical Nurses Association. The phone number is +1(303)918-9686 or *www.hyperbaricnurses.org*. The exam is administered by National Board of Diving and Hyperbaric Medical Technology (NBDHMT). They can be reached at +1(504)328-8871 or *www.nbdhmt.com*

Certified Hyperbaric Technologist. Nurses and technicians are eligible to take the Certified Hyperbaric Technologist (CHT) exam after 480 hours of hyperbaric medicine experience. Some physicians have also taken the exam. This exam is administered by the National Board of Diving and Hyperbaric Medical Technology (NBDHMT), which can be reached at +1(504)328-8871 or *www.nbdhmt.com*. Medicare intermediaries in certain states require that a nurse or technician be a CHT or CHRN before they will reimburse for the transcutaneous oxygen testing performed in the Wound Center.

Hyperbaric Department Considerations

If the Wound Center is contemplating including hyperbaric oxygen, the following considerations are important in making that decision.

Medicare Requirements. The Centers for Medicare and Medicaid Services (CMS) requires that a code team be available during the time hyperbaric patients are receiving hyperbaric therapy. As of this writing, Medicare will reimburse for hyperbaric oxygen therapy only if it is associated with a hospital. CMS has also published Provider Based Status Regulations which state that an outpatient department of the hospital must be located either in the hospital, next to the hospital, or no more than 250 yards from the hospital campus. Any distance further and CMS has to make the determination on being appropriate for Provider Based Status.

Time Table for Establishing a Wound Center. In general, the time table for opening a Wound Center with monoplace chambers may vary from three to six months depending on approval by state and local agencies, architect plans, administration approvals, etc. A multiplace chamber installation may take 6–12 months before patients can be treated in the chamber.

Room Design. Each state may have requirements that must be followed when building a wound care/hyperbaric medicine center. For example, in the State of Texas, certain requirements are outlined for Wound Centers that have hyperbaric facilities (21). Other states are taking note of the Texas requirements, and some are in the process of adopting these same requirements. The following is considered to be the minimum requirements for a hyperbaric suite:

1. Patient waiting area: The area should be out of traffic flow, under staff control, and contain enough seating capacity for patients and their relatives throughout the day. When the waiting area is for both inpatients and outpatients at the same time, separate areas shall be provided with privacy between both areas. A patient waiting area is not required for two or less individual (monoplace) hyperbaric chambers.
2. Control desk and reception area: A control desk and reception area should be provided to greet patients, fill out registration information, and serve as traffic control center throughout the day.
3. Holding area: This area should accommodate inpatients on stretchers or beds, and be out of the traffic flow. This area may be omitted for two or less monoplace hyperbaric chambers.
4. Patient toilet rooms: Toilet rooms shall be provided with hand washing fixtures that have hands-free operable controls with direct access from the hyperbaric suite.
5. Patients dressing rooms: Dressing rooms for outpatients should include a seat or bench, mirror, and provisions for hanging patient's clothing and for securing valuables. At least one patient dressing room should accommodate wheelchair patients.
6. Staff facilities: Toilets with hand-washing fixtures with hands-free operable controls may be outside the suite, but convenient for staff use.
7. Consultation room: An appropriate room for private consultations with wound care physicians shall be provided for outpatients.
8. Storage space: A clean storage space shall be provided for clean supplies and linens. Hand-washing fixtures shall be provided with

hands-free operable controls. When a separate storage room is provided, it may be shared with another department.

9. Soiled holding room: A soiled holding room shall be provided with waste receptacles and soiled linen receptacles.
10. Hand washing: A lavatory equipped for hand washing with hands-free operable controls shall be located in the room where the hyperbaric chambers are located.
11. Housekeeping room: The housekeeping room shall be nearby and contain a floor receptor or service sink, storage space for housekeeping supplies and equipment.
12. Hyperbaric chamber area: The hyperbaric area should be large enough to allow 2–4 monoplace chambers or one multiplace chamber plus room for stretchers and a console area where a technician or nurse can monitor the treatments and communicate with patients and/or staff inside the chamber. Space between monoplace chambers is as follows: chamber and sidewall, 5 feet; between chambers, 6 feet; and between the chamber headboard and wall, 3 feet. A minimum passage space of 4 feet shall exist at the head of the chamber. Typically, a monoplace operation may require between 2500-3000 ft^2 for all operations, while a multiplace chamber operation may require 3500–4000 ft^2.

Ordering and Installing Hyperbaric Chambers

1. Order chamber(s). Normally chamber manufacturers need six to eight weeks for construction, once the order is placed. Schedule chambers to arrive approximately at the same time as the final state inspection. A multiplace chamber can be available on the shelf, or it can be constructed to the specifications of your Center, which could require six months to a year for construction. Many times, building construction is done around a multiplace chamber, so coordination of this facility is much more involved.
2. Order the gas supply. Both oxygen and air are used. Monoplace chambers are usually pressurized with oxygen whereas multiplace chambers must be pressurized with air and the patient is delivered oxygen via mask or hood.
3. Connect chambers and perform safety checks to assure chambers are operational.
4. Conduct training of medical personnel to insure safe chamber operation.

National Fire Protection Association (NFPA) Considerations. NFPA 99, Standard for Health Care Facilities, refer to the chapter by Feldmeier entitled, "Problem Wounds: The Impact of Radiation Therapy and Chemotherapy," Hyperbaric Facilities contains the fire safety standards that must be met by any Wound Center that is equipped with hyperbaric oxygen therapy (22). NFPA 99 includes the following highlights:

1. Classification of multiplace, monoplace, or research hyperbaric chambers.
2. Housing for hyperbaric facilities: construction and equipment required.

3. Fabrication of the hyperbaric chamber: materials, flooring, finish, illumination, emergency lighting.
4. Chamber ventilation: flow rate, sources of air, oxygen, and other gases,
5. Fire protection: both multiplace and monoplace requirements.
6. Electrical systems: information on wiring, console requirements, lighting panels, etc., both inside and outside the chamber.
7. Grounding and ground fault protection.
8. Requirements for communications and monitoring inside and outside the chamber.
9. Chamber air supply monitoring.
10. Administration of the hyperbaric oxygen therapy program: recognition of hazards, training of personnel, safety director responsibilities, job descriptions, etc.
11. General requirements: open flames and hot objects, flammable gases and liquids, personnel (medical and patients), textiles allowed, equipment allowed, handling of gases.
12. Maintenance: documentation of activities, logs for maintenance, electrical safeguards, furniture in chamber, fire protection equipment, and house keeping.
13. Safety Director's Role
    a. Responsible for all hyperbaric equipment
    b. Participates with hospital and physicians in developing procedures for operation and maintenance of the hyperbaric facility.
    c. Makes recommendations on safety policies and procedures
    d. Has authority to restrict or remove potentially hazardous supply or equipment items from the chamber.
    e. Ensures that electrical monitoring, life support, protection, and ventilating arrangements in the hyperbaric chamber are inspected and tested as part of the routine maintenance program of the hospital.
14. The final authority for safety of the patients and personnel lies with the hospital.

MARKETING

Once the decision is made to have a wound healing program, education of the hospital staff should begin. Hospital nurses on the floors may provide referrals of wound care patients. Educational efforts may be in the form of literature on wound care, newsletters, videos, or scheduling wound care specialists to give talks on the subject. Providing continuing medical education (CME) credits will encourage attendance of physicians and nurses from outside the hospital. Home health agencies are a good target group, since they care for the majority of patients outside the hospital. Medical directors of the Wound Center should be called upon to talk with their colleagues, explaining their role in the Wound Center and encouraging those colleagues to make referrals of their problem wound patients. It is essential that the Wound Center return patients to the referring doctor once the wound is healed; otherwise, the Wound Center will get the reputation of keeping patients, and few other referrals will occur.

The general public should also be educated and made aware of this service in the community. The most common forms of advertisement include television, radio, billboards, and print ads. These ads may be aimed at certain populations, e.g., diabetic patients or patients with venous stasis disease. Scheduling of ads should be aimed at starting immediately before the Wound Center is ready to treat patients and should run until the Wound Center is well established. Certain agencies, such as the American Diabetes Association, should be contacted and a doctor or nurse from the Wound Center should set up a time when he or she can give a presentation to people with diabetes on the importance of early treatment for problem wounds that can lead to amputation if left untreated.

SUMMARY

Establishment of a successful wound care service is based on several factors: 1) A patient population that needs the service; 2) a hospital that is committed to providing the service to the community; 3) a multidisciplinary team of physicians and other trained professionals, nurses, and technologists committed to the cause of wound healing; and 4) having an organized program. Requirements for construction of the Wound Center will vary depending on local, county, state, and NFPA 99 requirements (22). Marketing the program will require identifying the medical community to educate and the public population that will ultimately benefit from the service in the community. The Wound Center can certainly impact the quality of life for patients who have previously found these wounds debilitating and costly to the health care system. Formation of a team of doctors and nurses dedicated to healing chronic wounds is key to the long-term success of the Wound Center. Finally, a Wound Center has to be profitable for the hospital and doctors who work there. Even in today's reimbursement environment, especially Medicare, a hospital can still generate positive financial results with a Wound Center. A full time medical director can also realize a good living by being associated with a hospital-based outpatient Wound Center.

ACKNOWLEDGMENTS

The authors thank Valerie Short, RN, ACHRN, CWOCN, CWS, CMBS for the information on hospital and physician reimbursement codes. We gratefully acknowledge the contribution of Toni Turner of Protia Health Services for the section on Electronic Documentation Systems.

REFERENCES

1. U.S. Department of Health and Human Services. Healthy People 2000: National Health Promotion and Disease Prevention Objectives. DHHS publ. No. 95-50213.Washington, DC: Government Printing Office, 1991; 73-177.
2. Mouton CP, Parker R. Wound healing in the geriatric patient. In: Sheffield, PJ, Smith APS, Fife CE, eds. *Wound Care Practice*. Flagstaff, AZ: Best Publishing, 2007.
3. Bakker K. Diabetes and the foot. *http://www.worlddiabetesday.org*/2005-campaign/diabetes-and-the-foot/
4. Division of Diabetes Translation. *Diabetes Surveillance*, 1980-87, Atlanta: Centers for Disease Control, April 1990.
5. Rith-Najarian, et al. Foot care in minorities: preventing amputations in high-risk populations. In: Levin ME, O'Neal LW, Bowker JH, eds.*The Diabetic Foot*, St Louis, Mo: Mosby Year Book, 1993; 577-586.
6. Jordan R. Etiology and treatment of venous leg ulcers, The Clinicians' Notebook 1998; 2(2):5.
7. Fife CE, Ethics in wound care and hyperbaric medicine. In: Sheffield PJ, Fife CE, Smith APS. *Wound Care Practice*, 2007.
8. Wysocki AB, Grinnel F. Fibronectin profiles in normal and chronic wound fluid. *Lab Invest*; 1990; 63:825-8315.
9. Lawrence WT. Clinical management of nonhealing wounds. In: Cohen IK, Dieglemann RF, Lindblad WJ. (eds) *Wound Healing: Biochemical & Clinical Aspects*. Philadelphia, PA: W B Saunders Co. 1992; 541-561.
10. Parving HH, et al. The effect of metabolic regulation on microvascular permeability to small and large molecules in short-term juvenile diabetes. *Diabetologia*, 1976; 12:161-169.
11. Palumbo PJ, Melton LJ III. Peripheral vascular disease and diabetes, In Harris MI, Hamman RF, eds, Diabetes in America, NIH Pub no 85-1468, Washington DC: US Government Printing Office, 1985. (Diabetes data compiled in 1984)
12. National Fire Protection Association. NFPA 101-2006, Life Safety Code. Quincy, MA: National Fire Protection, 2006.
13. Centers for Medicare and Medicaid Services. 2006 Medicare Outpatient Prospective Payment System (OPPS) Reimbursement rates for hospitals and physicians. *http://www.cms.hhs.gov/HospitalOutpatientPPS/* and *http://www.cms.hhs.gov/PhysicianFeeSched/*
14. Pai M, Hunt TK. Effect of varying oxygen tensions on healing open wounds. *Surg Gynecol.* 1972; 135: 756-758.
15. Knighton DR, et al. Oxygen tension regulates the expression of angiogenesis factor by macrophages. *Science* 1983; 221:1283-1285..
16. Mader JT, et al. Potentiation of tobramycin by hyperbaric oxygen in experimental Pseudomonas aeruginosa osteomyelitis. Presented at the 27th Interscience Conference on Antimicrobial *Agents and Chemotherapy*. New York: New York City, 1987.
17. Sheffield PJ. Tissue Oxygen measurements In: Problem Wounds: In: The Role of Oxygen. JC Davis and TK Hunt (Eds) New York: Elsevier, 1988; 17-51..
18. Zhao LL, Davidson JD, Wee SC, Roth SI, Mustoe TA. Effect of hyperbaric oxygen and growth factors on rabbit ear ischemic ulcers. *Arch Surg*, 1994; 129(10): 1043-9.
19. Mader JT, et al. A mechanism for the amelioration by hyperbaric oxygen of experimental staphylococcal osteomyelitis in rabbits, *J Infect Dis*. 1980; 142:915-922.
20. Cianci P, et al. Salvage of the problem wound and potential amputation with wound care and adjunctive hyperbaric oxygen therapy: an economic analysis. *J Hyperbaric Med.* 1988; 3:127-141.
21. Texas Dept of Health and Human Resources, Physical plant requirements for a hyperbaric center, 1988.
22. National Fire Protection Association. NFPA 99 - 2005, *Standard for Health Care Facilities*, Chapter 20, Hyperbaric Facilities Quincy, MA: National Fire Protection, 2005.

REVIEW QUESTIONS

1.) When deciding whether the hospital should have an organized Wound Center administrators and medical staff must first determine whether:
    a. it is congruent with the mission of the hospital
    b. there is a need for the service
    c. there is space available to house the service
    d. it is economically feasible to provide the service

2.) Opening a Wound Center may require inspection by which of the following:
    a. State Health Department
    b. Local Fire Marshall
    c. Centers for Medicare and Medicaid Services (CMS)
    d. A and B above
    e. B and C above

3.) National Fire Protection Association (NFPA) mandates that a hyperbaric facility have:
    a. Program Director
    b. Clinical Director
    c. Safety Director
    d. Medical Director

4.) The ideal location for the Wound Center is:
    a. On the hospital premises
    b. In a professional building adjacent to the hospital
    c. At a remote location away from the hospital
    d. Within the emergency room

5.) In the opinion of the author, a successful Wound Center depends on:
    a. A patient population that needs the service
    b. A team of physicians, nurses, and technicians committed to the cause of wound healing
    c. A hospital that is willing to commit the resources needed to provide the service to the community and surrounding areas
    d. All of the above

Answers: 1a, 2d, 3c, 4a, 5d

NOTES

CHAPTER 44

INFECTION CONTROL IN THE WOUND CARE SETTING

CHAPTER FORTY-FOUR OVERVIEW

Infection Control in the Wound Care Setting

Peggy Nakayama Coe, Jan J. Clark

INTRODUCTION

Infection control and healthcare go hand in hand in today's society. We have come a long way from Semmelweis' (1) discovery of chlorine-hand hygiene. Yet over 150 years since his discovery, healthcare continues struggling to enforce hand washing as the single, simple, and most effective way to stop the spread of infection. This chapter will provide insight into current, evidence-based infection control practices.

REASON FOR INFECTION CONTROL

Many patients come into clinics with wounds. Not all are infected, but all have the potential to become infected. Without proper infection control procedures in place these wounds can easily become sources for nosocomial infections within the clinic. Infection control practices are important in any health setting. Healthcare professionals not only heal wounds, but also provide education to patients on all aspects that enhance wound healing. These practices include education on personal hygiene, cleaning and disinfection of the environment, immunizations, disease surveillance, isolation and exclusion policies, transmission precautions, waste management and biohazardous waste management.

ARBITERS OF STANDARDS (AUTHORITIES)

Healthcare is facing overwhelming demands from multiple regulating authorities including Centers for Disease Control and Prevention (CDC), Occupational Safety and Health Administration (OSHA), National Institute for Occupational Safety and Health (NIOSH), The Joint Commission, local State Health Departments, and the multitude of professional organizations with expertise in infection control issues. Whether your wound clinic is a stand-alone clinic or connected with a hospital, all have guidelines, regulations and standards with which the clinic must comply. Functions of regulatory agencies such as OSHA, CDC, and NIOSH differ as described below.

OSHA

All healthcare organizations must abide with rulings from the Occupational Safety and Health Administration (OSHA). This is the agency responsible for such standards as the Occupational Exposure to Bloodborne Pathogens (29 CFR 1910.1030) (OSHA), and OSHA Respiratory Protection for M. Tuberculosis Standard (29 CFR 1910.139) are laws issued by the federal government. Healthcare agencies must comply with these standards. There is no choice. OSHA is responsible for creating and enforcing workplace safety and health regulations.

CDC

Centers for Disease Control and Prevention (CDC) is located in Atlanta, Georgia. The CDC is one of the major components of the Department of Health and Human Services. It is recognized as the lead federal agency for protecting the health and safety of people. The CDC provides credible information to further health decisions and promotes health. It serves as the national focus for developing and applying disease prevention and control, environmental health, and health promotion and education activities. The CDC is comprised of twelve different centers, institutes, and offices.

The CDC provides concise infection control guidelines on many health issues. It offers guidelines in such areas as tuberculosis control, HIV, and infection control for hospital personnel. The proposed OSHA TB Standard incorporates the CDC's TB guidelines into their standard, but OSHA added more stringency in the area of respiratory protection. The CDC has no power to sanction or force health facilities to follow its guidelines, but they are good suggestions and recommendations based on scientific data.

NIOSH

National Institute for Occupational Safety and Health (NIOSH) (2) is the federal agency responsible for conducting research and making recommendations for the prevention of work-related disease and injury. This institute is a part of the Centers for Disease Control and Prevention. The same Act of Congress created NIOSH and OSHA, but they are two separate agencies with separate responsibilities. Respirators used for TB protection must be NIOSH approved. NIOSH and OSHA often work together to protect worker safety and health.

JCAHO, now The Joint Commission

The Joint Commission is an independent, not-for-profit organization that was established over 50 years ago (3). The Joint Commision sets the standards by which healthcare quality is measured. The Joint Commission is the leader in raising the healthcare field to ever-higher standards. Accreditation by the Joint Commission is voluntary. Inspections occur every three years. Healthcare organizations seek accreditation for many reasons. Some of the reasons why organizations seek accreditation are: 1) Accreditation stimulates the organization's quality improvement efforts; 2) It is used to meet certain Medicare certification requirements; 3) It expedites third-party payment; and 4) It often fulfills state licensure requirements.

Since 1976 (4) when the Joint Commission published its first standard that dealt specifically with infection control, "Jayco" has intensified the importance of infection control. The surveillance, prevention, and control of infections are now considered to be as important as the other functions addressed in The Joint Commision manual.

APIC

The Association for Professionals in Infection Control and Epidemiology (APIC) is a multi-disciplinary voluntary international organization. APIC's purpose is to influence, support, and improve the quality of healthcare through the practice and management of infection control and the application of epidemiology in all health settings. APIC was born out of the recognized need for an organized, systematic approach to control nosocomial infections. Nosocomial infections are those which are a result of treatment in a hospital. APIC has assumed the responsibility for training programs for infection control personnel that were previously provided by the CDC. APIC provides excellent resources and guidelines on infection control issues for healthcare.

State Health Departments

Local state health departments also have requirements to which healthcare institutions must abide. Often these requirements follow CDC guidelines. The state requirements may be stricter, less strict, or equivalent to OSHA. When this is the case, you should follow the set of requirements that is necessary for compliance to all rules and regulations that your clinic must meet. Institutional policies will be based upon standards set by many if not all of these mentioned agencies that are considered authorities in infection control.

PRODUCTS

Alcohol Hand Antisepsis

As mentioned earlier, hand washing is the single most important means of preventing the spread of infection. Now we can add alcohol-based hand rub or alcohol hand gel as another important and approved means of preventing the spread of infection (5). Most alcohol-based hand antiseptics contain isopropanol, ethanol, n-propanol, or a combination of two of these products.

Alcohol's antimicrobial activity is attributed to its ability to denature proteins. Alcohols have bactericidal activity against most gram-positive and gram-negative microorganisms and good activity against the tubercle bacillus (6). Though they are not sporicidal, alcohols act against many fungi and viruses, including respiratory syncytial virus, hepatitis B virus, and HIV (7). In appropriate concentrations, alcohols provide the most rapid and greatest reduction in microbial counts on skin. Alcohol solutions of 60–95% alcohol are most effective, and higher concentrations are less potent because proteins are not easily denatured in the absence of water (7). Petroleum and petrolatum-based hand lotions are not compatible with alcohol hand gels (5). The interactions between these two products can render them ineffective. Also some lotions can break down latex gloves. It is important to check that your alcohol hand gel, hand lotion and gloves are compatible.

Alcohol hand wash as short as 15 seconds have been effective in preventing hand transmission of gram-negative bacteria. The most effective method for hand antisepsis is the one-minute alcohol hand wash, which is equivalent to a four to seven minute skin preparation with other antiseptics in reducing the number of skin bacteria (7, 8). A sufficient amount of alcohol to thoroughly wet the hands completely is required. Alcohol in impregnated pads used on the hands has less antimicrobial effects than those of liquid soaps with antiseptic ingredients.

Alcohol is not appropriate for use when hands are visibly dirty or contaminated with blood. When only small amounts of blood are present, ethanol and isopropanol may reduce viable bacterial counts on hands more than plain or antimicrobial soap (9). Alcohol-based products are more effective for standard hand washing or hand antisepsis by healthcare workers (HCWs) than soap or antimicrobial soaps. Alcohol-based products reduce the number of multidrug resistant pathogens recovered from the hands of HCWs more effectively than does handwashing with soap and water.

The major disadvantage of alcohol for skin antisepsis is its drying effect, but the newer preparations have additions of emollients to minimize skin drying. A second disadvantage of alcohol is that it is volatile and flammable and must be stored carefully, in flame cabinets, if kept in large quantities. Because of its flammability, before placing alcohol dispensers in hallways, the facility should check with the local Fire Marshall for possible fire code infractions.

OTHER HAND WASH PRODUCTS

Most hand soaps used in healthcare contain chlorhexidine, chloroxylenol (PCMX), hexachlorophene, iodine, or triclosan. Table 1 will give in a nutshell the pros and cons of these different hand wash products. Which product you choose to use will depend on your objective for hand antisepsis.

SINGLE-DOSE MEDICATION VS. MULTIPLE-DOSE VIALS

The use of multiple-dose vials (MDV) in an outpatient clinical setting is not an acceptable practice and should be discontinued. The personal use of a MDV by a single individual is acceptable, but it is not good practice when a MDV is used for several different individuals. The chance for contamination is very possible and the liability is even greater. Multi-dose vial contamination does occur and has been cited (10). The use of the contents of a MDV for different patients poses a risk of spreading or transferring infection in the event that the vial becomes contaminated. What expiration date should be applied to a multiple-dose medication vial after it has been first used? Given that some patients are immunocompromised, it may be prudent to consider policies and procedures that preclude or strictly control the use of multiple-dose vials for such patients. Similar considerations may be prudent in the case of patients with highly communicable diseases. The American Society of Health-System Pharmacists (ASHP) offers current practice standards concerning MDVs.

MDVs contain preservatives that assist with sterility of the product during its continued use. Single-dose vials do not contain preservatives, and as such should be immediately discarded once the vial is entered and medication removed. Other standard recommendations include: the use of aseptic technique when entering any medication vial, proper vial entry (wipe with

TABLE 1. PREPARATIONS USED FOR HAND HYGIENE

Product	Bactericidal	Viricidal	Residual Activity	Other
Plain soap	minimal, if any	minimal if any	None	• Can remove loosely adherent translent flora • Rapid acting
Alchols Isopropanol Ethonol n-propanol	Excellent against gram-positive and gram-negative, M. tuberculosis and fungi	Effective against herpes simplex, HIV, influenza virus, RSV vaccina, HBV and HCV	No appreciative persistent activity	• 60-95% solution most effective • Can be drying to hands • Less effective in presence of high protein load
Chlorohexidine gluconate (CHG)	Good against gram-positive, less against gram-negative bacteria and fungi, minimal against tubercle bacilli, not sporicidal	In vitro activity against HSV, HIV, CMV, influenza, RSV. Less against rotavirus, adenovirus and enterovirus	Good residual activity	• Slower acting than alcohols • Minimally affected by organic material • Good safty record when used as directed • Concentrations $\geq$1% can cause severe eye damage • Concentrations of 0.5–4% available
Chloroxlyene (PCMX)	Good against gram-positive, fair against gram-negative, mycobacteria and certain viruses	Fair activity against certain viruses	Residual activity dependent on concentration of PCMX, higher the Concentration The greater the residual activity, less residual than CHG	• Minimally affected by organic matter • Antimicrobial activity is slower than CHG & iodophors • Neutralized by monionic surfactants • Available in concentrations of 0.3–3.75%
Hexachlorophene	Good activity against S. aureaus, weak against gram-negative bacteria, fungi & mycobacteria	Effective against some but not all viruses	Good residual activity, its best feature	• Neurotoxicity limits its use, not for infant use • Slow-intermediate activity • Not for use on non-intact skin 0.3% formulations available by prescription only
Triclosan	Greater activity against gram-positive bacteria than gram-negative, reasonable activity against mycobacteria and Candida spp., limited against fungi	Good activity against viruses	Like chlorhexidine, good residual activity	• Minimally affected by organic matter • Affected by pH, surfactants & emollients • Well tolerated & seldom cause allergic reactions

70% alcohol and let the vial top dry before entry into the vial with a sterile needle), and the use of sterile syringe-needle for each entry into the vial. At any time a MDV is considered compromised, it should be discarded. Medication vials should be visually inspected before entry for visual impurities and vial integrity, and for medication expiration date.

Not all multi-dose medication vials require refrigeration once opened; check the manufacturer's recommendation for requirements. The arbitrary dating of opened vials does nothing for the guarantee of sterility. Studies have shown that after repeated vial entries using good aseptic technique MDVs remained sterile (11). The CDC still recommends writing entry dates on the labels of MDVs, as does The Joint Commision, and most state health departments. The bottom line is you must comply with all regulations and meet the strictest requirements.

EQUIPMENT AND THE INANIMATE ENVIRONMENT

Cleaning Surfaces, Counters, Tables, etc.

As patients are being sent home earlier from hospitals, more routine care will be delivered on an outpatient basis. Infection control measures will need to continue in the outpatient arena. Proper disinfection remains paramount in reducing nosocomial infections and the overall spread of disease. Nosocomial infections rank as one of the leading causes of death in the United States (12) and as more and more routine care is delivered on an outpatient basis, it comes to the reality that infections can also happen in outpatient areas.

Where bloodborne pathogens are of concern, there are very stringent disinfectant requirements. OSHA's Bloodborne Pathogen Standard states that the disinfectant must kill the Mycobacterium tuberculosis bacteria, the organism responsible for tuberculosis or the disinfectant must kill both the hepatitis B virus (HBV) and HIV-1, the virus responsible for AIDS.

The U.S. Environmental Protection Agency (EPA) requires each disinfectant to have a clearly defined label. The label will have directions for use, specific dilutions for certain procedures, required contact time for killing particular organisms, precautionary statements when using the disinfectant, specific steps to take in case of accidental contact or ingestion and storage and disposal for the product. All disinfectants must be given EPA approval and have the label reviewed to make sure the information is correct and the disinfectant does what its label states. Be sure to use the proper product for the job required. For floors and counter tops, surfaces that do not come in contact with non-intact skin or mucous membranes, a disinfectant is all that is required for cleaning. For equipment that will come into contact with mucous membranes or non-intact skin, high-level disinfection is required. For a normally sterile area of the body, sterile equipment is required.

If house-cleaning services are contracted out, make sure that you are hiring a firm that is aware of the regulations and can provide you with documentation that assures the firm is familiar and competent with the special needs of a clinic.

Non-critical patient care equipment can be a potential source of infection, but highly unlikely to do so. The public's perception of what causes infection may be incorrect and so visible contamination is undesirable in their eyes. Studies have documented hospital stethoscopes contaminated with gram-negative and gram-positive bacteria (13–15). These studies also showed that simple cleaning of stethoscopes with alcohol removes the bacterial contamination.

CHOICE OF STERILIZATION OR DISINFECTION LEVEL

Spaulding's classification scheme indicates the level of sterilization or disinfection required for various items.

- Critical items enter tissue or vascular space. Critical items require sterilization.
- Semi-critical items contact mucous membranes or non-intact skin. Semi-critical items require high-level disinfection and/or intermediate-level disinfection.
- Non-critical items contact intact skin. Non-critical items require intermediate or low-level disinfection.

Sterilization can be achieved through many methods: steam, dry heat, ethylene oxide (ETO) gas, 2% glutaraldehyde, hydrogen peroxide, and peracetic acid. High-level disinfection can be achieved by 2% glutaraldehyde, hydrogen peroxide, peracetic acid, and household bleach. Intermediate-level disinfection can be achieved with ethyl or isopropyl alcohol, household bleach, phenolic germicidal detergent or iodophor germicidal detergent. Low-level disinfection can be achieved with ethyl or isopropyl alcohol, phenolic germicidal detergent, iodophor germicidal detergent, quaternary ammonium germicidal detergent, or household bleach. To achieve any of these levels of disinfection, instruments must first be properly cleaned of any organic matter. All of these methods have very specific guidelines that must be followed to safely achieve the desired or required level of disinfection or sterility, but they are beyond the scope of this chapter. They can be found in textbooks written for these specific purposes.

Disposable vs. Re-useable Equipment

Whether you use disposable or re-useable equipment varies with your situation. If the clinic is located in a hospital the choice is easy, re-useable instruments are better quality and can easily be reprocessed by the central sterile department. Because the instruments will often be in contact with non-intact skin and tissue, these instruments require sterilization. Sterilization requires strict adherence to infection control, log books, quality control monitors, load-tracking methods, employee safety monitoring and much more. If your clinic is stand-alone, this may be more work than you are willing to do; disposables may be the route to take. Considerations that must be weighed against the cost of purchasing disposable equipment include: the cost of sterilizing instruments, the cost of the sterilization equipment, the work of keeping sterilization logs, and the time involved in instrument maintenance and wrapping of items for sterile processing.

STORAGE OF SUPPLIES

There must be separate areas for clean and dirty supplies, because the two cannot be mixed. Sterile products should not be stored directly under overhead sprinklers or plumbing junctures. This means no storage under sinks. No items should be stored closer than 18 inches from the ceiling. Sterile stock must be maintained at least 8 inches from the floor and storage shelves for these supplies must be solid bottomed or the supplies stored in bins on the shelves. Storage shelves must be 2–3 inches from any exterior wall. Rotation of supplies ensures that "old" supplies are used prior to "new" supplies. Identifying expired supplies and removing them from stock should be a routine task.

SPECIAL PRECAUTIONS IN CLINIC OR OFFICE

MRSA and VRE

Methicillin-resistant *S. aureus* (MRSA) and Vancomycin-resistant Enterococcus (VRE) are becoming more prevalent in today's healthcare arena so it is understandable that these organisms will appear in wounds of patients seen in clinics. Those at highest risk for developing MRSA colonization and infection are patients with a history of IV drug abuse, previous antibiotic therapy, have chronic disease, repeat hospitalizations, admission to an intensive care unit, received transplants, or a prolonged stay in a healthcare facility. The drug of choice for MRSA is intravenous vancomycin, while the drug of choice for VRE may be difficult to determine until cultures are complete.

Standard precautions and contact precautions should be adequate to protect healthcare workers and to prevent transmission to other patients. In the clinical setting, it is wise to designate one examination room (if there is more than one) for patients with VRE or MRSA. If there is only one examination room, scheduling that patient for the last appointment is a worthwhile precaution. Wearing gloves and hand washing are also very important to prevent the spread of any multi-resistant organism. Cleaning the environment between patients with an EPA approved disinfectant will work to successfully eliminate organisms, even multi-drug resistant strains. Areas that require cleaning between patients are those items with direct patient contact; the exam table or chair and the Mayo stand. No special cleaning procedures, wiping the walls or fogging the room, are required after treating a patient with multi-drug resistant strains. Terminal cleaning is done at the end of the clinic's day or prior to the beginning of the next day. Proper decontamination of equipment and judicious use of antibiotics is also instrumental in stopping multi-resistant organisms.

Artificial Fingernails

Artificial fingernails or extenders are not recommended for healthcare workers who do direct patient care. Natural fingernails should be kept short, as recommended from the Guideline for Hand Hygiene in Healthcare Settings. Artificial nails worn by healthcare workers can contribute to healthcare-associated infections and have been documented. Artificial nails have a higher rate of colonization when compared to natural nails (16, 17). Un-chipped polish on natural nails is not associated with increased colonization with micro-organisms (18).

Single-dose and Individually-Wrapped Supplies

Should you use individually wrapped supplies versus group-use bulk supplies? Studies show that multiple-group use supplies are easily contaminated and are often colonized (19). If you are not the only person taking from these supplies, you cannot guarantee the supplies have not been compromised. You may have proper infection control technique, but what about the person who used the supplies before you, or the person who followed you? Their technique is unknown. It is better to err on the side of safety and use single-dose, single wrapped items versus community-use supplies, such as gauze or cotton swabs, when it comes to dressings for wound care.

Engineering Controls

The Bloodborne Pathogens Standard was made mandatory for all of healthcare in 1991. In November of 2000, the Needlestick Safety and Prevention Act was signed into law. This updates the original Bloodborne Pathogens Standard and makes it mandatory that safety-engineered products have been evaluated and implemented and that this is also documented in their exposure control plan. The update also requires that exposure control plans be reviewed and updated at least annually to reflect changes in sharps safety technology. It requires each healthcare facility to maintain a sharps injury log with detailed information on percutaneous injuries to include the type and brand of device involved in the exposure incident, the department where the exposure occurred, and an explanation of how it occurred. Another important requirement mandates that employers solicit input from non-managerial health care workers (front-line workers) when identifying, evaluating and selecting safety-engineered sharps devices, and to document this process in the exposure control plan. The update also expands the definition of "engineering controls" to include devices with engineered sharps injury protection.

Other engineering controls remain unchanged. Used sharps must be placed into appropriately marked sharps containers; these containers must be conveniently placed, and must be marked with the biohazard label. Used needles must not be recapped. OSHA fines facilities during inspections for finding re-capped needles in sharps disposal containers. Filled sharps containers should also not be emptied into larger containers and re-used, the chance for injury is too great; and this is also a reason for OSHA fines.

Regulated Medical Waste

Regulated medical waste is also known as biohazardous waste, infectious waste or potentially infectious waste. By law it requires special treatment or handling. In the clinic setting regulated medical waste includes sharps, blood, blood products, laboratory wastes, pathological wastes, and isolation wastes. Regulated medical waste is generally considered capable of transmitting disease or causing injury.

This waste must be properly packaged for transport for disposal. If transport of the regulated medical waste entails that it will travel upon public roads, strict guidelines from the Department of Transportation (DOT), regulate how the waste is handled, transported on highways, and disposed of. Regulated medical waste ultimately ends up in red biohazardous containers before leaving a facility. If your clinic is within a hospital, disposal of your medical waste will not be a problem. It will be transported with the hospital's regulated medical waste. For stand-alone clinics, it becomes a bit more complicated. The best practice is to contract your regulated medical waste with a reputable company that will properly pick up, dispose of and maintain a good paper trail proof of disposal.

Exposure Follow-up (20)

All healthcare facilities must provide treatment and follow-up for bloodborne pathogen exposure. Prophylaxis actually begins when employment begins. The Bloodborne Pathogen Standard mandates that the employer offers free of charge the hepatitis B vaccine to those employees that have the chance of a Bloodborne pathogen exposure at least once a month. The Standard makes it mandatory that the hepatitis B vaccine is offered to the employee, but it is completely voluntary as to whether the employee takes the vaccine. Proof of the offering and proof of the refusal to take the vaccine should be documented in the employees health file. If an employee refuses to take the vaccine at the time of hiring, they also have the right at any time to change their mind and receive the vaccine free of charge.

If the employee has already received the vaccine, then the employee requires testing to make sure they have a positive antibody response (positive HbsAb). The Standard states that employers must know the antibody status of employees upon hiring. If upon testing the employee has no antibodies, the employee should receive a booster dose and be retested in four to six weeks. If antibody response remains negative, the employee should receive a repeat series of the vaccine, doses two and three should be completed at the appropriate time intervals as recommended according to the vaccine manufacturer.

If the clinic has a person working in an employee health capacity, they will be directing the required testing for new-hire and continue to keep the employee's health file current. Should an actual blood exposure occur, follow-up is mandatory by the employer and the follow-up required is explicitly spelled out in the Standard. Whether the clinic actually does the follow-up or contracts this service out to another facility is individual to each facility. If this service is contracted out to another facility or clinic, a written contract between the two facilities is recommended so that not only the initial testing is done, but the 6 week, 12 week, and 6 month follow-up testing is also completed for the exposed employee. The bottom line is this must be provided and must be provided free to the employee.

SUMMARY

Regulations for infection control practices are many, but the agencies that propose and enforce them do so to protect patients and healthcare workers. It is important that all healthcare workers use knowledge of wound care, aseptic and clean technique, and common sense to ensure a transmission-free environment.

REFERENCES

1. Semmelweis I. Etiology, concept, and prophylaxis of childbed fever. *Carter KC* ed. 1st ed. Madison, WI: The University of Wisconsin Press. 1983.
2. National Institute for Occupational Safety and Health. About NIOSH research and services. Retrieved on 4/16/03 from *http://www.cdc.gov/niosh/about.html.*
3. Joint Commission on Accreditation of Healthcare Organizations. Who is the joint commission? Retrieved on 4/16/03 from *http://www.jcaho.org/general+public/who+jc/index.htm.*
4. Russell B. APIC history. *Infection Control and Hospital Epidemiology* 1995; 16:522-525.
5. Boyce J, Pittet D. Guideline for hand hygiene in health-care settings, recommendations of the healthcare infection control practices advisory committee and the HICPAC/SHEA/APIC/IDSA hand hygiene task force. MMWR 2002:51(RR-16).
6. Larson E. APIC guideline for handwashing and hand antisepsis in health care settings. *Am J of Infect Control* 1995; 23:251-269.
7. Larson E, Morton H. Alcohol. In Block, SS. (Ed.), Disinfection, sterilization, and preservation 4th ed. Philadelphia, PA: Lea & Febiger. 1991; 191-203.
8. Geelhoed G, Sharpe K, Simon G. A comparative study of surgical skin preparation methods. *Surg Gynecol Obst* 1983; 157:265-268.
9. Larson E, Bobo L. Effective hand degerming in the presence of blood. *J Emerg Med* 1992; 10:7-11.
10. Levy M, Moff M, Jones B. Improper infection-control practices during employee vaccination program-District of Columbia and Pennsylvannia, *MMWR* 1993; 42(50):969-973.
11. Wilson J, Cobb D. Updating your multiple-dose vial policy: The background. 1998. Retrieved on 3/17/03 from http://libproxy-002.ouhsc.edu:2051/ovidweb.cgi.
12. Wenzel R, Edmunds M. The impact of hospital acquired infections. *Emerging Infectious Diseases* 2001; 7(2)175-178.
13. Bernard L, Kereveur A, Durand D, et al. Bacterial contamination of hospital physician's stethoscopes. *Infection Control & Hospital Epidemiology* 1999; 20(9):629-628.
14. Cohen H, Amir J, Matalon A, et al. Stethoscopes and otoscopes- a potential vector of infection? *Family Practice* 1997; 14(6):446-449.
15. Smith M, Mathewson J, Ulert I, et al. Contaminated stethoscopes revisited. 1996. Retrieved on 3/27/03 from http://libproxy-002.ouhsc.edu:2162/ovidweb.cgi.
16. Pottinger J, Burns S, Manke C. Bacterial carriage by artificial versus natural nails. *American Journal of Infection Control* 1989; 17:340-344.
17. Wynd C, Samstag D, Lapp A. Bacterial carriage on the fingernails of OR nurses. *AORN Journal* 1994; 60:796-805.
18. Hedderwick S, McNeil S, Lyons M, et al. Pathogenic organisms associated with artificial fingernails. *Infection Control and Hospital Epidemiology* 2000; 21:505-509.
19. Griffith C, Malik R, Cooper R, et al. Environmental surface cleanliness and the potential for contamination during handwashing. *Am J of Infect Control* 2003; 31:93-96.
20. Department of Labor. Occupational Safety and Health Administration. Occupational exposure to bloodborne pathogens (29 CFR part 1910.1030). *Federal Register* 1991; 56:64004–64182.

REVIEW QUESTIONS

1.) The single most important method for preventing the spread of infection is:
   a. washing with anti-microbial liquid soap
   b. washing with 70-95% alcohol products
   c. washing with 100% alcohol products
   d. washing with triclosan hand products

2.) The agency responsible for standards such as the Occupational Exposure to Bloodborne Pathogens and the M. tuberculosis Standard is:
   a. The CDC
   b. JCAHO
   c. OSHA
   d. NIOSH

3.) Infection control issues for clinics are governed by:
   a. the CDC
   b. your local State Health Department
   c. JCAHO
   d. The set of requirements that are necessary for compliance to all rules and regulations

4.) Those at highest risk for developing MRSA colonization and infection are patients with:
   a. History of IV drug abuse
   b. Repeat hospitalizations
   c. Admission to an intensive care unit
   d. Prolonged stay in a healthcare facility
   e. Any of the above

5.) Spaulding's classification scheme indicates the level of sterilization or disinfection required for various items. Critical items enter tissue or vascular space and require:
   a. Sterilization
   b. High-level disinfection and/or intermediate-level disinfection
   c. Intermediate or low-level disinfection
   d. Neither sterilization nor disinfection

Answers: 1b, 2c, 3d, 4e, 5a

CHAPTER 45

LATEX ALLERGY AND ADVANCED WOUND CARE

CHAPTER FORTY-FIVE OVERVIEW

NOTES

Latex Allergy and Advanced Wound Care

Jeffrey A. Niezgoda

INTRODUCTION

Why must latex allergies be discussed in an advanced wound care text? The skin and subcutaneous tissues are in and of themselves a system that interacts with and contains components of the respiratory, cardiovascular, immune, and nervous systems. The cascade of effects created by allergic reactions such as contact dermatitis, affects each of these systems and can halt or even reverse the healing process. Allergic reactions may be misdiagnosed as cellulitis, eczema, non-specific inflammation, fungal overgrowth, or venous stasis dermatitis. Latex allergy is one such reaction that must be considered in the differential diagnosis.

Many wound care products as well as some components of interventional modalities contain natural rubber latex (NRL). Early detection of latex sensitivity combined with appropriate treatment and secondary prevention interventions can decrease risk of adverse events and improve wound healing outcomes in this population. An in-depth literature review reveals that there is scant literature addressing the topic of wound healing and latex allergies, in fact one must extrapolate much of the data from dermatology and pathophysiology texts.

Wound healing is a complex biochemical process which can be broken down into four phases: hemostasis, inflammation, proliferation, and maturation. Allergic and hypersensitivity reactions such as those related to latex exposure, are caused by immune responses to environmental antigens that produce inflammation and may cause tissue injury. Differentiation between inflammation which is expected in the normal healing process and the inflammatory responses that the immune system mounts to fight pathogens and allergens is frequently a clinical and diagnostic dilemma.

LATEX

Natural rubber latex is manufactured from the sap of the Heva brasiliensis plant or "rubber tree" plant (1). Multiple chemicals are used in the production of the various forms of latex and rubber products including solvents, curing agents, and stabilizers. Allergic reactions to latex products can be triggered by the latex proteins themselves or the chemicals used in manufacturing.

Rubber or latex has revolutionized health care interventions and products. The first colostomy and urostomy patients used rags and other absorbent materials to contain their bodily fluids. Latex made it possible to create soft, pliable, moisture resistant appliances to collect and hold stool and urine. Red rubber catheters emptied distended neuropathic bladders gently without trauma. Elastic bandages supported weak joints and decreased the swelling of amputated limb stumps and edematous lower extremities. These latex containing devices improved healthcare dramatically. The list of healthcare products containing NRL include, but is not limited to: adhesive tape, Ambu bags, bulb syringes, condom catheters, condoms, elastic bandages, enema kits, gloves—examination and sterile, syringes, protective sheets, stethoscope tubing, GI tubes, tourniquets, and wound drains.

Late in the 1980's, a logarithmic increase in the use of NRL based latex products was seen following implementation of Universal or Standard Precautions to reduce the transmission of the Human Immunodeficiency Virus (HIV) and other blood-borne diseases in the health care setting. Rubber gloves were used universally by healthcare workers to provide protective barriers between the patient's blood and body fluids and the caregiver's skin. Latex gloves when compared to plastic, nitrile, and other synthetic products provide the most effective barrier between the skin integrity of the healthcare worker's hands and pathogen carrying body fluids. Latex gloves played a large role in sensitizing both the providers and the patients. Powdering latex gloves with talc or cornstarch makes them easier to don. Gloving and degloving aerosolizes the cornstarch or talc powder as well as the latex proteins that have bound to them. The dual routes of inhalation and topical exposure increased the prevalence of hypersensitivity reactions that occurred in healthcare environments.

Allergic and Hypersensitivity Reactions

The antigens or allergens involved in latex allergies include both the organic proteins contained in rubber and the chemicals used in manufacturing. Some allergens cause an immediate hypersensitivity reaction; others create delayed responses after repeated exposures to the noxious substance. There are three types of reactions to natural rubber latex: irritant contact dermatitis, Type IV (delayed) hypersensitivity, and Type I (immediate) hypersensitivity. It is useful to occasionally review the differences between the three, since latex avoidance is critical to those who have latex allergy.

Irritant Contact Dermatitis is a common reaction and is not an allergy. Itchy, dry, and irritated hands are the result of frequent hand washing and incomplete drying, use of hand sanitizers, and friction irritation from glove powder. Anyone who wears powdered latex gloves can develop this; however, in atopic individuals, contact dermatitis can be a sign of impending hypersensitivity if exposure to latex continues.

Type IV (delayed-type) Hypersensitivity is usually sensitivity to the chemicals used to make gloves, rather than to proteins from the natural rubber itself (1). Numerous chemicals are used in the manufacturing process, including emulsifiers, stabilizers, accelerators, stiffeners, colorants, and fragrances. Any of these can cause a contact dermatitis 24–48 hours after exposure, which can spread to other areas, including the face, if touched. Symptoms usually resolve spontaneously.

Type I (immediate-type) Hypersensitivity is an allergy to natural rubber latex (Hevea brasiliensis) proteins that occurs as a response to exposure. Type I reactions are a result of mast cell degranulation initiated by binding of the allergen to the immune globulin on the surface of the mast cell. Mast cells are tissue cells and are normally distributed in connective tissue, beneath the skin, in mucous membranes of the respiratory, gastrointestinal, and genitourinary tract, and along blood and lymph vessels. Exposure to topical and inhaled allergens is increased by the location of mast cells in the layers of the skin and mucous membranes. Mast cells are the primary mediators of the inflammatory response in these tissues.

Latex allergy (Type I hypersensitivity to latex proteins) can become a serious systemic allergic reaction. It usually begins within minutes of exposure but can sometimes occur hours later. Vasoactive mediators such as histamine are released producing varied symptoms, which commonly include runny nose, sneezing, itchy eyes, scratchy throat, hives, facial swelling and itching burning sensations. However, latex allergy can evolve into more severe symptoms including asthma; difficulty breathing, coughing and wheezing; cardiovascular and gastrointestinal ailments; and in rare cases, anaphylaxis and death. Emergency treatment for anaphylaxis may be required, and anyone who has experienced a Type I reaction attributable to latex exposure should wear a medical ID bracelet and carry an emergency epinephrine kit.

Inflammatory Response

In acute wound healing, the inflammatory phase begins immediately after the trauma or insult occurs and can last up to four days. Approximately 20 minutes after injury, vasodilatory hormones cause the capillary endothelial cells to relax their adhesion to adjacent cell walls allowing the plasma which contains fibrinogen, leukocytes, and monocytes to seep into the surrounding tissues. The additional fluid and proteins in the interstitium creates the swelling and edema usually associated with inflammation. Usually the area around the wound is red, warm, swollen and painful. The same clinical findings are noted in hypersensitivity reactions; however, they are mediated by the mast cell degranulation or by antigen-antibody complexes.

In normal wound healing, the leukocytes and monocytes differentiate into macrophages, which in turn scavenge for tissue debris, foreign matter and bacteria. The macrophage begins to produce chemotactic proteins called growth factors or cytokines that initiate the proliferative phase. Macrophages ingest microorganisms and release cytokines that stimulate angiogenesis and signal fibroblasts to synthesize collagen. The inflammatory phase is therefore an important component in normal wound healing. It is when inflammation causes further tissue damage or impedes the healing process, that anti-inflammatory interventions must take place. The clinician must be cognizant of these physiologic processes when prescribing treatment as the healing process can be suppressed if the patient is receiving corticosteroids, non-steroidal anti-inflammatory medications, anti-neoplastic drugs, anticoagulants, anti-prostaglandins, and immune system modulators.

Individuals at Risk

Those at highest risk for hypersensitivity to latex products used in wound care are health care workers and patients that have undergone multiple or repeated surgical procedures. The source of exposure to the latex allergen gives rise to the risk groups. Exposure may occur via skin, mucous membrane, respiratory tract linings, and intravenous/vascular access. The severity of the reaction to latex depends on the degree to which a person has been sensitized, the amount of latex protein to which a person is exposed, and the location of the contact.

Along with the healthcare providers, workers in the food processing and rubber industry are subject to occupational exposure to latex. Healthcare workers are no longer the only ones in need of protection to avoid exposure to body fluids. Police officers, teachers and daycare providers use latex gloves when dealing with injured people or coming in contact with body fluids like baby diapers and vomit.

Dermal Manifestations of Latex Allergy

Dermatitis

Dermatitis, also known as eczema, is characterized by inflammatory reactions involving, the epidermis, dermis, and mucous membranes. Causes are variable, and can be endogenous or exogenous (2). Acute forms of dermatitis are characterized by severe itching, erythema, and vesicle formation. Chronic forms are portrayed by pruritus, hyperkeratosis, trophic skin changes, and fissuring of the epidermis; or lichenification. Contact dermatitis is the most common type of reaction to latex in health care settings. This reaction is due to the Type IV delayed hypersensitivity reaction.

Venous stasis dermatitis

Venous insufficiency is an abnormal condition of the lower extremity venous circulation evidenced by a slowed or decreased return of blood from the legs and feet to the central venous system (3). This slowed return results in tissue changes including, but not limited to, swelling, discoloration, fibrosis, pain, ulceration, cellulitis, dermatitis, and decreased mobility. Current statistics about chronic wound incidence and prevalence illustrate the burden of this condition. More than 2.5 million Americans suffer from venous leg ulcers (4). Once venous insufficiency has progressed to the stage of ulceration it is most often slow to heal, recurrent, and lends the patient to a greater risk of repeated infection. The sequelae of venous disease range from a constant dull aching pain, oozing of serous fluid resulting in protein depletion, and localized soft tissue infections, and may progress to circumferential full thickness wounds, continuous severe pain, and limb threatening osteomyelitis.

Compression devices to decrease the edema or interstitial fluid accumulation are the foundation for treatment of venous insufficiency. Many of these compression therapies contain latex and therefore unfortunately create risk for allergic or sensitivity reactions in patients with venous disease. Unna's boots have been used since the late 1800's as a treatment for venous stasis ulcers. The boot consists of a gauze wrap impregnated with zinc oxide. This dressing is wrapped snugly around the leg from just above the toes to below the knee. A latex or elastic wrap typically provides additional support. Current therapies include three, four, and even five layer systems that exert compression both at rest and during ambulation through the implementation of both long stretch and short stretch wraps. These wraps have traditionally contained latex and thus serve as another source of latex exposure. Fortunately, the pharmaceutical industry has recognized this problem and responded with the development of compression dressings and devices that are latex-free.

Long standing venous insufficiency can lead to a condition known as venous stasis dermatitis. It is characterized by papules, vesicles, redness and intense pruritus. The dermatitis originates at the midsection of the region with edema but may after time extend beyond the borders of the lower extremity edema. Differential diagnoses associated with this erythematous rash accompanied by weeping of serous fluid, crusting, and ulceration located on an edematous lower extremity include, but are not limited to: bacterial infection (cellulitis) typically staphylococcal in origin, fungal infection, contact allergies to topical treatments such as neomycin or lanolin, a generalized inflammatory response, and hemosiderin staining.

In addition to the venous stasis dermatitis, other skin changes are noted with long standing venous hypertension. Lichenification or thickened plaques of skin, occurs in response to rubbing of dressings and persistent scratching in response to intense pruritus. Hyperpigmentation is a result of the build up of hemosiderin resulting from the decomposition of extravasated red blood cells, this actually the iron from the hemoglobin. Lipodermatosclerosis occurs when the deeper tissues become "woody" in texture due to chronic inflammation. Atrophie blanche appears as white scarred areas surrounded by enlarged capillarics. This tissue is often hypersensitive and very fragile. Hypersensitivities result from alteration in the immune system cells in the lower legs of persons with long standing venous hypertension. This places the patient with venous insufficiency at increased risk for developing contact allergies to substances to which they would not otherwise be allergic. The implementation of latex-free products and compression systems is mandatory in these at-risk patients.

TREATMENT OF LATEX DERMATITIS

As stated previously, proper diagnosis of the condition is paramount to providing the appropriate interventions. Prior to implementing treatment regimens for allergic or contact dermatitis, infections should be ruled out. A thorough medical history and complete patient assessment will yield valuable information to direct the diagnosis. If the cause of the symptoms eludes the practitioner, a biopsy may be necessary. Allergen patch testing may be conducted to determine the culprit causing an allergic contact dermatitis reaction. It may be necessary to refer the patient to a dermatologist or allergy specialist.

The first step in treatment is to determine the cause. Treatment of an underlying condition may be the ultimate cure of the dermatitis. If treatment of the erythematous rash is required to reduce skin and tissue damage, the following is a list recommended by the Mayo Clinic (5):

- Topical corticosteroids and newer topical immunosuppressive treatments
- Oral or topical antihistamines

- Avoidance of irritants or allergens
- Wet dressings: applying medicated cream to affected areas and then covering these areas with cotton material that has been soaked in a wetting solution
- Ultraviolet light treatments (UVA, UVB)
- Hospitalization for treatment of severe dermatitis that is not responding to the above treatments
- Immunosuppressive treatments

Considerations

Patients with a latex allergy should not have direct contact with latex-containing materials and should be treated in a "latex safe" environment. By obtaining complete patient health histories and preventing patients from having contact with potential allergens, health care professionals can minimize the possibility of patients having adverse reactions. Considerations in providing safe treatment for patients with possible or documented latex allergy include: screening for latex allergy, awareness of predisposing conditions such as spina bifida and urogenital anomalies, or individuals with multiple allergies or atopic dermatitis, providing a latex free treatment area, and communicating standardized latex allergy procedures including written policies and procedures.

If latex-related complications occur during or after the procedure, manage the reaction and seek emergency assistance as indicated. Follow current medical emergency response recommendations for management of anaphylaxis.

Prevention

The following recommendations are based on those issued by the National Institute for Occupational Health and Safety (NIOSH) (6):

If definitively diagnosed with allergy to natural rubber latex (NRL) protein:

- Avoid, as far as feasible, subsequent exposure to the protein and only use nonlatex (e.g., nitrile or vinyl) gloves.
- Make sure that other staff members wear either nonlatex or reduced protein, powder-free latex gloves.

Health care personnel can further reduce occupational exposure to NRL protein by taking the following steps:

- Use reduced protein, powder-free latex gloves.
- Frequently change ventilation filters and vacuum bags used in latex contaminated areas.
- Check ventilation systems to ensure they provide adequate fresh or recirculating air.
- Frequently clean all work areas contaminated with latex dust.

As with other potentially life-threatening allergies, the primary method of protection is avoiding contact with latex and being prepared to treat anaphylactic emergencies. Avoidance is crucial in guarding against further sensitization and severe allergic reactions to latex. People who have allergic symptoms after contact with latex should substitute latex-free versions of latex products in their homes and workplaces and should alert their health care providers that they have to be treated with latex-free equipment (7).

CONCLUSION

The reactions that are caused by exposure to latex products can lead to skin breakdown, tissue destruction, and impaired healing. Dermatitis that occurs in the advanced wound care population is often a clinical dilemma, accurate diagnosis is important to expedite positive healing outcomes. Latex allergy may masquerade as acute or subacute cellulitis, fungal infection of the skin, irritant dermatitis, or a variety of contact allergies. Awareness of latex allergy and its presentation will allow the practitioner to utilize this in the differential diagnosis. Prompt diagnosis and appropriate interventions including patient education will aid in preventing future reactions.

Wound care products and interventions include many products that contain latex. Over the past twenty years latex hypersensitivities have increased in prevalence due to the use of latex based products in healthcare. Reducing the number of rubber or latex products utilized in wound care will help to reduce sensitization and impending allergic reactions in this population that tends to be in need of long term medical treatment.

REFERENCES

1. Porth C. (2002) Alterations in the immune response in pathophysiology concepts of altered health states (6th ed.) Philadephia, PA: Lippincott Williams & Wilkins pp. 365-370
2. Porth C. (2002) Alterations in the Immune Response in Pathophysiology Concepts of Altered Health States (6th ed.) Philadephia, PA: Lippincott Williams & Wilkins pp. 371
3. Anderson D M, Keith J, & Novak PD, (2002). Mosby's Medical, Nursing, & Allied Health Dictionary (6th ed.). St. Louis, MO: Mosby.
4. Beitz J M, (2001). Overcoming barriers to quality wound care: A systems perspective. *Ostomy/Wound Management* 47 (3), 56-64
5. Treatment of Dermatitis at Mayo Clinic in Rochester. Retrieved January 4, 2007 from *http://www.mayoclinic.org/dermatitis-rst/index.html*
6. NIOSH Alert: Preventing Allergic Reactions to Natural Rubber Latex in the Workplace. US Dept. of Health and Human Services. August 1998:3.
7. Phillips P. (2001). A review of the expert opinion on latex allergy. Available at: *www.worldwidewounds.com*

REVIEW QUESTIONS

1.) The antigens and allergens involved in latex allergies include:
  a. Organic proteins contained in rubber
  b. Chemicals used in manufacturing
  c. Aerosols of cornstarch or talc powder
  d. Both a and b
  e. a, b, and c

2.) Which statement about allergic and hypersensitivity reactions is FALSE?
  a. Irritant contact dermatitis is a common reaction and is not an allergy.
  b. Type IV (delayed-type) hypersensitivity is usually sensitivity to the chemicals used to make gloves.
  c. Type I (intermediate-type) hypersensitivity is an allergy to natural rubber latex proteins.
  d. Latex allergy can never become a serious systemic allergic reaction.

3.) Those at least risk for hypersensitivity to latex products are
  a. Health care workers
  b. Food processing personnel
  c. Workers in the rubber industry
  d. People who have never been in contact with latex
  c. Patients who have undergone multiple or repeated surgical procedures

4.) If diagnosed with allergy to natural rubber latex, one should
  a. avoid subsequent exposure to natural rubber latex proteins
  b. use nonlatex (e.g., nitrile or vinyl) gloves
  c. make sure nearby persons wear either nonlatex or reduced protein, powder-free latex gloves
  d. All of the above

Answers: 1e, 2d, 3d, 4d.

NOTES

CHAPTER 46

DOCUMENTATION: TELLING THE STORY OF CARE

CHAPTER FORTY-SIX OVERVIEW

NOTES

DOCUMENTATION: TELLING THE STORY OF CARE

Edna Patricia Rios, Valerie Larson-Lohr

INTRODUCTION

Documentation is telling the story. The story of the treatment the patient has received while in the care of the practitioner. The story has multiple parts. Those parts include perspectives from physicians, nurses, therapists, nutritionists and all others that play a part in delivering care to the patient. The focus of this chapter is nursing documentation. Historically, nursing documentation was used to reflect physician orders that had been carried out. There would be cursory comments on how the patient ate, slept, presence or absence of pain, and how they performed activities of daily living. But all comments would focus off of the physicians' orders or notes.

In the 1970's and 80's, nurses began to develop their own language based on nursing diagnosis. The concept of nursing using the vocabulary of nursing diagnosis has had variable acceptance throughout the profession (1). While all agree we must have a common language, many times the format of nursing diagnosis becomes burdensome and instead of addressing a patient need, the need is made to fit within a specific category.

What has come from the work done on nursing diagnosis is the emphasis on the importance of clarity, conciseness and consistency. Clarity of the plan of care, what was accomplished this visit, and what needs to be done next visit. Conciseness or focusing of the topic, so the message is not lost in the words and the words that are present have meaning. Consistency in how the documentation is done from nurse to nurse and visit to visit.

NURSING DOCUMENTATION

In this chapter, we will narrow the focus of documentation even further to address care within a chronic wound environment: what are the requirements, how to evaluate and improve nursing documentation. Because patients at many wound centers have access to hyperbaric oxygen therapy we will briefly describe those documentation requirements as well.

Errors in Documentation

Errors commonly found in general nursing documentation include: blank spaces, missing key components, documentation of all health care providers with legible signatures, co-signatures for unlicensed personal by licensed staff who supervised care of patient, errors scratched out instead of a single mark through and use of blue ink instead of black ink (2). The general error areas are easy to repair and will need periodic maintenance to ensure staff compliance. In the specialty of wound care, documentation not only needs to "tell the story" of the patient encounter but many times must meet requirements of payers such as Medicare. While we will not specifically address documentation requirements of Medicare, we would advise all providers to know the documentation requirements of their Fiscal Intermediaries (Medicare payers for facilities).

Initial Nursing History

During the initial visit to the wound center, the registered nurse should obtain a complete history of the patient with a focus on the chronic wound and why it has failed to heal. Key questions should focus on how the wound occurred, how long the wound has been present, what is the current treatment, any previous treatment and has the wound ever healed. If the patient is diabetic, specific questions should be asked to obtain information on how much the patient understands their disease, do they regularly check their sugars, what are the results, how long have they had diabetes and do they use insulin. The balance of the assessment would include: social history, personal habits, past medical and surgical history, nutritional assessment, pain assessment and a review of systems (Figure 1). From the initial visit we move to the regular clinic visits to include hyperbaric oxygen therapy.

Documentation of wound assessment

Wound assessment components that should be addressed include: wound/graft appearance; presence/quantity of fibrin; granulation tissue texture & color; presence of exposed bone, tendon or ligament; presence of eschar; amount and color of drainage; assessment of pain; and any debridement or remodeling that is done to the wound. The wound care assessment should paint a picture of the wound to the next person who will provide care. Because the appearance of the wound may change from one visit to the next it is essential that the assessment be done accurately and completely on each visit. Any question on the assessment of the wound should be directed to either the physician or a senior staff member.

Included in the wound assessment is measuring the wound. This is a critical component and is used to determine healing rates. The key to wound measuring is consistency. Wound measurement is generally done as a wound volume which involves length, width and depth. Surface area measurement of wounds omits the critical component of depth and doesn't paint as accurate picture of the size of the wound. The definitions commonly used for measurement are:

1. Length - the orientation measured proximal to distal (from head to toe);
2. Width - the orientation measured along the perpendicular to the length, or finger tip to finger tip when the arms are extended out from the sides of the body;
3. Depth - taken at the deepest point in the wound.

Physical Assessment	ADDRESSOGRAPH

WOUND INFORMATION

1. Location of wound ______
2. How did it start? ______
3. When did your wound start? ______
4. Has it ever completely healed? ______
5. Where have you been treated for your wound? ______
6. Current wound care? ______
7. Historical wound care? ______
8. Have you ever received hyperbaric oxygen therapy? ______
9. If on dialysis, which days are you dialyzed Clinic

PERSONAL HABITS:

1. Tobacco Use Past: No/Yes Date Stopped: ______ Present: No/Yes Type: ______
   Per day for ______ Years
2. Alcohol Use Past: No/Yes Date Stopped: ______ Present: No/Yes Type: ______
   Drinks per week for ______ Years ______
3. Caffeine Use Past: No/Yes Date Stopped: ______ Present: No/Yes Type: ______
   Drinks per week for ______ Years ______
4. Describe your activities:
   [ ] Able to walk without assistance: [ ] Use Crutches: [ ] Use Cane:
   [ ] Confined to bed or wheelchair: [ ] Use Brace: [ ] Walker
5. Who will help care for you?

SOCIAL HISTORY:

Married [ ] Yes [ ] No Widowed [ ] Yes [ ] No Single [ ] Yes [ ] No Divorced [ ] Yes [ ] No

Children [ ] Yes [ ] No If yes, number of children ___ Children [ ] Yes [ ] No If yes, number of children ___
Do you have Home Health Care [ ] Yes [ ] No

If yes, Name of Home Health Agency ______

EDUCATION/LEARNING ASSESSMENT:

Ability to understand verbal instructions	[ ] Limited	[ ] Average	[ ] Good
Ability to understand written instructions	[ ] Limited	[ ] Average	[ ] Good
Knowledge of educational needs/treatment plan	[ ] Limited	[ ] Average	[ ] Good
Knowledge of educational needs/treatment plan	[ ] Limited	[ ] Average	[ ] Good

SPECIFIC BARRIERS TO LEARNING (Mark those appropriate) [ ] None

[ ] Physical [ ] Reading [ ] Language [ ] Sensory [ ] Motivational
[ ] Emotional [ ] Cultural [ ] Religious [ ] Cognitive

Primary Care Doctor		**Other physicians involved with care:**
Vascular:	**Orthopedic:**	**General Surgery:**
Podiatrist:	**Rehab:**	**Other:**

Figure 1. Initial Patient Assessment Form

PAST MEDICAL HISTORY:

		Month/Year of Diagnosis	Describe Problem
Diabetes Mellitus	☐ No ☐ Yes		
Lung Disease (asthma, COPD)	☐ No ☐ Yes		
Heart Disease	☐ No ☐ Yes		
Kidney Problems	☐ No ☐ Yes		
Eye Problems (cataract, retina)	☐ No ☐ Yes		
Hepatitis/Liver Problems	☐ No ☐ Yes		
High Blood Pressure	☐ No ☐ Yes		
Cancer	☐ No ☐ Yes		
Chemotherapy	☐ No ☐ Yes		
Radiation Therapy	☐ No ☐ Yes		
Collagen Vascular Disease	☐ No ☐ Yes		
(SLE, Scleroderma, Rheumatoid)	☐ No ☐ Yes		
Stroke	☐ No ☐ Yes		
Thyroid	☐ No ☐ Yes		
Osteomyelitis	☐ No ☐ Yes		

Diabetic Information:

I monitor my glucose regularly.

☐ No ☐ Yes

I test my blood ______ times a day/week

My glucose usually runs:

Morning ______ Noon ______ Dinner ______ Bedtime ______

Surgical History

Type of Surgery		Month/Year	Describe
Kidney Transplant	☐ No ☐ Yes	______	______
Amputation	☐ No ☐ Yes	______	______
Skin Grafts	☐ No ☐ Yes	______	______
Blood Vessel Surgery	☐ No ☐ Yes	______	______
Head/Neck Surgery	☐ No ☐ Yes	______	______

Other ____

____

____

System Review

Check and describe all that are appropriate

HEAD, EYES, EARS, NOSE THROAT:	√	**Description**
Head Injury	______	______
Seizures	______	______
Dizziness	______	______
Change in Hearing	______	______
Sinus Problems		

Figure 1. Initial Patient Assessment Form

RESPIRATORY	√	**Description**
Pneumothrorax		
Seasonal Allergies		
History of chest injury		
History of TB		
CARDIOVASCULAR	√	
Chest Pain		
Heart Irregular		
Use Oxygen at Home		
Pacemaker		
Swelling in Ankles		
Pedal Pulses		[ ] Palpable [ ] Doppler
Ankle Brachial Index		Right Left
DIGESTIVE	√	
Heartburn		
Recent weight loss/gain		
Recent change in appetite		
Diarrhea		
Constipation		
Incontinent of Stool		
BLADDER/KIDNEY	√	
Indwelling Catheter		
Difficulty with Urination		
Incontinent of Urine		
Dialysis (hemo, peritoneal)		
EXTREMITIES	√	
Leg Pain – at rest		
– with walking		
Joint Pain		
Varicose Veins		
Swelling of legs		
Seims-Weinstein Monofilament		[ ] Complete protection [ ] Partial protection [ ] No protection

Allergies to Medication:

Medication	Reaction

Current Medication	**Dose**	**Purpose**

Figure 1. Initial Patient Assessment Form

Nurtitional Assessment

Assessment Questions	YES	NO
1. Do you have an illness or condition that made you change the kind and/or amount of food you eat?	2	X
2. Do you eat fewer than 2 meals a day?	3	X
3. Do you eat only a few fruits or vegetables, or milk products per day?	2	X
4. Do you have 3 or more drinks of beer, liquor, or wine almost everyday?	2	X
5. Do you have tooth or mouth problems that make it hard for you to eat?	2	X
6. Are there times when you don't always have enough money to buy the food you need?	4	X
7. Do you eat alone most of the time?	1	X
8. Do you take 3 or more different prescribed or over-the-counter drugs per day?	1	X
9. Without wanting to, have you lost or gained 10 pounds in the last 6 months?	2	X
10. Are there times when you are not always physically able to shop, cook, and/or feed yourself.	2	X
11. Patients with the following current diagnosis: Malnutrition, Non-healing Chronic Wounds, Cancer, Failure to Thrive, Depression, Alzheimer's, or Alcoholism, shall automatically receive (1) point of each diagnosis.	2	X
TOTAL		X

Pt Category	YES Total	RISK LEVEL	PLAN OF CARE
	0 – 2	Low Nutritional risk	Re-evaluate in 8 weeks. Indicate in the ICMG to review during the 8-week Healing Assessment Review.
	3 – 5	Moderate Nutritional Risk	Educate the patient/family/care givers to improve the patient's eating habits and lifestyle. This may include consideration to patient's food perference and frequency of meals. Involve the Nutritionist/Physician as needed for educational materials or suggestion in improvement measures.
	6 or more	High Nutritional Risk	Nutritional consult indicated. Inform MD for further assesment/orders.

RN ______________________ Date ______________________

Figure 1. Initial Patient Assessment Form

Along with wound volume measurements any tunneling or undermining should be noted and documented based on the clock positions, with the 12 o'clock position being proximal.

Wounds should be properly labeled. New wounds require a photograph and a number. The same number will follow this wound until the wound is closed or converted. It is recommended that the numbers be sequential. Labeling terminology should be consistent. It is best to use appropriate medical terminology when labeling all wounds such as medial, proximal or distal. When labeling new wounds, it is recommended that each area be completely documented before moving to the next area. During subsequent visits, review several of the previous visits when seeing a patient. It is best to go back a few visits to make sure that an error has not occurred in numbering or identifying the wounds.

What about eschar? Many times a patient presents with eschar on a wound. When eschar is present, the wound cannot be completely visualized. The depth is unknown until the eschar is removed. When eschar is present, the wound can not be staged or graded. Staging or grading a wound provides a common language to describe the severity of the wound. Shea's Staging (I-IV) of pressure ulcer was the basis for modifications made by the International Society of Enterostomal Therapists (4,5). The two most frequently used methods to grade a wound is either Wagner's (6) or UTSA Diabetic Foot Classification (7). The nurse assessing the wound should have a good working knowledge and understanding of these systems in order to properly grade or stage a wound.

Documentation of wound dressings

The dressings or treatments applied to the wound and the assessment of effectiveness of the dressing should be documented. Facilities may choose to document dressings using generic terminology or by brand name. Either is acceptable as long as it is consistent and reflects the products that are used. One area of dressing documentation that needs attention is assessment of the effectiveness of the dressing. On the visit following the application of a dressing an assessment or evaluation of how well the dressing did should be documented. Was the dressing able to be maintained by the patient, did the dressing maintain the proper environment for wound healing, and was the dressing cost effective?

Documentation of hyperbaric visit

For those wound centers that have hyperbaric medicine capability, wound assessment may occur during the time of a hyperbaric treatment or may be completely independent. Documentation during a hyperbaric encounter should reflect the care of the patient, safety precautions, and accurately record the timing of the hyperbaric treatment (Table1) (3). These are considered to be baseline requirements that must be met, but other components may be added by the wound center.

Documentation of patient education

Patient education in the chronic wound setting is a critical component of wound healing and of maintaining the healed site after discharge. Prior to undertaking the education, assess the patient's willingness to learn, any barriers to learning, and the patient's preferred learning style. These three components will be combined to form a complete teaching plan for the patient and their significant others. When the healthcare provider undertakes the education, documentation should include what was taught, methods used, return demonstration if applicable, and an assessment of understanding on the part of the patient and/or significant other. Do not expect to teach everything at once. Begin by selecting a single component, provide the education and assessment of understanding then move to the next step when the patient is ready. In the authors' experience, consistent education has improved patient compliance with the wound healing program and has decreased the recidivism rates.

TABLE 1. HYPERBARIC DOCUMENTATION

Component	Frequency	Alerts
Vital signs to include: blood pressure, temperature, respiratory rate and pulse	Prior to each HBO2 treatment with increased frequency if vitals outside normal range	Elevated temperature, Other vitals outside of patient normals
Fingerstick glucose on diabetic patients	Prior to and post HBO2 treatment	Recommend: >120mg/dl prior to HBO2 and post-treatment glucose >100 md/dl (8).
Visualization of tympanic membranes	Prior to HBO2 treatment	Notify of any abnormal findings
Pulmonary Assessment	Prior to HBO2 treatment	Notify HBO2 physician of abnormal breath sounds such as wheezing, rales or rhonchi.
Condition of patient on arrival	Prior to HBO2 treatment	Notify physician of any deterioration in patient condition
Mode of arrival of patient	Prior to HBO2 treatment	No alerts
Safety assessment	Prior to HBO2 treatment	Notify safety director of any deviation of safety assessment
Medication administration	Prior to and post HBO2 treatment	Adverse reactions or ineffectiveness of medication
Adverse events	Post to HBO2 treatment	Notify covering physician of any event
Exact times of hyperbaric treatment	Post to HBO2 treatment	HBO2 manager should assure accurate math of dive times
Other patient care equipment	Prior to HBO2 treatment	Notify safety director and medical director of any equipment problems. All implantable equipment needs to be verified with manufacturer that it can be placed in HBO2 environment

Documentation of goals and discharge planning

A critical component of documentation and one that is frequently neglected is the plan of care/discharge planning. In this section the nurse should document the long term and short term goals of care. The long term goal for a venous ulcer patient may be to maximally reduce edema and fit for gradient compression stockings. The short term goal for the same patient is to keep the gradient compression dressing on between visits. Thoughtful documentation of the goals will provide the nurse who will be seeing the patient the following week an understanding of what the goals are and what needs to be addressed. This is an important source of communication necessary for continuity of care.

These key components to nursing documentation within a wound center are the foundation blocks to telling the story of the patient's care. The wound center might choose to add other components to the required documentation. This may be driven by an accrediting agency, a reimbursement source or identification of a necessary missing component. Whatever requirements are added, remember the three "Cs": clarity, conciseness, and consistency.

Maintaining quality documentation

The second part of good documentation is having a method in place to monitor the quality of the documentation. When reviewing the visit notes to assess the quality of the documentation, we should consider three key points: The note of each visit should paint a complete picture of the encounter, the record should read like a history of the care given, and the medical record is a legal document. This document one day could become your best friend or your worst enemy.

So how do we improve and maintain quality records? The incorporation of performance improvement is an essential part of any program. A good performance improvement program will facilitate the continuous monitoring

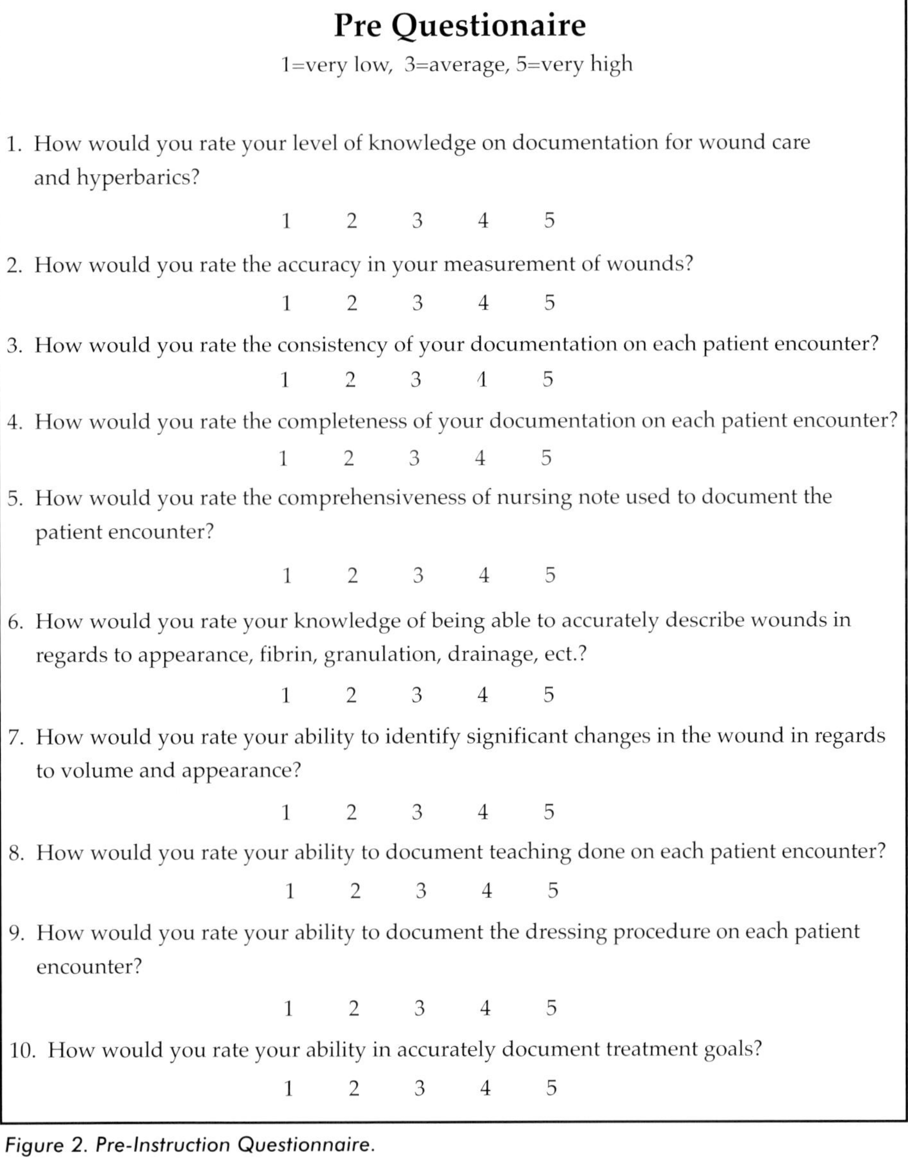

Pre Questionaire

1=very low, 3=average, 5=very high

1. How would you rate your level of knowledge on documentation for wound care and hyperbarics?

   1 2 3 4 5

2. How would you rate the accuracy in your measurement of wounds?

   1 2 3 4 5

3. How would you rate the consistency of your documentation on each patient encounter?

   1 2 3 4 5

4. How would you rate the completeness of your documentation on each patient encounter?

   1 2 3 4 5

5. How would you rate the comprehensiveness of nursing note used to document the patient encounter?

   1 2 3 4 5

6. How would you rate your knowledge of being able to accurately describe wounds in regards to appearance, fibrin, granulation, drainage, ect.?

   1 2 3 4 5

7. How would you rate your ability to identify significant changes in the wound in regards to volume and appearance?

   1 2 3 4 5

8. How would you rate your ability to document teaching done on each patient encounter?

   1 2 3 4 5

9. How would you rate your ability to document the dressing procedure on each patient encounter?

   1 2 3 4 5

10. How would you rate your ability in accurately document treatment goals?

    1 2 3 4 5

Figure 2. Pre-Instruction Questionnaire.

Wound Clinic/HBO Clinical Record Review

Patient ID#:__________ Age:________ Sex: ☐F ☐M Start Date:__________ Discharge Date:__________

Diagnosis(es):____________________________ Number of Center Visits:____________________________

Serivices Utilized: ☐WCC ☐HBO ☐Other:____________ Reason for Discharge:____________________________

Chart Documents	#Yes	#No	N/A	Comments
1. Patient demographics/registration sheet present?				
2. Consent for treatment completed?				
3. Consent for HBO treatment completed?				
4. HBO EKG present?				
5. HBO CXR present?				
6. Initial Wound Assessment form completed with picture?				
7. Physician dictated History and Physical present?				
8. Nurse History and Assessment completed?				
9. Neuropath Risk Assessment 5.07 Monofilament form completed?				
10. Pain Assessment form completed?				
11. Wound Location Sheet completed?				
Physician Orders	**#Yes**	**#No**	**N/A**	**Comments**
1. Physician signature/dated and noted line completed?				
2. Pain control documented?				
3. Lab section completed?				
4. Diagnostics section completed?				
5. General Consults section completed?				
6. Edema Control section completed?				
7. Off-Loading section completed?				
8. Dressing Orders section completed?				
9. Medications/Additional Orders section completed?				
10. Return Appointment section completed?				
Wound Treatment Record	**#Yes**	**#No**	**N/A**	**Comments**
1. Type of visit and date line completed?				
2. Arrival mode line completed?				
3. Vital Signs and Glucose line completed?				
4. Wounds documented with numbers and measurements?				
5. Pain Control line completed?				
6. Wound Characteristics completed?				
7. Compression Therapy section completed?				
8. home Health section completed?				
9. Discharge section completed?				
Wound Treatment Record	**#Yes**	**#No**	**N/A**	**Comments**
1. Nursing Progress Note section completed?				
2. Does Nursing Progress Note mention percent of chang in wound?				
3. Patient/Family Education section completed?				
4. Discharge Planning section completed?				
5. Are measurable goals and previous goals addressed in Discharge section?				

Areas For Improvement:____

____

Recommendations:____

____

Figure 3. Chart Auditing Tool

and evaluation of documentation. Prior to the implementation of a performance improvement program; however, it is essential to evaluate the areas that will require improvement as well as monitoring. A Pre instruction questionnaire (Figure 2) might be beneficial for evaluating the staff's initial knowledge levels and can serve as the initial building block for a performance improvement program., After obtaining a baseline assessment of staff's knowledge, a chart-auditing tool (Figure 3) can track areas of weakness in documentation and areas that may need improvement to meet current standards and guidelines. Following staff instruction on documentation, a Post Instruction survey (Figure 4) can be utilized to evaluate the effectiveness of the program. In addition, this survey can serve as an alert for previously unidentified areas that may need to be monitored.

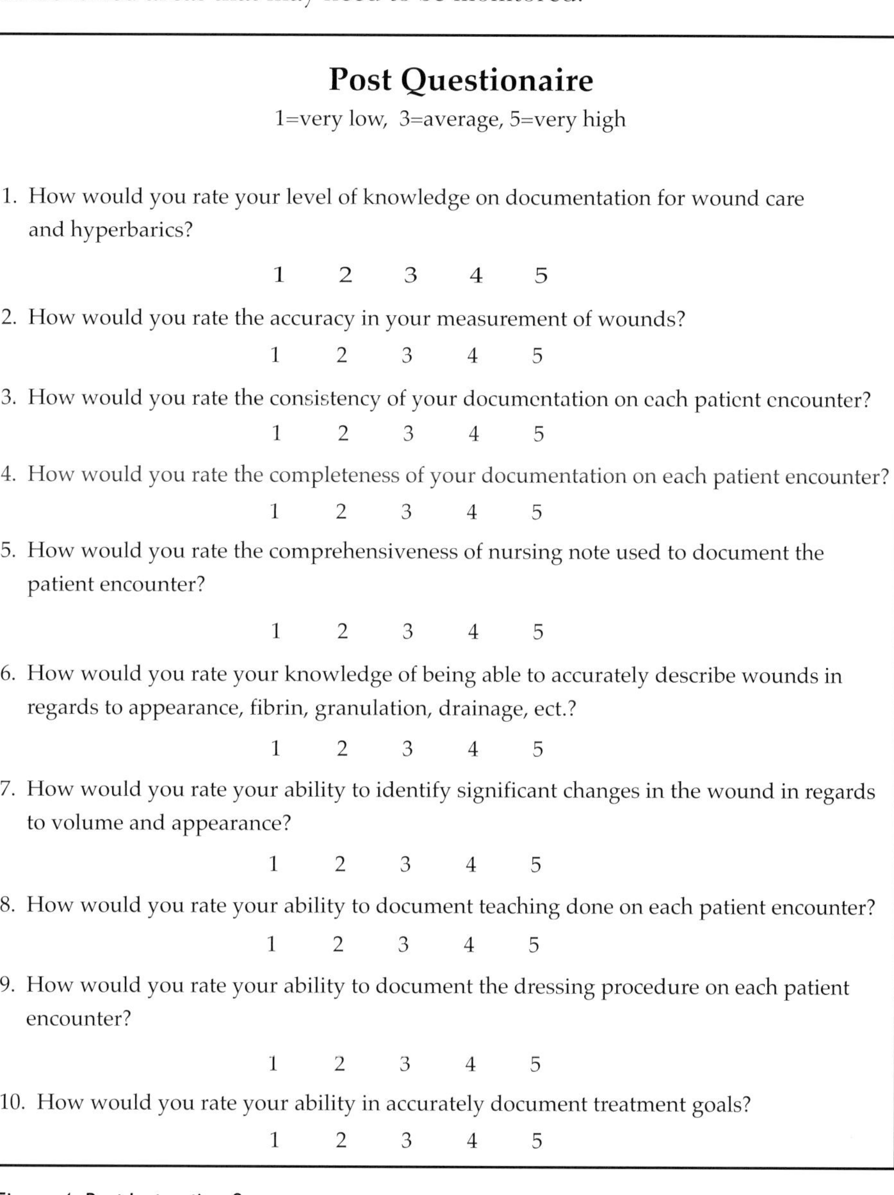

Post Questionaire

1=very low, 3=average, 5=very high

1. How would you rate your level of knowledge on documentation for wound care and hyperbarics?

   1 2 3 4 5

2. How would you rate the accuracy in your measurement of wounds?

   1 2 3 4 5

3. How would you rate the consistency of your documentation on each patient encounter?

   1 2 3 4 5

4. How would you rate the completeness of your documentation on each patient encounter?

   1 2 3 4 5

5. How would you rate the comprehensiveness of nursing note used to document the patient encounter?

   1 2 3 4 5

6. How would you rate your knowledge of being able to accurately describe wounds in regards to appearance, fibrin, granulation, drainage, ect.?

   1 2 3 4 5

7. How would you rate your ability to identify significant changes in the wound in regards to volume and appearance?

   1 2 3 4 5

8. How would you rate your ability to document teaching done on each patient encounter?

   1 2 3 4 5

9. How would you rate your ability to document the dressing procedure on each patient encounter?

   1 2 3 4 5

10. How would you rate your ability in accurately document treatment goals?

    1 2 3 4 5

Figure 4. Post Instruction Survey.

Performance improvement plan

Information collected from both chart audits and staff surveys are used to establish indicators. These indicators will serve as the structure of the performance improvement program. Once indicators have been established a threshold level will need to be set. This level should be based on the amount of improvement that is expected and necessary for documentation to be complete. Each quarter, or more frequently if necessary, information gathered from chart audits can be reviewed and if new indicators are needed they then can be established. As new indicators are identified, staff members will require in-service training in the areas that need improvement. Data collected from routine chart audits can be easily tracked and the information used to determine if established thresholds are being met or if further in-service training is required. This plan will allow continuous monitoring of documentation and performance improvement.

This is one example of a performance improvement plan. There are others which can be equally effective. It is important to have a method by which to monitor documentation. Frequency of monitoring should be guided by identified needs, consistent incompleteness of documentation, lack of understanding by staff on how to do documentation, and hospital guidelines.

REFERENCES

1. Bellack JP, Edlund BJ. Nursing assessment and diagnosis. 2nd Edition, Jones and Bartlett Publishers, Sudberry, MA.
2. Joint Commission on Accreditation of Healthcare Organizations. Section I, Patient focused functions, comprehensive accreditation manual for hosptials. November 2000.
3. Shea J. Pressure sores: classification and management. Clin Orthopaedics Related Res. 1975;112:89–100.
4. International Association of Enterostomal Therapy. Dermal Wounds: Pressure Sores. Laguna Beach, Calif: IAET; 1988
5. Wagner FW. The dysvascular foot: A system for diagnosis and treatment. Foot Ankle 1981; 2: 64-122.
6. Armstrong DG, Harkless LB. Validation of a diabetic wound classification system. The conribution of depth, infection and ischemia to risk of amputation. Diabetes Care 1998 May; 21(5): 855-9.
7. McHowell W. Care of the patient receiving hyperbaric oxygen therapy. In: Hyperbaric Nursing (Larson-Lohr V, Norvell HC, eds) Best Publishing Company, Flagstaff, AZ, 2002.
8. Parker K, Fife C. Effects of HBO2 on glucose measurement: Implications for care. In: Hyperbaric Nursing (Larson-Lohr V, Norvell HC, eds) Best Publishing Company, Flagstaff, AZ, 2002.

REVIEW QUESTIONS

1.) The "three Cs" of documentation are:
   a. Constant, Comprehensive, Complete
   b. Claim, Claimant, Collector
   c. Cool, Calm, Collected
   d. Clarity, Conciseness, Consistency

2.) Painting a complete picture when documenting includes:
   a. Clarity of the plan of care
   b. Conciseness or focusing of the topic
   c. Consistency in how the documentation is done
   d. All of the above

3.) The components of an adequate wound assessment include all of the following EXCEPT:
   a. Wound/graft appearance
   b. Granulation tissue texture & color
   c. Presence of exposed bone, tendon or ligament
   d. Amount and color of drainage
   e. The surgical plan

4.) Indicators that serve as the structure of the performance improvement program are obtained from:
   a. Chart audits
   b. Staff surveys
   c. Pre-instruction questionnaire
   d. Both a and b

5.) According to the authors a critical component of documentation that is frequently neglected is the plan of care/discharge planning.
   a.True
   b. False

Answers: 1d, 2d, 3e, 4d, 5a

CHAPTER 47

Coding, Charging, Billing and Collecting for Wound Care and Hyperbaric Medicine Services: Getting Paid for the Work You Do

CHAPTER FORTY-SEVEN OVERVIEW

Coding, Charging, Billing and Collecting for Wound Care and Hyperbaric Medicine Services: Getting Paid for the Work You Do

Ronald P. Bangasser, Thomas M. Bozzuto

On May 3, 2007, Dr. Ronald P. Bangasser, who served as California Medical Association president passed away. Ron, a family practitioner, was always an example of what a doctor should be, operating his wound care clinic, his practice, all the while serving his patients and colleagues through his advocacy for the CMA.

This chapter is dedicated to Ron's contribution to hyperbaric medicine.

INTRODUCTION

This chapter will help Wound Care and Hyperbaric Departments be successful by suggesting ways to correctly code, bill, and collect on the services provided. The system of coding, billing, and collecting is specific to the United States and is based on the payment scheme set up by the Centers for Medicare and Medicaid Services (CMS), formerly known as the Health Care Finance Administration (HCFA). CMS sets up the system for paying the bills for Medicare and Medicaid recipients in the United States. The Federal Government pays for over 50% of all money spent on health care in the United States. Private insurance companies collect premiums from businesses and individuals and pay for most of the rest of the health care delivered in this country. Patients pay less than 20% of the cost of health care in cash out of their own pockets. This system of coding, billing, and collecting for services may be different in other countries, but some of the ideas and principles will be similar and should be helpful.

BILLING, CODING, AND COLLECTING FOR ACTUAL SERVICE PROVIDED

Being able to provide premier wound care services is only the first step in the practice of Wound Care and Hyperbaric Medicine in the United States. Insurance issues, including understanding the complex International Classification of Diseases, Ninth Revision, Clinical Modification (ICD-9-CM) and Current Procedural Terminology (CPT 2007) systems for coding and billing correctly, negotiating contracts, and finally getting money to continue business operations, can cause many physicians and their staff members to rush for the exits looking for easier ways to make a living. Hassles abound in this area, in which most physicians have very little training and even less experience.

There are actually only a few common CPT codes that are used in Wound Care and Hyperbaric Medicine. If you know these codes and their descriptors, there is little chance for error in CPT coding. Table 1 is a short list of the most often used Evaluation and Management (E/M) codes:

TABLE 1. EVALUATION MANAGEMENT CODES

E/M Code	Descriptor	Complexity	Time (average)
99201	New Patient Office or Other Outpatient Visit	Problem focused	10 min
99202	New Patient Office or Other Outpatient Visit	Expanded	20 min
99203	New Patient Office or Other Outpatient Visit	Detailed	30 min
99204	New Patient Office or Other Outpatient Visit	Comprehensive	45 min
99205	New Patient Office or Other Outpatient Visit	Comprehensive—high complexity	60 min
99211	Established Patient Office or Other Outpatient Visit	Minimal	5 min
99212	Established Patient Office or Other Outpatient Visit	Problem focused	10 min
99213	Established Patient Office or Other Outpatient Visit	Expanded	15 min
99214	Established Patient Office or Other Outpatient Visit	Detailed	25 min
99215	Established Patient Office or Other Outpatient Visit	Comprehensive	40 min
99251	New or Established Patient Impatient Consultation	Problem focused	20 min
99252	New or Established Patient Impatient Consultation	Expanded	40 min
99253	New or Established Patient Impatient Consultation	Detailed	55 min
99254	New or Established Patient Impatient Consultation	Comprehensive	80 min
99255	New or Established Patient Impatient Consultation	Comprehensive—high complexity	110 min
99183	Physician Attendance/Supervision of HBO2 per session		

The levels of E/M services include examination, evaluations, and treatments. Medical screening includes the history, examination and medical decision-making required to determine the type of appropriate care of the patient. The levels of E/M services cover a wide variation in skill, effort, time, responsibility and medical knowledge required for diagnosing and treating patients.

The key components in selecting a level of E/M service are history, examination, and medical decision-making. When counseling and/or coordination of care diminates (50%) of the patient and/or family encounter (face-to-face time), the time may be considered the key or controlling factor to qualify for a particular level of E/M service. The extent of counseling/coordination of care must be documented in the medical record. Contributory factors include counseling, coordination of care, and nature of the presenting problem. Time is to be used as an indicator and an average. Time of a visit may represent a range, which may be higher or lower depending on actual clinical circumstances. Time in the office setting is defined as face-to-face with the patient or the family. In the inpatient setting, total time spent with the patient at the bedside and on the patient's hospital floor or unit is used.

Other CPT codes need to be coded as accurately as possible. Common codes for debridement are in Table 2.

TABLE 2. COMMON CPT CODES FOR DEBRIDEMENT

11040	Partial thickness skin debridement
11041	Full thickness skin debridement
11042	Debridement of skin and subcutaneous tissue
11043	Debridement of skin, subcutaneous tissue and muscle
11044	Debridement of skin, subcutaneous tissue, muscle, and bone

If there are multiple surgical procedures performed during the same patient care session (other than E/M), you must report the most significant procedure first, with all other procedures listed with a –51 modifier.

Entire courses are given on CPT coding and the current CPT 2007 text is more than 500 pages long. Further details in this chapter exceed the scope of this work. It is important to use these classes and text to avoid errors in coding which in the most extreme circumstance could result in an investigation by federal authorities.

Proper diagnosis coding using the International Classification of Disease, Ninth Revision, Clinical Modification (ICD-9-CM) is critical for proper billing and collecting of fees for services rendered to patients. The text for physician codes also exceeds 500 pages. Many thousands of diagnostic codes exist and more than one may be needed to describe a patient's specific medical condition or conditions. Patients often have many medical problems and therefore many ICD-9-CM codes may be used. When procedures and/or ancillary services are rendered in addition to an E/M code on the same day, the physician must link the appropriate diagnosis code to each service rendered to avoid medical necessity denials that result in payment delays.

In an effort to promote proper utilization of established wound care management codes, the AMA revised the active wound management CPT codes and correlating descriptions as of January 2006. In addition, The Centers for Medicare and Medicaid Services (CMS) assigned CPT codes to three Ambulatory Payment Classification Groups (APC's) which have payment rates for Hospital-Owned Outpatient Wound Care Departments (HOPDs). These codes are to be used to indicate the removal of devitalized and/or necrotic tissue to promote healing in selective non-selective debridement cases when a patient's wound does not require surgical debridement.

One Medicare Carrier recently released a wound debridement guidance document and Local Carrier Determination (LCD). Among the key points in this directive area:

- Surgical debridement codes 11040–11044 must be based on the type of tissue removed, not the depth of grade of the ulcer or wound
- Surgical debridement will be considered "not medical necessary" when documentation indicates that the wound is without
  - infection
  - necrosis
  - non-viable tissue

  and has pink or red granulation tissue
- CPT cde 11042 is defined as debridement; *skin and subcutaneous tissue.* Wound care providers are using this code incorrectly when they are removing *fibrin* which is not not skin. To bill 11042, the Carrier expects the provider to debride the skin and subcutaneous tissue—only when necrotic or subcutaneous tissue removed, even though the ulcer or wound may extend to bone.
- The Carrier states that an individual wound would not be expected to be repeatedly debrided of skin and subcutaneous tissue because these tissues do not regrow very quickly.

Several years ago, the AMA released active wound management codes to be used by nurses and physical therapists when they removed devitalized and/or necrotic tissue from wound to promote healing. However these codes did not have payment rages for HOPD's. Therefore HOPD's had two choices:

- include this work into their clincial visit levels, or
- request that physicians perform active debridements*

Effective January 2006, the AMA revised the active wound management CPT codes and their descriptions. Simultaneously, CMS assigned the CPT codes to APC groups which have payment rates for HOPD's. The new CPT codes are:

97597	Removal of devitalized tissue from wound(s), selective debridement, without anesthesia (e.g., high pressure water jet with/without suction, sharp selective dridement with scissors, scalpel and forceps), with or without topical application(s), wound assesssment, and instruction(s) for ongoing care, may include use of a whirlpool, per session; total wound(s) surface area ≤ 20 square centimeters
97598	Removal of devitalizd tissue from wound(s), selective debridement, without anesthesia (e.g., high pressure waterjet with/without suction, sharp selective debridement with scissors, scalpel and forceps), with or without topical application(s), wound assessment, and instruction(s) for ongoing care, may include use of a whirlpool, per session; total wound(s) surface area > 20 square centimeters

* Shaum KD. Newly Funded Selective and Non-Selective Debridement Codes: Impact on Hospital Owned Outpatient Wound Care Departments. HMP Communications, Healthpoint, Ltd. Malvern PA, 2006.

97062 Removal of devitalized tissue from wound(s), non-selective debridement, without anesthesia (e.g., wet-to-moist dressings, enzymatic, abrasion), including topical application(s), wound assessment, and instruction(s) for ongoing care, per session

It is suggested that physicians and HOPD's contact their local Fiscal Intermediary (FI) for Medicare to determine their particular LCD for debridement(s).

For proper billing, the medical code that best describes the cause for the patient's visit to your office is the first or primary code used for billing for the visit. Other codes should be added to the bill if other disease processes are addressed during the visit, as these add complexity to the visit and may help qualify for a higher CPT code and therefore higher reimbursement.

Changes in CPT Codes for 2006

The most significant changes in the CPT codes in 2006 (Table 3) for physicians practicing wound care are the changes in the codes for bioengineered tissue grafts. The other important change is that debridement codes (15000, 1104x) cannot be billed on the same day as application of the above tissue grafts.

TABLE 3. EXAMPLES OF CHANGES IN 2006 CPT CODES

CPT Code	Descriptor
15340	Tissue cultured allogeneic skin substitute; first 25 sq cm or less
15341	Tissue cultured allogeneic skin substitute; each additional 25 sq cm (The Global Period is 10 days, meaning one cannot bill for additional services related to follow-up of the application for a 10 day period after the application.)
15330	Acellular dermal allograft, trunk, arms, legs; first 100 sq cm or less, or one percent of body area of infants and children
15331	Acellular dermal allograft, trunk, arms, legs; each additional 100 sq cm, or each additional one percent of body area of infants and children, or part thereof. (List separately in addition to code for primary procedure) (The Global Period for application of acellular tissue in 90 days)
15400	Xenograft, skin (dermal), for temporary wound closure; truck, arms, legs; first 100 sq cm or less, or one percent of body area of infants and children
15401	Xenograft, skin (dermal), for temporary wound closure; each addditional 100 sq cm, or each additional one percent of body area of infants and children, or part thereof (List separately in addition to code for primary procedure.)
15420	Xenograft skin (dermal), for temporary wound closure, face, scalp, eyelids, mouth, neck, ears, orbits, genitalia, hands, feet, and/or multiple digits; first 100 sq cm or less, or one percent of body area of infants and children
15421	Xenograft skin (dermal), for temporary wound closure, face, scalp, eyelids, mouth, neck, ears, orbits, genitalia, hands, feet and/or multiple digits; each additional 100 sq cm, or each additional one percent of body area of infants and children, or part thereof (List separately in addition to code for primary procedure.) (The Global Period for xenografts is 90 days.)

Medicare through the Centers for Medicare and Medical Services (CMS) has determined that some medical conditions qualify for Hyperbaric Oxygen services.

These are included in Table 4.

Most of the above diagnoses require a 5th digit to the right of the other four to define the area of the body being described, such as 923.10 to describe a crush injury to the forearm.

TABLE 4. COMMON ICD-9 CM CODES FOR MEDICARE COVERED INDICATION FOR HBO2

ICD-9 CM Code	Diagnosis
040.0	Gas Gangrene
986	Toxic effect of carbon monoxide
993.3	Decompression sickness
958.0	Air embulis
900 to 904	Various areas of injury to blood vessels
958.8	Compartment syndrome
996.9	Complications of reattached extremity or body part
922 to 929	Crush injury of specific body areas
996.52	Compromised skin grafts with plans for preparation or preservation
730.1	Chronic osteomyelitis
526.89	Osteoradionecrosis of the mandible
444.89	Acute retinal vessel occlusion or central retinal artery occlusion
250.8	Diabetic foot ulcer with osteomyelitis

It is important to realize that although CMS recognizes the above codes for payment for Hyperbaric Oxygen (HBO2) services; this is often not true for commercial insurance companies. It is crucial to check and get prior authorization in advance for these HBO2 services. You must also check on fee schedules in advance of providing these services. Some insurance companies may have contract language to cover the areas of authorization and payment, but many will not.

Hyperbaric Oxygen Therapy Billing

Many wound care centers are now incorporating hyperbaric oxygen therapy into their armamentarium of services. To a physician beginning a hyperbaric practice the intricacies of proper billing may seem staggering even though there is only one CPT code for hyperbaric oxygen therapy.

99183 Physician attendance and supervision of hyperbaric oxygen therapy, per session

There have been years of discussion with representatives of Medicare over exactly what that phrase means. Without going into all the fine points and counterpoints about where the physician has to be and when, an excerpt from a communication from Coverage and Analysis Group, Office of Clinical Standards and Quality of CMS states:

> *HBO2 falls under the benefit category of "incident to" physician service and the level of supervision is direct supervision. That means that the physician must be readily available. That generally means that the supervising physician must be in the suite or department but does not have to be right at the chamber during the dive.*
>
> *As for billing, CMS does not preclude the physician from carrying on other duties as long as he/she is able to directly supervise the person administering HBO2. They must be readily available on, not off-site.*

There is also significant confusion about the wording of Coverage Issues Manual (CIM) §35-10 that lists the "covered" indications for hyperbaric oxygen therapy under Medicare. A short history will be explanatory. When the forefathers in the Undersea Medical Society took the first Hyperbaric Oxygen Committee Report to Social Security (who was responsible for administering Medicare prior to HFCA), the descriptors in the Committee Report were accepted as the covered indications. At this time, ICD-9 codes did not exist. At the inception of the ICD-9 codes, the wording of the hyperbaric indications did not exactly match many of the codes, so the code closest to the descriptor in the Committee Report was chosen to represent that indication. The Medicare Coverage for Hyperbaric Oxygen Therapy is listed in the Appendix of this chapter. Be aware that some states fiscal intermediaries (FI's) for Medicare have modified the national coverage policy, so it behooves each physician to know the local coverage determination (LCD). Some states have added descriptors under each ICD-9 code and diagnosis to better explain their interpretation of the codes.

When the physician initially sees the patient, a consultation or initial patient visit can be billed similar to a wound care patient. The consultation for hyperbaric therapy should be complete, discuss the chief complaint, history of present illness, medical, surgical, social and family histories, allergies, physical examination, discussion of any laboratory or imaging studies reviewed, interpretation of any testing done in the department, list the diagnoses, and a plan of care. Although listing multiple diagnoses may justify the complexity of the consultation or patient visit, be aware that the CMS-1500 (the billing form used to bill Medicare for physician services) has only four lines to list diagnoses. Because you are being consulted for hyperbaric services, the diagnosis justifying the hyperbaric oxygen therapy should be listed first. If it is too far down the list in your diagnoses, it will 'fall off' the CMS-1500 form and the hyperbaric therapy will be denied because none of the diagnoses listed on the form meet coverage criteria for hyperbaric oxygen therapy.

Make sure your coders and billers are aware of the narrow range of covered ICD-9 codes for hyperbaric oxygen therapy so that no latitude is taken in interpreting other codes for the diagnosis.

Since 99183 is procedure code, an evaluation and management code (E&M) cannot be billed at the same encounter unless it is for a distinct and separately identifiable service that is unrelated to the supervision of the patient's hyperbaric therapy. In addition, a -25 modifier must be added to the E/M CPT code to avoid bundling issues.

It is useful to list in your plan of therapy documents that support the treatment of the patient for the condition listed (such as the UHMS Hyperbaric Oxygen Therapy Committee Report, The American College of Hyperbaric Medicine's Preferred Practice Protocols, or the National Cancer Institute's Position Statement, if applicable). Mentioning in your consultation that based on the patient's history, review of systems, physical examination, and testing that the treatment with hyperbaric oxygen therapy is both reasonable and medically necessary will save hours of having to write letters of medical necessity to insurers (not only Medicare), and will give you an indication of whether your consult was really read by them prior to requesting additional information! Having an accurate dictation and a compete consultation is your best chance of receiving reimbursement with minimal requests for medical necessity or additional information. For most diagnoses, Medicare requires that conservative treatment either precede or be performed along with the hyperbaric oxygen therapy. Therefore, it is essential in your consultation to dictate any previous or adjunctive therapy that is being done and whether it is being successful or not in order to justify the addition of hyperbaric therapy. A dictation template for consultation, wound care follow-up visits, and discharge summaries is listed in the Appendix C to this chapter.

UNDERSTANDING SITE OF CARE AND PROFESSIONAL AND TECHNICAL COMPONENTS OF CODING

Payment for services is dependent on the site where the service is delivered. If care is delivered in an office setting, payment for a 99213 (established patient-limited) will be greater than if the same service is performed in an outpatient hospital setting where the hospital bills a fee for bed usage.

Some procedures and tests (lab and x-ray) have two components to the care. There is the physician component of the care called the Professional Component. There is also the equipment fee for the care called the Technical Component. If a physician owns the lab or the equipment used, that physician will receive payment for the Professional and the Technical Component of the care. If, however, the equipment is owned by another party, say the hospital, the Technical Component of the care will be paid to the hospital and only the Professional Component of the care will be paid to the physician. These component payments may be described in contracts, so the payments methods need to be recognized and scrutinized in advance of final contract arrangements with the hospital and/or with the insurance plans.

CODING AND BILLING WOUND CARE DRESSINGS

Many Wound Care and Hyperbaric Oxygen Medicine Departments are combined. Patients often have their dressings changed during treatments. Proper coding and billing for these dressing changes is necessary because the dressings are very expensive. Use the CPT and ICD-9 books as references for the proper codes, and use a cost plus basis for billing the dressings.

USE OF IV ANTIBIOTICS—INPATIENT VERSUS OUTPATIENT

Many of our patients require the use of IV antibiotics during the course of their treatment. Medicare patients have coverage for inpatient IV antibiotics only. They do not have payment coverage for outpatient IV antibiotics. Some Medicare+Choice programs will cover outpatient IV antibiotics if medical necessity is documented. Medicaid programs vary from state to state. In California, for example, outpatient IV antibiotics are covered if the patient is "case managed." Commercial insurances will usually cover outpatient IV antibiotics, again based on documented medical necessity.

APPROPRIATE PAYMENT FOR ANCILLARY SERVICES RELATED TO RESEARCH

If you are involved in research projects of any type, it is important to know if other services, such as lab, x-rays, MRI's, and related procedures performed in your office are covered by the research grant. If they are not, ancillary services related to the research project may be billed to the insurance plan for payment in most states. Many states have laws that require these services to be paid by the patient's insurance.

INFORMATION ON STATE INSURANCE LAWS FOR PAYMENT

In most states, payment requirements for health plans can be found on websites for the department of insurance or, in California, for Health Maintenance Organizations (HMO's), the Department of Managed Health Care (DMHC). Also, the American Medical Association (AMA) website at *www.ama-assn.org* includes details of state-specific insurance rules with coverage details. Many state medical society sites have details of laws and regulations related to payment requirements.

Besides websites, most of the above referral services have 1-800 telephone numbers for questions related to laws and regulations relating to insurance company requirements for coverage and payment.

THE NEED FOR PROPER DOCUMENTATION

Proper written documentation of the condition of the wound/s and the overall condition of the patient cannot be emphasized enough. The adage that "If it is not documented, it did not happen" applies to Wound Care and HBO2 units just as it does to any other medical office or inpatient setting. Vital signs, wound size and depth measurements, description of the color and condition of the wound, arterial pulses near the wound area, and overall condition of the patient with appropriate organ system exams need to documented at each visit. "A picture is worth a thousand words" works well for wounds. Pictures taken initially and periodically during the treatment process help the physician, the patient and their family, and the insurance company recall in vivid detail how the wound is progressing or not. It has helped this author collect tens of thousands of contested dollars for services rendered. It also helps in getting authorization for initial and continued care. A final picture of the closed and healed wound is helpful also. Photos, with permission, can be used to educate others to the value of your Wound Care and Hyperbaric Medicine Department. Digital photography is the best way to see the results immediately and keep a file on each patient for future use. It is also very forgiving if you are not a professional photographer.

STEPS TO APPEAL DENIED OR UNDERPAID CLAIMS

When you receive an EOB (Explanation of Benefits) from an insurance company or the state or federal government, there are several steps you need to take to make sure you are paid properly. First, verify that your billing was correct, including the CPT codes and the ICD-9-CM codes. Make sure that the bill was sent to the correct address and for the correct patient. Make sure the patient had insurance coverage at the time of the visits. Check to make certain that authorization had been obtained in advance for services rendered. If you have a contract with an insurance plan, confirm that the service is covered and how much you should receive for that service.

Rebilling costs a lot of money, so be certain that all of the above is covered before you or your billing service sends another bill. If the EOB comes back without a check or if the check is less that you believe you are due, it is time to appeal.

Most insurance companies, third party payers, and Medicaid and Medicare intermediaries have clearly established policies dealing with the appeals process. State and federal laws and regulations protect physicians and can help with collecting the correct fees for services. Often a phone call will clear up the issue, but when that fails, a written appeal to the insurance plan is required. If the plan requests patient information, be sure that you have authorization to send the information to the plan. Only send the specific information requested by the plan and nothing more or less. Most states have laws related to turnaround time on these payment and appeals issues. You must take the time to become familiar with them. The AMA's Private Sector Advocacy (PSA) Unit has developed many tools to help physicians navigate the maze of claims submission processes. You can access this information at *www.ama-assn.org/ama/pub/catetory/11410.html*

TECHNIQUES IN CONTRACTING WITH INSURANCE COMPANIES

Firstly, and most importantly, READ THE CONTRACT. Everyone is very busy and there is little time in and out of the office to read a contract. The language is difficult to read and the terms that are used are not easily understood. But, the contract will determine how and when you will be paid, so someone has to study it carefully. The contract spells out how multiple surgeries will be paid. The contract states where services will be bundled or left unbundled. The contract states how bills are to be submitted and to whom. The contract has attachments that tell you how much you will get paid for each unit of work you perform. The contract will tell you if you will be listed on other panels of physicians with other companies. The contract may include an "all products" clause. This clause says that you must take all the companies insurance products, if you take one. The contract will also contain information about how to appeal a claim. There will also be information about how to terminate a contract, both from the insurance side and from your side. There may be language that forces you to continue to see patients for the company, even after the agreement is terminated, either with or without compensation for that care. The time period for this "run-out" of continued care could be as much as 180 days after termination. There are many other pages of contract language that you or your staff or an outside expert need to understand before you sign the contract. Often, if there is specific language that you wish removed from the contract, just crossing out the unwanted language will stop its implementation. However, if there are large sections of language that need to be changed or removed, you or your designee will have to negotiate with the insurance company's representative.

Negotiating a contract is difficult and time consuming. You need some background and expertise in this area to get a good outcome. If you are interested in pursuing this yourself, take classes in negotiating and practice the techniques you learn before going into a real negotiating session. If, as with most of us, there is neither the time nor the energy to take classes to learn negotiating skills, you need to use an expert to help. Sometimes you may have a staff person who has had experience in negotiating, but most often, you will need to get outside help. Many state medical societies and some specialty societies have information about common contracting pitfalls. They will know some of what to look out for. But federal anti-trust laws limit these societies. They cannot take your specific contract and analyze it for you. You need an expert whom you will pay for his or her services. There are many experts available in this area. Some may be attorneys, or accountants, or previous insurance company employees who worked in the area of contract negotiation. Check references and plan to pay for the expertise. A relatively small amount of money spent getting the contract right before signing it will save you many hassles and much money in the long run. The better the contract analysis, the better the income. The AMA's advocacy efforts include resources for managed care contracting. This information includes a format for contracting which favors the physician. This can be accessed at *www.ama-assn.org/ama/pub/category/19876.html.*

USING OUTCOMES DATA TO ADD VALUE IN CONTRACTING

Showing how well you take care of your Wound Care and Hyperbaric Medicine patients can help improve your contract negotiations. Gathering outcomes on your patients and showing how effective limb-saving techniques can be will allow you to negotiate higher fees and reduce authorization requirements. There is no question that salvaging a limb rather than amputating that limb results in decreased mortality and morbidity. It is also vastly less expensive for the insurance company because of the added costs of physical therapy and prosthetic devices. Early referral to Wound Care and Hyperbaric Medicine Departments, for appropriate diagnoses and treatment, saves limbs, improves patient outcomes and satisfaction, and ultimately, saves the insurance company money. Having outcomes data for your department, showing true patient care successes and failures, can result in better payments for your department and less difficulty in getting authorizations. Bills are paid more quickly and with less hassle. Ultimately, you and your staff and your patients will all feel better, leading to even better outcomes.

CONTRACTING WITH IPA'S AND MEDICAL GROUPS

In some states, you will need to contract with physician groups for Wound Care and Hyperbaric Medical Care. All of the previous comments apply in negotiating techniques. The contracts are usually much less complex and more straightforward. There is often little more than authorization requirements and payment plans in these contracts and therefore negotiations are shorter and easier. Outcome information and data, both from your department and from national peer-reviewed articles, will help in improving results in these negotiations. CMS Medicare coverage diagnoses will provide helpful contracting parameters for Hyperbaric Oxygen therapy payment. Earlier lists of E/M codes provide the basis for payment for Wound Care services.

OTHER TECHNIQUES THAT MAY ADD VALUE IN CONTRACT NEGOTIATIONS

Documentation of certification and training in Wound Care and Hyperbaric Medicine will add value in contract negotiations. This information can be contained in a short biography and detailed in a curriculum vita (CV). Support staff certification will also be beneficial. Getting the unit accredited by the Undersea and Hyperbaric Medical Society or other nationally recognized organization adds credibility to your negotiation for better compensation and less authorization requirements.

Another technique that can give you added clout in negotiations is active support from the physicians in your area and even support from the community you serve. This support can be gained by simply being available to local physicians when consulted and giving those physicians good feedback about their patients. Continuing Medical Education (CME) lectures for the local physician community can also add support for your department. Community involvement, by offering to give lectures and by participating in community affairs like clubs or activities, will gain active community support for your patient care work. Getting to know members of the city council and the board of supervisors before you need their help will add value for your department.

Hospital medical staff privileges are very important for adding value in contract negotiations. Being on the medical staff will also add direct referrals to your practice and will add physician support for the patient care work you deliver. Attending General Staff meetings and being on a committee or two will add contracts and add more support for your program.

ROLE OF ORGANIZED MEDICINE IN ADDING COVERED SERVICES TO LEGISLATION AND REGULATION

Adding value in contracting depends on coverage for services by CMS Medicare and other legislative and regulatory bodies at both the federal and state level. A single individual is unlikely to be able to carry an issue at these levels. It takes organizations of physicians and other providers to be able to get coverage for added services when the science clearly shows the value of those services. Medical specialty societies, like the Undersea and Hyperbaric Medical Society (UHMS), can promote for this added coverage at both the state and federal levels. The American Medical Association (AMA) and state medical societies can also assess coverage issues to help get the proper legislation passed and the proper regulations written and implemented. Getting the proper regulation implemented can often be more difficult than passing the original legislation passed.

Knowing your local representatives at the state and federal levels can help in getting legislation passed. They can also help if there are problems that occur related to their local area constituents. It is very important to meet these legislators before there is a problem. It is often easier to meet them in their local community when they are home for a break in their session.

POSTSCRIPT

Because of a significant increase in Medicare paments for wound care and debridements, the Office of the Inspector General (OIG) of Department of Health and Human Services has determined that it will begin an audit of all facilities and physicians billing for wound care services (similar to the audit conducted on Hyperbaric Oxygen Therapy in 2000) as part of its Work Plan for 2007.

This work plan states:

> **Wound Care Services**
> We will determine whether claims for wound care services were medically necessary and billed in accordance with Medicare requirements. Medicare allowed amounts of certain wound care services billed by physicians increased from approximately $98 million in 1998 to $147 million in 2002. We will also examine the adequacy of controls to prevent inappropriate payments for wound care services. *(OEI; 02-04-00410; expected issue date: FY 2007; work in progress).*

Therefore, physician knowlege of appropriate billing and coding for wound care services is of paramount importance. In addition to recoupment of payments for services found to be paid in error, physicians and hospitals could be found guilty of fraudulent billing practices which could incur civil monetary penalties in addition to recoupment.

ACKNOWLEDGMENTS

One of the authors (TMB) would like to thank Cindy G. Distafano, CPC for her review and assistance with coding issues discussed in this chapter.

REFERENCES

1. Practice Management Information Corporation. International Classification of Diseases, Ninth Revision, Clinical Modification, Sixth Edition (ICD-9-CM), Los Angeles, CA: *Practice Management Information Corporation* 2002.

2. INGENIX. 2003 ICD-9-CM International Classification of Diseases, 9th Revision, Clinical Modification, Professional for Physicians, Volumes 1 and 2. Edited by Anita C Hart, and Catherine A Hopkins. Salt Lake City, UT: INGENIX, 2003. [INGENIX, 2525 Lake Park Blvd, Salt Lake City, UT 84120].

3. American Medical Association. CPT 2007, Current Procedural Terminology, Standard Edition. Edited by Michael Beehe, et al. Chicago, IL: AMA Press, 2007. [AMA Press, 515 N State St, Chicago, IL, 60610].

4. Centers for Medicare and Medicaid Services. CIM 35-10 and NCD 20.29. Hyperbaric Oxygen Therapy

5. Florida Medicare LCD (Local Coverage Decision) Hyperbaric Oxygen Therapy

REVIEW QUESTIONS

1.) The system for paying the bills for Medicare and Medicaid recipients in the United States is set up by:
    a. US Federal Government
    b. Private insurance companies
    c. Employers
    d. Patients

2.) Over 50% of all money spent on health care in the United States is paid by:
    a. US Federal Government
    b. Private insurance companies
    c. Employers
    d. Patients

3.) The key components in selecting the appropriate level of Evaluation and Management (E/M) service are:
    a. History
    b. Examination
    c. Medical decision-making
    d. All of the above
    e. a and b, but not c

4.) When treating Medicare patients, higher complexity in the patient visit justifies a higher level of E/M service and therefore larger reimbursement for the physician.
    a. True
    b. False

5.) Reimbursement is dependent on
    a. Physician documentation
    b. Interpretation by the payer
    c. Accurate coding
    d. All of the above
    e. a and c, but not b

Answers: 1a, 2a, 3d, 4a, 5d.

NOTES

APPENDIX A

National Coverage Determination for Hyperbaric Oxygen Therapy (CMS)

NATIONAL 20.29—HYPERBARIC OXYGEN THERAPY

(Rev. 48, Issued: 03-17-06; Effective/Implementation Dates: 06-19-06)

CIM 35-10

For purposes of coverage under Medicare, hyperbaric oxygen (HBO) therapy is a modality in which the entire body is exposed to oxygen under increased atmospheric pressure.

A. Covered Conditions

Program reimbursement for HBO therapy will be limited to that which is administered in a chamber (including the one man unit) and is limited to the following conditions:

1. Acute carbon monoxide intoxication,
2. Decompression illness,
3. Gas embolism,
4. Gas gangrene,
5. Acute traumatic peripheral ischemia. HBO therapy is a valuable adjunctive treatment to be used in combination with accepted standard therapeutic measures when loss of function, limb, or life is threatened.
6. Crush injuries and suturing of severed limbs. As in the previous conditions, HBO therapy would be an adjunctive treatment when loss of function, limb, or life is threatened.
7. Progressive necrotizing infections (necrotizing fasciitis),
8. Acute peripheral arterial insufficiency,
9. Preparation and preservation of compromised skin grafts (not for primary management of wounds),
10. Chronic refractory osteomyelitis, unresponsive to conventional medical and surgical management,
11. Osteoradionecrosis as an adjunct to conventional treatment,
12. Soft tissue radionecrosis as an adjunct to conventional treatment,

13. Cyanide poisoning,
14. Actinomycosis, only as an adjunct to conventional therapy when the disease process is refractory to antibiotics and surgical treatment,
15. Diabetic wounds of the lower extremities in patients who meet the following three criteria:
    a. Patient has type I or type II diabetes and has a lower extremity wound that is due to diabetes;
    b. Patient has a wound classified as Wagner grade III or higher; and
    c. Patient has failed an adequate course of standard wound therapy.

The use of HBO therapy is covered as adjunctive therapy only after there are no measurable signs of healing for at least 30 days of treatment with standard wound therapy and must be used in addition to standard wound care. Standard wound care in patients with diabetic wounds includes: assessment of a patient's vascular status and correction of any vascular problems in the affected limb if possible, optimization of nutritional status, optimization of glucose control, debridement by any means to remove devitalized tissue, maintenance of a clean, moist bed of granulation tissue with appropriate moist dressings, appropriate off-loading, and necessary treatment to resolve any infection that might be present. Failure to respond to standard wound care occurs when there are no measurable signs of healing for at least 30 consecutive days. Wounds must be evaluated at least every 30 days during administration of HBO therapy. Continued treatment with HBO therapy is not covered if measurable signs of healing have not been demonstrated within any 30-day period of treatment.

B. Noncovered Conditions

All other indications not specified under §270.4(A) are not covered under the Medicare program. No program payment may be made for any conditions other than those listed in §270.4(A).

No program payment may be made for HBO in the treatment of the following conditions:

1. Cutaneous, decubitus, and stasis ulcers
2. Chronic peripheral vascular insufficiency
3. Anaerobic septicemia and infection other than clostridial
4. Skin burns (thermal)
5. Senility
6. Myocardial infarction
7. Cardiogenic shock
8. Sickle cell anemia
9. Acute thermal and chemical pulmonary damage, i.e., smoke inhalation with pulmonary
10. Acute or chronic cerebral vascular insufficiency
11. Hepatic necrosis
12. Aerobic septicemia
13. Nonvascular causes of chronic brain syndrome (Pick's disease, Alzheimer's disease, Korsakoff's disease)
14. Tetanus
15. Systemic aerobic infection

16. Organ transplantation
17. Organ storage
18. Pulmonary emphysema
19. Exceptional blood loss anemia
20. Multiple Sclerosis
21. Arthritic Diseases
22. Acute cerebral edema

C. Topical Application of Oxygen

This method of administering oxygen does not meet the definition of HBO therapy as stated above. Also, its clinical efficacy has not been established. Therefore, no Medicare reimbursement may be made for the topical application of oxygen.

Cross reference: §270.5 of this manual.

NOTES

APPENDIX B

MEDICARE COVERAGE POLICY FOR HYPERBARIC OXYGEN THERAPY LCD FOR FLORIDA

Hyperbaric Oxygen Therapy is a medical treatment in which the patient is entirely enclosed in a pressure chamber breathing 100% oxygen (O_2) at greater than one atmosphere (atm) pressure. Either a monoplace chamber pressurized with pure O_2 or a larger multiplace chamber pressurized with compressed air where the patient receives pure O_2 by mask, head tent, or endotracheal tube may be used.

In order to receive Medicare reimbursement for HBO therapy, services must be rendered under the direct supervision of the physician.

Indications and Limitations of Coverage and/or Medical Necessity

HBO therapy is covered by Medicare for the following conditions:

1. Acute carbon monoxide intoxication induces hypoxic stress. The cardiac and central nervous systems are the most susceptible to injury from carbon monoxide. The administration of supplemental oxygen is essential treatment. Hyperbaric oxygen causes a higher rate of dissociation of carbon monoxide from hemoglobin than can occur breathing pure air at sea level pressure. The chamber compressions should be between 2.5 and 3.0 ATA. It is not uncommon in patients with persistent neurological dysfunction to require subsequent treatments within six to eight hours, continuing once or twice daily until there is no further improvement in cognitive functioning.
2. Decompression illness arises from the formation of gas bubbles in tissue or blood in volumes sufficient enough to interfere with the function of an organ or to cause alteration in sensation. The cause of this enucleated gas is rapid decompression during ascent. The clinical manifestations range from skin eruptions to shock and death. The circulating gas emboli may be heard with a doppler device. Treatment of choice for decompression illness is HBO with mixed gases. The result is immediate reduction in the volume of bubbles. The treatment prescription is highly variable and case specific.

The depths could range between 60 to 165 feet of sea water for durations of 1.5 to over 14 hours. The patient may or may not require repeat dives.

3. Gas embolism occurs when gases enter the venous or arterial vasculature embolizing in a large enough volume to compromise the function of an organ or body part. This occlusive process results in ischemia to the affected areas. Air emboli may occur as a result of surgical procedures (e.g., cardiovascular surgery, intra-aortic balloons, arthroplasties, or endoscopies), use of monitoring devices (e.g., Swan-Ganz introducer, infusion pumps), in nonsurgical patients (e.g., diving, ruptured lung in respirator-dependent patient, injection of fluids into tissue space), or traumatic injuries (e.g., gunshot wounds, penetrating chest injuries). Hyperbaric oxygen therapy is the treatment of choice. It is most effective when initiated early. Therapy is directed toward reducing the volume of gas bubbles and increasing the diffusion gradient of the embolized gas. Treatment modalities range from high pressure to low pressure mixed gas dives.
4. Gas gangrene is an infection caused by the clostridium bacillus, the most common being clostridium perfringens. Clostridial myositis and myonecrosis (gas gangrene) is an acute, rapidly growing invasive infection of the muscle. It is characterized by profound toxemia, extensive edema, massive death of tissue and variable degree of gas production. The most prevalent toxin is the alpha-toxin which in itself is hemolytic, tissue-necrotizing and lethal. The diagnosis of gas gangrene is based on clinical data supported by a positive gram-stained smear obtained from tissue fluids. X-ray radiographs, if obtained, can visualize tissue gas.

   The onset of gangrene can occur one to six hours after injury and presents with severe and sudden pain at the infected area. The skin overlying the wound progresses from shiny and tense, to dusky, then bronze in color. The infection can progress as rapidly as six inches per hour. Hemorrhagic vesicles may be noted. A thin, sweet-odored exudate is present. Swelling and edema occur. The noncontractile muscles progress to dark red to black in color.

   The acute problem in gas gangrene is to stop the rapidly advancing infection caused by alpha-toxin. Medical treatment is aimed at stopping the production of alpha-toxin and to continue treatment until the advancement of the disease process has been arrested. The goal of HBO therapy is to stop alpha-toxin production thereby inhibiting further bacterial growth at which point the body can use its own host defense mechanisms. HBO treatment starts as soon as the clinical picture presents and is supported by a positive gram-stained smear. A treatment approach utilizing HBO, is adjunct to antibiotic therapy and surgery. Initial surgery may be limited to opening the wound. Debridement of necrotic tissue can be performed between HBO treatments when clear demarcation between dead and viable tissue is evident. The usual treatment consists of oxygen administered at 3.0 ATA pressure for 90 minutes three times in the first 24 hours. Over the next four to five days, treatment sessions twice a day are usual. The sooner HBO treatment is initiated, the better the outcome in terms of life, limb and tissue saving.

5. Crush injuries and suturing of severed limbs, acute traumatic peripheral ischemia (ATI), and acute peripheral arterial insufficiency: Acute traumatic ischemia is the result of injury by external force or violence compromising circulation to an extremity. The extremity is then at risk for necrosis or amputation. Secondary complications are frequently seen: infection, non-healing wounds, and non-united fractures.

   The goal of HBO therapy is to enhance oxygen at the tissue level to support viability. When tissue oxygen tensions fall below 30 mm Hg , the body's ability to respond to infection and wound repair is compromised. Using HBO at 2–2.4 atm, the tissue oxygen tension is raised to a level such that the body's responses can become functional again. The benefits of HBO therapy for this indication are enhanced tissue oxygenation, edema reduction and increased oxygen delivery per unit of blood flow thereby reducing the complication rates for infection, nonunion and amputation.

   The usual treatment schedule is three 1.5 hour treatment periods daily for the first 48 hours. Additionally, two 1.5 hour treatment sessions daily for the next 48 hours may be required. On the fifth and sixth days of treatment, one 1.5 hour session would typically be utilized. At this point in treatment, outcomes of restored perfusion, edema reduction and either demarcation or recovery would be sufficient to guide discontinuing further treatments.

   For acute traumatic peripheral ischemia, crush injuries and suturing of severed limbs, Hyperbaric Oxygen Therapy is a valuable adjunctive treatment to be used in combination with accepted standard therapeutic measures, when loss of function, limb, or life is threatened. Arterial insufficiency ulcers may be treated by HBO therapy if they are persistent after reconstructive surgery has restored large vessel function.

6. The principal treatment for progressive necrotizing infections (necrotizing fasciitis) is surgical debridement and systemic antibiotics. HBO therapy is recommended as an adjunct only in those settings where mortality and morbidity are expected to be high despite aggressive standard treatment. Progressive necrotizing fasciitis is a relatively rare infection. It is usually a result of a group A streptococcal infection beginning with severe or extensive cellulitis that spreads to involve the superficial and deep fascia, producing thrombosis of the subcutaneous vessels and gangrene of the underlying tissues. A cutaneous lesion usually serves as a portal of entry for the infection, but sometimes no such lesion is found.

7. Preparation and preservation of compromised skin grafts utilizes HBO therapy for graft or flap salvage in cases where hypoxia or decreased perfusion have compromised viability. This indication is not for primary management of wounds.

HBO therapy enhances flap survival. Treatments are given at a pressure of 2.0 to 2.5 ATA lasting from 90–120 minutes. It is not unusual to receive treatments twice a day. When the graft or flap appears stable, treatments are reduced to daily. Should a graft or flap fail, HBO therapy may be used to prepare the already compromised recipient site for a new graft or flap. It does not apply to the initial preparation of the body site for a graft. HBO therapy is not necessary for normal, uncompromised skin grafts or flaps. Medicare's coverage does not apply to artificial skin grafts.

8. Chronic refractory osteomyelitis persists or recurs following appropriate interventions. These interventions include the use of antibiotics, aspiration of the abscess, immobilization of the affected extremity, and surgery. HBO therapy is an adjunctive therapy used with the appropriate antibiotics. Antibiotics are chosen on the basis of bone culture and sensitivity studies. HBO therapy can elevate the oxygen tensions found in infected bone to normal or above normal levels. This mechanism enhances healing and the body's antimicrobial defenses. It is believed that HBO therapy augments the efficacy of certain antibiotics (gentamicin, tobramycin, and amikacin). Finally, the body's osteoclast function of removing necrotic bone is dependent on a proper oxygen tension environment. HBO therapy provides this environment. HBO treatments are delivered at a pressure of 2.0 to 2.5 ATA for a duration of 90–120 minutes. It is not unusual to receive daily treatments following major debridement surgery. The number of treatments required vary on an individual basis. Medicare can cover the use of HBO therapy for chronic refractory osteomyelitis that has been demonstrated to be unresponsive to conventional medical and surgical management.
9. HBO's use in the treatment of osteoradionecrosis and soft tissue radionecrosis is one part of an overall plan of care. Also included in this plan of care are debridement or resection of nonviable tissues in conjunction with antibiotic therapy. Soft tissue flap reconstruction and bone grafting may also be indicated. HBO treatment can be indicated both preoperatively and postoperatively.

   The patients who suffer from soft tissue damage or bone necrosis present with disabling, progressive, painful tissue breakdown. They may present with wound dehiscence, infection, tissue loss and graft or flap loss. The goal of HBO treatment is to increase the oxygen tension in both hypoxic bone and tissue to stimulate growth in functioning capillaries, fibroblastic proliferation and collagen synthesis. The recommended daily treatments last 90–120 minutes at 2.0 to 2.5 ATA. The duration of HBO therapy is highly individualized.
10. Cyanide poisoning carries a high risk of mortality. Victims of smoke inhalation frequently suffer from both carbon monoxide and cyanide poisoning. The traditional antidote for cyanide poisoning is the infusion of sodium nitrite. This treatment can potentially

impair the oxygen carrying capacity of hemoglobin. Using HBO therapy as an adjunct therapy adds the benefit of increased plasma dissolved oxygen. HBO's benefit for the pulmonary injury related to smoke inhalation remains experimental. The HBO treatment protocol is to administer oxygen at 2.5 to 3.0 ATA for up to 120 minutes during the initial treatment. Most patients with combination cyanide and carbon monoxide poisoning will receive only one treatment.

11. Actinomycosis is a bacterial infection caused by Actinomyces israelii. Its symptoms include slow growing granulomas that later breakdown, discharging viscid pus containing minute yellowish granules. The treatment includes prolonged administration of antibiotics (penicillin and tetracycline). Surgical incision and draining of accessible lesions is also helpful. Only after the disease process has shown refractory to antibiotics and surgery, could HBO therapy be covered by Medicare. HBO therapy must be utilized adjunct to conventional therapy.
12. Treatment of diabetic wounds of the lower extremities in patients who meet the following criteria:
    - Patient has type I or type II diabetes and has a lower extremity wound that is due to diabetes.
    - Patient has a wound classified as Wagner grade III or higher; and
    - Patient has failed an adequate course of standard wound therapy.

The use of HBO therapy will be covered as adjunctive therapy only after there are no measurable signs of healing for at least 30 days of treatment with standard wound therapy and must be used in addition to standard wound care. Standard wound care in patients with diabetic wounds includes: assessment of a patient's vascular status and correction of any vascular problems in the affected limb if possible, optimization of nutritional status, optimization of glucose control, debridement by any means to remove devitalized tissue, maintenance of clean, moist bed of granulation tissue with appropriate moist dressings, appropriate off-loading, and necessary treatment to resolve any infection that might be present. Failure to respond to standard wound care occurs when there are no measurable signs of healing for at least 30 consecutive days. Wounds must be evaluated at least every 30 days during administration of HBO therapy.

Prior to the initiation of HBO therapy, it is expected in most cases that the diagnosis will be established by the referring or treating physician.

Indications of effective treatment outcomes for HBO include:

- Improvement or healing of wounds.
- Improvement of tissue perfusion.
- New epithelial tissue growth and granulation.
- Tissue PO_2 of at least 30 mm Hg of oxygen is necessary for oxidative function to occur.
- Mechanical reduction in the bubble size of air emboli alleviates decompression sickness and gas/ air emboli.

- Tissue PO_2 of 40 or greater defines resolved hypoxia. The body can now resume host functions of wound healing and anti-microbial defenses without the need of HBO therapy.

HBO therapy should not be a replacement for other standard successful therapeutic measures; however, it is the treatment of choice and standard of care for decompression sickness and arterial gas embolism. Traumatic or spontaneous pneumothorax constitute contraindications to adjunctive HBO therapy only if untreated. Pregnancy is considered a contraindication to HBO therapy except in the case of carbon monoxide poisoning where it is specifically indicated.

CPT/HCPCS Section & Benefit Category

Medicine/Other Services and Procedures

CPT/HCPCS Codes

99183	Physician attendance and supervision of hyperbaric oxygen therapy, per session
G0167	Hyperbaric oxygen treatment not requiring physician attendance, per treatment session

Not Otherwise Classified Codes (NOC)

N/A

ICD-9 Codes that Support Medical Necessity

For services prior to 04/01/2003:

039.0-039.9	Actinomycotic infections
040.0	Gas gangrene
444.21-444.22	Arterial embolism and thrombus of arteries of the extremities
444.81	Arterial embolism and thrombosis of iliac artery
526.89	Other specified diseases of the jaws
728.86	Necrotizing fasciitis
730.10-730.19	Chronic osteomyelitis
902.53	Injury to blood vessels of iliac artery
903.01	Injury to blood vessels of axillary artery
903.1	Injury to brachial blood vessels
904.0	Injury to blood vessels of common femoral artery
904.41	Injury to blood vessels of popliteal artery
927.00-927.09	Crushing injury of shoulder and upper arm
927.10-927.11	Crushing injury of elbow and forearm
927.20-927.21	Crushing injury of wrist and hand(s) except finger(s) alone
927.8	Crushing injury of multiple sites of upper limb
927.9	Crushing injury of unspecified site of upper limb
928.00-928.01	Crushing injury of hip and thigh
928.10-928.11	Crushing injury of knee and lower leg
928.20-928.21	Crushing injury of ankle and foot, excluding toe(s) alone

928.3	Crushing injury of toe(s)
928.8-928.9	Crushing injury of multiple sites and unspecified site of lower limb
929.0-929.9	Crushing injury of multiple and unspecified sites
958.0	Early complication of trauma, air embolism
986	Toxic effect of carbon monoxide
987.7	Toxic effect of hydrocyanic acid gas
989.0	Toxic effect of hydrocyanic acid and cyanides
990	Effects of radiation, unspecified
993.2	Other and unspecified effects of high altitude
993.3	Caisson disease
996.52	Mechanical complication due to graft of other tissue, not elsewhere classified
996.90-996.99	Complications of reattached extremity or body part
999.1	Complications of medical care, embolism

For services on or after 04/01/2003:

039.0-039.9	Actinomycotic infections
040.0	Gas gangrene
250.70-250.73	Diabetes with peripheral circulation disorders
250.80-250.83	Diabetes with other specified manifestations
444.21-444.22	Arterial embolism and thrombosis of arteries of the extremities
444.81	Arterial embolism and thrombosis of iliac artery
526.89	Other specified diseases of the jaws
707.10	Ulcer of lower limb, unspecified
707.12	Ulcer of calf
707.13	Ulcer of ankle
707.14	Ulcer of heel and midfoot
707.15	Ulcer of other part of foot
707.19	Ulcer of other part of lower limb
728.86	Necrotizing fasciitis
730.10-730.19	Chronic osteomyelitis
902.53	Injury to blood vessels of iliac artery
903.01	Injury to blood vessels of axillary artery
903.1	Injury to brachial blood vessels
904.0	Injury to blood vessels of common femoral artery
904.41	Injury to blood vessels of popliteal artery
927.00-927.09	Crushing injury of shoulder and upper arm
927.10-927.11	Crushing injury of elbow and forearm
927.20-927.21	Crushing injury of wrist and hand(s) except finger(s) alone
927.8	Crushing injury of multiple sites of upper limb
927.9	Crushing injury of unspecified site of upper limb
928.00-928.01	Crushing injury of hip and thigh
928.10-928.11	Crushing injury of knee and lower leg
928.20-928.21	Crushing injury of ankle and foot, excluding toe(s) alone

928.3	Crushing injury of toe(s)
928.8-928.9	Crushing injury of multiple sites and unspecified site of lower limb
929.0-929.9	Crushing injury of multiple and unspecified sites
958.0	Early complication of trauma, air embolism
986	Toxic effect of carbon monoxide
987.7	Toxic effect of hydrocyanic acid gas
989.0	Toxic effect of hydrocyanic acid and cyanides
990	Effects of radiation, unspecified
993.2	Other and unspecified effects of high altitude
993.3	Caisson disease
996.52	Mechanical complication due to graft of other tissue, not elsewhere classified
996.90-996.99	Complications of reattached extremity or body part
999.1	Complications of medical care, air embolis

Diagnoses that Support Medical Necessity

N/A

ICD-9 Codes that DO NOT Support Medical Necessity

N/A

Diagnoses that DO NOT Support Medical Necessity

N/A

Reasons for Denials

When performed for indications other than those listed in the "Indications and Limitations of Coverage and/or Medical Necessity" section of this policy.

Topical application of oxygen (Topox) does not meet the definition of HBO therapy. Also, its clinical efficacy has not been established; therefore, no reimbursement may be made.

Local coverage policy for HBO therapy requires that a physician be in direct supervision during an HBO therapy session. Services performed in the absence of a physician will not be reimbursed (G0167).

No program payment may be made for HBO in the treatment of the following conditions (per CIM 35-10):

- Cutaneous, decubitus and stasis ulcers
- Chronic peripheral vascular insufficiency
- Anaerobic septicemia and infection other than clostridial
- Skin burns (thermal)
- Senility
- Myocardial infarction
- Cardiogenic shock
- Sickle cell anemia
- Acute thermal and chemical pulmonary damage, i.e., smoke inhalation with pulmonary insufficiency
- Acute or chronic cerebral vascular insufficiency
- Hepatic necrosis

- Aerobic septicemia
- Nonvascular causes of chronic brain syndrome (Pick's disease Alzheimer's disease Korsakoff's disease)
- Tetanus
- Systemic aerobic infection
- Organ transplantation
- Organ storage
- Pulmonary emphysema
- Exceptional blood loss anemia
- Multiple Sclerosis
- Arthritic Diseases
- Acute cerebral edema

Noncovered ICD-9 Codes

Any diagnosis codes not listed in the "ICD-9 Codes That Support Medical Necessity" section of this policy.

Noncovered Diagnosis

N/A

Coding Guidelines

Evaluation and management services and/or procedures (e.g., wound debridement, transcutaneous PO_2 determinations) provided in a hyperbaric oxygen treatment facility in conjunction with a hyperbaric oxygen therapy session may be reported separately.

This code reflects a per session descriptor, therefore, regardless of the time HBO therapy is performed (e.g., 1 hour, 2 hours) during each session, each unit billed equals one session.

For each of the fifteen covered conditions, the following diagnosis should be utilized:

- Acute carbon monoxide intoxication—Diagnosis 986
- Decompression illness—Diagnosis 993.2, or 993.3
- Gas embolism—Diagnosis 958.0, or 999.1
- Gas gangrene—Diagnosis 040.0
- Acute traumatic peripheral ischemia—Diagnosis 902.53, 903.01, 903.1, 904.0 or 904.41
- Crush injuries and suturing of severed limbs—Diagnosis 927.00-927.09, 927.10-927.11, 927.20-927.21, 927.8, 927.9, 928.00-928.01, 928.10-928.11, 928.20-928.21, 928.3, 928.8-928.9, 929.0-929.9, or 996.90-996.99
- Progressive necrotizing infections:(necrotizing fasciitis)—Diagnosis 728.86
- Acute peripheral arterial insufficiency—Diagnosis 444.21, 444.22, 444.81
- Preparation and preservation of compromised skin grafts (flaps)—Diagnosis 996.52
- Chronic refractory osteomyelitis, unresponsive to conventional medical and surgical management—Diagnosis 730.10-730.19
- Osteoradionecrosis as an adjunct to conventional treatment—Diagnosis 526.89

- Soft tissue radionecrosis as an adjunct to conventional treatment—Diagnosis 990
- Cyanide poisoning—Diagnosis 987.7 or 989.0
- Actinomycosis, only as an adjunct to conventional therapy when the disease process is refractory to antibiotics and surgical treatment—Diagnosis 039.0-039.9
- Treatment of diabetic wounds of the lower extremities—Diagnosis 250.70-250.73, 250.80-250.83, 707.10, 707.12-707.15, and 707.19.

Documentation Requirements

There must be medical documentation to support the condition for which HBO therapy is being given. Documentation for all services should be maintained on file (e.g., progress notes and treatment record) to substantiate medical necessity for HBO treatment.

This medical documentation must include:

- An initial assessment which will include a medical history detailing the condition requiring HBO therapy. The medical history should list prior treatments and their results including antibiotic therapy and surgical interventions. This assessment should also contain information about adjunctive treatment currently being rendered;
- Physician progress notes;
- Any communication between physicians detailing past or future (proposed) treatments;
- Positive gram-stain smear is required to support the diagnosis of gas gangrene;
- Definitive radiographic evidence and bone culture with sensitivity studies are required to confirm the diagnosis of osteomyelitis; and
- HBO treatment records describing the physical findings, the treatment rendered and the effect of the treatment upon the established goals for therapy.

Utilization Guidelines

Payment will be made for HBO therapy when it is clinically practical. HBO therapy should not be a replacement for other standard successful therapeutic measures. Depending on the response of the individual patient and the severity of the original problem, treatment may range from less than one week to several months duration, the average being 2–4 weeks. The use of hyperbaric oxygen for more than two months, (30 days for the treatment of diabetic wounds) regardless of the condition of the patient, will be reviewed for medical necessity before further reimbursement is made.

Sources of Information and Basis for Decision

- American College of Hyperbaric Medicine (1997). Preferred practice protocols for hyperbaric medicine. Houston, TX: Author.
- Dorlands Illustrated Medical Dictionary, 28th edition. Philadelphia. W.B. Saunders Co.
- Undersea and Hyperbaric Medical Society. (1996, 1999). Hyperbaric Oxygen Therapy: A committee report.

APPENDIX C

DICTATION TEMPLATES

CONSULTATION

Patient name
Medical Record Number
Date of Consult
Referring Physician
Chief Complaint
History of Present Illness
    Narrative of how problem developed
    How long problem has been present
Past Medical History
    Medical
    Surgical
    Social (Smoking/EtOH)
    Drugs (Medicinal/recreational)
    Allergies
    Family History
Review of Systems
Review of Previous Treatments for Present
    Condition (and outcomes)
Physical Examination
    Address systemic **AND** local factors contributing to problem
Labs
CBC, SMAC, GlycoHgb if diabetic, ESR, C&S,
    Biopsy, UCG if childbearing age, TCOM on every patient with
    extremity wound (HBO consult if hypoxic)
Imaging
    X-ray, Bone Scan, CT, MRI, Doppler, Arteriogram
Diagnosis
Treatment Plan (Plan of Care)
    Discuss results of all labs/imaging and impact on patient treatment
    Debridement(s)
    Dressings
    Ancillary Services (PT, OT, Home Health, Dietary, Diabetic Counseling)
Is patient candidate for growth factor or bioengineered tissue,
    compression therapy, or other advanced wound care?
    Anticipated time in Wound Care Service
    Anticipated Result/Therapeutic Endpoint of therapy
    Discussion of Risks/Complications of Therapy

If hyperbaric candidate:
- Number of anticipated treatments
- Treatment protocol (time & pressure)
- Discussion of rationale and complications
- Anticipated result/endpoint
- Statement about medical necessity

Copy to Referring **AND** Primary Physician(s)
Orders Written if Patient Receiving Home Health or Nursing Home OR Admitted

DISCHARGE

Patient Name
Medical Record Number
Date of First Visit (Treatment)
Date of Last Visit (Treatment)
Total Number of visits (Treatments)
Diagnosis
Significant Labs or Imaging
Course of Therapy
- Debridements
- Dressings
- Ancillary Treatments
- Tolerance to Therapy
- Interruptions in Therapy
- Additional Consultations
- HBO Treatments

Additional Procedures/Treatments
Response to Therapy
Condition on Discharge
Discharge Instructions given to Patient/Family
Copy to Referring and Primary Physician

WOUND CARE VISIT

Patient Name
Medical Record Number
Date of Visit & Visit Number
Date of Last Visit
Vital Signs
Reason for Visit
Complaints (pain/drainage)
Location of Wound
Dressings intact/drainage on dressings?
Strikethrough/Tracking
Size of Wound (Length/Width/Depth)
Appearance of Wound (granulation tissue, erythema, amount of drainage on wound/Type of drainage)

Associated Symptoms (Swelling/Lymphangitis/Lymphedema)
Odor
Necrotic Tissue
Staging of Ulcer (AHCPR/Wagner-Harris/PEDIS)
Treatment Plan
    Wound Photography/Planometry Done?
    Debridement/Procedure Note
    Cleansing Agent
    Irrigating Agent
    Type of Debridement and Material Debrided
    Primary Dressing
    Secondary Dressing
    Bandage
Discussion of Any Lab(s)/Imaging Performed at last visit
    Any New Tests Ordered?
    New Prescriptions Written?
    Next Follow-Up Visit
Written Orders for Home Health, Nursing Home, OR Discussion of home care orders given to family until next visit
Copy to Referring AND Primary Physician

NOTES

INDEX

Volume One: pages 1–601 • Volume Two: pages 603–1210

C

D

F

G

H

J

K

L

M

Q

R

S

T

U

V

W

X, Y, Z

NOTES